NEPHROLOGY

SECRETS

NEPHROLOGY

SECRETS

Third Edition

Edgar V. Lerma, MD, FACP, FASN, FAHA, FASH, FNLA
Clinical Associate Professor of Medicine
Section of Nephrology
Department of Medicine
University of Illinois at Chicago College of Medicine
Associates in Nephrology, S.C.
Chicago, Illinois

Allen R. Nissenson, MD, FACP, FASN
Emeritus Professor of Medicine
David Geffen School of Medicine at the University of California, Los Angeles
Los Angeles, California
Chief Medical Office
DaVita, Inc.
El Segundo, California

ELSEVIER
MOSBY

1600 John F. Kennedy Blvd.
Ste 1800
Philadelphia, PA 19103-2899

NEPHROLOGY SECRETS, THIRD EDITION

ISBN: 978-1-4160-3362-2

Notices

Knowledge and best practice in this field are constantly changing. As new research and experience broaden our understanding, changes in research methods, professional practices, or medical treatment may become necessary.

Practitioners and researchers must always rely on their own experience and knowledge in evaluating and using any information, methods, compounds, or experiments described herein. In using such information or methods, they should be mindful of their own safety and the safety of others, including parties for whom they have a professional responsibility.

With respect to any drug or pharmaceutical products identified, readers are advised to check the most current information provided (i) on procedures featured or (ii) by the manufacturer of each product to be administered, to verify the recommended dose or formula, the method and duration of administration, and contraindications. It is the responsibility of practitioners, relying on their own experience and knowledge of their patients, to make diagnoses, to determine dosages and the best treatment for each individual patient, and to take all appropriate safety precautions.

To the fullest extent of the law, neither the Publisher nor the authors, contributors, or editors, assume any liability for any injury and/or damage to persons or property as a matter of products liability, negligence or otherwise, or from any use or operation of any methods, products, instructions, or ideas contained in the material herein.

Library of Congress Cataloging-in-Publication Data

Nephrology secrets.—3rd ed. / [edited by] Edgar V. Lerma, Allen R. Nissenson.
   p. ; cm.
Includes bibliographical references and index.
ISBN 978-1-4160-3362-2 (pbk. : alk. paper)
1. Kidneys—Diseases—Miscellanea. 2. Nephrology—Miscellanea. I. Lerma, Edgar V. II. Nissenson, Allen R.
[DNLM: 1. Kidney Diseases—Examination Questions. WJ 18.2]
 RC903.N477 2012
 616.6′1—dc22

2011009371

Senior Acquisitions Editor: James Merritt
Developmental Editor: Andrea Vosburgh
Publishing Services Manager: Patricia Tannian
Senior Project Manager: Claire Kramer

Printed in the United States of America

Last digit is the print number: 9 8 7 6 5 4 3 2 1

To my mentors, colleagues, and friends at the University of Santo Tomas Faculty of Medicine and Surgery in Manila, Philippines, and Mercy Hospital and Medical Center/ University of Illinois at Chicago, who have molded me as an individual and as a physician, and have guided me to where I am right now.

To my mentors and colleagues at Northwestern University Feinberg School of Medicine, particularly Drs. Daniel Batlle, Robert Rosa, William Schlueter, Murray Levin, Cybele Ghossein, and David Roxe, all of whom have profoundly influenced my decision to be actively involved in the teaching profession.

To all the medical students, interns and residents who at one time or another have crossed paths with me at Advocate Christ Medical Center/University of Illinois at Chicago, from whom I have learned so much.

To my parents and my brothers, without whose unremitting love and care, and never-ending support through thick and thin, I would not have reached my goals in life.

Most especially, to my two lovely daughters Anastasia Zofia and Isabella Ann, and my ever dearest wife Michelle, a truly admirable and unique individual, who sacrificed a lot of time and exhibited unparalleled patience as I devoted a significant amount of time and effort to this project. Truly, they are my inspiration.

EL

CONTRIBUTORS

Rajiv Agarwal, MD, FAHA, FASN
Professor of Medicine, Division of Nephrology,
Department of Medicine, Indiana University School
of Medicine and Roudebush VA Medical Center,
Indianapolis, Indiana

Martin J. Andersen, DO
Assistant Professor of Clinical Medicine, Division
of Nephrology, Department of Medicine, Indiana
University Medical Center, Indianapolis, Indiana

John R. Asplin, MD, FASN
Clinical Associate, Section of Nephrology,
Department of Medicine, University of Chicago
Pritzker School of Medicine; Medical Director,
Litholink Corporation, Chicago, Illinois

George L. Bakris, MD
Professor of Medicine, Department of Medicine,
Section of Adult and Pediatric Endocrinology,
Diabetes and Metabolism, The University of
Chicago; Director, Hypertensive Diseases Unit,
Department of Medicine, Section of Adult and
Pediatric Endocrinology, Diabetes and Metabolism,
The University of Chicago Medical Center,
Chicago, Illinois

Daniel Batlle, MD
Earle, del Greco, and Levin Professor of
Nephrology/Hypertension, Professor of Medicine,
Division of Nephrology/Hypertension,
Northwestern University/Feinberg School of
Medicine, Chicago, Illinois

Tomas Berl, MD
Professor of Medicine, Department of Medicine,
Division of Renal Diseases and Hypertension,
University of Colorado Denver, Aurora, Colorado

Scott D. Bieber, DO
Fellow, Division of Nephrology, University of
Washington, Seattle, Washington

Daniel C. Cattran, MD, FRCPC, FACP
Professor of Medicine, University of Toronto;
Senior Scientist, Toronto General Research
Institute, University Health Network, Toronto,
Ontario, Canada

Devasmita Choudhury, MD
Associate Professor, Department of Medicine,
University of Texas Southwestern Medical Center;
Director, In-Center and Home Dialysis, Department
of Medicine, Dallas VA Medical Center, Dallas, Texas

Rolando Claure-Del Granado, MD
Postdoctoral Fellow, Department of Medicine,
Division of Nephrology, University of California,
San Diego, San Diego, California

Byron P. Croker, MD, PhD
Chief, Pathology and Laboratory Medicine Service,
North Florida/South Georgia Veterans Health
System; Professor, Pathology, Immunology, and
Laboratory Medicine, University of Florida,
Gainesville, Florida

Bradley M. Denker, MD
Associate Professor of Medicine, Harvard Medical
School; Physician, Renal Division, Brigham and
Women's Hospital; Chief of Nephrology, Harvard
Vanguard Medical Associates, Boston, Massachusetts

Vimal K. Derebail, MD, MPH
Assistant Professor of Medicine, Division of
Nephrology and Hypertension, Department of
Internal Medicine, University of North Carolina at
Chapel Hill, Chapel Hill, North Carolina

Robert J. Desnick, PhD, MD
Dean for Genetics and Genomics, Professor and
Chairman, Department of Genetics and Genomic
Sciences, Mount Sinai School of Medicine,
New York, New York

Christiane Drechsler, MD, PhD
Fellow, Nephrology and Clinical Research,
Department of Medicine, Division of Nephrology,
University Hospital Würzburg, Würzburg, Germany

Alfonso Eirin, MD
Research Fellow, Division of Nephrology and
Hypertension, Mayo Clinic, Rochester, Minnesota

Garabed Eknoyan, MD
Professor of Medicine, Department of Medicine,
Baylor College of Medicine, Houston, Texas

Mohsen El Kossi, MBBCh, MSc, MD,
MRCP(UK)
Consultant Renal Physician, Renal Unit, Doncaster
Royal Infirmary, Doncaster, United Kingdom

Meguid El Nahas, MD, PhD, FRCP
Professor, Department of Nephrology, Sheffield
Kidney Institute, University of Sheffield, Sheffield,
United Kingdom

William J. Elliott, MD, PhD
Professor of Preventive Medicine, Internal Medicine,
and Pharmacology; Head, Division of Pharmacology,
Pacific Northwest University of Health Sciences,
Yakima, Washington

David H. Ellison, MD
Professor of Medicine and Physiology and
Pharmacology, Division of Nephrology and
Hypertension, Oregon Health and Science University,
Portland, Oregon

Uta Erdbruegger, MD
Assistant Professor, Division of Nephrology,
Department of Medicine, University of Virginia Health
System, Charlottesville, Virginia

Angela Alonso Esteve, MD
Clinical Fellow in Adult Nephrology, Department of
Medicine, University of Toronto; Clinical Fellow in
Adult Nephrology, Toronto General Hospital,
University Health Network, Toronto, Ontario, Canada

Fernando C. Fervenza, MD, PhD
Professor of Medicine, Division of Nephrology and
Hypertension, Mayo Clinic, Rochester, Minnesota

Robert A. Figlin, MD, FACP
Chair, Division of Hematology/Oncology, Department
of Medicine, Cedars-Sinai Medical Center, Samuel
Oschin Comprehensive Cancer Institute; Department
of Medicine, David Geffen School of Medicine at the
University of California, Los Angeles, Los Angeles,
California

Mony Fraer, MD, FACP, FASN
Assistant Professor, Division of Nephrology,
Department of Internal Medicine, University of Iowa
Hospitals and Clinics, Iowa City, Iowa

Eli A. Friedman, MD, MRCP
Distinguished Teaching Professor of Medicine,
State University of New York Downstate Medical
Center, Brooklyn, New York

Debbie S. Gipson, MD, MS
Associate Professor, Department of Pediatrics,
University of Michigan, Ann Arbor, Michigan

Patrick E. Gipson, MD
Clinical Assistant Professor, Department of Internal
Medicine and Pediatrics, University of Michigan, Ann
Arbor, Michigan

Stanley Goldfarb, MD
Professor of Medicine, Department of Medicine,
University of Pennsylvania School of Medicine,
Philadelphia, Pennsylvania

Joyce M. Gonin, MD
Associate Professor of Medicine, Division of
Nephrology and Hypertension, Georgetown
University Medical Center, Washington, DC

Ryan S. Griffiths, MD
Nephrologist, Department of Medicine, Providence
St. Vincent's Hospital, Portland, Oregon;
Nephrologist, Department of Medicine, Legacy
Meridian Park Hospital, Tualatin, Oregon;
Nephrologist, Oregon Kidney and Hypertension
Clinic, Portland, Oregon

Mitchell L. Halperin, MD, FRCP(C), FRS
Emeritus Professor of Medicine, Department of
Medicine/Nephrology, University of Toronto and
St. Michaels Hospital; Attending Staff, Department of
Medicine/Nephrology, Keenan Research Centre in the
Li Ka Shing Knowledge Institute, Toronto, Ontario,
Canada

Marie C. Hogan, MD, PhD, FACP
Assistant Professor of Medicine, Division of
Nephrology and Hypertension, Department of Internal
Medicine, Mayo Clinic, Rochester, Minnesota

Edward J. Horwitz, MD
Assistant Professor of Medicine, Case Western
Reserve University School of Medicine; Assistant
Professor of Medicine, Department of Medicine,
MetroHealth Medical Center, Cleveland, Ohio

Susan Hou, MD, FACP
Professor of Medicine, Department of Medicine,
Division of Nephrology and Hypertension, Loyola
University Stritch School of Medicine; Medical
Director, Kidney Transplant Program, Department of
Medicine, Loyola University Medical Center,
Maywood, Illinois

Ashley B. Irish, MBBS, FRACP
Clinical Associate Professor, Faculty of Medicine and
Pharmacology, University of Western Australia;
Consultant Nephrologist, Department of Nephrology
and Renal Transplantation, Royal Perth Hospital,
Perth, Western Australia, Australia

J. Ashley Jefferson, MD, FRCP
Associate Professor, Division of Nephrology,
University of Washington, Seattle, Washington

Kamyar Kalantar-Zadeh, MD, MPH, PhD
Professor, Departments of Medicine, Pediatrics, and
Epidemiology, University of California, Los Angeles,
Los Angeles, California; Attending Nephrologist,
Department of Medicine, Harbor UCLA, Torrance,
California

Kamel S. Kamel, MD, FRCP(C)
Professor, Department of Medicine, University of
Toronto; Head, Division of Nephrology, Department
of Medicine, St. Michael's Hospital, Toronto, Ontario,
Canada

Elaine S. Kamil, MD
Professor of Pediatrics, Department of Pediatrics,
David Geffen School of Medicine at University of
California, Los Angeles; Clinical Director, Department
of Pediatric Nephrology, Cedars-Sinai Medical
Center, Los Angeles, California

B.S. Kawar, MBBS, MD, MRCP(UK)
Honorary Senior Lecturer, University of Sheffield;
Consultant Nephrologist, Sheffield Kidney Institute,
Sheffield Teaching Hospitals NHS Foundation Trust,
Sheffield, United Kingdom

Brian Kirmse, MD
Assistant Professor, Department of Genetics and
Genomic Sciences, Mount Sinai School of Medicine
and Mount Sinai Hospital, New York, New York

Csaba P. Kovesdy, MD
Clinical Associate Professor of Medicine, Division of
Nephrology, University of Virginia, Charlottesville,
Virginia; Chief of Nephrology, Salem Veterans Affairs
Medical Center, Salem, Virginia

Warren Kupin, MD, FACP
Professor of Medicine, Division of Nephrology and
Hypertension, University of Miami Miller School of
Medicine; Associate Director of Transplant Nephrology,
Division of Nephrology and Hypertension, Jackson
Memorial Hospital, Miami, Florida

Michael R. Lattanzio, DO
Fellow, Division of Nephrology, Department of
Medicine, University of Maryland School of
Medicine, Baltimore, Maryland

Edgar V. Lerma, MD, FACP, FASN,
FAHA, FASH, FNLA
Clinical Associate Professor of Medicine, Section of
Nephrology, Department of Medicine, University of
Illinois at Chicago College of Medicine; Associates
in Nephrology, S.C., Chicago, Illinois

Moshe Levi, MD
Professor of Medicine, Physiology, and Biophysics;
Vice Chair of Medicine for Research, Division of
Renal Diseases and Hypertension, University of
Colorado, Denver, Colorado

Edmund J. Lewis, MD
Muehrcke Family Professor of Nephrology, Director, Section of Nephrology, Department of Internal Medicine, Rush University Medical Center, Chicago, Illinois

Stuart L. Linas, MD
Professor, Department of Medicine, University of Colorado Denver School of Medicine; Chief of Nephrology, Denver Health, Denver, Colorado

Etienne Macedo, MD, MAS, PhD
Associate Professor, Division of Nephrology, Department of Medicine, University of Sao Paulo, Sao Paulo, Brazil

Supriya Maddirala, MD
Assistant Professor of Medicine, Medical Director, OHSU Acute Unit, Department of Medicine, Division of Nephrology, Oregon Health and Science University, Portland, Oregon

David Martins, MD, MS
Assistant Professor of Medicine, College of Medicine, Charles Drew University of Medicine and Science, Los Angeles, California

Rajnish Mehrotra, MBBS, MD
Professor of Medicine, Department of Medicine, David Geffen School of Medicine at the University of California, Los Angeles; Associate Chief, Division of Nephrology and Hypertension, Department of Medicine, Harbor-UCLA Medical Center, Los Angeles, California

Ravindra L. Mehta, MD, DM, FACP, FASN
Professor of Clinical Medicine, Associate Chair of Clinical Research, Director, UCSD, CREST, and MAS in Clinical Research Program, Department of Medicine, University of California, San Diego; Nephrologist, UCSD Medical Center Thornton Hospital, La Jolla, California; Nephrologist, UCSD Medical Center Hillcrest, San Diego, California

Maria Valentina Irazabal Mira, MD
Research Fellow, Division of Nephrology and Hypertension, Mayo Clinic, Rochester, Minnesota

Snesha Modi, MD
Resident Physician, Department of Internal Medicine, University of Illinois at Chicago-Advocate Christ Medical Center, Oak Lawn, Illinois

Rebecca Moore, MD
Assistant Professor, Department of Medicine, University of Colorado Denver School of Medicine, Denver, Colorado

Patrick H. Nachman, MD, FASN
Professor of Medicine, UNC Kidney Center, University of North Carolina, Chapel Hill, North Carolina

Lavinia A. Negrea, MD
Assistant Professor, Department of Medicine, Case Western Reserve University School of Medicine, University Hospitals Case Medical Center, Cleveland, Ohio

Lindsay E. Nicolle, MD, FRCPC
Professor, Department of Internal Medicine and Medical Microbiology, University of Manitoba; Department of Internal Medicine, Health Sciences Centre, Winnipeg, Manitoba, Canada

Marina Noris, PhD
Head, Transplant Research Center "Chiara Cucchi de Alessandri & Gilberto Crespi," Mario Negri Institute for Pharmacological Research, Ranica, Bergamo, Italy

Keith C. Norris, MD
Professor and Interim President, Department of Medicine, Charles Drew University; Assistant Dean for Translational Science, Department of Medicine, David Geffen School of Medicine at the University of California, Los Angeles, Los Angeles, California

Anna Oliveras, MD, PhD
Chief, Hypertension and Vascular Risk Unit, Department of Nephrology, Hospital Universitari del Mar, Parc de Salut Mar; Member, HERACLES Cardiovascular Research Network, Program of Research in Inflammatory and Cardiovascular Disorders (RICAD), IMIM, Hospital del Mar, Barcelona Biomedical Research Park, Barcelona, Spain

Ali J. Olyaei, PharmD
Professor of Medicine and Pharmacotherapy, Oregon State University/Oregon Health and Science University, Portland, Oregon

Sumanta Kumar Pal, MD
Assistant Professor, Department of Medical Oncology
and Experimental Therapeutics, City of Hope
Comprehensive Cancer Center, Duarte, California

Paul M. Palevsky, MD
Chief, Renal Section, VA Pittsburgh Healthcare
System; Professor of Medicine, Department of
Medicine, University of Pittsburgh School of
Medicine, Pittsburgh, Pennsylvania

Biff F. Palmer, MD
Professor of Internal Medicine, Director, Renal
Fellowship Training Program, Division of
Nephrology, Department of Internal Medicine,
University of Texas Southwestern Medical Center,
Dallas, Texas

Ami M. Patel, MD
Assistant Professor of Medicine, Division of
Nephrology and Hypertension, Drexel University
College of Medicine; Academic Nephrologist,
Hahnemann University Hospital, Philadelphia,
Pennsylvania

Mark A. Perazella, MD, FASN
Professor of Medicine, Director, Nephrology
Fellowship Training Program; Medical Director,
Physician Associate Program, Section of Nephrology,
Department of Medicine, Yale University School of
Medicine, New Haven, Connecticut

Sarah Prichard, MD, FRCP(C)
Vice President, Global Medical, Clinical, Scientific
Affairs and Research, Renal Division, Baxter
Healthcare, Deerfield, Illinois

Mahboob Rahman, MD, MS
Associate Professor, Department of Medicine, Case
Western Reserve University; Staff Nephrologist,
University Hospitals Case Medical Center; Staff
Nephrologist, Louis Stokes VA Medical Center,
Cleveland, Ohio

C. Venkata S. Ram, MD, MACP, FACC
Director, Texas Blood Pressure Institute; Director,
Medical Education and Clinical Research,
DNA; Clinical Professor of Internal Medicine,
University of Texas Southwestern Medical
School, Dallas, Texas

Madhav V. Rao, MD
Staff Physician, Section of Nephrology, Department
of Medicine, Advocate Illinois Masonic Hospital;
Weiss Memorial Hospital; Associates in Nephrology,
Chicago, Illinois

Vijaykumar M. Rao, MD, FACP, FASN
Adjunct Professor of Surgery, Northwestern
University/Feinberg School of Medicine; Assistant
Professor of Clinical Medicine, Rush University;
President, Associates in Nephrology, Chicago,
Illinois

Guiseppe Remuzzi, MD, FRCP
Director, Department of Immunology and
Transplantation, Azienda Ospedaliera Ospedali Riuniti
di Bergamo; Director, Negri Bergamo Laboratories,
Mario Negri Institute for Pharmacological Research,
Bergamo, Italy

Michael V. Rocco, MD, MSCE
Vardaman M. Buckalew, Jr. Professor of Medicine/
Nephrology, Department of Internal Medicine, Section
on Nephrology, Wake Forest University School of
Medicine, Winston-Salem, North Carolina

Claudio Ronco, MD
Director, Department of Nephrology Dialysis and
Transplantation, International Renal Research
Institute, San Bartolo Hospital, Vicenza, Italy

Ally Rosen, MD
Assistant Professor of Radiology, Mount Sinai
Medical Center, New York, New York

Mitchell H. Rosner, MD
Associate Professor and Vice Chairman, Department
of Medicine, University of Virginia, Charlottesville,
Virginia

Michael R. Rudnick, MD, FACP, FASN
Associate Professor of Medicine, Department of
Medicine, University of Pennsylvania School of
Medicine, Philadelphia, Pennsylvania

Earl H. Rudolph, DO
Nephrology Fellow, Department of Nephrology and
Hypertension, Georgetown University Medical Center,
Washington, DC

Jose F. Rueda, MD
Clinical Associate Professor, Department of Medicine, Division of Nephrology and Hypertension, Oregon Health and Science University, Portland, Oregon

Ernesto Sabath, MD
Hemodialysis Unit, Department of Nephrology, Hospital General de Queretaro, Queretaro, Mexico

John R. Sedor, MD
MetroHealth Research Endowment Professor, Department of Medicine, Case Western Reserve University; Department of Medicine, MetroHealth System, Cleveland, Ohio

Anuja Pradip Shah, MD
Clinical Instructor of Medicine, Department of Medicine, David Geffen School of Medicine at the University of California, Los Angeles; Clinical Instructor and Research Fellow, Division of Nephrology and Hypertension, Department of Medicine, Harbor-UCLA Medical Center, Torrance, California

William L. Simpson Jr., MD
Assistant Professor, Department of Radiology, Mount Sinai Medical Center; Attending Radiologist, Department of Radiology, Mount Sinai Hospital, New York, New York

Rajalingam Sinniah, DSc, MD, PhD, FRCPI, FRCPA, FRCPath
Clinical Professor of Pathology, School of Pathology and Laboratory Medicine, The University of Western Australia; Consultant Pathologist, Anatomic Pathology, Pathwest Laboratory Medicine, Royal Perth Hospital, Perth, Western Australia, Australia

James A. Sloand, MD, FACP
Adjunct Professor of Medicine, Department of Medicine, Nephrology Division, University of Rochester School of Medicine, Rochester, New York; Senior Medical Director, Medical Affairs, North American Renal Division, Baxter Healthcare Corporation, McGaw Park, Illinois

Mathew D. Sorensen, MD, MS
Clinical Fellow, Department of Urology, University of California San Francisco, San Francisco, California

Stuart M. Sprague, DO
Professor, Department of Medicine, University of Chicago Pritzker School of Medicine, Chicago, Illinois; Chief, Division of Nephrology and Hypertension, NorthShore University Health System, Evanston, Illinois

Lesley A. Stevens, MD, MS
Assistant Professor of Medicine, Department of Medicine, Tufts University School of Medicine; Attending Physician, William B. Schwartz Division of Nephrology, Tufts Medical Center, Boston, Massachusetts

John B. Stokes, MD
Professor and Director, Nephrology Division, Department of Internal Medicine, University of Iowa; Department of Veterans Affairs, Iowa City VA Medical Center, Iowa City, Iowa

Marshall L. Stoller, MD
Professor and Vice Chairman, Department of Urology, University of California, San Francisco, San Francisco, California

Lynda Anne M. Szczech, MD, MSCE
Associate Professor of Medicine, Department of Medicine/Nephrology, Duke University School of Medicine and Duke University Medical Center, Durham, North Carolina

Jeffrey Thomas, MD
Renal Fellow, Department of Nephrology, University of Colorado Health Sciences Center, Denver, Colorado

C. Craig Tisher, MD
Professor Emeritus, Department of Medicine, University of Florida College of Medicine; Attending Physician, Department of Medicine/Nephrology, Shands Hospital, Gainesville, Florida

Vicente Torres, MD, PhD
Professor of Medicine, Division of Nephrology and Hypertension, Mayo Clinic, Rochester, Minnesota

Howard Trachtman, MD, FASN
Professor of Pediatrics, Albert Einstein College of Medicine, Bronx, New York; Chief, Division of Nephrology, Department of Pediatrics, Cohen Children's Medical Center of New York, New Hyde Park, New York

Cynthia Tsien, MD, CM
Postgraduate Research Fellow, Department of Medicine, Division of Gastroenterology, Toronto General Hospital, Toronto, Ontario, Canada

Meryem Tuncel, MD
Assistant Professor, Department of Internal Medicine, Texas Tech University Health Sciences Center, Lubbock, Texas

Neil Turner, PhD, FRCP
Professor of Nephrology, Department of Renal Medicine, University of Edinburgh; Hon Consultant, Department of Renal Medicine, Royal Infirmary, Edinburgh, United Kingdom

Suneel M. Udani, MD, MPH
Fellow, Department of Nephrology, University of Chicago Medical Center, Chicago, Illinois

Beth A. Vogt, MD
Associate Professor, Department of Pediatrics, Case Western Reserve University; Attending Physician, Department of Pediatric Nephrology, Rainbow Babies and Children's Hospital, Cleveland, Ohio

Christoph Wanner, MD
Professor of Medicine, Department of Medicine, Division of Nephrology, University Hospital, Würzburg, Germany

Matthew R. Weir, MD
Professor and Director, Division of Nephrology, Department of Medicine, University of Maryland School of Medicine, Baltimore, Maryland

William L. Whittier, MD
Assistant Professor of Medicine, Department of Internal Medicine, Division of Nephrology, Rush University Medical Center, Chicago, Illinois

Eleri Williams, MRCP
University of Edinburgh, Renal Medicine, Royal Infirmary, Edinburgh, United Kingdom

Jay B. Wish, MD
Professor, Department of Medicine, Case Western Reserve University; Medical Director, Dialysis Program, University Hospitals Case Medical Center, Cleveland, Ohio

Florence Wong, MBBS, MD, FRACP, FRCPC
Associate Professor, Department of Medicine, University of Toronto; Staff Hepatologist, Department of Medicine, Toronto General Hospital, University Health Network, Toronto, Ontario, Canada

†Yalemzewd Woredekal, MD
Assistant Professor of Medicine, State University of New York Downstate Medical Center; Director, Hemodialysis, Kings County Hospital Center, Brooklyn, New York

†Deceased.

PREFACE

In medicine, the time-honored Socratic method has been the predominant influence in the teaching styles used by various institutions of higher learning, both locally and internationally. In keeping with this very effective teaching method, the first edition of Anthony Zollo's *Medical Secrets* was published in 1991. The subtitle was "Questions you will be asked on rounds, in the clinic, and on oral exams." The book was very successful, as it appealed not only to the learners but also to the teachers. Subsequently, various fields of medicine came out with their own editions, with particular focus on individual specialties.

In 2009 we gathered a select group of highly motivated individuals who were well-renowned authoritative figures in the various fields of nephrology, hypertension, and kidney transplantation and who had exemplary reputations with regard to the profession of teaching medicine. In keeping with the design of the original *Medical Secrets*, we have included questions on everyday topics in addition to some "zebras" with particular academic interest.

We hope that this book will be used not only by nephrologists and nephrology fellows, medical residents and interns, and medical students, but also by primary care providers with particular interest in this very exciting field of medicine.

From personal experience, we know that very few people read a textbook from cover to cover. For a variety of reasons, the majority would read only one or a few chapters at any given time. Therefore, we tried to ensure that each chapter would be complete in itself. As a consequence, there is unavoidable overlap among some of the information provided in some chapters; we, however, feel that this was truly necessary, at least from an information-retrieving standpoint, and in this way it will not be necessary for readers to read bits of information between one or more chapters just to get complete information regarding a particular subject.

Certainly this book would not have been possible were it not for so many people. First, we would like to thank the contributing authors, who have spent countless hours in producing high-quality, up-to-the-last-minute information that we would characterize as "edutaining." We spent a significant amount of time communicating via telephone and e-mail as we reviewed the chapters and discussed recommendations, most of which were agreed upon, but, on occasion, disputed. We express our sincere gratitude for their openness to this very collegial collaboration, which has been a truly rewarding learning experience for us. In particular, I would like to thank Dr. Jon Scheinman for his valuable review of the chapter on Sickle Cell Nephropathy. We appreciate the help and support of all the staff of Elsevier, most especially Andrea Vosburgh, our Developmental Editor; James Merritt, our Senior Acquisitions Editor; and Cassie Carey, our Production Editor, all of whom have been very patient with our procrastinations and stubbornness at times.

We thank our teachers and mentors, who devoted their own time to educate and train us to become who we are. We thank all the medical students, residents, and fellows who in one way or another have given us inspiration to persevere in the teaching profession. Mostly, we thank all of our patients, who have been truly instrumental in our learning and devotion to medicine. On behalf of all the contributors to this book, we fervently hope that all our efforts will contribute to relieving your suffering and perhaps lead to your recovery.

Dr. Yalem Woredekal, who died while this work was in preparation, exemplified courage and dedication sustaining academic purpose. Afflicted with renal failure requiring support by maintenance hemodialysis, she nevertheless was able to perform her duties as director of a university dialysis facility, including publishing insightful papers. We were proud to have Yalem's participation and will miss her wisdom, humanity, and empathy for the sick.

Edgar V. Lerma, MD
Allen R. Nissenson, MD

CONTENTS

III. CHRONIC KIDNEY DISEASE

IV. PRIMARY GLOMERULAR DISORDERS

VIII. RENAL DISEASES IN SPECIAL POPULATIONS

IX. TREATMENT OPTIONS

X. TRANSPLANTATION

XI. HYPERTENSION

XII. ACID–BASE AND ELECTROLYTE DISORDERS

TOP 100 SECRETS

These secrets are 100 of the top board alerts. They summarize the concepts, principles, and most salient details of nephrology.

1. Tobacco abuse confers a significant increase in the risk for progression of kidney dysfunction, regardless of the underlying cause of the kidney disease.

2. The urine protein-to-creatinine (using a random urine specimen) ratio has been shown to have a good correlation with the 24-hour urine protein determination.

3. All estimates of glomerular filtration rate (GFR) based on serum creatinine will be less accurate in patients not in a steady state of creatinine balance (in whom serum creatinine is changing), patients at the extremes of muscle mass (such as the frail elderly, critically ill, or those with cancer or, conversely, body builders), or those with unusual diets. Confirmatory tests with measured creatinine clearance should be performed for people in whom the estimates may be inaccurate.

4. Acute kidney injury (AKI), a term that is now replacing the older term acute renal failure (ARF), describes a sudden decrease in renal function occurring over a period of hours to days.

5. The most important risk factor for the development of AKI is the presence of pre-existing chronic kidney disease (CKD).

6. Use of loop diuretics should be limited to the management of patients with volume overload and not for AKI or oliguria per se.

7. It is not necessary to wait until severe uremia develops to initiate dialytic support; renal replacement therapy should be used as a supportive therapy in the presence of progressive azotemia and oliguria, rather than a rescue therapy for late manifestation of AKI.

8. In hospitalized patients with cirrhosis, prerenal azotemia is the most common cause of acute renal failure, followed by acute tubular necrosis, hepatorenal syndrome, and postrenal failure.

9. Patients with impaired left ventricular ejection fraction (LVEF) seem to be more prone to severe AKI compared to those with preserved LVEF, and the severity of left ventricular dysfunction correlates with the severity of AKI.

10. It is well established that individuals with CKD have a 10- to 20-fold increased risk for cardiac death compared to age-matched and gender-matched controls without CKD.

11. Patients with CKD have higher levels of BNP (b-type natriuretic peptide) and NT-proBNP (N-terminal pro b-type natriuretic peptide) than age- and gender-matched subjects without reduced renal function, even in the absence of clinical congestive heart failure (CHF).

12. More than two thirds of patients who developed acute phosphate nephropathy had three or more of the following risk factors: (1) age >60 years, (2) female gender, (3) GFR <60 mL/min, (4) hypertension, (5) angiotensin-converting enzyme (ACE) inhibitor/angiotensin-receptor blocker (ARB) use, and (6) diuretic use.

13. The proton pump inhibitors (PPIs) are associated primarily with acute interstitial nephritis; however, less common adverse renal effects include hyponatremia, impaired calcineurin inhibitor metabolism, and hypomagnesemia.

14. The weight loss drug orlistat rarely may cause acute kidney injury and nephrolithiasis because its use may lead to intestinal malabsorption and enteric hyperoxaluria.

15. The antiseizure and migraine drug topiramate is a carbonic anhydrase inhibitor that is associated with proximal renal tubular acidosis and calcium phosphate stone formation.

16. AKI resulting from sepsis occurs early in the course of the disease. Of patients presenting with septic shock, investigators found 64% had evidence of AKI, defined by the RIFLE criteria, within 24 hours of onset of shock.

17. Patients with septic AKI have a mortality rate of approximately 70% compared to 20% for patients with severe sepsis or 49% for patients with septic shock in the absence of AKI.

18. Rasburicase, a recombinant uric oxidase, rapidly lowers uric acid levels and, although expensive, is an effective therapy in the prevention and treatment of AKI associated with tumor lysis syndrome.

19. Another prophylactic treatment is N-acetylcysteine (also known as Mucomyst), which can be used for its antioxidative properties. Although results about its effectiveness are debatable, N-acetylcysteine is generally recommended because it is safe and inexpensive.

20. The natural history of the primary nephrotic syndrome depends on the underlying cause. Thus, patients with minimal change nephrotic syndrome (MCNS) have an excellent long-term prognosis, in contrast to those with primary focal segmental glomerulosclerosis (FSGS), in whom nearly 50% will progress to end-stage renal disease (ESRD) over 5 to 10 years of follow-up, and 25% to 30% of these patients may experience recurrent disease in a kidney transplant.

21. Corticosteroids are generally considered the first agent to be tried to reduce proteinuria in all patients with nephrotic syndrome, unless there is a clinical contraindication to their use.

22. Most patients with CKD die from cardiovascular disease before reaching ESRD.

23. Many patients with CKD not receiving hemodialysis and most patients receiving hemodialysis are iron deficient and require iron supplementation.

24. The FDA has determined that the target hemoglobin (Hb) level for patients with anemia and receiving erythrocyte-stimulating agents (ESAs) is 10 to 12 g/dL, but this has become a matter of some controversy.

25. Randomized controlled studies consistently demonstrate that normalizing the Hb level of patients with CKD with ESAs is associated with poorer outcomes than a Hb target in the 9.0 to 11.5 g/dL range.

26. The characteristic lipid profile of patients with chronic kidney disease consists of high triglycerides and low high-density lipoprotein (HDL) cholesterol concentrations, whereas total and low-density lipoprotein (LDL) cholesterol are normal or even low.

27. Post hoc analyses of statin trials support the administration of statins in patients with early stages of chronic kidney disease (CKD stage 1–3).

28. Patients with advanced chronic kidney disease do not benefit to the same extent from lipid-lowering therapy as do patients with early stages of CKD.

29. Although hemoglobin A1c is a sufficient marker of blood sugar control in a patient with kidney disease who does not yet require dialysis, this parameter has limited utility in patients who are receiving dialysis. Studies suggest little correlation between average blood glucose level and hemoglobin A1c as a result of nonenzymatic glycosylation of hemoglobin in the uremic serum and therefore little correlation with clinical outcomes.

30. Minimal change disease (MCD) is the cause of nephrotic syndrome in about 90% of children younger than age 6, in about 65% of older children, and in about 20% to 30% of adolescents. In adults, only about 10% to 25% of nephrotic syndrome results from MCD, but it represents the third most common cause of nephrotic syndrome in adults after membranous nephropathy and focal, segmental glomerulosclerosis.

31. The vast majority of children with MCD have a very favorable prognosis. In children a prompt remission within 7 to 9 days of steroid therapy, the absence of microhematuria, and age older than 4 years at presentation predict fewer relapses.

32. In adults, focal segmental glomerulosclerosis (FSGS) is the fourth most common cause of ESRD.

33. Primary FSGS has a high incidence of recurrence in allografts, and recurrence may lead to loss of the allograft.

34. Membranous nephropathy (MN) remains the leading cause of nephrotic syndrome in white adults. Patients who remain nephrotic are at an increased risk for thromboembolic and cardiovascular events.

35. Membranous nephropathy occurs as an idiopathic (75% of cases) or secondary disease (autoimmune diseases, infection, and malignancies), where up to 70% of patients will have nephrotic syndrome at the time of presentation. It is a chronic disease, with spontaneous remission and relapses clearly documented.

36. Current data suggest that new therapeutic agents such as rituximab and synthetic adrenocorticotropic hormone (ACTH) are effective in reducing proteinuria while having few adverse effects.

37. MN can recur after kidney transplantation in approximately 42% of patients, causing proteinuria, allograft dysfunction, and graft failure. Recurrence most often occurs during the first year.

38. Immunoglobulin A (IgA) nephropathy is the most common biopsy-proven primary glomerulonephritis in the world.

39. The classical presentation is painless gross hematuria 2 to 3 days after an upper respiratory infection.

40. When accompanied only by microscopic hematuria, the long-term prognosis of IgA nephropathy is excellent.

41. Primary membranoproliferative glomerulonephritis (MPGN) is one of the least common causes of idiopathic nephrotic syndrome, accounting for at most 5% to 10% of cases and an incidence in the range of 1 to 2 per million population per year.

42. Diabetic retinopathy is present in more than 95% of individuals with diabetic nephropathy.

43. A urinalysis should be performed on every patient with systemic lupus erythematosus (SLE) at each visit, and abnormalities in the urine should be confirmed and evaluated by a nephrologist. Immunologic serology for SLE and serum chemistries are also useful to determine whether lupus nephritis is present.

44. Urinalysis, although important, may be misleading because the increased urinary excretion of light chains associated with myeloma is not detected by testing for albumin (e.g., Albustix) but only for total protein (e.g., sulfosalicylic acid test) or by specific urine electrophoresis and immunofixation.

45. Myeloma cast nephropathy is a medical emergency and requires immediate diagnosis and early institution of therapy to prevent irreversible renal failure.

46. Dexamethasone, 20 mg bid, which induces apoptosis of plasma cells, can be immediately commenced to rapidly reduce the serum light-chain load while additional chemotherapy agents are considered.

47. Kidney injury is principally related to the light-chain component of myeloma because, unlike immunoglobulins, light chains are freely filtered at the glomerulus and reabsorbed in the proximal tubule.

48. The measurement of serum free light-chain (FLC) by nephelometry is rapid (hours); is more sensitive (1–3 mg/L); and, along with a serum panel of protein electrophoresis (SPE) (to determine the presence or a whole immunoglobulin component), will diagnose the majority of patients with myeloma, amyloidosis, and other monoclonal Ig deposition disease.

49. Goodpasture's disease is the most aggressive and rapidly progressive glomerulonephritis encountered in clinical practice. Crescentic nephritis may be accompanied by life-threatening pulmonary hemorrhage.

50. Treatment with cyclophosphamide, steroids, and plasma exchange can arrest the disease, but renal damage may be irrecoverable.

51. In small-vessel vasculitis, the mainstay of therapy consists of corticosteroids and cyclophosphamide.

52. In antineutrophil cytoplasmic autoantibody (ANCA) vasculitis, plasma exchange is presently recommended in addition to corticosteroids and cyclophosphamide for patients presenting with advanced renal failure and/or pulmonary hemorrhage.

53. A high rate of venous thromboembolism has been reported in ANCA vasculitis, with about 10% of patients developing symptomatic events.

54. In both atypical hemolytic uremic syndrome (HUS) and in thrombotic thrombocytopenic purpura (TTP), the clinical outcome; response to therapy; and, in atypical HUS, the outcome of kidney transplantation are greatly influenced by the specific underlying defect.

55. Identification of the specific genetic defect underlying atypical hemolytic uremic syndrome is critical to predict outcome, response to therapy, and outcome of kidney transplantation.

56. The course of poststreptococcal glomerulonephritis (PSGN) has been well documented for both the pharyngitis and skin infection sites of streptococcal infection; renal disease begins 10 to 14 days after the onset of streptococcal pharyngitis, whereas it takes about 21 days for the development of glomerulonephritis after a skin infection. These time patterns are critical because usually the infection has healed and only later on does the patient present with renal disease.

57. The typical serum creatinine level is usually 0.5 to 0.6 mg/dL in patients with cirrhosis, which is well below the normal expected maximum range for the general population—1.2 mg/dL for women and 1.5 mg/dL for men. Patients with liver disease can have a significant loss of GFR with a serum creatinine level within "the normal range" for the general population.

58. Patients with HIV are frequently coinfected with hepatitis C and/or B and may develop renal disease from these infections.

59. Highly active antiretroviral therapy (HAART) is the primary treatment only for HIV-associated nephropathy (HIVAN) and is not as successful in HIV immune-complex kidney (HIVICK).

60. Dialysis and transplantation are viable options for patients with HIV.

61. Guidelines require all patients with HIV to be regularly screened for renal disease with a GFR and urinalysis for proteinuria.

62. Patients receiving hemodialysis may have unrecognized Fabry disease, a treatable X-linked renal disease. The plasma α-galactosidase A assay reliably diagnoses affected males but not heterozygous females, who require mutation analysis for accurate diagnosis.

63. Enzyme replacement therapy in Fabry disease can clear the renal glycolipid accumulation and stabilize renal function; early treatment and adequate dose (1 mg/kg every other week) are important.

64. The classical triad of fever, maculopapular rash, and peripheral eosinophilia is seen in only a minority of cases (<10%) of acute tubulointerstitial nephritis (ATIN).

65. Drug-induced ATIN is not dose dependent. A repeat exposure to the same drug can potentially lead to recurrence of the disease process.

66. Pyuria is not, by itself, diagnostic of urinary tract infection or an indication for antimicrobial therapy. However, the absence of pyuria has a high negative predictive value to exclude urinary tract infection.

67. Asymptomatic bacteriuria should be screened for and treated only in pregnant women or individuals who are to undergo an invasive genitourinary procedure likely to be associated with mucosal bleeding.

68. There is a high rate of fetal loss among pregnant patients receiving dialysis, but the outcome of pregnancy in transplant recipients with stable, well-preserved renal function is good despite immunosuppressive medication.

69. Patients with sickle cell nephropathy may be particularly vulnerable to develop acute tubular necrosis as a result of hemodynamic insults or toxins, acute pyelonephritis, and urinary tract obstruction.

70. When possible, initial treatment with peritoneal dialysis has the potential benefit of improving early survival outcome, improving renal transplant results, preserving vascular access, and maintaining more downstream renal replacement options.

71. New policies have been proposed that would favor the allocation of kidney transplants from younger donors to younger recipients. This allocation schema would increase allocation of kidneys to patients more likely to benefit from transplantation, resulting in many thousands of additional life-years saved.

72. In 2004 the median time until any type of kidney transplant was 1219 days or approximately 3.3 years. The length of time until kidney transplantation has changed little between 1998 and 2004.

73. Quantification of BK virus DNA in plasma by polymerase chain reaction has a sensitivity and specificity of 100% and 88%, respectively; however, not all patients with viremia have nephritis (positive predictive value of 50%).

74. The goal in treating BK-associated nephropathy is to eradicate the virus while maintaining renal function and preventing acute or chronic rejection.

75. Those who are cytomegalovirus (CMV) donor positive and CMV recipient negative (CMV D+/R−) are at greatest risk for severe "primary" infection during the first 3 months post-transplantation. Data, however, demonstrated that the CMV D+/R+ group and not the D+/R− group has a worst graft and patient survival at 3 years.

76. The ALERT study demonstrated that statin use among patients who have had renal transplant conferred significant reductions in cardiovascular mortality.

77. Kidney/Disease Outcomes Quality Initiative (K/DOQI) guidelines suggest goal blood pressure less than 130/80 mm Hg for all recipients of renal transplant with a decreased goal of less than 125/75 mm Hg being considered in patients with significant proteinuria.

78. Reduction in cardiovascular risk and kidney disease progression is achieved by blood pressures (BP) substantially <140/90 mm Hg, approaching 130/80 mm Hg.

79. Indiscriminate sodium (salt) use or intake is a common cause of resistant hypertension and need for additional BP medications.

80. Home BP recordings, compared to clinic BP recordings, provide more information regarding cardiovascular and renal risk. Goal BPs are <135/85 mm Hg for patients with essential hypertension and <130/80 mm Hg for patients with diabetes or CKD.

81. For most patients with CKD, an ACE inhibitor or ARB is an appropriate first choice. With the epidemics of obesity, diabetes mellitus, and CKD, nearly all patients with hypertension will need multiple medications—many will require three or more.

82. No randomized trials to date have demonstrated a clear benefit for revascularization over medical management alone in the treatment of atherosclerotic renal artery stenosis.

83. Obstructive sleep apnea is becoming a more widely recognized cause of hypertension because we now have methods for efficient screening (with the Berlin questionnaire), diagnosis (with overnight polysomnographic testing, often in the home), and treatment (typically involving aldosterone antagonists), in addition to continuous positive airway pressure during sleep.

84. The most common cause of drug-induced hypertension is the (often self-) administration of nonsteroidal anti-inflammatory drugs; steroids, cyclosporine, erythropoietin, and tacrolimus are taken by fewer patients, but more antihypertensive drugs are usually prescribed when the patient taking these drugs experiences elevated blood pressures.

85. The JNC-VII guidelines recommend thiazide-type diuretics as initial drug therapy for most patients with isolated systolic hypertension (ISH) unless there are specific contraindications for their use.

86. The standard recommendation for lowering blood pressure in the setting of a hypertensive emergency is to lower mean arterial pressure by about 10% in the first hour and a further 10% to 15% in the next hour—NOT <140/90 mm Hg.

87. Although many intravenous antihypertensive drugs can be used for hypertensive emergencies, the pharmacokinetic advantages of sodium nitroprusside (very short onset of action, very short elimination half-life) usually outweigh the risk of cyanide or thiocyanate poisoning, which are more common with high doses or long durations of therapy.

88. Acute aortic dissection differs from all other hypertensive emergencies because the blood pressure target is <120/80 mm Hg within 20 minutes of diagnosis and it uses an intravenous β-blocker to decrease the shear stress on the ruptured intimal flap.

89. Although traditionally an acceptable first-line therapy for hypertension, β-blockers (particularly atenolol, which has ~72% of the clinical trial data) are not currently recommended in either U.S. or U.K. guidelines as initial therapy for uncomplicated hypertensives.

90. Limiting dietary sodium from 3 g/day to 1.5 g/day reduces BP both in hypertensive and nonhypertensive populations and can protect from cardiovascular disease.

91. Patients with obstructive sleep apnea (OSA) have a >2-fold higher risk for hypertension. Continuous positive airway therapy may improve BP, particularly in those patients with severe OSA.

92. Both weight loss and exercise can improve BP control. Moderate intensity exercise (e.g., walking) for a minimum of 30 minutes 5 days a week or vigorous activity (e.g., jogging) for a minimum of 20 minutes 3 days a week can improve BP even among older people.

93. A high salt intake can negate the beneficial effects of diuretics.

94. Abnormalities in serum sodium concentration reflect disturbances in water, not sodium homeostasis. Thus, disorders of serum sodium occur with low, normal, or high total body sodium.

95. Although every patient with hypernatremia is hypertonic, not every patient with hypo-natremia is hypotonic. Hyponatremia can coexist with normal or even high tonicity as in pseudohyponatremia and translocational hyponatremia.

96. Duration of hyponatremia and the presence of symptoms determine the correction of hyponatremia. In acute symptomatic hyponatremia, increasing serum sodium rapidly with hypertonic saline by 4 to 6 mEq/L may be sufficient to prevent tentorial herniation. In patients with chronic hyponatremia, correction limits are 12 mEq/L in 24 hours and 18 mEq/L in 48 hours to decrease the risk for osmotic demyelination. When these are exceeded, serum sodium should be lowered again.

97. Calcium will work within minutes to counteract the cardiac arrhythmias of hyperkalemia; however, it only lasts for minutes, so other more definitive treatments must be used after this initial life-saving measure.

98. The current recommendation not to use metformin in patients with renal insufficiency with a serum creatinine of 1.4 mg/dL (124 umol/L) in women or 1.5 mg dL (132 umol/L) in men is widely disregarded by most physicians because the incidence of lactic acido-sis remains extremely low; because it is not very soluble in lipids, it is a weak uncoupler of oxidative phosphorylation and hence rarely (in the absence of an acute overdose) is the sole cause of lactic acidosis.

99. Measuring the concentration of Cl^- in the urine in an excellent first step in the clinical approach to patients with metabolic acidosis.

100. Respiratory alkalosis is the most common acid–base abnormality in patients hospital-ized in intensive care units, occurring either as the simple disorder or as a component of mixed disturbances.

I. PATIENT ASSESSMENT

HISTORY AND PHYSICAL DIAGNOSIS

Edgar V. Lerma, MD, and Snesha Modi, MD

1. **How do patients with kidney disease typically present?**
   Patients with kidney disease typically present in several ways:
   - Abnormal laboratory studies (e.g., elevated blood urea nitrogen [BUN] and serum creatinine, decreased estimated glomerular filtration rate, or abnormal serum electrolyte values)
   - Asymptomatic urinary abnormalities (e.g., gross or microscopic hematuria, proteinuria, microalbuminuria)
   - Changes in urinary frequency or problems with urination (e.g., polyuria, nocturia, urgency)
   - New-onset hypertension
   - Worsening edema in dependent areas
   - Nonspecific symptomatologies (e.g., nausea, vomiting, malaise)
   - At times symptoms can be specific (e.g., ipsilateral flank pain in those with obstructing nephrolithiasis)
   - Incidental discovery of anatomic renal abnormalities on routine imaging studies (e.g., horseshoe kidney, congenitally absent or ptotic kidney, asymmetric kidneys, angiomyolipoma, renal mass, polycystic kidneys)

2. **What important features need to be elicited during history taking in patients referred for kidney disease evaluation?**
   - Previous diagnosis of kidney disease (e.g., previous documentation of BUN and serum creatinine values)
   - History of asymptomatic urinary abnormalities (e.g., hematuria, proteinuria)
   - History of alterations in urinary frequency or urgency, etc.
   - History of diabetes
   - History of hypertension (including cardiac history)
   - Previous exposure to nephrotoxic medications (e.g., NSAIDs, COXIBs)
   - Previous adverse reactions to renin-angiotensin-aldosterone system blocking agents (e.g., angiotensin-converting enzyme inhibitors, angiotensin receptor antagonists)
   - Recent gastrointestinal endoscopic procedures requiring bowel cleansing (risk of acute phosphate nephropathy in those who use phosphate-containing enema)
   - Recent exposure to contrast-requiring procedures (risk of contrast-induced nephropathy)
   - Recent systemic infections or intercurrent illnesses
   - Family history of kidney disease or any relative requiring some form of renal replacement therapy (e.g., polycystic kidney disease, Alport's syndrome)

3. **Why is smoking history important in patients with kidney disease?**
   Chronic kidney disease has been shown to be closely related to cardiovascular disease and smoking. The concept of smoking as an "independent" progression factor in kidney disease has been a subject of interest in numerous investigations. Since 2003 several publications of clinical and experimental data concerning the adverse renal effects of smoking have drawn interest, including large, prospective, population-based, observational studies. These studies

clearly demonstrate that smoking is a relevant risk factor, and it does confer a significant increase in the risk for progression of kidney dysfunction (i.e., elevation of serum creatinine) regardless of the underlying cause of the kidney disease.

It has been suggested that urinary cotinine, a metabolite of nicotine, can potentially be utilized as an objective measure of smoking exposure. Its use has not been studied in the population with chronic kidney disease.

4. **What familial diseases are characterized by kidney involvement?**
    - Polycystic kidney disease (PKD)
    - Focal segmental glomerulosclerosis (linked to chromosome 11)
    - Hypertension
    - Diabetes mellitus
    - Fabry's disease
    - Alport's syndrome
    - Sickle cell nephropathy
    - Familial hyperuricemic nephropathy
    - Hereditary interstitial kidney disease (HISK; linked to chromosome 1)
    - Familial hypercalcemic hypocalciuria
    - Cystinuria
    - HDR syndrome (syndrome of hypoparathyroidism, sensorineural hearing loss, and renal disease; also called Barakat syndrome; mapped to chromosome 10p)

5. **What are the common symptoms and signs that are seen in patients with advanced kidney disease?**
    Chronic kidney disease is usually characterized by nonspecific signs and symptoms in the earlier stages and can only be detected by an increase in serum creatinine.

    Symptoms
    - Loss or decreased appetite
    - Easy fatigability
    - Generalized weakness
    - Involuntary weight loss (resulting from cachexia) or gain (resulting from fluid retention)
    - Alterations in mentation (e.g., lethargy, coma, difficulty concentrating)
    - Nausea and vomiting; dyspepsia
    - Metallic taste
    - Generalized itching or pruritus
    - Seizures
    - Difficulty breathing
    - Edema
    - Intractable hiccups
    - "Frothy" appearance of urine
    - Decreased sexual interest (e.g., erectile dysfunction)
    - Restless legs

    Signs
    - Elevated blood pressure
    - Pallor (from anemia)
    - Volume overload (jugular venous distention, peripheral edema, pulmonary edema, anasarca)
    - Friction rub (pericarditis)
    - Asterixis and myoclonus

6. **What is a bedside diagnostic test that will suggest the presence of underlying diabetic nephropathy?**
    Funduscopy. It is believed that the similarities in the vascularization between the retina and the kidneys account for the correlation of the typical microvascular complications commonly seen in patients with diabetes mellitus.

    Patients with type 2 diabetes with proliferative retinopathy often present with renal involvement, manifested by either microalbuminuria (in the earlier stages) or overt proteinuria. It is, therefore, recommended that all patients with diabetes and proliferative retinopathy undergo an evaluation of renal function including testing for microalbuminuria.

    It must be remembered that although the presence of retinopathy does support a diabetic source of proteinuria, the lack of diabetic retinopathy does not rule out diabetic nephropathy. Such type 2 diabetics who do not have retinopathy frequently exhibit nondiabetic glomerular disease. However, in those with type 1 diabetes, only a minority of patients with advanced retinopathy have histologic changes in the glomeruli and microalbuminuria, and most have little or no renal disease.

7. **What are the common extrarenal manifestations associated with kidney diseases?**

Dermatologic (see Question 8)

Arthritis
- Lupus nephritis
- Rheumatoid arthritis
- Henoch-Schönlein purpura
- Cryoglobulinemia
- Sarcoidosis
- Amyloidosis
- Multiple myeloma
- Gout nephropathy

Hemoptysis
- Pulmonary renal syndome (PRS)
  Goodpasture's syndrome (also called anti-GBM disease)
  Henoch-Schönlein purpura
  Immunoglobulin A nephropathy
  Pauci-immune crescentic glomerulonephritis
  Wegener's granulomatosis
  Churg-Strauss syndrome
  Microscopic polyarteritis
  Cryoglobulinemia

- Lupus nephritis with pneumonitis
- Pulmonary thromboembolism/infarction related to hypercoagulability (membranous nephropathy)
- Volume overload (congestive heart failure, mitral stenosis)

Hearing Loss
- Alport's syndrome
- HDR syndrome (hypoparathyroidism, sensorineural hearing loss, and renal disease; also called Barakat syndrome)

Abdominal Discomfort
- Henoch-Schönlein purpura
- Cryoglobulinemia
- Microscopic polyarteritis

Intracerebral aneurysms: Autosomal-dominant polycystic kidney disease (also with mitral valve prolapse)

KEY POINTS: HISTORY AND PHYSICAL DIAGNOSIS

1. The similarities in the vascularization between the retina and the kidneys account for the correlation of the typical microvascular complications commonly seen in patients with diabetes mellitus.

2. Tobacco abuse confers a significant increase in the risk for progression of kidney dysfunction, regardless of the underlying cause of the kidney disease.

3. In patients with calciphylaxis, those with proximal lesions (trunk, buttocks, and thighs) tend to have worse prognosis compared with those with more distal lesions (forearms and fingers; calves and toes).

8. **What are common dermatologic manifestations of kidney disease?**
Xerosis or dryness of the skin, especially on the extensor surfaces of the extremities, is common among patients receiving dialysis. It can lead to generalized pruritus and can be extremely uncomfortable.

    Pruritus or itching is among the most common symptom of end-stage renal disease. In severe cases, it can be unrelenting. Although mostly benign in etiology (see xerosis, previous), it can lead to secondary complications, such as excoriations and lichen simplex chronicus, which may be disfiguring in extreme cases.

    The use of emollients, moisturizing lotions, keratolytic agents, and hydration have been commonly recommended as conservative treatment.

In some cases, phototherapy (ultraviolet B radiation [UBV] administered as total-body irradiation three times a week for a total of 8–10 sessions) has been shown to be helpful. It has been suggested that UBV (wavelength 280–315 nm) inactivates certain pruritogenic chemicals and induces the formation of metabolites with antipruritic effects. The risk of malignancy is fairly significant, especially in fair-skinned individuals.

Topical capsaicin (0.025%), by reducing the levels of substance P in cutaneous type C sensory nerve endings, has been useful for localized pruritus.

Topical tacrolimus (0.03% for 3 weeks, followed by 0.01% for another 3 weeks) has also been described to be of benefit but can predispose to dermatologic malignancies. For this reason it is not recommended as a first-line therapy and is not for prolonged use.

Gabapentin (100–300 mg after each dialysis treatment), a known anticonvulsant, also has antipruritic effects. Prominent side effects include depression of the central nervous system.

μ-opioid receptor antagonists, such as PO naltrexone, have also been used with some success. In the same family, intranasal butorphanol (a κ-opioid receptor agonist and μ-opioid receptor antagonist) has also been shown to be another option.

Other treatment options that have been tried in severe cases include PO-activated charcoal, selective 5-HT_3 antagonists (ondansetron and granisetron), oral cromolyn, cholestyramine, thalidomide, erythropoietin, and intravenous lidocaine.

Changes in pigmentation—in particular, hyperpigmentation—have been attributed to the increased levels of melanocyte-stimulating hormone (MSH) and the subsequent deposition of melanin in the basal layer of the epidermis.

Some patients may have a "sallow" discoloration of the skin believed to be caused by deposition of lipochrome pigment and carotenoids in the dermis and subcutaneous tissues.

Pallor is commonly associated with varying degrees of anemia as a result of chronic kidney disease.

Uremic frost refers to the deposition of crystallized urea that is excreted from sweat in the epidermis.

Ecchymoses are commonly associated with uremic platelet dysfunction.

Lindsay's nails, also known as "half and half nails," refer to the whitish discoloration of the proximal half of fingernails, believed to be a result of edema of the nail bed and underlying capillary network.

Calcific uremic arteriolopathy (CUA), also known as calciphylaxis, is characterized by painful, subcutaneous purpuric plaques and nodules that become necrosed in advanced stages. When the extremities are involved, the lesions tend to be bilateral and symmetric in distribution and often are described as a mottled or violaceous discoloration with a reticular pattern, similar to livedo reticularis (seen in atheroembolic renal disease). Of note, those with proximal lesions (trunk, buttocks, and thighs) tend to have a worse prognosis compared to those with more distal lesions (forearms and fingers; calves and toes).

Several known risk factors predispose to CUA—namely, poorly controlled secondary hyperparathyroidism, uncontrolled diabetes mellitus, female gender, duration of renal replacement therapy, and use of Coumadin (warfarin).

The increased expression of osteopontin and bone morphogenic protein 4 suggests the pivotal role that inducers of vascular calcification play in its pathogenesis.

Suspicion is the key to early diagnosis. When identified in its earlier stages (nonulcerative), initiation of therapeutic measures has been shown to improve prognosis.

Prevention is the key to management of CUA. Aggressive control of secondary hyperparathyroidism (see Chapter 21) is pivotal.

Sodium thiosulfate has two mechanisms of action—namely, it chelates Ca from soft tissues and it acts as an antioxidant, inducing endothelial nitric oxide synthesis, thereby improving local blood flow and soft tissue oxygenation. A commonly utilized regimen consists of IV Na thiosulfate 5 to 25 g administered during dialysis for several weeks to months.

Bisphosphonates (IV pamidronate and ibandronate and PO etidronate) are believed to be effective in altering ectopic deposition of calcium phosphate and directly inhibiting calcification via the nuclear factor κB cascade, although there are limited data.

Hyperbaric oxygen therapy improves oxygen delivery to damaged tissues by increasing the partial pressure of oxygen; it also promotes wound healing by supporting phagocytosis and angiogenesis while decreasing tissue edema.

Acquired perforating dermatosis (Kyrle disease) is predominantly seen in African Americans with diabetes mellitus. It is usually characterized by a linear confluence of papules with a central, oyster shell–like keratotic plug, distributed on the trunk, proximal extremities, scalp, and face, and the lesions are pruritic. Possible etiologies include an inflammatory skin reaction secondary to the presence of uremic toxins, uric-acid deposits, or scratching-induced trauma.

Porphyria cutanea tarda (PCT) commonly presents as a vesicobullous disease commonly involving the dorsum of both hands and feet but can affect any sun-exposed areas. It is commonly accompanied by sclerodermoid plaques (facial hyperpigmentation) and hypertrichosis. It is usually secondary to increased levels of uroporphyrins.

Avoidance of sun exposure is the cornerstone of management. Other measures to decrease uroporphyrin levels include the use of high flux dialysis membranes (to improve dialysis efficacy) and small-volume weekly phlebotomies in extreme, rare cases.

Common precipitating factors are alcohol intake, use of estrogen and iron supplementations, and chronic infections (e.g., hepatitis B or C virus, HIV).

One common differential diagnosis is pseudoporphyria, which is clinically similar to PCT with the exception of normal uroporphyrin levels.

Nephrogenic systemic fibrosis (NSF) is characterized by progressive fibrosis and thickening of the skin (similar to scleroderma), which is particularly painful. The lesions appear as plaques, papules, or nodules distributed in an asymmetric fashion over the distal extremities.

Recently, the pathogenetic role of gadolinium (contrast material used in magnetic resonance studies) has been the subject of interest. The interval between exposure to gadolinium and the early manifestations of NSF can range from 2 days to 18 months, and this wide range of variability has been attributed to the mobilization of gadolinium from bone stores over time.

No effective treatment is known to date. Preventive measures are often the main keys. Prophylactic measures that have been described include the use of hemodialysis (HD; eliminates 92% of gadolinium after two HD sessions; 99% after three HD sessions) in patients with advanced stages of chronic kidney disease. Peritoneal dialysis is not effective in eliminating gadolinium from the body.

REFERENCES

1. Abu-Alfa A. The impact of NSF on the care of patients with kidney disease. *J Am Coll Radiol* 2008;5:42–52.

2. Glynne P, Deacon A, Goldsmith D, Pusey C, Clutterbuck E. Bullous dermatoses in end-stage renal failure: Porphyria or pseudoporphyria? *Am J Kidney Dis* 1999;34:155–160.

3. Jones-Burton C, Vessal G, Brown J, Dowling TC, Fink JC. Urinary cotinine as an objective measure of cigarette smoking in chronic kidney disease. *Nephrol Dial Transplant* 2007;22(7):1950–1954.

4. Kuypers D. Skin problems in chronic kidney disease. *Nat Clin Pract Nephrol* 2010;5:157–170.

5. National Kidney Foundation. K/DOQI clinical practice guidelines for chronic kidney disease: Evaluation, classification, and stratification. *Am J Kidney Dis* 2002;39(2 Suppl 1):S1–266.

6. Orth SR, Hallan SI. Smoking: A risk factor for progression of chronic kidney disease and for cardiovascular morbidity and mortality in renal patients—Absence of evidence or evidence of absence? *Clin J Am Soc Nephrol* 2008;3:226–236.

7. Penfield JG, Reilly RF Jr. What nephrologists need to know about gadolinium. *Nat Clin Pract Nephrol* 2007;3:654–668.

CHAPTER 2

URINALYSIS

Edgar V. Lerma, MD, and Mitchell H. Rosner, MD

1. **What is uroscopy?**

   Uroscopy comes from the word "uroscopia" meaning scientific examination of the urine. It is derived from the Greek words *ouron* meaning urine and *skopeo* meaning to behold, contemplate, examine, or inspect. Such analysis of the urine has been historically called uroscopy until the 17th century, and now it is called "urinalysis."

2. **What is the proper way of collecting and handling a urine specimen for analysis?**

   When collecting the urine specimen, the first 200 mL of early-morning voided urine should be discarded. In men a simple midstream urine collection should suffice, whereas in women the external genitalia should be cleaned first, to avoid contamination with secretions, before collecting the urine specimen in midstream. The specimen should be collected in a clean, but not necessarily sterile, container.

   Thereafter, the urine specimen should be analyzed within the first 30 to 60 minutes of voiding; the initially uncentrifuged specimen is examined under the microscope for various elements, such as red blood cells (RBCs) and RBC casts, white blood cells (WBCs) and WBC casts, squamous epithelial cells, hyaline and granular casts, and so on. Subsequently, it is centrifuged at 3000 rpm for approximately 3 to 5 minutes. The resulting supernatant is collected in a test tube and analyzed for color, pH, specific gravity, blood, protein, and glucose.

3. **What are the typical elements in a routine urinalysis? What are the possible interpretations of the findings?**

   See Table 2-1.

   - **Color:** Normal urine color can vary from pale or light yellow to deep amber or dark yellow, and color is a result of the presence of a pigment called urochrome. Two important characteristics that influence urine color are its chemical composition and urine concentration. In a subject who is volume depleted, urine concentration tends to be elevated, giving rise to a highly darker-yellow urine. However, in a patient with diabetes insipidus, urine-concentrating ability is impaired, thereby making the urine lighter yellow in color. Certain medications and foods also can alter the urine color (Table 2-2). In porphyria cutanea tarda, the urine turns into the color of port wine.
   - **Clarity or turbidity:** The degree of turbidity or cloudiness is usually influenced by excess amounts of cellular debris and casts but can also be secondary to excess proteinuria and/ or crystals or contamination with vaginal discharge.
   - **pH:** Normal urine pH ranges between 4.5 and 8.0. In a normal individual, the daily average endogenous acid production is 1 mEq/kg, and this entails an obligate renal H ion excretion to maintain acid balance, thereby keeping urine pH lower or slightly acidic. It is useful in differentiating the different types of renal tubular acidosis (RTA), which is characterized by the inability to acidify urine to a pH <3.5 (i.e., despite an overnight fast and acid loading). Similarly, it also provides a clue to certain disease states (e.g., nephrolithiasis). Alkaline urine is usually seen in urinary tract infection (UTI) caused by urea-splitting organisms

TABLE 2-1.	URINE DIPSTICK TESTING	
Measured	False-Negative Results	False-Positive Results
Specific gravity	Reduced values in the presence of glucose, urea, alkaline urate	Increased values in the presence of protein >1 g/L, ketoacids
pH	Reduced values in the presence of formaldehyde	—
Hemoglobin	Ascorbic acid, high nitrite concentration, delayed examination, high density of urine, formaldehyde (0.5 g/L)	Myoglobin, microbial peroxidases, oxidizing detergents, hydrochloric acid
Glucose	Ascorbic acid, urinary tract infection	Oxidizing detergents, hydrochloric acid
Albumin	Immunoglobulin light chains, hydrochloric acid, tubular proteins, globulins, colored urine	Alkaline urine (pH 9), quaternary ammonium detergents, chlorhexidine, polyvinylpyrrolidone
Leukocyte esterase	Isotonic urine, vitamin C (intake g/day), protein >5 g/L, glucose >20 g/L, mucous specimen, cephalosporins, nitrofurantoin; mercuric salts, trypsin inhibitor oxalate, 1% boric acid	Oxidizing detergents, formaldehyde (0.4 g/L), sodium azide, colored urine from beet ingestion, or bilirubin
Nitrites	No vegetables in diet, short bladder incubation time, vitamin C, Gram-positive bacteria	Colored urine
Ketones	Improper storage	Free sulfhydryl groups (e.g., captopril), L-dopa, colored urine

From Johnson RJ, Feehally J. *Comprehensive clinical nephrology,* 2nd ed. Philadelphia: Mosby, 2003.

(*Proteus mirabilis*), associated with magnesium–ammonium phosphate crystals and staghorn calculi, whereas acidic urine is seen with uric acid calculi. In rhabdomyolysis, some investigators recommend that urine should be alkalinized (pH >6.5) to prevent myoglobin from forming potentially obstructing tubular casts.

- **Specific gravity:** The urine-specific gravity (1.005–1.025) reflects the ability of the kidneys to concentrate urine. In patients with impaired urinary-concentrating ability (acute tubular necrosis, sickle cell nephropathy, diabetes insipidus), the specific gravity tends to be low. Although imprecise at times, it can reflect a person's hydration status.
- **Blood:** The urinary dipstick test for blood detects the peroxidase activity of RBCs. In the presence of positive hematuria on dipstick analysis, the concomitant presence of RBCs on urine microscopy confirms the presence of hematuria as opposed to hemoglobinuria (paroxysmal nocturnal hemoglobinuria, transfusion-related reactions, infection with *Plasmodium falciparum,* infection with *Clostridium welchii)* and myoglobinuria (rhabdomyolysis or myoglobinuric renal failure).
- **Protein:** Normal urinary protein should not exceed 150 mg/day. Among these urinary proteins are albumin and Tamm-Horsfall mucoproteins (also called uromodulin). Urinary

TABLE 2-2.	POSSIBLE CAUSES OF ALTERED URINE COLOR
Urine Color	**Possible Causes**
Red	Foods: beets, blackberries, rhubarb Medications: laxatives, antipsychotics (chlorpromazine, thioridazine), Anesthetics (propofol) Toxins: lead, mercury Conditions: urinary tract infections, nephrolithiasis, porphyria, hemoglobinuria (rhabdomyolysis); see Question 7
Orange	Foods: vitamin C, carrots Medications: rifampin, phenazopyridine
Green	Foods: asparagus Medications: vitamin B, propofol Conditions: *Pseudomonas* urinary tract infection
Blue	Medications: amitriptyline, indomethacin, IV cimetidine, IV promethazine, triamterene, methylene blue Conditions: blue diaper syndrome (see Question 5)
Brown	Foods: fava beans Medications: antimalarials (chloroquine, primaquine), antimicrobials (metronidazole, nitrofurantoin), laxatives (senna), methocarbamol, levodopa Conditions: hepatobiliary diseases (obstructive and nonobstructive), tyrosinemia, Gilbert's syndrome
Purple	See Question 4
Black	Conditions: malignant melanoma, porphyria, alkaptonuria (ochronosis)

dipsticks only detect the presence of albumin; however, they are notorious for being poor indicators of the presence of urinary globulins and Bence Jones proteins (commonly seen in multiple myeloma). It is important to recognize that the dipstick measurement of urine protein is dependent on the concentration of the urine specimen so that a patient with a small volume of concentrated urine may test 2+ for protein, but when a 24-hour urine collection is obtained the actual daily concentration is much smaller. However, a patient with a large volume of dilute urine may test trace positive for protein but may have a larger amount of total 24-hour urine protein excretion. Thus, it is important to quantitate the amount of proteinuria found on dipstick testing (Table 2-3). A more reliable test for the presence of nonalbumin proteins is called the sulfosalicylic acid test (SSA), which is more reliable in detecting the presence of albumin, globulin, and Bence Jones proteins in the urine, even in low amounts (Table 2-4). See Questions 14–16 for more on proteinuria.

- **Glucose:** Normal urinary glucose should not exceed 130 mg/day. Glucosuria commonly indicates the presence of diabetes mellitus. Urinary dipsticks (utilize the glucose oxidase reaction) only detect the presence of glucose. For pediatric patients with suspected inborn errors of metabolism, other semi-quantitative tests are used, such as Clinitest and Benedict's test.
- **Ketones:** The presence of ketones in the urine is abnormal. Three common ketones detected include acetone, acetoacetic acid, and β-hydroxybutyric acid. Conditions whereby ketonuria may be present include poorly controlled diabetes, pregnancy, and starvation.

TABLE 2-3. URINARY DIPSTICKS

Dipstick	Proteinuria (mg/dL)
Trace	10–30
1+	30
2+	100
3+	300
4+	≥1,000

TABLE 2-4. SULFOSALICYLIC ACID TEST

Sulfosalicylic Acid Test	Appearance/Result	Proteinuria (mgs/dL)
Trace	Slight turbidity	20
1+	Print visible through specimen	50
2+	Print invisible	200
3+	Flocculation	500
4+	Dense precipitate	≥1000

- **Nitrite:** Urinary nitrates are converted by certain bacterial species (*Escherichia coli, Klebsiella, Proteus, Pseudomonas, Enterobacter, Citrobacter*) into nitrite. Therefore, a positive nitrite is an indication of the presence of such bacteria. Certain bacteria (*Haemophilus, Staphylococcus, Streptococcus*) do not have the ability to convert nitrate to nitrite. Therefore, this test is considered specific but not very sensitive, whereas a positive nitrite may be suggestive of an active urinary tract infection; a negative result does not necessarily rule it out.
- **Leukocyte esterase:** When WBCs in the urine undergo lysis, esterases are released. Therefore, a positive leukocyte esterase test generally implies the presence of underlying pyuria and urinary tract infection. Sterile pyuria is usually seen in analgesic nephropathy and in urinary tract infections caused by *Chlamydia, Ureaplasma urealyticum,* and *Mycobacterium tuberculosis.*
- **Bacteria:** In the appropriate clinical scenario, positive tests for nitrite, leukocyte esterase, and bacteria further strengthen the diagnosis of underlying urinary tract infection. However, despite this, one has to also consider the presence of squamous epithelial cells, which if abundant (≥15–20/hpf) may indicate primarily a contaminated urine specimen.
- **Bilirubin and urobilinogen:** Normally, bilirubin in the urine should be undetectable. The presence of significant amounts of water-soluble, conjugated bilirubin in the urine may be a clue to underlying liver disease or obstructive hepatobiliary conditions. Conjugated bilirubin is normally metabolized into urobilinogen, which is reabsorbed via the portal circulation, with a small amount being filtered by the glomerulus. Increased levels of urobilinogen are seen in conditions characterized by excessive hemolysis of RBCs and liver parenchymal diseases. In obstructive biliary disease, urobilinogen levels are decreased.
- **Microscopy:**
  Cells: The presence of >15–20 squamous epithelial cells/hpf is usually an indication that the urine specimen is contaminated. The presence of dysmorphic RBCs (also called acanthocytes) and/or RBC casts is the *sine qua non* of glomerulonephritis. The presence of

increased WBCs and/or WBC casts points to underlying urinary tract infections or tubulointerstitial diseases. The presence of <2–5 WBCs/hpf is considered normal.

Casts: Urinary casts are cylindrical particles that are formed from coagulated protein (Tamm-Horsfall protein) secreted by tubular cells. As their name implies, they are usually formed in the long, thin, hollow renal tubules and they take the shape of the tubule. They are formed only in the distal convoluted tubule or the collecting duct. The proximal convoluted tubule and loop of Henle are not locations for cast formation. Factors known to promote cast formation include low urine flow rate, high urinary salt concentration, and low urine pH, all of which favor protein denaturation and precipitation, particularly that of the Tamm-Horsfall protein (which serves as the organic matrix that glues or cements casts together) (Table 2-5; Fig. 2-1).

Crystals: See Table 2-6 and Figure 2-2.

Bacteria: Because of the abundance of normal microbial flora in the vagina and/or external urethral meatus, it is not uncommon to see bacteria in urine specimens. Similarly, if the urine specimen is left standing at room temperature for a considerable period, such bacteria can multiply rapidly. Therefore, the identification of various microbial organisms (on Gram staining) in any urine specimen should be interpreted with regard to concomitant symptomatology. (See Chapter 47 for discussion regarding asymptomatic bacteriuria.) Therefore, the diagnosis of bacteriuria in those with suspected urinary tract infection should be followed immediately by a culture and sensitivity study. In general, the presence of ≥100,000/mL of a single organism reflects significant bacteriuria. The presence of multiple organisms may reflect polymicrobial contamination. However, the presence of any organism in catheterized or suprapubic tap obtained specimens should be considered significant.

Yeasts: The presence of yeast cells may represent either contamination or true infection. They are often difficult to distinguish from red cells and amorphous crystals but are distinguished by their tendency to bud. Most often they are *Candida,* which may colonize the bladder, urethra, or vagina.

Pus cells: Pyuria may be indicative of underlying urinary tract infection. However, when associated with other cellular elements, or debris, it may have very limited diagnostic value.

TABLE 2-5. CASTS	
Urinary Casts	**Disease Associations**
Hyaline	May be nonspecific; seen in normal individuals or during severe intra-vascular volume depletion (after strenuous exercise or with diuretic use)
Granular	Acute tubular necrosis ("muddy-brown" granular casts)
Waxy and broad	Advanced kidney disease
Red blood cell	Glomerulonephritis
White blood cell	Urinary tract infections (pyelonephritis, cystitis), tubulointerstitial nephritis, renal tuberculosis, vaginal infections
Fatty	Nephrotic syndrome ("Maltese-cross" appearance under polarized light)

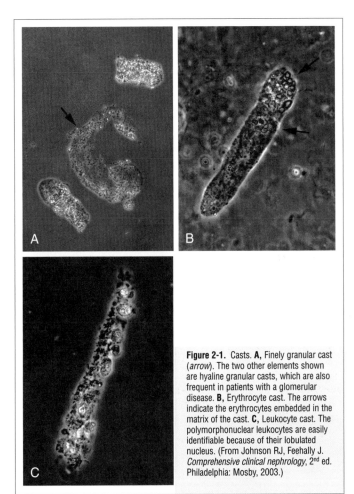

Figure 2-1. Casts. **A,** Finely granular cast (*arrow*). The two other elements shown are hyaline granular casts, which are also frequent in patients with a glomerular disease. **B,** Erythrocyte cast. The arrows indicate the erythrocytes embedded in the matrix of the cast. **C,** Leukocyte cast. The polymorphonuclear leukocytes are easily identifiable because of their lobulated nucleus. (From Johnson RJ, Feehally J. *Comprehensive clinical nephrology*, 2nd ed. Philadelphia: Mosby, 2003.)

TABLE 2-6.   CRYSTALS

Urinary Crystals	Description	Disease Association
Calcium oxalate	"Envelope-shaped"	Ethylene glycol toxicity
Uric acid	"Diamond" or "Barrel-shaped"	Hyperuricosuria
Triple phosphate (also called struvite) or magnesium ammonium phosphate	"Coffin-lid"	Urinary tract infection caused by urea-splitting organisms (*Proteus, Klebsiella*)
Cystine	"Hexagonal"	Cystinuria
Flat rectangular crystal plates	"Fan" or "starburst" pattern	Indinavir

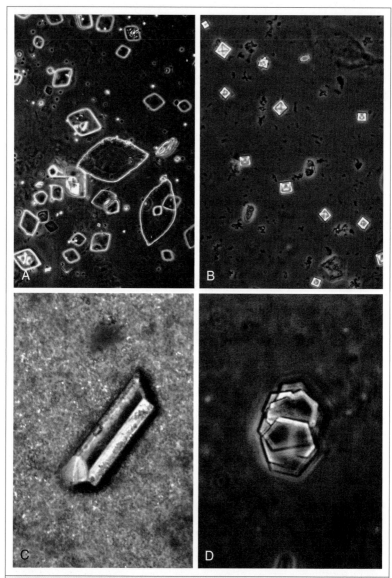

Figure 2-2. Crystals. **A,** Uric acid crystals. This rhomboid shape is the most frequent. **B,** Bihydrated calcium oxalate crystals. They have the typical appearance of a letter envelope. **C,** Triple phosphate crystal. On the background of a massive amount of amorphous phosphates particles. **D,** Cystine crystals. (From Johnson RJ, Feehally J. *Comprehensive clinical nephrology*, 2nd ed. Philadelphia: Mosby, 2003.)

4. **What is the purple urine bag syndrome?**

   Initially described in medical literature in 1978, purple urine bag syndrome (PUBS) is a rare condition associated with alkaline urine and urinary tract infections caused by sulphatase- and phosphatase-producing bacteria (*Providencia, E. coli, Proteus, Pseudomonas, Klebsiella*). It is commonly observed in institutionalized elderly females with chronic indwelling catheters who are also constipated. The etiology remains unclear, although it is believed that the presence of indigo and indirubin pigments (which are metabolites of tryptophan) react with the synthetic material composition of the urinary catheter and bag and are responsible for the purple discoloration of the urine.

   Of interest, from a historical perspective, England's "Mad" King George III was described by his physicians in 1812 to have a blue-tinged urine.

5. **What is the blue diaper syndrome?**

   This is another name for familial hypercalcemia with nephrocalcinosis and indicanuria, a rare, autosomal recessive disease caused by a metabolic defect in the reabsorption of tryptophan in the basolateral membrane of the proximal tubule. Bacterial degradation of tryptophan in the intestine leads to an excessive production of indole, thereby leading to indicanuria, which, during oxidation to indigo blue, causes a peculiar bluish discoloration of the urine staining the diaper. Symptoms generally involve the alimentary tract and include vision problems and fevers.

6. **What is red diaper syndrome?**

   It is seen in infants and is caused by prodigiosin, which is a red pigment produced by many strains of the Gram-negative bacillus *Serratia marcescens*.

7. **What is black urine disease?**

   Also called alkaptonuria or homogentisuria, it is a rare, autosomal-recessive condition, secondary to a defect in the enzyme homogentisate 1,2-dioxygenase, which is involved in the degradation of tyrosine. As a result, homogentisic acid is formed and excreted in the urine in excessive amounts. Excessive homogentisic acid causes ochronosis, pigmented sclerae, aortic and mitral regurgitation, and formation of kidney stones and prostatic stones.

   Of interest, most cases in literature are in patients who are either from Slovakia or the Dominican Republic.

8. **Does the odor of the urine have any diagnostic significance?**

   The ammonia odor of normal urine is usually a result of bacterial (normal flora) breakdown of urea. The odor of urine is influenced by consumption of certain foods and medications. For instance, consumption of asparagus and curry can cause a strong odor to urine.

9. **What is the significance of hematuria?**

   Hematuria can be either gross or microscopic.
   - Gross hematuria is the presence of red or brown urine that is visible to the naked eye. The degree of discoloration has limited value because as little as 1 mL of blood per liter of urine can cause varying degrees of urine discoloration. In the initial evaluation of a patient with gross hematuria, it must be determined whether the urine discoloration is truly secondary to pathologic bleeding within the urinary tract. In patients who are menstruating or in the postpartum states, it is not ideal to evaluate them for hematuria. Conditions whereby the urine may appear grossly red, in the absence of actual bleeding, include intake of certain medications, such as rifampin, phenothiazine, or phenazopyridine (analgesic), or intake of beets in certain predisposed individuals. It is also important to differentiate hematuria from other causes of red urine such as hemoglobinuria and myoglobinuria. The latter is usually seen in those with acute rhabdomyolysis.
   - Microscopic hematuria is defined as the presence of three or more RBCs/hpf in two of three urine samples. Often, it is detected incidentally by urine dipstick examination.

Careful history taking is of paramount importance in the evaluation of patients with hematuria. Important historical information usually provides diagnostic clues. For instance, the occurrence of concomitant flank pain with radiation to the ipsilateral testicle or labia suggests underlying nephrolithiasis; burning on urination or dysuria may point to possible urinary tract infection; a recent bout of upper respiratory tract infection may suggest either postinfectious glomerulonephritis or immunoglobulin A nephropathy. A family history of hematuria is also vital because certain diseases tend to run in families, such as polycystic kidney disease or sickle cell nephropathy. Likewise, thin basement membrane nephropathy (TBMN; also known as benign familial hematuria) tends to occur in families and is notable for having a rather benign course despite the presentation. Exercise-induced hematuria is a benign condition seen in adolescents who exercise vigorously (e.g., long-distance runners).

In elderly individuals (those older than age 50) the finding of gross or microscopic (even transient) hematuria should trigger an extensive evaluation to rule out malignancy involving the genitourinary tract. The incidence of bladder cancer and other malignancies involving the kidneys and the ureters is significantly elevated, particularly in those with a prolonged history of chronic smoking and analgesic use. The occurrence of symptoms of increased urgency and frequency with hematuria in this population should suggest urinary tract obstruction secondary to either benign prostatic hypertrophy (BPH) or prostatic malignancy.

At times, the presence of asymptomatic hyperuricosuria or hypercalciuria (spot urine calcium-to-urine creatinine ratio >2.0 mg/kg) can also cause hematuria, and this is common in children.

An important aspect of the evaluation of patients with hematuria is to differentiate glomerular from nonglomerular bleeding (Table 2-7). For those with glomerular bleeding, especially in the presence of progressive renal decline, a percutaneous renal biopsy may be necessary.

TABLE 2-7. GLOMERULAR VERSUS NONGLOMERULAR BLEEDING

Glomerular	Nonglomerular
Associated with: Proteinuria >500 mg/day Red blood cell (RBC) casts Dysmorphic RBCs	Associated with: Proteinuria >500 mg/day Absent RBC casts Absent dysmorphic RBCs
Usually seen in acute glomerulonephritis, thin basement membrane nephropathy (TBMN)	**Renal Causes:** Tubulointerstitial nephritis Polycystic kidney disease Sickle cell disease or trait Renovascular disease (atheroembolic renal disease, renal vein thrombosis, arteriovenous malformations, nutcracker syndrome)
	Urologic Causes: Tumors or malignancies Stones Infections (urethritis, prostatitis, cystitis, pyelonephritis)
	Medications: Chemotherapeutic agents (cyclophosphamide, ifosfamide, mitotane) Anticoagulants

10. **What is the "three tube test" for hematuria?**
The three tube test (also called three container method) is performed to determine the location of bleeding in the urinary tract. Three consecutive samples of the urine stream are collected: the first 10–15 mL, midstream 30–40 mL, and the last 5–10 mL. Hematuria (or predominance of RBCs on urine microscopy) primarily in the first sample (initial hematuria) is suggestive of an anterior urethral source of bleeding, whereas hematuria primarily at the end of the urine stream (terminal hematuria) points to a lesion at the bladder trigone (bladder neck) or a posterior urethra. Hematuria in all three samples is seen in lesions that may be anywhere above the bladder neck (bladder, ureters, or kidneys).

11. **What is cyclic hematuria?**
It is commonly seen in women in the reproductive age group, in whom the onset of hematuria correlates with menstrual periods, suggesting the possibility of endometriosis involving the urinary tract. It is also seen in vesicouterine fistulas that arise as a complication of previous cesarean sections (Youssef's syndrome).

12. **What is the loin pain hematuria syndrome?**
Considered as a diagnosis of exclusion in patients with hematuria, loin pain hematuria syndrome (LPHS) is characterized by the presence of recurrent or persistent, severe, unilateral or bilateral flank pain accompanied by gross or microscopic hematuria. Commonly seen in young, white females, it has been associated with chronic pelvic pain and with thin basement membrane nephropathy.

13. **What is the nutcracker syndrome?**
Nutcracker syndrome is also known as left renal vein entrapment syndrome. It is believed to be secondary to compression of the left renal vein as it passes through the angle between the abdominal aorta and the superior mesenteric artery. Common presentations include hematuria (resulting from varices within the renal pelvis and ureter), left-sided varicocele, and left flank discomfort. Diagnosis is established by performing a left renal venography. Treatment is primarily surgical (e.g., endovascular stenting, renal vein reimplantation, and gonadal vein embolization).

14. **What is the significance of proteinuria?**
Proteinuria usually implies that there is a defect in glomerular permeability. In general, proteinuria can be classified into persistent or transient. Among the causes of persistent proteinuria, there are three types: (1) glomerular, (2) tubular, or (3) overflow.
- Glomerular proteinuria includes diabetic nephropathy and other common glomerular disorders. It is usually caused by increased filtration of albumin across the glomerular capillary wall. Other causes of glomerular proteinuria have a rather benign course, such as orthostatic and exercise-induced proteinuria. These latter causes are characterized by significantly lesser degrees of proteinuria, ranging <2 g/day.
- Tubular proteinuria is usually seen in those with underlying tubulointerstitial diseases. They usually have defective reabsorptive capacities in the proximal tubules, such that, instead of the proteins being normally reabsorbed, they are excreted in the urine. In contrast to glomerular proteinuria, whereby macromolecules such as albumin are leaked out, in tubular proteinuria it is mostly low molecular weight proteins, such as immunoglobulin light chains, etc.
- Overflow proteinuria (also called overproduction proteinuria) is exemplified by multiple myeloma, in which there is an overabundance of immunoglobulin light chains secondary to overproduction. Simply put, proteinuria occurs as a result of the amount of protein produced basically exceeding the maximum threshold for reabsorption in the tubules.
  Whereas both glomerular and tubular proteinuria are secondary to abnormalities involving the glomerular capillary and tubular walls, respectively, in overflow proteinuria, the problem lies in overproduction of certain proteins.

Quantification of the degree of proteinuria is accomplished by performing a 24-hour urine collection, which can be cumbersome, especially in elderly individuals or in those with concomitant fecal or urinary incontinence.

The urine protein-to-creatinine (using a random urine specimen) ratio has been shown to have a good correlation with the 24-hour urine protein determination.

In transient proteinuria conditions, there is a transient change in glomerular hemodynamics causing increased excretion of urinary protein. These are usually benign and self-limited. Examples include congestive heart failure, fevers, strenuous exercise, seizure disorders, and even extremes of stress. Orthostatic proteinuria (see Question 14) falls under this category.

KEY POINTS: URINALYSIS

1. Normal urine color can vary from pale or light yellow to deep amber or dark yellow and is the result of the presence of a pigment called urochrome.

2. Urinary dipsticks only detect the presence of albumin; however, they are notorious for being poor indicators of the presence of urinary globulins and Bence Jones proteins.

3. The presence of ketones in the urine is abnormal.

4. Careful history taking is of paramount importance in the evaluation of patients with hematuria.

5. The urine protein-to-creatinine (using a random urine specimen) ratio has been shown to have a good correlation with the 24-hour urine protein determination.

14. **What is orthostatic proteinuria?**
Orthostatic or postural proteinuria, by definition, is demonstration of increased urine protein excretion in the upright position and normal urine protein excretion in the supine position. It is a benign condition, mostly seen among adolescents, the mechanism of which is not clearly understood. The diagnosis is established by performing a split urine collection. The protocol for a split urine collection is as follows: (1) The first morning void is discarded. (2) A 16-hour upright collection is obtained between 7 AM and 11 PM, with the patient performing normal activities and finishing the collection by voiding just before 11 PM. (The times can be adjusted according to the normal times at which the patient awakens and goes to sleep.) (3) The patient should assume the recumbent position 2 hours before the upright collection is finished to avoid contamination of the supine collection with urine formed when in the upright position. (4) A separate overnight 8-hour collection is obtained between 11 PM and 7 AM.

Patients with orthostatic proteinuria do not progress to end-stage renal disease; in fact, proteinuria resolves spontaneously in the majority of affected patients.

15. **What is the difference between a 24-hour protein excretion and a protein–creatinine ratio on a random urine sample?**
The 24-hour urine protein excretion represents the reference (gold-standard) method. It is used universally, averages the variation in proteinuria caused by circadian rhythm, and is the most accurate for monitoring proteinuria during treatment. However, it is influenced largely by the rate of diuresis, requires detailed instructions for urine collection, and can be impractical in some circumstances (e.g., outpatient setting and elderly patients). Moreover, during collection, urine can undergo contamination and rough preanalytic errors can occur (e.g., incorrect collection and incorrect calculation of urinary volume).

The protein–creatinine ratio on a random urine sample is a recommended alternative to 24-hour urine collection. It is easy to obtain, is not influenced by variation in water intake and rate of diuresis, greatly reduces preanalytic errors, and the same sample can be used for microscopic investigation.

A review of the literature showed sufficient evidence of a strong correlation between protein–creatinine ratio in a random urine sample and 24-hour protein excretion. However, it should be remembered that a normal protein–creatinine ratio is sufficient to rule out the presence of pathologic proteinuria (which decreases the number of unnecessary 24-hour urine collections), whereas in the case of a protein–creatinine ratio greater than the cutoff value, a full 24-hour quantification is indicated. Moreover, correlation between protein–creatinine ratio and 24-hour protein excretion may be not accurate at protein levels greater than 1 g/L (>0.1 g/dL), and the reliability of protein–creatinine ratio for monitoring proteinuria during treatment is still not proven.

BIBLIOGRAPHY

1. Armstrong JA. Urinalysis in western culture: A brief history. *Kidney Int* 2007;71:384.
2. Lerma EV. Approach to the patient with renal disease. In Lerma EV, Berns JR, Nissenson AR (eds.). *Current diagnosis and treatment in nephrology and hypertension.* New York: McGraw-Hill, 2008.
3. Pillai BP, Chong VH, Yong AML. Purple urine bag syndrome. *Singapore Med J* 2009;50(5):e193–194.
4. Simerville JA, Maxted WC, Pahira JJ. Urinalysis: A comprehensive review. *Am Fam Phys* 2005;71(6):1153–1162.
5. Simonson MS. Measurement of urinary protein. In Hricik D, Miller TR, Sedor JR (eds.). *Nephrology secrets,* 2nd ed. Philadelphia: Hanley & Belfus, 2003, pp. 11–14.

CHAPTER 3

MEASUREMENT OF GLOMERULAR FILTRATION RATE

Lesley A. Stevens, MD

1. **What is the glomerular filtration rate (GFR)?**
   The GFR is the amount of plasma filtered through glomeruli per unit of time. Although the term can refer to the function of a single nephron, GFR most often refers to the sum filtration rate of all functioning nephrons.

2. **What is the difference between single-nephron GFR and total GFR?**
   The single-nephron GFR refers to the work performed by a single functioning nephron. It can be affected by hemodynamic alterations or structural damage. As part of the adaptation of the kidney to injury, uninjured nephrons undergo hypertrophy and hyperfiltration to compensate for the loss of functioning nephrons (compensatory hyperfiltration). Thus, total GFR remains relatively normal despite a decrease in functioning nephrons. As such, the GFR is dependent on the number of nephrons (N) and the single-nephron glomerular filtration rate (SNGFR):

$$GFR = N \times SNGFR$$

3. **What is the clinical significance of the GFR?**
   The level of GFR is accepted as the most useful index of kidney function in health and disease. A decrease in GFR precedes the onset of kidney failure; therefore a persistently reduced GFR is a specific diagnostic criterion for chronic kidney disease (CKD). CKD is defined as GFR <60 mL/min per 1.73 m^2 in addition to markers of kidney damage. The severity of CKD is also determined by the level of GFR. Kidney failure is defined as GFR <15 mL/min per 1.73 m^2. Kidney failure is associated with uremic symptoms and laboratory findings, such as anemia, malnutrition, bone and mineral disorders, neuropathy, and decreased quality of life. There is a graded relationship between the severity of these signs and symptoms at intermediate reductions in GFR in patients with kidney disease. The level of GFR is also associated with progression to kidney failure and cardiovascular disease. In addition, drug dosages will need to be adjusted for the level of GFR.

4. **What are normal values for GFR in adults?**
   Normal GFR varies according to age, sex, and body size. In young adults it is approximately 120–130 mL/min/1.73 m^2, and it declines with age.

5. **How is GFR measured?**
   The gold-standard method to measure GFR is urinary clearance of an ideal filtration marker. An ideal filtration marker is one that is (1) freely filtered at the glomerulus; (2) present at a stable plasma concentration; and (3) not reabsorbed, secreted, or metabolized by the kidney. The ideal filtration marker is inulin. However, this is rarely used and alterative markers such as iohexol and iothalamate are more commonly used.

   For a substance that is cleared by urinary excretion, the clearance formula may be written as follows:

$$Cx = Ux \times V/Px$$

where Ux is the urinary concentration of x and V is the urine flow rate. The term $U_x \times V$ represents the urinary excretion rate of x. If substance x is freely filtered at the glomerulus, then urinary excretion represents the net effects of glomerular filtration, tubular reabsorption, and secretion.

As an alternative to urinary clearance, GFR can be calculated from plasma clearance following a bolus intravenous injection of an exogenous filtration marker computed from:

$$C_x = A_x / P_x$$

where Ax is the amount of the marker administered and Px is computed from the entire area under the disappearance curve.

6. **What is the relationship between creatinine clearance and measured GFR?**
A timed urinary collection for creatinine can be performed to estimate the measured GFR. Creatinine clearance is usually determined by using venous blood for serum creatinine and a 24-hour urine collection. In practice, several problems can severely compromise the utility of creatinine clearance. Because the renal tubules secrete creatinine, measurements of creatinine clearance can significantly overestimate true GFR, particularly in patients with kidney disease. Accurate measurements of creatine clearance also require complete and carefully timed urine collections; inadequate urine collections yield spurious results. Repeated measurements of creatinine clearance may overcome some of the errors.

7. **How is GFR estimated in routine clinical practice?**
GFR is usually estimated from endogenous filtration markers. The level of all known endogenous filtration markers is determined by factors other than GFR, including generation from muscle mass and diet, tubular secretion, and extrarenal elimination. GFR estimating equations use the filtration marker in combination with demographic variables to overcome some of the limitations from non-GFR determinants. The most commonly used filtration marker is serum creatinine. Currently, many laboratories report estimated GFR whenever a serum creatinine is ordered. The most commonly used equation is the MDRD Study equation, but a more accurate equation, the CKD-EPI equation, has recently been published.

8. **What are the major limitations of serum creatinine as a clinical index of kidney disease?**
Creatinine is a 113 dalton amino acid derivative generated from the breakdown of creatine in muscle, distributed throughout total body water, and excreted by the kidneys primarily by glomerular filtration. Although the serum level is affected primarily by the level of GFR, it is also affected by other physiologic processes, such as tubular secretion, generation, and extrarenal excretion of creatinine (Table 3-1). As a result of variation in these processes individuals and over time within individuals, especially creatinine generation, the cutoff for normal versus abnormal serum creatinine concentration differs among groups. In addition, assays for serum creatinine vary across clinical laboratories, leading to differences in GFR estimates for the same patient when creatinine is measured in different labs. Because of the wide range of normal for serum creatinine in most clinical laboratories, GFR must decline to approximately half the normal level before the serum creatinine concentration rises above the upper limit of normal.

9. **What are GFR estimating equations?**
Estimating equations combine the endogenous filtration marker(s) with other variables, such as age, sex, race, and body size, as surrogates for non-GFR determinants of the filtration markers and, therefore, can overcome some of the limitations of the filtration marker alone. An estimating equation is derived using regression techniques to model the observed relationship between the serum level of the marker and measured GFR in a study population.

10. **What is the Cockcroft-Gault formula?**
The Cockcroft-Gault formula was developed in 1973 using data from 249 men with creatinine clearance (Ccr) from approximately 30–130 mL per minute. It is not adjusted for body surface area.

TABLE 3-1. FACTORS AFFECTING SERUM CREATININE CONCENTRATION

Factor	Effect on Serum Creatinine	Mechanism/Comment
Older age	Decrease	Reduced creatinine generation from age-related decline in muscle mass
Female sex	Decrease	Reduced creatinine generation from reduced muscle mass
African American race	Increase	Higher creatinine generation rate as a result of higher average muscle mass in African Americans compared to Caucasians; not known how muscle mass in other races compares to that of African Americans or Caucasians
Diet:		
Vegetarian diet	Decrease	Decrease in creatinine generation
Ingestion of cooked meats	Increase	Transient increase in creatinine generation; however, this may be blunted by transient increase in GFR
Body habitus:		
Muscular	Increase	Increased muscle generation as a result of increased muscle mass ± increased protein intake
Malnutrition/ muscle wasting/ amputation	Decrease	Reduced creatinine generation from reduced muscle mass ± reduced protein intake
Obesity	No change	Excess mass is fat, not muscle mass, and does not contribute to increased creatinine generation

$$Ccr = \{[(140 - age) \times weight]/(72\ Scr)\} \times 0.85\ if\ female$$

where Ccr is expressed in milliliters per minute, age in years, weight in kilograms, and serum creatinine (Scr) in milligrams per deciliter.

Modifications of the Cockcroft and Gault equation using ideal body weight instead of actual body weight are sometimes used but have not been validated.

11. **What is the MDRD Study equation?**

The four-variable MDRD Study equation was developed in 1999 using data from 1628 patients with CKD and GFR from approximately 5–90 mL/min/1.73 m². It estimates GFR adjusted for body surface area and is more accurate than measured creatinine clearance from 24-hour urine collections or estimated by the Cockcroft-Gault formula. The equation is as follows:

$$GFR = 186 \times Scr^{-1.154} \times age^{-0.203} \times 0.742\ if\ female \times 1.210\ if\ African\ American$$

The equation was re-expressed in 2005 for use with a standardized serum creatinine assay, which yields 5% lower values for serum creatinine concentration:

$$GFR = 175 \times Standardized\ Scr^{-1.154} \times age^{-0.203} \times 0.742\ if\ female \times 1.210$$
$$if\ African\ American$$

GFR is expressed in mL/min/1.73 m², Scr is serum creatinine expressed in mg/dL, and age is expressed in years.

12. **What is the CKD-EPI equation?**
The CKD-EPI equation is a new equation to estimate GFR from serum creatinine, age, sex, and race. It was developed in a cohort of 8254 subjects pooled together from 10 research studies and clinical populations with diverse characteristics, including people with and without kidney diseases, and across the range of GFR (2–198 mL/min/1.73 m²) and age range (18–97 years). The equation was validated in a separate cohort of 3896 people from 16 separate studies, GFR range 2–200 mL/min/1.73 m² and age range 18–93 years. The CKD-EPI equation was as accurate as the MDRD Study equation in the subgroup with estimated GFR less than 60 mL/min/1.73 m² and substantially more accurate in the subgroup with estimated GFR greater than 60 mL/min/1.73 m².

13. **When should GFR be measured instead of estimated?**
A clearance measurement using exogenous markers or creatinine should be performed when estimates based on serum creatinine are likely to be inaccurate. The indications for a clearance measurement include the following:
- Extremes of age and body size
- Severe malnutrition or obesity
- Disease of skeletal muscle
- Paraplegia or quadriplegia
- Vegetarian diet
- Rapidly changing kidney function
- Pregnancy

14. **Can measurements of blood urea nitrogen (BUN) serve as an index of GFR?**
BUN is not a reliable index of GFR. The renal tubules reabsorb urea in quantities that vary depending on the state of hydration, thus rendering the BUN an inaccurate marker for GFR. BUN concentration is also strongly affected by changes in catabolism and protein intake.

KEY POINTS: GLOMERULAR FILTRATION RATE

1. The level of glomerular filtration rate (GFR) is accepted as the most useful index of kidney function in health and disease. A persistently reduced GFR is a specific diagnostic criterion for chronic kidney disease (CKD), and the severity of CKD is also determined by the level of GFR. For drugs cleared by the kidney, dosages need to be adjusted for the level of GFR.

2. GFR is usually estimated from endogenous filtration markers, most commonly serum creatinine. The level of all known endogenous filtration markers is determined by factors other than GFR, including generation from metabolism and diet, tubular secretion, or reabsorption and extrarenal elimination. GFR estimating equations use the filtration marker in combination with demographic variables to overcome some of the limitations from non-GFR determinants. Two creatinine-based estimating equations are the MDRD Study equation and CKD-EPI equation.

3. All estimates of GFR based on serum creatinine will be less accurate in patients not in a steady state of creatinine balance (in whom serum creatinine is changing), in patients at the extremes of muscle mass (such as the frail elderly, critically ill, or those with cancer or, conversely, body builders), or those with unusual diets. Confirmatory tests with measured creatinine clearance should be performed for people in whom the estimates may be inaccurate.

15. **What is cystatin C?**
Cystatin C is a 13 kDalton nonglycosylated basic protein that is produced by all nucleated cells. It is freely filtered by the glomerulus and then reabsorbed and catabolized by the tubular

epithelial cells, with only small amounts excreted in the urine. Its urinary clearance cannot be measured, which makes it difficult to study factors affecting its clearance and generation. The generation of cystatin C appears to be less variable and less affected by age and sex than serum creatinine. However, some studies have reported increased cystatin C levels associated with higher levels of C-reactive protein or body mass index, hyperthyroidism, and steroid use. In addition, other studies suggest extrarenal elimination at high levels of cystatin C and higher intraindividual variation compared to serum creatinine, particularly among transplant patients.

16. **Is cystatin C a more accurate filtration marker than creatinine?**
Some but not all studies show that serum levels of cystatin C estimate GFR better than serum creatinine alone. Estimating equations based on serum levels of cystatin C, either alone or in combination with serum creatinine, have been developed. These equations have variable performance compared to serum creatinine and variable performance among populations. These equations need to be validated in other studies prior to use in clinical practice.

Recent studies have clearly demonstrated that cystatin C is a better predictor of adverse events in the elderly, including mortality, heart failure, bone loss, peripheral arterial disease, and cognitive impairment, than either serum creatinine or estimated GFR. These findings may be because cystatin C is a better filtration marker than creatinine, particularly in the elderly. An alternative explanation is that factors other than GFR that affect serum levels of creatinine and cystatin C differentially confound the relationships between these measures and outcomes.

17. **Can estimated GFR be used in patients with rapidly changing kidney function?**
Serum levels of endogenous filtration markers and estimated GFR derived from these markers can only be an accurate index of measured GFR in the steady state. In patients with rapidly changing kidney function, the rate and direction of change in the level of the filtration marker and in estimated GFR reflect the magnitude and direction of the change in measured GFR but do not accurately reflect the level of GFR. With an acute decline in true GFR, the observed decrease in estimated GFR is less than the decline in GFR, thus estimated GFR is greater than true GFR. Conversely, after an increase in GFR, the observed increase in estimated GFR is greater than the increase in true GFR and estimated GFR is thus less than GFR.

BIBLIOGRAPHY

1. Cockcroft D, Gault M. Prediction of creatinine clearance from serum creatinine. *Nephron* 1976;16(1):31–41.

2. Levey AS. Assessing the effectiveness of therapy to prevent the progression of renal disease. *Am J Kidney Dis* 1993;22(1):207–214.

3. Levey AS, Coresh J, Greene T, Stevens LA, Zhang Y, Hendriksen S, Kusek JW, Van Lente F, for the Chronic Kidney Disease Epidemiology Collaboration. Using standardized serum creatinine values in the modification of diet in renal disease study equation for estimating glomerular filtration rate. *Ann Intern Med* 2006;145(4):247–254.

4. Levey AS, Stevens LA, Schmid CH, Zhang YL, Castro AF 3rd, Feldman HI, Kusek JW, Eggers P, Van Lente F, Greene T, Coresh J. A new equation to estimate glomerular filtration rate. *Ann Intern Med* 2009;150(9):604–612.

5. Shlipak MG, Sarnak MJ, Katz R, Fried LF, Seliger SL, Newman AB, Siscovick DS, Stehman-Breen C. Cystatin C and the risk of death and cardiovascular events among elderly persons. *N Engl J Med* 2005;352(20):2049–2060.

6. Stevens LA, Coresh J, Greene T, Levey AS. Assessing kidney function—Measured and estimated glomerular filtration rate. *N Engl J Med* 2006;354(23):2473–2483.

7. Stevens LA, Coresh J, Schmid CH, Feldman HI, Froissart M, Kusek J, Rossert J, Van Lente F, Bruce RD, Zhang Y, Greene T, Levey AS. Estimating glomerular filtration rate using cystatin C alone and in combination with serum creatinine: A pooled analysis of 3418. individuals. *Am J Kidney Dis* 2008;51(3):395–406.

8. Stevens LA, Lafayette LA, Perrone RD, Levey AS. Laboratory evaluation of kidney disease. In Schrier R (ed.). *Disease of the kidney and urinary tract*, 8th ed. Philadelphia: Lippincott Williams & Wilkins, 2006, pp. 299–336.

9. Stevens LA, Levey AS. Measured GFR as a confirmatory test for estimated GFR. *J Am Soc Nephrol* 2009;20(11):2305–2313.

10. Stevens LA, Schmid CH, Greene T, Li L, Beck GJ, Joffe MM, Froissart M, Kusek JW, Zhang YL, Coresh J, Levey AS. Factors other than glomerular filtration rate affect serum cystatin C levels. *Kidney Int* 2009;75(6):652–660.

RENAL IMAGING TECHNIQUES

Ally Rosen, MD, and William L. Simpson Jr., MD

CHAPTER 4

1. **List the most commonly used imaging modalities for the kidneys.**
   - Radiography (plain film, excretory urography, retrograde pyelography, cystography)
   - Ultrasonography (US)
   - Computed tomography (CT) scan
   - Magnetic resonance imaging (MRI) and magnetic resonance angiography (MRA)
   - Radionuclide imaging
   - Renal angiography

2. **Describe the information that can be provided about the urinary tract on the plain abdominal radiograph.**
   The plain abdominal radiograph, also called kidneys, ureters, bladder (KUB), can show the following:
   - Calcifications: renal calculus, calcified neoplasm, sloughed papilla, medullary or cortical nephrocalcinosis, ureteric or bladder calculus/tumor
   - Air: air within or adjacent to the kidneys from severe infection, such as in diabetes
   - Soft tissue changes: obliteration of the psoas or renal outline may indicate inflammation or tumor
   - Bone: changes of renal osteodystrophy and either lytic or blastic metastasis

3. **What is the current role of excretory urography (EU)?**
   - Had been the initial modality for upper tract imaging in patients with hematuria, flank pain, and other urologic disease for the past five decades
   - Replaced by CT urography in most medical centers
   - Less sensitive in detecting renal masses than US, CT, or MRI
   - EU does not allow reliable differentiation of solid masses from cysts

4. **What are the components of a CT urogram?**
   Comprehensive upper tract imaging includes the following:
   - Unenhanced axial CT of the kidneys—detection of calcification and baseline density measurement to determine enhancement of masses
   - Enhanced CT of the abdomen and pelvis (corticomedullary and nephrographic phase)—detection of enhancement of renal masses
   - Excretory phase imaging of the abdomen and pelvis obtained with projection urography and/or axial CT images—essential for assessing subtle urothelial abnormalities including urothelial tumors; papillary necrosis; calyceal deformity; ureteral stricture; and inflammatory changes of the renal collecting systems, ureters, and bladder
   - CT images may be reviewed as two-dimensional (2D) and three-dimensional (3D) reformatted images

5. **What are the relative contraindications to intravenous (IV) contrast administration?**
   - Previous allergic reaction to contrast media
   - Concern about contrast-induced nephrotoxicity
   - Multiple myeloma

- Asthma
- Multiple allergies
- Volume depletion
- Pregnancy
- Metformin use

6. **What is retrograde pyelography?**

The injection of contrast material directly into the distal ureter or the ureteral orifice of the bladder for visualization of the collecting system and ureter, without relying on the ability of the kidneys to excrete contrast media. The primary use of retrograde pyelography is to evaluate suspected ureteral obstruction in the patient in whom the ability to excrete contrast material is significantly impaired.

This is an adjunctive technique when conventional imaging studies fail to adequately demonstrate the suspected pathology. Retrograde pyelography offers no evaluation of the renal parenchyma and is relatively invasive because cystoscopy is required for placement of the catheters.

7. **List the strengths of ultrasonography in the evaluation of renal disease.**

- Sensitive for detection of perirenal fluid collections, pelvicalyceal dilatation, and cysts
- Differentiates cortex and medulla
- Differentiates cystic and solid masses
- Shows the renal contour and perinephric space
- Demonstrates renal blood flow by Doppler technique
- Provides good renal imaging irrespective of renal function; may be used in patients with elevated serum creatinine
- Can be used portably at the bedside in the intensive care unit
- Safe: uses no ionizing radiation or nephrotoxic contrast medium
- Low cost

8. **List the weaknesses of ultrasonography in the evaluation of renal disease.**

- Does not show fine pelvicalyceal detail
- Does not show the entire normal ureter; may occasionally see proximal or distal ureters
- Does not show the entire retroperitoneum
- Can miss small renal calculi and most ureteral calculi
- Gives no functional information
- Operator dependent

9. **What is the diagnostic utility of ultrasound?**

- Estimating kidney size
- Assessing the echogenicity of the kidney (increased echogenicity may indicate chronic renal disease but is nonspecific)
- Preferred screening modality for suspected obstruction because it is very sensitive to dilatation of the collecting system, such as from obstruction in renal failure, pelvic neoplasm, in renal transplant, and in acute urinary tract infection with pyonephrosis
- Complete ureteral obstruction can be excluded by documenting the presence of a ureteral jet (color flow seen on Doppler ultrasound as urine passes into the bladder from the ureteral orifice)
- Calculi are seen as echogenic foci with shadowing
- Can differentiate solid mass from cystic mass
- Diagnosing adult polycystic kidney disease and screening involved families
- Guiding interventional procedures such as renal biopsy and cyst aspiration
- Detecting perinephric fluid collections
- Evaluating renal transplant allograph to assess suspected fluid collection (lymphocele, hematoma, urinoma); evaluating for parenchymal disease or detecting vascular complications

10. **When is CT scan superior to ultrasound for evaluation of renal disease?**
   - For evaluation of an indeterminate mass on US or a solid mass when neoplasm is suspected
   - CT can define the extent of the neoplasm and lymph node involvement, give a more comprehensive view of the perirenal and pararenal spaces and Gerota's fascia, evaluate vasculature (renal vein/inferior vena cava involvement), and stage neoplasms
   - CT is the imaging method of choice in evaluation of suspected renal trauma (additional information about other organ injuries can be obtained at the same time)
   - CT is more efficacious for visualization of the retroperitoneum and adrenal glands

11. **What is the Bosniak classification?**
   In 1986 Bosniak proposed a classification to characterize cystic renal masses as "nonsurgical" (i.e., benign) or "surgical" (i.e., requiring surgery). In his original classification, there were four categories:
   - Category I: simple benign cysts (fluid-filled, no perceptible wall)
   - Category II: benign cystic lesions that are minimally complicated (mural calcifications, few thin septations)
   - Category III: more complicated cystic lesions (calcifications, thickened or numerous septations, enhancement of the septations, mural nodules, thickened, irregular wall)
   - Category IV: lesions that are clearly malignant cystic carcinomas (mural nodules with vascularization, enhancement of solid components)

   Categories I and II are considered nonsurgical, whereas categories III and IV are surgical.
   In 1993 in another landmark article, Bosniak revised the classification system to include a subset of minimally complicated lesions that could be managed with follow-up imaging: category IIF (more numerous thin septations, slight cyst wall thickening, totally intrarenal, nonenhancing, high-density lesions, i.e., hyperdense cysts).
   From a review of the literature, the risk that a "surgical" lesion is malignant is approximately 50% (range 25%–100%). The risk of malignancy in a cystic lesion that is being followed up (Bosniak IIF) is approximately 5%. A septated cyst is considered surgical if the septa are thick, irregular, or nodular or demonstrate significant enhancement (i.e., category III).

12. **What is the inexpensive first step in evaluating a patient with suspected ureteral stone?**
   Radiography is often used as an inexpensive first step in examining a patient suspected of having urolithiasis because the majority (90%) of urinary calculi are radiopaque. Large calculi can easily be seen; confounding factors such as overlying bowel gas, gallstones, or fecal material and osseous structures such as transverse processes or the sacrum can easily hide small calculi.

13. **What is the test of choice for the examination of patient with acute flank pain?**
   Unenhanced CT scan of the abdomen and pelvis is the preferred imaging modality because virtually all stones are of sufficient attenuation to be detected on CT, with the exception of a stone that consists entirely of protease inhibitors, such as indinavir sulfate (Crixivan, Merck, Rahway, NJ). In addition to the direct visualization of a stone in the lumen of the ureter, secondary signs of obstruction on CT are commonly present. Unenhanced CT can also reveal many other causes of acute flank pain unrelated to the urinary system, such as pelvic masses, appendicitis, and diverticulitis.
   Ureteral dilatation has a sensitivity of approximately 90% for use in making a diagnosis of acute ureteral obstruction. Stranding of the perinephric fat and stranding of the periureteral fat both have sensitivities of approximately 85%.

14. **Which cross-sectional imaging techniques are useful for the comprehensive evaluation of the genitourinary tract?**
   Computed tomographic urography (CTU) and magnetic resonance urography (MRU) provide an assessment of the renal parenchyma, urinary collecting system, bladder, and surrounding

structures. MRU is an evolving group of techniques with the potential to noninvasively provide a comprehensive and specific imaging test for many urinary tract abnormalities without the use of ionizing radiation.

15. **What are the limitations of MRU?**
   - Relative insensitivity for renal calculi
   - Relatively long imaging times
   - Sensitivity to motion and lower spatial resolution compared with CT and radiography

16. **What is nephrogenic systemic fibrosis (NSF)?**
   A rare but potentially debilitating or even fatal fibrosing condition that most often affects the skin but is now also recognized to involve multiple organs. NSF is associated with renal failure and the administration of large amounts of gadolinium-based MR contrast agent. It was first described in 1997 and was called nephrogenic fibrosing dermopathy; the nomenclature was changed to nephrogenic systemic fibrosis in 2005.

17. **What are the risk factors for developing NSF?**
   - High doses of gadolinium-based contrast agents
   - Both acute and chronic renal failure
   - Vascular injury
   - Venous thrombosis
   - Coagulopathy

   In patients with acute kidney injury, the use of gadolinium-based contrast agent should be avoided. For patients with chronic renal failure, the FDA has determined that the risk is greatest when the estimated glomerular filtration rate is less than 30 mL/min/1.73 m^2. In this setting, it should be determined whether use of a gadolinium-based contrast agent is essential for diagnosis, and alternative imaging techniques and tests should be considered. If use of a gadolinium-based contrast agent is essential, informed patient consent should be obtained and the radiologist should consider techniques aimed at reducing the dose.

   For patients receiving hemodialysis when MR imaging is essential, it is recommended that hemodialysis be performed immediately after gadolinium-based contrast agent administration and again 24 hours later.

   Use of gadolinium-based contrast agents should especially be avoided in patients undergoing peritoneal dialysis, in whom plasma clearance of such agents is prolonged.

   When use of gadolinium-based contrast material is necessary for diagnosis, it is possible to reduce total gadolinium administration through the use of agents with higher relaxivity. Management of NSF requires an understanding of the risk factors of this disease and developing an institutional policy for identifying and testing at-risk patients.

18. **What are some of the clinical applications of MRA?**
   - Accurately evaluating patients suspected to have renal artery stenosis without the risks associated with nephrotoxic contrast agents, ionizing radiation, or arterial catheterization
   - Mapping the vascular anatomy for planning renal revascularization
   - Planning repair of abdominal aortic aneurysms
   - Assessing renal bypass grafts and renal transplant anastomoses
   - Evaluating vascular involvement by renal tumors

19. **Which is the study of choice for evaluating renal trauma?**
   The primary role of imaging in renal trauma is to accurately assess the severity and extent of injury, evaluate the injured kidney for underlying disorders, evaluate the anatomy and function of the opposite kidney, and assess for other associated injuries. Contrast-enhanced CT scan is the imaging technique of choice to evaluate the entire urinary tract, including the renal vasculature, renal parenchyma, and the collecting system.

   When a renal laceration is detected on CT, a 10-minute delayed scan (excretory phase) should be obtained to assess the collecting system and evaluate for urinary extravasation.

Delayed images are also helpful for characterizing the nature of a perinephric fluid collection and for distinguishing a hematoma from a urinoma.

In patients with blunt trauma and suspected utereropelvic junction injury, CT with excretory phase imaging is a reliable tool for evaluation.

20. **What are the clinical indications for radionuclide renal imaging?**
    - Estimation of quantitative glomerular filtration rate and effective renal plasma flow
    - Measurement of "split" renal function to determine whether nephrectomy is warranted or safe
    - Evaluation of renal function to aid in diagnosis of acute tubular necrosis, urinary tract obstruction, renal transplant rejection, or impaired blood flow at renal arterial anastomotic site
    - Evaluation for urinary extravasation (leak)
    - Diuretic renogram is useful in differentiating functionally insignificant urinary tract dilatation from obstruction

21. **List the indications for renal angiography.**
    - Evaluation and treatment of renovascular hypertension via balloon angioplasty
    - Preoperative evaluation of complicated donor kidney
    - Evaluation and treatment of renal transplant for renal artery occlusion or stenosis
    - Evaluation and treatment of renal vein thrombosis
    - Complex renal masses or complications of polycystic disease or trauma (possibly)

22. **What are the criteria for diagnosing contrast nephropathy?**
    Although there is no universally accepted definition, an increase in serum creatinine level of 0.5 to 1.0 mg/dL or 25% to 50% from baseline is used.

23. **What are risk factors for contrast nephropathy?**
    - Pre-existing renal insufficiency (creatinine level >1.5 mg/dL)
    - Diabetes
    - Age >75 years
    - Concurrent use of nephrotoxic drugs
    - Large volume of contrast
    - Hyperuricemia
    - Use of ionic, high osmolar contrast media
    - Greatest risk in patients with renal impairment and diabetes

24. **What is the typical time course of renal impairment in a patient with contrast nephropathy?**
    Serum creatinine level rises over 1 to 2 days after contrast administration, peaks 4 to 7 days after contrast administration, and returns to normal 10 to 14 days after contrast administration.

25. **What are the advantages and disadvantages of the various imaging methods used to diagnose renal artery stenosis?**
    See Table 4-1.

26. **What is the diagnostic utility of ultrasound in the evaluation of a renal transplant?**
    - Parenchymal echogenicity and masses
    - Perinephric collections (seroma, hematoma, urinoma, lymphocele)
    - Hydronephrosis
    - Ureteral obstruction/stenosis
    - Vascular compromise/complications
    - Guide for intervention (biopsy/aspiration/drainage)

TABLE 4-1. IMAGING METHODS FOR THE DIAGNOSIS OF RENAL ARTERY STENOSIS

Method	Advantages	Disadvantages
Doppler ultrasound	■ Low cost	■ Operator dependent ■ Bowel obscures visualization of entire artery ■ Can be limited by body habitus ■ Low sensitivity for detection of accessory renal arteries
Computed tomography angiography	■ Sensitivity and specificity near 100% ■ Accurate depiction of accessory renal arteries ■ Rapid acquisition	■ Ionizing radiation ■ Requires contrast administration
Magnetic resonance angiography	■ 95% sensitivity ■ Lack of radiation	■ Can miss small accessory arteries ■ Lower spatial resolution than computed tomography angiography ■ Risk of nephrogenic systemic fibrosis with contrast enhanced techniques
Digital subtraction angiography	■ Allows for interventional treatment	■ Ionizing radiation ■ Requires contrast administration ■ Potential complication of groin puncture/vascular access

27. **What are the categories of radiotracers used in renal imaging?**
    Glomerular filtration agents measure glomerular filtration rate:
    ■ Technetium 99 diethylenetriamine pentaacetic acid, 99mTc-DTPA
    ■ Technetium 99 mercaptoacetyl triglycine, 99mTc-MAG3
    ■ Iodine 131 o-iodohippurate, 131I-OIH
    ■ 99mTc-MAG3 and 131I-OIH are superior to 99mTc-DTPA in patient with poor renal function
    Tubular secretion agents estimate effective renal plasma flow:
    ■ Technetium 99 mercaptoacetyl triglycine, 99mTc-MAG3
    ■ Iodine 131 o-iodohippurate, 131I-OIH
    Tubular retention agents used for cortical imaging:
    ■ Technetium 99 dimercaptosuccinate, 99mTc-DMSA
    ■ Technetium 99 glucoheptonate, 99mTc-GH

KEY POINTS: RENAL IMAGING TECHNIQUES

1. Computed tomography (CT) urography has replaced excretory urography for evaluation of hematuria in most medical centers.

2. Ultrasound provides good renal imaging irrespective of renal function.

3. Unenhanced CT scan is the preferred imaging modality for a patient with acute flank pain.

4. The greatest risk of contrast nephropathy is in patients with pre-existing renal impairment and diabetes.

5. Radionuclide renal imaging provides both functional and anatomic information about the kidneys.

BIBLIOGRAPHY

1. Brenner BM. *Brenner and Rector's The Kidney*, 8th ed. Philadelphia: Saunders, 2008.

2. Hartman DS, Choyke PL, Hartman MS. From the RSNA Refresher Course: A practical approach to cystic renal mass. *Radiographics* 2004;24:S101–S115.

3. Dunnick NR, Sandler CM, Amis ES, Newhouse JH (eds.). *Textbook of Uroradiology*, 3rd ed. Philadelphia: Lippincott, Williams & Wilkins, 2001.

4. Johnson RJ, Floege J, Feehaly J (eds.). *Comprehensive Clinical Nephrology*, 3rd ed. Philadelphia: Mosby, 2003.

5. Kawashima A, Vrtiska TJ, LeRoy AJ, Hartman RP, McCollough CH, King BF. CT urography. *Radiographics* 2004;24:S35–S54.

CHAPTER 5

RENAL BIOPSY

C. Craig Tisher, MD, and Byron P. Croker, MD, PhD

1. **What are the major clinical uses for a renal biopsy?**
   - To diagnose kidney disease
   - To assess prognosis
   - To monitor disease progression
   - To aid in the selection of a rational approach to therapy
   - To monitor and assess response to treatment

2. **In which clinical settings is a renal biopsy most useful as an aid in the evaluation and management of a patient with undiagnosed kidney disease?**
   - **Acute kidney injury (AKI):** In the absence of an explanation for AKI when the patient is evaluated initially or when recovery of renal function has not occurred after 3 to 4 weeks of supportive therapy that may include acute dialysis, a kidney biopsy is recommended to distinguish between acute tubular necrosis and those diseases that may require a different therapeutic approach.
   - **Chronic renal failure (CRF):** A renal biopsy may be useful in patients with unexplained CRF and normal-sized kidneys. In contrast, a biopsy is not recommended in the presence of undersized kidneys that have severe parenchymal damage including glomerulosclerosis, chronic vascular injury, and interstitial fibrosis. Kidneys with this degree of disease have a greater propensity for biopsy-induced bleeding.
   - **Nephrotic syndrome:** A renal biopsy is generally indicated in infants younger than 1 year of age (possible congenital nephrotic syndrome) and in adults with the nephrotic syndrome and no evidence of systemic disease before therapy is initiated. Children with the nephrotic syndrome are likely to have steroid-responsive disease; thus, biopsy is reserved for those who are unresponsive to a short course of steroids.
   - **Proteinuria:** In the presence of persistent proteinuria of 2 g/24 hours/1.73 m² or more and especially when associated with an abnormal urine sediment or documented functional deterioration, a renal biopsy may be useful to detect an underlying kidney disease. Isolated orthostatic proteinuria is not an indication for biopsy.
   - **Hematuria:** Renal biopsy should be reserved for those individuals with microscopic hematuria that has persisted beyond 6 months; in patients with episodic gross hematuria; or in individuals with a family history of hematuria, particularly when associated with proteinuria and/or an abnormal urine sediment. Diagnostic possibilities include immunoglobulin A nephropathy, benign essential hematuria, thin basement membrane disease, and Alport syndrome. Renal biopsy is rarely helpful in the clinical setting of short-term, isolated microscopic hematuria. Secondary causes of hematuria such as those resulting from abnormalities in the lower urinary tract must be excluded.
   - **Systemic disease:** Disorders such as systemic lupus erythematosus, diabetes mellitus, Schönlein-Henoch purpura, Goodpasture's syndrome, polyarteritis nodosa, various dysproteinemias, and Wegener granulomatosis often manifest kidney involvement. Renal biopsy is frequently useful to establish or confirm a diagnosis and guide subsequent treatment.
   - **Transplant allograft:** Renal biopsy is used extensively to differentiate between the various forms of rejection and other causes of kidney failure such as acute tubular necrosis,

hemorrhagic infarction, drug-induced tubulointerstitial nephritis or nephrotoxicity, and de novo or recurrent glomerulonephritis. Baseline (time zero or donor biopsies) and stable functioning graft biopsies are being used increasingly to detect subclinical disease.

3. **What are the relative and absolute contraindications to a percutaneous renal biopsy?**
Most nephrologists would agree there are several absolute contraindications to renal biopsy (Table 5-1). There is potential for increased risk of morbidity or mortality in the presence of sepsis, severe uncontrolled hypertension, a hemorrhagic diathesis, known or suspected renal parenchymal infection or malignancy, solitary ectopic or horseshoe kidney (except the transplanted kidney), and a patient who is uncooperative. Platelet dysfunction as a result of anemia is a relative contraindication that often can be corrected with a combination of dialysis and administration of desmopressin (DDAVP). The latter is a vasopressin analogue that stimulates platelet aggregation. Likewise, hypertension may represent a relative contraindication, assuming it is brought under adequate control before the biopsy procedure.

4. **What risks and complications are associated with a renal biopsy?**
Percutaneous renal biopsy performed by an experienced operator using ultrasonography, computed tomography, or image-amplification fluoroscopy is a safe and reliable technique. The most common complication is bleeding, which occurs in the majority of patients. However, it is usually self-limited and rarely requires blood replacement or operative intervention. Other complications include arteriovenous fistulas and small aneurysms that are rarely significant clinically. Mortality is in the range of 0.1% to 0.2% or less.

KEY POINTS: RENAL BIOPSY

1. The renal biopsy is often useful to diagnose kidney disease, assess prognosis, monitor disease progression, aid in the selection of therapy, and follow the response to treatment.

2. Absolute contraindications to a percutaneous renal biopsy include the presence of sepsis, uncontrolled hypertension, a hemorrhagic diathesis, parenchymal infection or malignancy, solitary or horseshoe kidney (except the transplanted kidney), and a patient who is uncooperative.

3. The most common complication of a percutaneous renal biopsy is bleeding, which is usually self-limited and rarely requires blood replacement or operative intervention.

TABLE 5-1. CONTRAINDICATIONS TO RENAL BIOPSY*	
Kidney Status	**Patient Status**
Multiple cysts	Uncontrolled blood pressure
Solitary kidney	Uncontrolled bleeding diathesis
Acute pyelonephritis/perinephritic abscess	Uremia
Renal neoplasm	Obesity
	Patient who is uncooperative

*Most contraindications to renal biopsy are relative rather than absolute; when clinical circumstances necessitate urgent biopsy, they may be overridden, apart from uncontrolled bleeding diathesis.
From Johnson RJ, Feehally J. *Comprehensive Clinical Nephrology*, 2nd ed. Philadelphia: Mosby, 2003.

5. **What laboratory data should be obtained before undertaking a renal biopsy?**
   Routine laboratory tests that should be obtained before biopsy include a prothrombin time,
   a partial thromboplastin time, complete blood count, platelet count, blood type, an antibody
   screen for possible cross-matching should a transfusion be necessary, and a urinalysis to
   exclude a urinary tract infection. A bleeding time is only necessary if there are abnormal
   coagulation tests (Fig. 5-1). Patients should be instructed to avoid ingestion of aspirin and
   nonsteroidal anti-inflammatory agents in the week preceding the biopsy.

6. **What does the biopsy procedure involve?**
   The percutaneous renal biopsy is usually performed on the left kidney using a posterolateral
   approach under real-time ultrasound or fluoroscopic guidance with the patient in the supine
   position. Mild sedation is an option that depends largely on the preference of the patient and
   nephrologist. Today most operators prefer to use one of the spring-loaded automatic or semi-
   automatic biopsy guns that vary in size from 14 to 18 gauge. Local anesthesia is applied to
   the skin at the biopsy site and along the anticipated biopsy tract as determined through
   preliminary imaging. Most operators prefer to biopsy the cortex in the lower pole of the
   kidney. Two or three samples of tissue constitute an adequate biopsy in most patients.

   After completion of the procedure, which is usually performed in a hospital setting, the
   patient is maintained on bed rest for 18 to 24 hours. Vital signs are obtained frequently to look
   for evidence of hypovolemia as a result of excessive bleeding. Hematocrit level is obtained
   approximately 4 hours after biopsy and before discharge. Many nephrologists recommend
   evaluation of aliquots of each voided urine to observe for gross hematuria. In those patients in
   whom a percutaneous biopsy is not feasible and a histopathologic diagnosis is critical, strong
   consideration should be given to proceeding with a laparoscopic or open biopsy.

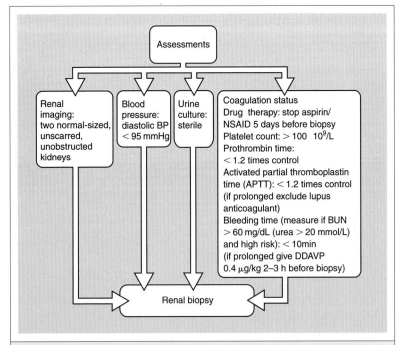

Figure 5-1. Workup for renal biopsy. (From Johnson RJ, Feehally J. *Comprehensive Clinical Nephrology,* 2nd ed. Philadelphia: Mosby, 2003.)

In carefully selected patients, percutaneous needle biopsy of the kidney is being performed with increased frequency as an outpatient procedure. Individuals who are free of pain at the biopsy site, have clear urine, and have stable cardiovascular signs for a minimum of 4 to 6 hours after the procedure can be safely discharged.

7. **How should the kidney tissue be handled following the biopsy procedure?**
The tissue specimens should be sent to the laboratory in a timely fashion (30 minutes); submitted for light, immunofluorescence, and transmission electron microscopy; and evaluated by a pathologist who is experienced in the interpretation of kidney biopsies. Proper evaluation of the biopsy material includes both gross and histologic examination of the specimen. Gross examination can be performed with either a dissecting microscope or a handheld lens. Cortical tissue can be identified by the presence of red, punctuate glomeruli. Areas of cortical infarction, necrosis, or pyogenic inflammation are often pale and surrounded by a hyperemic border. Older kidney allografts may have a distinct pale "rind" of fibrous tissue on the surface of the cortex. In contrast, the surface of newer grafts may be deeply colored as a result of the presence of recent hemorrhage.

Identification of the cortex allows the operator to divide the cortical tissue into three parts that can then be processed separately for light, electron, and immunofluorescence microscopy. Exact proportions of this division depend on the total amount of cortex that is available. In most instances 8 to 12 glomeruli are sufficient to render a light microscopic diagnosis and often less if the disease is generalized and diffuse. After the cortex is divided, any remaining tissue such as medulla is also processed for light microscopy. If only a few millimeters of cortical tissue are available, it is usually best to process the entire specimen for electron microscopy.

Less frequently used techniques for evaluation of a kidney biopsy include microbiologic cultures, chemical analyses, enzyme assays, and molecular pathology. The use of these additional techniques is dictated largely by the clinical situation.

BIBLIOGRAPHY

1. Faulk RJ, Jennette JC. Renal biopsy and treatment of glomerular disease. In Humes HD (ed.). *Kelley's Textbook of Internal Medicine*, 4th ed. Philadelphia: Lippincott Williams & Wilkins, 2000, pp. 1273–1290.

2. Hergesell O, Felten H, Andrassy K, et al. Safety of ultrasound-guided percutaneous renal biopsy—Retrospective analysis of 1090. consecutive cases. *Nephrol Dial Transplant* 1998;13:975–977.

3. Korbet SM. Percutaneous renal biopsy. *Semin Nephrol* 2002;22:254–267.

4. Nicholson ML, Wheatley TJ, Doughman TM, et al. A prospective randomized trial of three different sizes of core-cutting needle for renal transplant biopsy. *Kidney Int* 2000;58:390–395.

5. Parrish AE. Complications of percutaneous renal biopsy: A review of 37 years' experience. *Clin Nephrol* 1992;38:135–141.

6. Ravenscraft MD, Weaver ME, Jandrisak MD. Ambulatory transplant biopsy: Safe and effective. *J Am Soc Nephrol* 1994;5:1032 (abstract).

7. Tisher CC, Croker BP. Indications for and interpretation of the renal biopsy: Evaluation by light, electron and immunohistologic microscopy. In Schrier RW (ed.). *Diseases of the Kidney and Urinary Tract*, 8th ed. Philadelphia: Lippincott Williams & Wilkins, 2007, pp. 420–447.

8. Whittier WL, Korbet SM. Timing of complications in percutaneous renal biopsy. *J Am Soc Nephrol* 2004;15:142–147.

EPIDEMIOLOGY, ETIOLOGY, PATHOPHYSIOLOGY, AND DIAGNOSIS OF ACUTE KIDNEY INJURY

Paul M. Palevsky, MD

CHAPTER 6

1. **What is acute renal failure?**
    Acute renal failure (ARF) is a sudden decrease in renal function occurring over a period of hours to days. The acute decrease in glomerular filtration rate is usually manifested by the accumulation of nitrogenous waste products including urea and creatinine in the blood (azotemia) and is sometimes accompanied by oliguria.

2. **What is the difference between acute renal failure and acute kidney injury?**
    Although the terms acute kidney injury (AKI) and acute renal failure both describe the sudden decrease in kidney function, the term AKI has gained increasing usage over the past 5 to 10 years because it reflects the importance of smaller decrements in kidney function that do not result in complete loss of kidney function. This terminology parallels the similar replacement of the older terminology of chronic renal failure with chronic kidney disease.

3. **What is oliguria?**
    Oliguria (literally "small urine") is a reduction in urine volume to a volume that is insufficient to excrete the necessary solute load. Oliguria is generally defined as a urine volume of <0.5 mL/kg per hour in children or a urine volume of <20 mL/hour or <400 mL/day in adults. Anuria is defined as a urine output of <100 mL/day.

4. **What are the RIFLE and AKIN criteria?**
    RIFLE (**r**isk, **i**njury, **f**ailure, **l**oss, and **e**nd stage) and AKIN (Acute Kidney Injury Network) are staging criteria used to assess the severity of AKI. The RIFLE staging system stratified AKI into three strata of severity (risk, injury, and failure) on the basis of either change in serum creatinine (50%, 100%, or 200% increase) or duration of oliguria (6 hours, 12 hours, or 24 hours) and two outcome stages based on duration of kidney failure (Table 6-1). The subsequent AKIN criteria revised the RIFLE staging system by defining AKI as a 50% increase in serum creatinine or a 0.3 mg/dL increase over baseline occurring within 48 hours and by dropping the two outcome stages (see Table 6-1). In both classification systems, increasing severity of AKI is associated with increasing risk of death. Although these classification systems are important for epidemiologic studies and clinical trials, their utility in clinical practice is uncertain.

5. **How common is acute kidney injury?**
    Estimates of the incidence of AKI depend on the definition used for case finding and the population studied. It is estimated that 5% to 10% of hospitalized patients develop AKI. AKI is much more common in patients who are critically ill; 35% to 40% of patients who are critically ill will develop AKI based on the RIFLE or AKIN criteria, and 5% will develop severe AKI requiring renal replacement therapy. Epidemiologic studies have demonstrated that AKI is becoming more common, with an almost 20-fold increase over the past quarter century.

TABLE 6-1	RIFLE AND AKIN STAGING SYSTEMS FOR ACUTE KIDNEY INJURY			
RIFLE Stages	Increase in Serum Creatinine* in RIFLE Criteria	Urine Output* RIFLE and AKIN Criteria	Increase in Serum Creatinine* in AKIN Criteria	AKIN Stages
Risk	≥150% of baseline	<0.5 mL/kg/hour for >6 hours	≥0.3 mg/dL over baseline; or ≥150% of baseline	Stage 1
Injury	≥200% of baseline	<0.5 mL/kg/hour for >12 hours	≥200% of baseline	Stage 2
Failure	≥300% of baseline; or ≥0.5 mg/dL to a level >4.0 mg/dL	<0.3 mL/kg/hour for >24 hours; or Anuria for >12 hours	≥300% of baseline; or ≥0.5 mg/dL to a level >4.0 mg/dL	Stage 3
Loss	Need for renal replacement therapy as a result of acute kidney injury for >4 weeks			
End stage	Need for renal replacement therapy as a result of acute kidney injury for >3 months			

*Stage determined by highest severity of serum creatinine and urine output criteria.

6. **What are the causes of acute kidney injury?**
   AKI encompasses any process that causes an abrupt decrease in kidney function. The differential diagnosis includes prerenal azotemia (approximately 50% to 70% of cases), obstructive nephropathy (approximately 5% of cases; see Chapter 17), and intrinsic forms of AKI.

7. **Is acute tubular necrosis the same as acute kidney injury?**
   Acute tubular necrosis (ATN) is the most common form of intrinsic AKI. However, there are multiple other etiologies of AKI, as described previously, and the two terms are not synonymous.

8. **Which patients are at risk for the development of acute kidney injury?**
   The most important risk factor for the development of AKI is the presence of pre-existing chronic kidney disease. Elderly patients are at increased risk for development of AKI because they often have unrecognized diminished kidney function. Other risk factors include diabetes mellitus and volume depletion. Medications that cause intrarenal vasoconstriction, such as nonsteroidal anti-inflammatory drugs (NSAIDs), also predispose to the development of AKI.

9. **What is prerenal azotemia?**
   Prerenal azotemia is a functional form of AKI that results from diminished renal perfusion. Because there is no parenchymal injury, the hallmark of prerenal azotemia is the rapid normalization of kidney function when renal perfusion is restored. Common etiologies of prerenal azotemia include intravascular volume depletion, congestive heart failure (cardiorenal syndrome, see Chapter 9), and advanced liver disease. The hepatorenal syndrome (see Chapter 8) is a severe form of prerenal azotemia in patients with cirrhosis of the liver and severe portal hypertension. Patients with prerenal azotemia are often (although not always) oliguric and generally manifest increased sodium reabsorption if not being treated with diuretics.

10. **How can prerenal azotemia be differentiated from acute tubular necrosis?**
    It is important to differentiate between prerenal azotemia and intrinsic forms of AKI
    because prerenal azotemia will generally improve with correction of the underlying
    hemodynamic disturbance. In contrast, volume loading of patients with ATN or other forms
    of intrinsic AKI will not result in improved kidney function and may exacerbate volume
    overload. Characteristic laboratory findings that help to differentiate between prerenal
    azotemia and ATN reflect the preservation of tubular function with increased sodium
    reabsorption and urinary concentration in prerenal azotemia (Table 6-2). Pre-existing
    chronic kidney disease or diuretic use may limit the usefulness of these indices.

11. **What are the fractional excretions of sodium and urea and how are they
    calculated?**
    The fractional excretions of sodium and urea are indices of tubular function that are useful in
    differentiating between prerenal azotemia and acute tubular necrosis, particularly in patients
    with oliguric AKI. In prerenal states, the renal tubular response to decreased effective
    perfusion is to increase tubular sodium reabsorption. The fractional excretion of sodium
    (FE_{Na}), which is the percentage of the sodium filtered at the glomerulus that is excreted in the
    urine, will decrease from a normal value of slightly less than 1% and will be significantly less
    than 1%. In contrast, in many forms of ATN, impaired tubular function will result in elevated
    values of FE_{Na} (>23%).
    The FE_{Na} is calculated by dividing the urine sodium excretion by the filtered sodium load:
    - The excreted $Na^+ = U_{Na} \times V$, where U_{Na} is the urine sodium concentration and V is the
      urine volume
    - The filtered $Na^+ = P_{Na} \times GFR$, where P_{Na} is the plasma sodium concentration and GFR is
      the glomerular filtration rate
    - The GFR can be estimated as the creatinine clearance, $U_{creat} \times V/P_{creat}$, where U_{creat} and
      P_{creat} are the urine and plasma creatinine concentrations, respectively.
    - Thus, $FE_{Na} = (U_{Na} \times V)/(P_{Na} \times GFR) = (U_{Na} \times V)/[(P_{Na} \times U_{creat} \times V)/P_{creat}]$
    - $= (U_{Na}/P_{Na})/(U_{creat}/P_{creat})$
    Although the FE_{Na} is helpful in differentiating between prerenal azotemia and ATN, it is not
    completely reliable. Patients who develop ATN in the setting of volume depletion, or as the result
    of contrast-induced nephropathy or rhabdomyolysis, may have an FE_{Na} <1%. Conversely, the

TABLE 6-2 LABORATORY DIFFERENTIATION BETWEEN PRERENAL AZOTEMIA AND ACUTE TUBULAR NECROSIS		
	Prerenal Azotemia	**Acute Tubular Necrosis**
Serum blood urea nitrogen:creatinine ratio	>20:1	10:1
Urine-specific gravity	>1.015	~1.010
Urine sodium	<20 mmol/L	>40 mmol/L
Fractional excretion of sodium	<1%	>2%
Fractional excretion of urea	<35%	>50%
Urine osmolality	>500 mOsm/kg	~300 mOsm/kg
Urine sediment	Normal or hyaline casts	Renal tubular cells and "muddy brown" granular casts

FE_{Na} may be $>1\%$ in patients with prerenal azotemia who are taking diuretics or who have underlying chronic kidney disease. In these patients, the fractional excretion of urea (FE_{urea}) may be helpful in differentiating between prerenal azotemia and ATN. The FE_{urea} is calculated in a fashion analogous to the FE_{Na}:

$$FE_{urea} = (U_{urea}/P_{urea})/(U_{creat}/P_{creat})$$

In prerenal azotemia FE_{urea} is usually $<35\%$; in ATN, values are typically $>50\%$.

12. What is abdominal compartment syndrome?

Abdominal compartment syndrome is caused by an increase in intra-abdominal pressure resulting in dysfunction of multiple organ systems including decreased cardiac output and hypotension, increased thoracic pressure, decreased pulmonary compliance and increased airway pressures leading to impaired ventilation, and decreased visceral perfusion that may lead to intestinal ischemia and infarction and AKI. It is thought that increased renal venous pressure rather than increased intra-parenchymal pressure is the primary cause of AKI in the abdominal compartment syndrome. Common causes of abdominal compartment syndrome include trauma with intra-abdominal hemorrhage, abdominal surgery, retroperitoneal hemorrhage, peritonitis, pancreatitis, massive fluid resuscitation, abdominal banding, repair of large incisional hernia, laparoscopy and pneumoperitoneum, and ileus. It has been suggested that abdominal compartment syndrome may contribute to as many as 30% of cases of AKI in patients who are critically ill.

13. How is the abdominal compartment syndrome diagnosed?

The hallmark of abdominal compartment syndrome is an intra-abdominal pressure >20 mm Hg or greater associated with a single or multiple organ system failure that was not previously present. Intra-abdominal pressure may be assessed by transduction of urinary bladder pressure.

14. What is obstructive (postrenal) acute kidney injury?

Obstructive (postrenal) AKI results from blockage to urine flow at the level of the ureters (upper tract) or the bladder outlet or urethra (see Chapter 17). For upper tract obstruction to cause AKI, the obstruction must be bilateral or unilateral with an absent or nonfunctional contralateral kidney.

15. What are the causes of intrinsic acute kidney injury?

A variety of renal parenchymal diseases can cause AKI, including acute and rapidly progressive forms of glomerulonephritis (see Chapter 15), acute interstitial nephritis (Chapter 46), acute tubular necrosis (ATN), acute vascular diseases (e.g., renal artery thromboembolism, atheroembolic disease), and intratubular deposition of crystals (e.g., calcium oxalate in ethylene glycol positioning, uric acid in tumor lysis syndrome, acyclovir and indinavir) or paraproteins (myeloma cast nephropathy). ATN is the most common etiology of intrinsic AKI.

16. How can the different causes of intrinsic acute kidney injury be differentiated?

Although there are no specific therapies for the treatment of ATN, specific therapies are available for many of the other forms of intrinsic AKI. Diagnostic clues may be apparent from the history and physical examination, paying careful attention to the history of medication use and medical procedures and careful examination of the skin for evidence of vasculitis, drug eruption, and atheroembolism. Examination of the urine often provides key findings for differentiating among etiologies of intrinsic AKI (Table 6-3). Definitive diagnosis may require kidney biopsy.

17. What is acute interstitial nephritis?

Acute interstitial nephritis (AIN) is a form of AKI that results from immunologically mediated lymphocytic infiltration of the renal parenchymal interstitium, often with accompanying eosinophils. Although the classic presentation consists of AKI accompanied by a triad of fever, rash, and eosinophilia, the complete triad is observed in only a small minority of patients.

TABLE 6-3   URINE FINDINGS IN INTRINSIC AKI

AGN/RPGN	AIN	ATN	Crystal Nephropathies	Myeloma Kidney
Dysmorphic RBCs RBC casts	RBCs WBCs WBC casts Eosinophiluria	Tubular epithelial cells Coarse granular casts ("muddy brown" casts)	Crystaluria Oxalate—ethylene glycol Urate—tumor lysis syndrome Drug—acyclovir, indinavir	Bence-Jones proteinuria Free urinary light chains

AKI = acute kidney injury; AGN = acute glomerulonephritis; RPGN = rapidly progressive glomerulonephritis; AIN = acute interstitial nephritis; ATN = acute tubular necrosis; RBC = red blood cell; WBC = white blood cell.

18. **What are the causes of acute interstitial nephritis?**
    Although AIN may develop as the result of infections, malignancy, and immunologically mediated systemic disease, it is most often associated with medication use (Table 6-4). The most common medications include antibiotics, particularly penicillins, cephalosporins, sulfonamides and rifampin, and proton pump inhibitors. NSAIDs are associated with an atypical form or interstitial nephritis, usually not associated with fever, rash, or eosinophilia, and often associated with nephrotic proteinuria.

19. **Does the presence of eosinophiluria mean a patient has acute interstitial nephritis?**
    Although eosinophiluria has been considered a hallmark finding, it is not specific because it may be seen in pyelonephritis, prostatitis, cystitis, and atheroembolic disease.

TABLE 6-4   ETIOLOGIES OF ACUTE INTERSTITIAL NEPHRITIS

MEDICATIONS
Penicillins
Cephalosporins
Sulfonamides
Rifampin
Proton pump inhibitors
Phenytoin
Furosemide
Nonsteroidal anti-inflammatory drugs (NSAIDs)

INFECTIONS
Bacterial
Viral
Rickettsial
Tuberculosis

SYSTEMIC DISEASES
Systemic lupus erythematosus
Sarcoidosis
Sjögren's syndrome
Tubulointerstitial nephritis and uveitis
Malignancy
Idiopathic

20. **What are the causes of acute tubular necrosis?**
    Acute tubular necrosis may develop as the result of hypotension and renal ischemia, in the setting of sepsis with or without overt hypotension, or as the result of nephrotoxin exposure. Ischemia contributes to approximately 60% to 70% of cases of ATN, sepsis to 50% to 60% of cases, and nephrotoxins to 30% to 40% of cases. The nephrotoxins commonly associated with development of ATN are listed in Table 6-5.

21. **What is the pathophysiology of acute tubular necrosis?**
    Although ATN is characterized by a profound decrease in glomerular filtration rate, the connection between the tubular injury and the loss of glomerular function is not entirely understood. Three major mechanisms are thought to underlie the loss of renal function in ATN:
    - **Intratubular obstruction:** Following an ischemic or nephrotoxic injury, tubular epithelial cells and cellular debris are sloughed from the tubular epithelium and occlude the tubular lumen distally. These sloughed cells and debris form the granular casts seen in the urine sediment.
    - **Tubular backleak:** The sloughing of apoptotic and necrotic tubular epithelial cells results in denuding of the tubular basement membrane and unregulated backleak of glomerular filtrate. The combination of tubular obstruction and backleak results in increased urine flow through the tubular lumen.
    - **Vasoconstriction and microvascular injury:** Although the pathognomonic injury in ATN is to the tubular epithelium, there is both reactive vasoconstriction and endothelial injury in the microvasculature that results in decreased glomerular perfusion, reducing the GFR directly and contributing to extension of the initial injury.

22. **What is the clinical course of acute tubular necrosis?**
    Clinically, four phases of ATN can be described. In the **initiation phase,** exposure to the nephrotoxic agent, ischemia, or sepsis initiates the injury to the kidney. In clinical practice, there are often multiple exposures whose cumulative effect results in initiation of ATN. The initiation phase is then followed by an **extension phase,** during which there is continued cellular injury mediated by continued microvascular injury and activation of inflammatory mediators despite the fact that the triggering exposure has resolved. This is then followed by a **maintenance phase,** which may last from days to 6 weeks or longer. During the maintenance phase, the glomerular filtration rate remains markedly depressed, often accompanied by oliguria. During this phase patients are often dependent on some form of renal replacement therapy (dialysis or continuous hemofiltration). With time, the patient may enter the **recovery phase,** during which there is regeneration of the tubular epithelium and an improvement in kidney function. This phase is often characterized by a brisk increase in urine

TABLE 6-5 ETIOLOGIES OF ACUTE TUBULAR NECROSIS	
NEPHROTOXIC	**ISCHEMIC**
Exogenous	Prolonged prerenal azotemia
Radiocontrast agents	Hypotension
Aminoglycosides	Hypovolemic shock
Amphotericin B	Cardiopulmonary arrest
Cisplatinum	Cardiopulmonary bypass
Acetaminophen	Aortic surgery
Endogenous	**SEPSIS**
Hemoglobin	
Myoglobin	

output and is often referred to as the **diuretic phase.** Although the glomerular filtration rate may recover to near normal levels, there is often residual renal injury manifested by a decrease in glomerular filtration rate from baseline, a loss of renal functional reserve, or evidence of tubular dysfunction that may persist for months or years.

23. **What are the risk factors for the development of acute tubular necrosis?**
Pre-existing kidney disease with a decrease in glomerular filtration rate is the most significant risk factor for the development of ATN. Patients with diabetic nephropathy are at increased risk as compared to patients with nondiabetic kidney disease of equal severity. Other factors that predispose to the development of ATN include volume depletion and the use of pharmacologic agents that decrease renal perfusion, particularly nonselective NSAIDs and selective cyclo-oxygenase-2 (COX-2) inhibitors.

24. **Can acute kidney injury be prevented?**
Unfortunately, other than good medical care with avoidance of volume contraction, prevention of hypotension, and avoidance of nephrotoxic agents, no specific interventions have been reliably demonstrated to prevent the development of AKI. The best model for prevention of AKI is prevention of contrast-induced nephropathy following administration of iodinated contrast agents for angiography and computed tomography. Although multiple agents such as N-acetylcysteine and sodium bicarbonate have been evaluated, the efficacy of these agents beyond volume expansion with isotonic saline remains controversial.

KEY POINTS: ACUTE KIDNEY INJURY

1. Acute kidney injury (AKI), a term that is now replacing the older term acute renal failure (ARF), describes a sudden decrease in renal function occurring over a period of hours to days.

2. The differential diagnosis of AKI includes prerenal azotemia, obstructive nephropathy, and intrinsic forms of AKI.

3. Prerenal azotemia is a functional form of AKI that results from diminished renal perfusion. Because there is no parenchymal injury, the hallmark of prerenal azotemia is the rapid normalization of kidney function when renal perfusion is restored.

4. A variety of renal parenchymal diseases can cause intrinsic AKI, including acute tubular necrosis (ATN), acute interstitial nephritis, acute and rapidly progressive forms of glomerulonephritis, acute vascular diseases, and intratubular deposition of crystals or paraproteins. ATN is the most common etiology of intrinsic AKI.

5. The most important risk factor for the development of AKI is the presence of pre-existing chronic kidney disease.

6. Other than good medical care with avoidance of volume contraction, prevention of hypotension, and avoidance of nephrotoxic agents, no specific interventions have been reliably demonstrated to prevent the development of AKI.

25. **What is the treatment of acute kidney injury?**
The treatment of AKI is dependent on the specific cause. Prerenal states need to be treated with correction of intravascular volume depletion and optimization of cardiac function. AKI from urinary tract obstruction needs to be treated with decompression of the urinary tract. AIN is treated with discontinuation of the offending agent; the role of glucocorticoids therapy remains controversial. Acute glomerular syndromes need to be treated based on the specific

etiology. The management of ATN is entirely supportive. There are no effective pharmacologic agents. Renal replacement therapy is used to support patients while anticipating recovery of kidney function.

26. **What are the outcomes of acute kidney injury?**
Acute kidney injury is associated with high rates of morbidity and mortality. In patients who are critically ill and have severe ATN requiring dialytic support, hospital mortality rates are in the range of 40% to 70%. Even prerenal azotemia is associated with increased mortality, with mortality rates as high as 30% in some series. Recovery of kidney function in survivors is often incomplete, and there is a markedly increased risk of progressive chronic kidney disease and development of dialysis-requiring end-stage renal disease after an episode of AKI.

BIBLIOGRAPHY

1. Abdel-Kader K, Palevsky PM. Acute kidney injury in the elderly. *Clin Geriatr Med* 2009;25:331–358.
2. Bellomo R, Ronco C, Kellum JA, et al. Acute renal failure—Definition, outcome measures, animal models, fluid therapy and information technology needs: The Second International Consensus Conference of the Acute Dialysis Quality Initiative (ADQI) Group. *Crit Care* 2004;8:R204–212.
3. Hsu CY, McCulloch CE, Fan D, et al. Community-based incidence of acute renal failure. *Kidney Int* 2007;72:208–212.
4. Mehta R, Kellum J, Shah S, et al. Acute Kidney Injury Network: Report of an initiative to improve outcomes in acute kidney injury. *Crit Care* 2007;11:R31.
5. Nash K, Hafeez A, Hou S. Hospital-acquired renal insufficiency. *Am J Kidney Dis* 2002;39:930–936.
6. Sharfuddin AA, Molitoris BA. Pathophysiology of ischemic acute kidney injury. *Nature Reviews Nephrology* 2011;7:189–200.
7. Thadhani R, Pascual M, Bonventre JV. Acute renal failure. *N Engl J Med* 1996;334:1448–1460.
8. Wald R, Quinn RR, Luo J, et al. Chronic dialysis and death among survivors of acute kidney injury requiring dialysis. *JAMA* 2009;302:1179–1185.

CHAPTER 7

MANAGEMENT OPTIONS: CONTINUOUS RENAL REPLACEMENT THERAPY

Rolando Claure-Del Granado, MD; Etienne Macedo, MD, PhD; and Ravindra L. Mehta, MD

1. **What are the main treatment strategies of nonpharmacologic management of acute kidney injury (AKI)?**

   There is no established effective treatment for AKI, and the most important strategy for avoiding the development and progression of AKI is prevention. The preventive strategies include identifying high-risk populations, assuring euvolemia, maintaining renal perfusion pressure, and minimizing nephrotoxin exposure. For all these strategies to be effective, adequate early intervention is a requirement.

   - Adequate volume status is critical for maintaining hemodynamic stability, tissue perfusion, and organ function. On established AKI, volume expansion has not shown to increase glomerular filtration or improve renal function; however, hypovolemia remains the main risk factor associated with the onset and the progression of AKI. Fluid challenge is often required during episodes of hypotension and/or oliguria to restore cardiac output, systemic blood pressure, and renal perfusion to promote diuresis. However, recent evidence suggests that positive fluid balance is associated with worse outcomes in patients who are critically ill.

   - There are no evidence-based recommendations regarding the level of mean arterial pressure (MAP) that should be maintained to assure adequate renal perfusion pressure (RPP). The main cause of inadequate RPP is systemic hypotension; however, intra-abdominal hypertension and abdominal compartmental syndrome are underappreciated complications of medical and surgical illnesses that compromise RPP and can result in AKI. It is important to closely monitor and intervene in cases of elevated intra-abdominal pressure, especially in patients who are postabdominal surgery and in those with volume overload.

   - For minimizing nephrotoxins exposure the following points should be considered: patient risk factors for drug toxicity, possible drug interactions, daily assessment of renal function, and monitoring of drug levels when possible. A search for alternative non-nephrotoxic therapies should always be done.

2. **What type of fluid should be chosen for preventing AKI?**

   There is currently no ideal type of fluid for preventing AKI; one must consider that the several fluids available for treating hypovolemia have different effects on volume expansion, fluid, and electrolyte balance; acid–base control; and renal function (although this last point is controversial). In patients who are critically ill there is no evidence that resuscitation with colloids is associated with better outcomes than crystalloids, although in some specific clinical scenarios, the type of fluid used during AKI can affect patient's renal function and outcomes. In patients with spontaneous bacterial peritonitis, the use of albumin has shown to reduce incidence of AKI. Compared with normal saline, lactate ringer infusion in kidney transplant recipients may favor early diuresis. The risk of developing hyperkalemia and metabolic acidosis with the use of lactate ringer in kidney transplant recipients is also lower.

   The use of high molecular weight hyperoncotic starches is associated with an increased risk of AKI, especially in patients who are septic or post-transplant. Several studies have shown a beneficial effect of isotonic bicarbonate solution compared to isotonic NaCl solution to reduce the incidence of contrast-induced AKI in patients at high risk. However, a recent systematic review and meta-analysis found no evidence of hydration with sodium bicarbonate. The benefit of sodium bicarbonate for the prevention of contrast-induced AKI is limited to small trials. In summary, the type of fluid chosen should be individualized for each patient.

3. **Is there a specific target of mean arterial blood pressure that should be reached in patients with AKI?**

There is no evidence-based recommendation regarding the level of MAP that should be maintained to assure adequate RPP (RPP = MAP − renal venous pressure, which approximates to central venous pressure). Therapeutic trials in sepsis have proved that a target MAP between 60 and 65 mm Hg is associated with improved patient outcomes, although renal function has not been reported on these studies. Data derived from animal studies demonstrated that the lower autoregulatory MAP threshold in the renal circulation is 80 mm Hg; but there are limited human data consistent with this experimental finding. Renal autoregulation appears to be a more efficient protective mechanism of renal perfusion associated with hypertensive renal injury rather than in decreased renal perfusion pressure in hypotensive episodes.

Experimental data suggested that during AKI the autoregulation is lost and renal blood flow becomes linearly pressure dependent, resulting in recurrent episodes of AKI with subsequent hypotension. Therefore, the maintenance of an adequate MAP is considered an important goal for preventing and managing AKI.

Based on current literature, in patients with an adequate cardiac output and vasodilatory shock, the target MAP should be ≥65 mm Hg. Patients with ventricular dysfunction may require lower MAP targets, whereas patients with previous hypertension require higher MAP targets. Adjustment of vasoconstrictor agents should be individualized.

4. **How could exposure to nephrotoxins be prevented during AKI?**

Surveillance for nephrotoxicity risk factors is the first step to avoid the development of AKI and prevent and minimize post-AKI exposure to nephrotoxins. Risk factors can be classified as patient specific, such as female gender, old age (>65 years old), or presence of nephrotic syndrome or chronic kidney disease; kidney specific, such as proximal tubular uptake of toxins or biotransformation; and drug specific, such as combinations of toxins, drugs that promote enhanced nephrotoxicity, and water-insoluble parental compounds. Usually more than one risk factor is present.

Some recommendations should be considered to prevent nephrotoxins exposure during AKI:

- Find alternative therapies for drugs with significant nephrotoxic potential
- Conduct appropriate monitoring of renal function
- Ensure drug dosing and correction of dosage are in accordance with pre-existing organ dysfunction (besides AKI)
- Consider the specific aspects of the drug pharmacokinetics
- Maintain adequate volume status and sodium repletion
- Continuously reassess concomitant medications for possible interactions
- Select diagnostic tests that do not require use of a nephrotoxic agent in patients at higher risk for renal injury.

The use of estimating equations (MDRD Study and Cockroft-Gault) in AKI is associated with the limitation of serum creatinine as a filtration marker. Serum creatinine is affected by factors other than GFR, such as muscle mass, diet, and drugs, which are factors frequently present in patients who are critically ill. In addition, the nonlinear relationship between serum creatinine and GFR results in overestimation of renal function during the development phase of AKI and underestimation during the recovery phase. Considering the inaccuracy of all creatinine-based estimation of GFR, the risk of toxicity with a higher dose should be weighed against the risk of treatment failure with a lower dose.

5. **Is there an ideal vasopressor for use in patients with AKI?**

There is clinical evidence that continuous infusion of norepinephrine may increase urine output and improve creatinine clearance in hyperdynamic septic shock. Clinical studies have shown that the use of norepinephrine (1 μm/kg minute) as compared to dopamine (up to 50 μm/kg minute) restores normotension (MAP target $\geq$80 mm Hg) in all patients, whereas the use of dopamine (up to 50 μm/kg minute) restores normotension in only one third of the patients. These studies also showed an improvement in urinary output in patients treated with norepinephrine. In patients with septic shock, treatment with norepinephrine was associated with a lower mortality rate compared to patients treated with dopamine. Norepinephrine use was also identified as a predictor of survival on the multivariate logistic regression analysis. Finally, two recent studies have compared the effects of terlipressin and norepinephrine in patients with hepatorenal syndrome (HRS). Taken together these small studies suggest that norepinephrine is an alternative therapy for patients with HRS.

No controlled studies have been conducted to compare phenylephrine or epinephrine with norepinephrine; still, they are not recommended as a first-line vasopressor during AKI because of the uncontrolled alpha-adrenergic effect of phenylephrine and epinephrine secondary effects (hyperlactatemia, hyperglycemia, acidosis, and tachycardia). The VASST study has compared the effects of vasopressin (0.01–0.03 U/min) to norepinephrine (5–15 μg/min) infusion on the outcome of patients with septic shock. In patients in the RIFLE "Risk" category, vasopressin was associated with a lower rate of progression of AKI and a lower rate of need for renal replacement therapy when compared with norepinephrine. However, low-dose vasopressin did not reduce mortality rates as compared with norepinephrine.

6. **Could dopamine prevent or treat AKI?**

Four recent meta-analyses and one large multicenter, double-blinded, placebo-controlled, randomized clinical trial have explored the use of the "renal dose" (low-dose) of dopamine in patients with AKI. These studies have failed to show that low-dose dopamine can improve renal function, reduce mortality, or prevent renal dysfunction in patients with AKI.

In a more recent study, the use of low-dose dopamine (2 μg/kg per min) in patients in the intensive care unit (ICU) with AKI increased renal vascular resistance measured by Doppler ultrasound and did not modify the urine output or hemodynamic parameters, such as blood pressure and heart rate. If low-dose dopamine has any beneficial effect, it is not sustained and consists of a transiently increase in urine output that usually lasts 24 hours.

7. **Is fenoldopam effective in treating patients with AKI?**

The use of fenoldopam has shown to improve renal function in patients with septic AKI. New data from experimental AKI models suggest that fenoldopam may have additional protective effects on AKI, including anti-inflammatory effects independent of its vasodilator action. One of these anti-inflammatory effects is the inhibition of the nuclear translocation of nuclear factor-κB, a cellular promoter of cytokine production. The intrarenal administration of fenoldopam showed it was not associated with drops in the systolic blood pressure, as compared with the intravenous administration, and it had a clear dose-dependent effect. The rates of contrast nephropathy among patients receiving 0.4 mg/kg/min of intrarenal fenoldopam were significantly lower than for those receiving 0.2 mg/kg/min of intravenous fenoldopam. Further investigation in a large, multicenter, randomized controlled trial will be required to determine the use of fenoldopam as an effective renoprotective agent.

8. **What is the role of loop diuretics in patients with AKI?**

Loop diuretics inhibit the Na$^+$ K$^+$ 2Cl$^-$ cotransporter in the apical membrane of the ascending loop of Henle, responsible for the reabsorption of 25% to 40% of the Na$^+$. They inhibit the prostaglandin dehydrogenase, resulting in reduction of renal vascular resistance and increasing renal blood flow. They decrease metabolic demand of renal tubular cells with concomitant reduction in oxygen consumption by blocking the Na$^+$ K$^+$ 2Cl$^-$ cotransporter. By increasing urine flow, they "wash out" renal tubules and could reduce the necrotic debris that causes backleakage of glomerular filtrate into renal interstitium. Their use in early or established AKI facilitates the management of hyperkalemia, hypercalcemia, and fluid balance.

Patients with AKI and other comorbidities such as heart failure, cirrhosis, and/or nephrotic syndrome may be resistant to the effect of bolus administration of loop diuretics, resulting from avid sodium retention after plasma concentration has decreased below the effective level. Long-term tolerance can occur associated with factors that affect pharmacokinetics such as reduced bioavailability, reduced renal blood flow, albuminuria, and hypoalbuminemia, or factors that affect pharmacodynamics, such as increased distal sodium reabsorption, distal tubular hypertrophy, and increased $Na^+ K^+ 2Cl^-$ cotransporter expression. Loop diuretic responsiveness could be improved by the optimization of blood pressure to restore renal blood flow, the correction of acidosis, the use of thiazide diuretics, and the coadministration of albumin.

A Cochrane Database systematic review showed greater diuresis and a better safety profile when loop diuretics were given as continuous infusion. Despite some theoretical advantages, loop diuretics did not show any benefit in the prevention or treatment of AKI. None of the available evidence shows that loop diuretics increase the recovery of renal function nor reduce the need for renal replacement therapy, days on replacement treatment, length of ICU or hospital stay, or mortality. Although still controversial, some recent studies have associated this type of diuretics with worse outcomes. The increase in urine output and correction of hyperkalemia could delay nephrology consultation and dialysis indication. Use of loop diuretics should be limited to the management of patients who are volume overloaded and not for AKI or oliguria per se. The use of high doses (1–3.4 g per day) of furosemide is associated with temporary deafness and tinnitus.

9. **What is the role of osmotic diuretics in patients with AKI?**
    Osmotic diuretics are freely filtered at the glomerulus and undergo limited reabsorption in the tubules. They act on the proximal tubule and at the loop of Henle. They expand the extracellular fluid volume, decrease blood viscosity, and inhibit renin release, resulting in increased renal blood flow and reduction in medullary tonicity. Although prophylactic mannitol is effective in animal models of acute tubular necrosis, the clinical efficacy of mannitol is less well established. In many centers, mannitol has been used during AKI related to rhabdomyolysis associated with crush syndrome. No evidence supports the use of mannitol in preventing or treating AKI.

10. **What is the role of thiazide diuretics in patients with AKI?**
    Thiazide diuretics inhibit Na^+ reabsorption in the early distal convoluted tubule by inhibiting the NaCl cotransporter. This transporter is a major mechanism of sodium reabsorption in the distal collecting tubule and is responsible for reuptake of 5% to 8% of the Na^+ load under normal conditions. Thiazide diuretics are usually used in association with loop diuretics to increase natriuresis and have no role in the prevention or treatment of AKI of any cause.

11. **What is the value of natriuretic peptides as an early intervention in AKI?**
    Natriuretic peptides like atrial natriuretic peptide (ANP) suppress the synthesis of angiotensin II and aldosterone; it has also been shown in experimental studies that ANP dilates the afferent arteriole and constricts the efferent arteriole of the glomerulus, potentially maintaining the glomerular filtration rate. ANP also has anti-inflammatory and antiapoptotic effects. All these effects together could attenuate both vascular and tubular effects that play major roles in the pathophysiology of AKI.

    Experimental studies have demonstrated protective effects of ANP in ischemic models of AKI; additional in vivo studies have demonstrated AKI protection despite a significant decrease in mean arterial blood pressure. Studies in humans have shown that, in patients with early ischemic or cyclosporine-induced AKI, ANP improves both glomerular filtration rate and renal blood flow. A small study suggests that low-dose ANP infusion reduces the probability of dialysis and improves dialysis-free survival in early ischemic AKI after cardiac surgery complicated by circulatory shock. A similar study shows that ANP may decrease the need for dialysis after liver transplantation. A large, prospective, double-blind, placebo-controlled, randomized study showed that a greater number of patients in the ANP arm achieved improvement in creatinine clearance than controls, especially in patients with oliguria. The concern with this drug is the potential decrease of blood pressure associated with their systemic vasodilator effect. The development of more selective forms of ANP could be a promising agent in early intervention in AKI.

A multicenter, randomized, double-blinded, placebo-controlled trial (NAPA study) evaluated the effects of nesiritide in 303 patients with chronic left ventricular dysfunction who were undergoing coronary artery bypass graft using cardiopulmonary bypass with or without mitral valve surgery. The NAPA study results demonstrated short-term benefits of nesiritide on perioperative renal function as assessed by lower increments in serum creatinine levels, a lower reduction in estimated GFR, and a greater urine output 24 hours after surgery.

12. **In which setting is the use of adenosine antagonists indicated?**
Adenosine is a renal vasoconstrictor; it has been shown to be a mediator of the intrarenal hemodynamic changes that lead to AKI after radiocontrast agent administration and after other insults by binding to A_1 receptors. Two of these adenosine antagonists, theophylline and aminophylline, have been specifically evaluated after vascular surgery and after radiocontrast agent administration. After radiocontrast administration, a meta-analysis showed a decreased degree of change in serum creatinine but no difference in relevant clinical outcomes. No benefit was found in studies evaluating the effect of theophylline after cardiac surgery. Use of theophylline in certain patients at high risk in whom adequate hydration is not possible (e.g., patients in heart failure) could be useful; however, based on current data available, routine use of theophylline to prevent AKI cannot be recommended.

13. **What is the actual role of insulin therapy and glycemic control?**
Hyperglycemia is an important factor associated with outcomes in patients who are critically ill, including those with AKI. In a multicenter randomized controlled trial, intensive insulin treatment to reduce serum glucose to less than 110 mg/dL was associated with a significant reduction in ICU mortality and in the incidence of AKI. Hyperglycemia has direct and indirect effects on renal function; hyperglycemia increases acute inflammatory response and oxidative stress and increases the incidence of some complications such as sepsis-associated AKI. Insulin therapy may prevent renal injury through positive effects on serum lipids, acting as scavengers of endotoxins, by modulation of aberrant endothelial activation, and deranged endothelial nitric oxide synthesis.

In a subsequent study, including a more broad population of patients who were critically ill, the reduction in mortality associated with insulin therapy could not be replicated. But insulin use still was associated with a reduction in newly acquired kidney injury. A more recent study showed that there was no effect of intensive insulin therapy on the incidence of some renal outcomes such as need for renal replacement therapy or oliguria, except in the surgical subset of patients. This study also showed that insulin therapy reduces the incidence of AKI.

Based on current evidence, thigh glycemic control with insulin in patients with AKI remains a controversial intervention. A recent systematic review has concluded that there is no evidence that supports the use of intensive insulin therapy in general medical–surgical ICU patients who are fed according to the current guidelines. Thigh glycemic control is associated with a high incidence of hypoglycemia and a high rate of death in patients not receiving parental nutrition. Until the result of a new large multicenter randomized trial is available, intensive insulin therapy should be used with caution.

14. **Erythropoietin: What is new?**
Erythropoietin (EPO) receptors have been identified in several tissues including endothelial cells, myocytes, vascular smooth cells, mesangial cells, and renal proximal tubular cells. EPO has many pleiotropic effects and, in experimental models of acute kidney ischemia, EPO has

shown to modulate mitogenesis, vascular repair, oxidative stress, inflammation, and apoptosis. Numerous in vitro and in vivo studies have examined the role of EPO as a preconditioning treatment to prevent AKI. In a small randomized clinical trial in patients scheduled for elective coronary artery bypass graft surgery, the prophylactic administration of EPO (300 U/kg) before surgery prevented AKI and improved postoperative renal function as compared with the administration of placebo. EPO could potentially be used in established AKI as an accelerant of renal recovery through its vascular and anti-inflammatory effects. An open-label, randomized controlled clinical trial exploring this potential role of EPO in accelerating the recovery phase of AKI is ongoing.

15. **What is the role of nutrition in the management of patients with AKI?**
Patients with AKI often have protein-energy wasting syndrome (PEW), which could be present as a pre-existing (chronic kidney disease) and/or hospital-acquired condition. PEW constitutes a major negative prognostic factor associated with increased mortality in the setting of AKI. Thus, nutritional support is fundamental; when the gastrointestinal tract cannot be used for enteral feeding, or when enteral nutrition is not enough to reach nutrient intake goals, parental nutrition should be instituted. The main goals of nutritional support in patients with AKI are to ensure the delivery of adequate amounts of nutrients, prevent PEW and its inherited metabolic complications, promote wound healing and tissue reparation, support immune system function, and reduce mortality. Patients with AKI receiving renal replacement therapy (RRT) should receive at least 1.5 g/kg per day of proteins and not more than 30 Kcal/kg per day nonprotein calories, with lipid supply representing about 30% to 35% of energy. To compensate for amino acid losses during RRT, protein supply should be increased by 0.2 g/kg per day. Unfortunately, the accurate assessment of a patient with AKI's nutritional indices is often difficult and inaccurate in the setting of critical illness. A close integration between nutritional support and RRT is required in AKI, with the aim of carefully tailoring both therapies during patients' changing needs.

16. **When should renal replacement therapy be initiated?**
There is no doubt among physicians that RRT should be started when absolute indications are present (blood urea nitrogen [BUN] >100 mg/dL, hyperkalemia >6 mEq/L with electrocardiogram changes, hypermagnesemia >8 mEq/L plus anuria plus hyporeflexia, pH <7.15, and diuretic therapy resistance volume overload). Difficulties arise when indications are not absolute (progressive azotemia but BUN <100 mg/dL, hyperkalemia >6 mEq/L without electrocardiogram changes, isolated hypermagnesemia, pH >7.15, oliguria). Although the maintenance of serum creatinine and BUN concentrations below arbitrarily set levels is usually a reference for starting dialysis treatment, neither creatinine nor BUN should be used to absolutely determine when to initiate dialysis. BUN reflects factors not directly associated with kidney function such as catabolic rate and volume status; serum creatinine is influenced by age, race, muscle mass, and catabolic rate, and its volume of distribution varies in patients with fluid overload. Other factors such as fluid balance control, nutrition needs, severity of the underlying disease, and acid–base and electrolyte balance should guide the decision to start dialysis. However, there are some potential safety concerns regarding earlier initiation of dialysis, including increased risk for infection from an in-dwelling dialysis catheter, hypotension, potential for delayed renal recovery, and leukocyte activation from contact with dialysis membranes, among others.

Timing of RRT, a potentially modifiable factor, might exert an important influence on patient survival. We favor utilizing an approach that recognizes that the strategy in treating AKI is to minimize and avoid uremic and volume-overload complications. Thus, it is not necessary to wait for progressive uremia to initiate dialytic support; it is better to use RRT as a supportive therapy in the presence of progressive azotemia and oliguria, rather than a rescue therapy for late manifestation of AKI. Current data are inadequate to define the optimal timing of RRT initiation in AKI; adequately powered randomized controlled trials are required to properly answer this question.

17. **What modalities of renal replacement therapy are available for treating patients with AKI?**

The modalities that can be use in the treatment of patients with AKI include the following:

- Conventional intermittent hemodialysis (IHD)
- Various types of continuous renal replacement therapies (CRRT) such as continuous venovenous hemofiltration (CVVH), continuous venovenous hemodialysis (CVVHD), and continuous venovenous hemodiafiltration (CVVHDF).
- Hybrid modalities that combine aspects of both IHD and CRRT, like slow low-efficiency dialysis (SLED), slow continuous ultrafiltration (SCUF), or extended daily diafiltration
- Peritoneal dialysis

Removal of solutes can be achieved by convection (hemofiltration), diffusion (hemodialysis), or the combination of the two methods (hemodiafiltration). The amount of solute transported per unit of time (clearance) depends on the molecular weight of the solute, the characteristics of the membrane, and the dialysate and blood flows. Intermittent hemodialysis (IHD) has been used widely for the past four decades to treat end-stage renal disease and AKI. Diffusive clearance is more effective for small molecular weight solutes such as potassium, urea, and creatinine. Solutes with higher molecular weight (between 500 and 60,000 Daltons), so-called "middle molecules," are better removed by convection, where hydrostatic pressure provides the driving force for plasma across a membrane. Whereas ultrafiltration implies fluid removal, hemofiltration necessitates partial or complete replacement of the fluid removed. The composition of the hemofiltration solution can vary, and the solution can be infused pre-filter or post-filter. Intermittent ultrafiltration, in contrast to intermittent hemodiafiltration, can be done with the same machines as IHD but is used specifically for volume removal. Most nephrologists use isolated ultrafiltration as a method of rapid fluid removal when the major indication for renal replacement or support is pulmonary edema or refractory congestive cardiomyopathy. Extended daily dialysis (EDD) or SLED differs from IHD in that dialysate and blood flow are intentionally kept low but the duration of the treatment is extended. These hybrid modalities can be performed at night for 8 to 12 hours using ICU staff, thereby eliminating interruption of therapy, reducing staff requirements, and avoiding scheduling conflicts. Studies comparing hybrid modalities to CRRT have revealed favorable hemodynamic tolerance in patients who were critically ill while achieving dialysis adequacy and ultrafiltration targets because the fluid removal and the solute clearance are more gradual.

Because RRT can be provided in various forms, as shown previously, the choice of a specific type of RRT should be based on the availability of resources, the needs of the patient, and the expertise of the staff.

18. **What type of vascular access should be used?**

Guidelines recommend that for acute hemodialysis access should be obtain by percutaneous placement of a double lumen catheter in the internal jugular, femoral, or subclavian vein. If renal replacement therapy is expected to extend beyond several days, consideration should be given to early placement of a tunneled catheter in the internal jugular vein.

Catheter malfunction has an important impact on the delivered dialysis dose as observed by the investigators of the ATN study; of interest, one study has shown that twin tunneled catheters in the femoral vein provide better function than conventional femoral vein catheters. The femoral vein is technically easiest to access; nevertheless, the concern of the risk of infection by using this type of access has limited its use over jugular or subclavian. One recent randomized controlled trial showed that femoral catheters were not associated with an increased risk of infections as compared with jugular catheters, except in patients with high body mass indexes. Thoracic catheters have the advantage of lower recirculation. However, it should be kept in mind that subclavian vein cannulation is associated with higher rates of both short-term (e.g., pneumothorax and hemorrhage) and long-term complications (e.g., stenosis). Subclavian catheters should be placed only if all the other options are not viable. Use of portable ultrasound machines has improved the success rate of cannulation and decreased rates of complications, and they should be routinely used if available.

19. Which factors could affect the modality selection of RRT?

It is debated whether continuous modalities are better than intermittent modalities in treatment of patients with AKI. Intermittent hemodialysis has several advantages that have made this therapy widely used. Among these advantages, the short duration of therapy with rapid correction of electrolyte and acid–base disturbances and fluid removal provide the therapy great efficacy. The availability of intermittent hemodialysis machines and trained nurses allows the dialysis in patients with AKI where machines for continuous therapies are not available. However, the duration of the procedure, 3 to 5 hours, limits the control of fluid regulation and acid–base and electrolyte balance. Patients with hemodynamic instability may not tolerate the high ultrafiltration rates necessary to achieve a fluid balance control. CRRT can offer advantages over IHD, which include slower fluid removal, allowing the elimination of a greater amount of fluids without compromising hemodynamic stability, better solute clearance and correction of acid–base and electrolyte abnormalities, and better metabolic control. Some data had suggested that intradialytic hypotensive episodes during IHD could decrease the rate of recovery of renal function, but CRRT can also have some limitations and disadvantages, such as need for continuous anticoagulation, patient immobilization, and greater human resource requirement including the need for ICU monitoring. Although there are many arguments that favor the use of CRRT in patients who are critically ill with AKI, current evidence has not shown any benefit of using CRRT instead of IHD in this group of patients. The hybrid modalities, SLED and EDD, can provide adequate solute control (as IHD does) and require less intensive monitoring and time in comparison to CRRT.

It is now recognized that more than one therapy can be utilized for managing patients with AKI. Transitions in therapy are common and reflect the changing needs of patients during their hospital course. For instance, patients in the ICU may initially start on CRRT when they are hemodynamically unstable, transition to SLED-EDD when they improve, and leave the ICU receiving IHD.

20. Is there an ideal dose of dialysis?

Since 2000 multiple studies in intermittent hemodialysis and in CRRTs have suggested that higher doses of renal replacement therapy (RRT) are associated with improved outcomes; however, two recent large, multicenter, randomized control trials (ATN study and RENAL study) do not support the hypothesis that a higher dose of RRT will improve outcomes. It appears that the relationship between dose administered by RRT and survival has two regions: a dosage-dependent region where increases in intensity of dose are associated with improved survival and a dosage-independent region where after a threshold is reached, further increment on the intensity of dose is not associated with better outcomes. These two studies, rather than implying that dose is not important in the treatment of patients who are critically ill with AKI, suggest that dose should be measured. The influence on solute clearance of some operational characteristics of RRT such as frequent filter clotting and protein fouling of the membrane can translate into a lower dose of delivered dialysis; that is why simply prescribing a target dose or adjusting for treatment interruptions is not enough for finding an ideal dose of dialysis.

Besides small solute clearance, other aspects of dosing should be considered (volume control, acid–base, nutritional status, etc.) to find an ideal dose of dialysis during AKI.

21. How should dose be measured?

Because the establishment of a link between dialysis dose measured by urea clearance and clinical outcomes in patients with end-stage renal disease, the clearance of urea adjusted for the volume of distribution of water has been used as an index of dialysis adequacy (Kt/V). Although widely used for chronic patients, the use of this dose-assessment parameter in AKI is not clear. In AKI the changes in body water volumes and urea generation rates result in inaccuracy of these formulas. The calculated Kt/V in patients with AKI has been shown to be 30% higher than the measured clearance in the dialysate as a result of episodes of hypotension, dialyzer clotting, and vascular access recirculation. In

CRRT, we also overestimate the true solute clearance by using the effluent volume as surrogate markers of delivered dose. Progressive decline in filter efficacy reduces clearance over time, which results in a gap between prescribed and delivered dialysis dose. The use of dialysate-side measurements provided more accurate dose information (actual solute removal) because it accounts for the loss of filter efficacy. Thus, measuring the actual solute removal in the effluent and calculating the clearance based on the mass extracted could dramatically improve the way we assess the effect of dose on outcomes in patients who are critically ill.

KEY POINTS: CONTINUOUS RENAL REPLACEMENT THERAPY

1. There is no established effective treatment for acute kidney injury (AKI), and the most important strategy for avoiding the development and progression of AKI is prevention.

2. Use of loop diuretics should be limited to the management of patients who are volume overloaded and not for those with AKI or oliguria per se.

3. It is not necessary to wait until severe uremia develops to initiate dialytic support; renal replacement therapy should be used as a supportive therapy in the presence of progressive azotemia and oliguria, rather than as a rescue therapy for late manifestation of AKI.

4. Recent studies did not show benefit of higher dose of dialysis in patients who were critically ill. However, these results do not mean that dose is not important, but they imply that delivered dose should be measured.

22. **What are the advantages of CRRT in a patient with sepsis and AKI?**
The use of hemofiltration in CRRT techniques may have an immunomodulatory effect. Some of the inflammatory mediators are water-soluble cytokines—interleukin (IL) 6, IL-8, IL-1, and tumor necrosis factor—and can be removed by convection according to their molecular weight and degree of plasma protein binding. The membrane characteristics such as molecular weight cut off, structure, and charge also affect the ability of a solute to convectively cross a membrane and the adsorption capacity.
   Despite some encouraging results, the clinical benefit of conventional CRRT in sepsis has been disappointing. Consequently, efforts have been made to improve the efficiency of soluble mediator removal by increasing ultrafiltration rates and enlarging the pore size of membranes.

23. **How is clotting of the dialyzer prevented?**
The contact of blood with the extracorporal circuit, lines, and membrane activates platelets and the production of a variety of inflammatory and prothrombotic mediators. The result is the induction of fibrin deposition and filter clotting. Clotting of the dialyzer reduces its longevity and, more important, reduces the efficiency of solute clearance. Inefficient anticoagulation reduces the dialyzer performance by diminishing the surface of the membrane available for diffusion or convection.
   The anticoagulation for RRT can be systemic or regional when only the dialysis circuit is anticoagulated. Systemic anticoagulation with unfractionated heparin is the most commonly used method. Heparin is usually administrated as a bolus, followed by a continuous infusion into the arterial line. The optimal dose for patients with AKI is not established. The target is to maintain a partial thromboplastin time of 1.5 to 2 times the normal level. The use of low molecular weight heparin requires the monitoring of factor Xa levels, as it is excreted mainly by the kidney. In patients at high risk of bleeding, systemic anticoagulation should be avoided. Although intermittent hemodialysis can often be performed without anticoagulation using intermittent saline flushes every 15 to 30 minutes in the arterial line. In CRRT regional anticoagulation with citrate is the alternative method; citrate is infused continuously in the

arterial line and chelates the free calcium in the circuit, inhibiting the coagulation cascade. Part of the complex calcium-citrate is removed by dialysis clearance and part is metabolized in the liver. Serum calcium concentrations (preferably ionized) should be monitored and continuous, or intermittent calcium infusion should be performed as necessary. The use of regional citrate anticoagulation increases the buffer load during the treatment as citrate is converted to bicarbonate in the liver. The possibility of metabolic alkalosis requires modifications in the hemofiltration solution or dialysate.

24. **What complications should be expected when using RRT?**
The most common complications include hypotension, bleeding, electrolyte imbalances, infection, and hypothermia. Hypotension is the most common complication of dialysis, occurring in around 30% of the treatments. Several factors associated with the dialysis treatment can cause hypotension: cardiac events, electrolyte imbalances, elevated dialysate temperature, bacterial contamination of system, low dialysate sodium concentration, clearance of vasoactive drugs, and intake of antihypertensive medications prior to treatment, among others. However, hypotension is most often related to imbalance between fluid removal and fluid replacement by the extravascular compartment. A large amount of fluid removal is a major risk factor for hypotension, especially in patients with compromised refilling capacity, as in diabetic neuropathy, low cardiac ejection fraction, diastolic dysfunction, and sepsis. Although CRRT has been demonstrated to reduce the episodes of hypotension and allow better acid–base and electrolyte control, the prolonged time of therapy can increase the risk of volume and electrolyte depletion. In spite of the expected safety of obtaining fluid removal over a longer period with CRRT, careful monitoring is mandatory. Hypotension and hemodynamic instability are still frequent in CRRT. In intensive and/or prolonged treatment, CRRT results in overcorrection of electrolyte imbalances, especially when nonphysiologic solutions are used as dialysate or replacement fluids. Hypocalcemia, hypophosphatemia, and hypokalemia are common complications associated with higher doses of CRRT, requiring careful electrolyte monitoring during the procedure. The use of peritoneal dialysate fluids for CRRT can cause hyperglycemia, demanding special attention with potassium imbalance. Patients receiving CRRT are at increased risk for hypothermia as blood circulates in the extracorporeal circulation for a prolonged time. Dialysate and replacement fluids should be warmed prior to administration, and body temperature should be frequently monitored. Because CRRT requires anticoagulation for a longer time, the risk of bleeding complications is also increased and monitoring of hemoglobin and hematocrit is important to detect hidden bleeding. Patients receiving RRT are vulnerable to catheter-related infections, including local to the vascular access site and systemic. The cooling effect of prolonged extracorporeal circulation in CRRT may be masked fever and special monitoring for other signs of infection is mandatory.

BIBLIOGRAPHY

1. Baldwin I, Bellomo R, Naka T, et al. A pilot randomized controlled comparison of extended daily dialysis with filtration and continuous veno-venous hemofiltration: Fluid removal and hemodynamics. *Int J Artif Organs* 2007;30(12):1083–1089.

2. Bellomo R, Egi M. Glycemic control in the intensive care unit: why we should wait for NICE-SUGAR. *Mayo Clin Proc* 2005;80(12):1546–1548.

3. RENAL Replacement Therapy Study Investigators, Bellomo R, Cass A, et al. Intensity of continuous renal-replacement therapy in critically ill patients. *N Engl J Med* 2009;361(17):1627–1638.

4. Berbece AN, Richardson RM. Sustained low-efficiency dialysis in the ICU: cost, anticoagulation, and solute removal. *Kidney Int* 2006;70(5):963–968.

5. Crowley ST, Peixoto AJ. Acute kidney injury in the intensive care unit. *Clin Chest Med* 2009;30(1):29–43, vii–viii.

6. Fiaccadori E, Cremaschi E. Nutritional assessment and support in acute kidney injury. *Curr Opin Crit Care* 2009;15(6):474–480.

7. Finfer S, Bellomo R, Boyce N, et al. A comparison of albumin and saline for fluid resuscitation in the intensive care unit. *N Engl J Med* 2004;350(22):2247–2256.

8. Himmelfarb J. Continuous dialysis is not superior to intermittent dialysis in acute kidney injury of the critically ill patient. *Nat Clin Pract Nephrol* 2007;3(3):120–121.

9. Himmelfarb J. Continuous renal replacement therapy in the treatment of acute renal failure: critical assessment is required. *Clin J Am Soc Nephrol* 2007;2(2):385–389.

10. Ho KM, Sheridan DJ. Meta-analysis of frusemide to prevent or treat acute renal failure. *BMJ* 2006;333(7565):420

11. Holt BG, White JJ, Kuthiala A, et al. Sustained low-efficiency daily dialysis with hemofiltration for acute kidney injury in the presence of sepsis. *Clin Nephrol* 2008;69(1):40–46.

12. Huang PP, Stucky FS, Dimick AR, et al. Hypertonic sodium resuscitation is associated with renal failure and death. *Ann Surg* 1995;221(5):543–554; discussion 554–557.

13. Kellum JA, Cerda J, Kaplan LJ, et al. Fluids for prevention and management of acute kidney injury. *Int J Artif Organs* 2008;31(2):96–110.

14. Kellum JA, Leblanc M, Gibney RT, et al. Primary prevention of acute renal failure in the critically ill. *Curr Opin Crit Care* 2005;11(6):537–541.

15. Kramer BK, Preuner J, Ebenburger A, et al. Lack of renoprotective effect of theophylline during aortocoronary bypass surgery. *Nephrol Dial Transplant* 2002;17(5):910–915.

16. Lauschke A, Teichgräber UK, Frei U, et al. "Low-dose" dopamine worsens renal perfusion in patients with acute renal failure. *Kidney Int* 2006;69(9):1669–1674.

17. Lee RW, Di Giantomasso D, May C, et al. Vasoactive drugs and the kidney. *Best Pract Res Clin Anaesthesiol* 2004;18(1):53–74.

18. Liao Z, Zhang W, Hardy PA, et al. Kinetic comparison of different acute dialysis therapies. *Artif Organs* 2003;27(9):802–807.

19. Malbrain ML, Deeren D, De Potter TJ. Intra-abdominal hypertension in the critically ill: it is time to pay attention. *Curr Opin Crit Care* 2005;11(2):156–171.

20. Marshall MR. Current status of dosing and quantification of acute renal replacement therapy. Part 2: dosing paradigms and clinical implementation. *Nephrology* (Carlton) 2006;11(3):181–191.

21. O'Malley CM, Frumento RJ, Hardy MA, et al. A randomized, double-blind comparison of lactated Ringer's solution and 0.9% NaCl during renal transplantation. *Anesth Analg* 2005;100(5):1518–1524, Table of Contents.

22. Palevsky PM. Renal support in acute kidney injury—How much is enough? *N Engl J Med* 2009;361(17):1699–1701.

23. Pannu N, Gibney RN. Renal replacement therapy in the intensive care unit. *Ther Clin Risk Manag* 2005;1(2):141–150.

24. Parienti JJ, Thirion M, Mégarbane B, et al. Femoral vs jugular venous catheterization and risk of nosocomial events in adults requiring acute renal replacement therapy: a randomized controlled trial. *JAMA* 2008;299(20):2413–2422.

25. Ragaller MJ, Theilen H, Koch T. Volume replacement in critically ill patients with acute renal failure. *J Am Soc Nephrol* 2001;12(Suppl 17):S33–39.

26. Ratanarat R, Permpikul C, Ronco C. Renal replacement therapy in acute renal failure: which index is best for dialysis dose quantification? *Int J Artif Organs* 2007;30(3):235–243.

27. Riou B, Cittanova ML. An international review of HES. *Intens Care Med* 1999;25(11):1340–1341.

28. Ronco C. Continuous dialysis is superior to intermittent dialysis in acute kidney injury of the critically ill patient. *Nat Clin Pract Nephrol* 2007;3(3):118–119.

29. Ronco C, Bellomo R, Homel P, et al. Effects of different doses in continuous veno-venous haemofiltration on outcomes of acute renal failure: A prospective randomised trial. *Lancet* 2000;356(9223):26–30.

30. Saudan P, Niederberger M, De Seigneux S, et al. Adding a dialysis dose to continuous hemofiltration increases survival in patients with acute renal failure. *Kidney Int* 2006;70(7):1312–1317.

31. Schetz M. Vasopressors and the kidney. *Blood Purif* 2002;20(3):243–251.

32. Schrier RW. Early intervention in acute kidney injury. *Nat Rev Nephrol* 2010;6(1):56–59.

33. Seabra VF, Balk EM, Liangos O, et al. Timing of renal replacement therapy initiation in acute renal failure: a meta-analysis. *Am J Kidney Dis* 2008;52(2):272–284.

34. Sturiale A, Campo S, Crasci E, et al. Experimental models of acute renal failure and erythropoietin: what evidence of a direct effect? *Ren Fail* 2007;29(3):379–386.

35. Tolwani AJ, Wille KM. Anticoagulation for continuous renal replacement therapy. *Semin Dial* 2009;22(2):141–145.

36. van den Berghe G, Wouters P, Weekers F, et al. Intensive insulin therapy in the critically ill patients. *N Engl J Med* 2001;345(19):1359–1367.

CHAPTER 8

HEPATORENAL SYNDROME

Cynthia Tsien, MD, and Florence Wong, MBBS, MD

1. **What is hepatorenal syndrome?**

   The International Ascites Club defines hepatorenal syndrome (HRS) as "a potentially reversible syndrome that occurs in patients with cirrhosis, ascites and liver failure, consisting of impaired renal function, marked abnormalities in cardiovascular function, and intense over-activity of the endogenous vasoactive systems."

   It is important to emphasize that HRS is a form of functional renal failure; kidney biopsy reveals normal histology.

   Salerno F, Gerbes A, Gines P, et al. Diagnosis, prevention and treatment of hepatorenal syndrome in cirrhosis. *Gut* 2007;56:1310–1318.

2. **What is the incidence of HRS?**

   The annual incidence of HRS in patients with cirrhosis and ascites is 8%. The probability of developing HRS is 18% in 1 year and 39% at 5 years.

   Gines A, Escorsell A, Gines P, et al. Incidence, predictive factors, and prognosis of the hepatorenal syndrome in cirrhosis with ascites. *Gastroenterology* 1993;105:229–236.

3. **What is the pathophysiology of HRS?**

   - **Reduction in the effective arterial blood volume:** Hemodynamic changes occur in advanced cirrhosis that result in significant arterial vasodilatation. The vasodilatation occurs preferentially in the splanchnic circulation with consequent pooling of blood in the splanchnic vascular bed. This splanchnic steal syndrome results in relatively insufficient blood volume in many other vascular compartments, including the systemic circulation, known as a reduction in the effective arterial blood volume.
   - **Excess renal vasoconstriction:** The reduction in the effective arterial blood volume causes activation of various compensatory vasoconstrictor systems, including the renin-angiotensin-aldosterone system (RAAS), the sympathetic nervous system, and the nonosmotic release of vasopressin. The renal circulation is particularly sensitive to vasoconstrictors, resulting in a decrease in renal blood flow with consequent reduction in glomerular filtration rate (GFR).
   - **Abnormal renal autoregulation in advanced cirrhosis:** Renal autoregulation is the process whereby regulatory mechanisms ensure that the kidneys receive an approximately constant blood supply regardless of the day-to-day fluctuations in blood pressure. In cirrhosis, the autoregulation curve is shifted to the right (Fig. 8-1). That is, for any given renal perfusion pressure, there is less renal blood flow than in a healthy individual, so the patient with advanced cirrhosis is more vulnerable to developing renal failure. This is thought to be related to the excess sympathetic drive seen in cirrhosis.
   - **Portal hypertension:** Increased portal pressure is associated with reduced renal blood flow, mediated via increased sympathetic nervous activity to the renal vessels. This is known as the hepatorenal reflex. Therefore, insertion of a transjugular intrahepatic portosystemic shunt (TIPS), which eliminates portal hypertension, is able to improve renal blood flow.

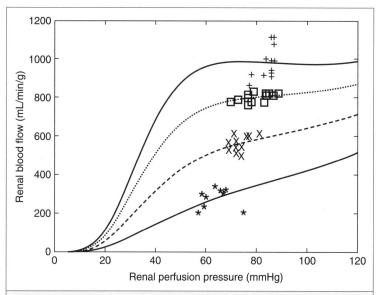

Figure 8-1. Autoregulation curve in cirrhosis. +, pre-ascites; □, diuretic sensitive ascites; X, diuretic resistant ascites; *, hepatorenal syndrome. (From Stadlbauer VP, Wright GA, Banaji M, et al. Relationship between activation of the sympathetic nervous system and renal blood flow autoregulation in cirrhosis. *Gastroenterology* 2008;134:111–119.)

- **Abnormal cardiac function in cirrhosis:** The presence of systemic arterial vasodilatation in advanced cirrhosis leads to a hyperdynamic circulation with tachycardia, high cardiac output, and low systemic vascular resistance. In addition, there is a newly recognized condition known as cirrhotic cardiomyopathy, consisting of myocardial thickening, diastolic dysfunction at rest, and systolic dysfunction under conditions of stress. Because of these factors, the heart is unable to further increase its cardiac output in periods of stress (e.g., sepsis), resulting in further compromise of the renal circulation and a predisposition to the development of HRS.

Arroyo V, Terra C, Gines P. Advances in the pathogenesis and treatment of type-1 and type-2 hepatorenal syndrome. *J Hepatol* 2007;46:935–946.

Ruiz del Arbol L, Urman J, Fernandez J, et al. Systemic, renal, and hepatic hemodynamic derangement in cirrhotic patients with spontaneous bacterial peritonitis. *Hepatology* 2003;38:1210–1218.

Stadlbauer VP, Wright GA, Banaji M, et al. Relationship between activation of the sympathetic nervous system and renal blood flow autoregulation in cirrhosis. *Gastroenterology* 2008;134:111–119.

Wong F. Hepatorenal syndrome. In: Lerma EV, Nissenson AR, Berns JS (eds.). *Current Diagnosis and Treatment in Nephrology and Hypertension.* New York: McGraw Hill, 2009.

Wong F, Pantea L, Sniderman K. The use of midodrine, octreotide and transjugular intrahepatic portosystemic stent shunt in the treatment of cirrhotic patients with ascites and renal dysfunction including hepatorenal syndrome. *Hepatology* 2004;40:55–64.

4. **What is the clinical presentation of HRS?**
   HRS is a form of renal failure, so patients present with increased serum creatinine, reduced creatinine clearance, and low urine output—not unlike the clinical picture of renal failure in patients who are noncirrhotic. Clinically, there are two types of HRS.

   Type 1 HRS is characterized by a rapidly progressive renal failure, defined as doubling of the initial serum creatinine to a level >2.5 mg/dL in less than 2 weeks. It usually develops following a precipitating event but can occur spontaneously. Patients are usually very ill, with severe jaundice, coagulopathy, and liver failure.

Type 2 HRS is characterized by moderate renal failure, with a serum creatinine between 1.5 and 2.5 mg/dL. It usually evolves slowly over weeks to months, typically in patients with ascites refractory to diuretic therapy. Type 2 HRS is felt to be an extension of refractory ascites when hemodynamic changes worsen over time. Patients with type 2 HRS are usually less ill than those with type 1 HRS, with a milder degree of jaundice and coagulopathy.

5. **What factors can precipitate the development of HRS?**
Any condition that causes a further reduction of the effective arterial blood volume can potentially precipitate type 1 HRS.

Therefore, conditions that reduce arterial blood volume such as overdiuresis, large-volume paracentesis ($\geq$5 liters) without intravascular volume replacement in patients with refractory ascites, and gastrointestinal bleeding are well-known precipitants of type 1 HRS.

Other triggers are conditions that worsen the arterial vasodilatation, such as sepsis with any infection (but especially spontaneous bacterial peritonitis) or surgical jaundice (bile acids are vasodilators).

Fasolato S, Angeli P, Dallagnese L, et al. Renal failure and bacterial infections in patients with cirrhosis: Epidemiology and clinical features. *Hepatology* 2007;45:223–229.

6. **How do you diagnose HRS?**
HRS is a diagnosis of exclusion. The following are the acceptable diagnostic criteria for HRS:
- Cirrhosis and ascites
- Serum creatinine >1.5 mg/dL
- No improvement of serum creatinine after at least 48 hours of diuretic withdrawal and volume expansion with albumin (1 g/kg body weight/day) up to 100 g maximum
- Absence of shock
- No current or recent treatment with nephrotoxic drugs
- Absence of parenchymal kidney disease as indicated by proteinuria >500 mg/day, microhematuria (>50 red blood cells/high power field), and/or abnormal renal ultrasonography

Urinary electrolyte criteria are not required for the diagnosis of HRS. The presence of infection does not preclude the diagnosis of HRS.

7. **What diagnostic workup should be performed in the patient with cirrhosis and acute renal failure?**
A trial of diuretic withdrawal, together with intravascular volume replacement, can replenish the effective arterial blood volume. The intravascular volume replacement can be blood if the patient is anemic or albumin at the dose of 1 g/kg of body weight up to a maximum of 100 gm per day.

The workup should consist of a full septic workup, including blood cultures, chest x-ray, urine and sputum cultures, a diagnostic paracentesis to exclude spontaneous bacterial peritonitis, and swabbing any possible skin sources of infection. Treat all proven sources of infection. A urinalysis to assess for casts, proteinuria, and hematuria should be done to exclude organic renal disease. An abdominal ultrasound should be performed to exclude small kidneys or structural abnormalities in the kidneys.

8. **What is the differential diagnosis of acute renal failure in the patient with cirrhosis?**
Similar to the patient without cirrhosis, there are three major categories of acute renal failure, also known as acute kidney injury (AKI).

Prerenal azotemia occurs secondary to renal hypoperfusion, with no evidence of glomerular or tubular lesions. Common causes are overdiuresis, large-volume paracentesis without intravascular volume replacement, or gastrointestinal bleeding. HRS can be considered a form of prerenal azotemia, which is not volume responsive.

Intrinsic renal failure is a result of structural damage to the kidney; examples include acute tubular necrosis and glomerulonephritis.

Finally, postrenal failure results from obstruction to the passage of urine, as seen in a bladder neck obstruction.

In hospitalized patients with cirrhosis, prerenal azotemia is the most common cause of acute renal failure, accounting for 70% of all cases, followed by acute tubular necrosis (30%), hepatorenal syndrome (17%), and postrenal failure (<1%).

Moreau R, Durand F, Poynard T, et al. Terlipressin in patients with cirrhosis and type 1 hepatorenal syndrome: A retrospective multicenter study. *Gastroenterology* 2002;122:923–930.

Peron JM, Bureau C, Gonzalez L, et al. Treatment of hepatorenal syndrome as defined by the international ascites club by albumin and furosemide infusion according to the central venous pressure: A prospective pilot study. *Am J Gastroenterol* 2005;100:2702–2707.

9. **Can biomarkers assist in the diagnosis of HRS?**
   Current guidelines for the diagnosis of HRS use elevated levels of serum creatinine to diagnose renal impairment; however, the use of serum creatinine is suboptimal for several reasons. Its levels vary widely with age, sex, and muscle mass, which is diminished in patients with cirrhosis. The presence of jaundice can interfere with its measurement. Therefore, serum creatinine can still be within the normal limits even when the GFR is significantly reduced. Furthermore, changes in serum creatinine can lag several days behind acute changes in GFR, until new steady-state equilibrium is reached.

   Therefore, several biomarkers have been proposed as diagnostic tools for acute kidney injury. These include liver fatty acid binding protein (L-FABP) and neutrophil gelatinase-associated lipocalin (NGAL), which are proteins expressed in the renal tubule epithelium. Elevated levels of urinary L-FABP and NGAL have been shown to correlate well with established cases of AKI. However, levels do not differ among the different etiologies of AKI, and they have not been confirmed in cirrhosis as accurate markers of HRS. A recent systematic review and meta-analysis found NGAL levels to be a predictor of the early development of AKI and correlating with clinical outcomes, such as the need for dialysis and mortality. Thus, the future role of these biomarkers in patients with cirrhosis may be in the early diagnosis of AKI, rather than the specific diagnosis of HRS, although this has yet to be demonstrated.

Devarajan P. Neutrophil gelatinase-associated lipocalin (NGAL): A new marker of kidney disease. *Scand J Clin Lab Invest Suppl* 2008;241:89–94.

Ferguson M, Vaidya V, Waikar S, et al. Urinary liver-type fatty acid-binding protein predicts adverse outcomes in acute kidney injury. *Kidney Int* 2010;77:708–714.

Haase M, Bellomo R, Devarajan P, et al. Accuracy of neutrophil gelatinase-associated lipocalin (NGAL) in diagnosis and prognosis in acute kidney injury: A systematic review and meta-analysis. *Am J Kidney Dis* 2009;54:1012–1024.

Silkensen JR, Kasiske BL. Laboratory assessment of renal disease: Clearance, urinalysis, and renal biopsy. In: Brenner BM (ed.). *Brenner and Rector's The Kidney,* 7th ed. Philadelphia: Saunders, 2004, pp. 1107–1150.

10. **What is the rationale for the various treatment options for HRS?**
    The recent development of various treatments for HRS (mostly for type 1 HRS) is based on correcting the different aspects of pathophysiology of HRS.
    1. Improving the effective arterial blood volume: Volume expanders
    2. Reducing the extent of splanchnic and/or systemic arterial vasodilatation: Vasoconstrictors
    3. Eliminating portal hypertension: TIPS shunt
    4. Removal of toxins, some of which are vasodilators: MARS
    5. Correcting liver dysfunction and eliminating portal hypertension: Liver transplantation

11. **What are some general treatment measures for type 1 HRS?**
    - Treat any source of infection.
    - Discontinue any nephrotoxic medications, including diuretics and nonsteroidal anti-inflammatories.
    - Discontinue antihypertensive agents such as angiotensin-converting enzyme (ACE) inhibitors and angiotensin II antagonists. In patients with decompensated cirrhosis, the

RAAS is vital to the maintenance of arterial pressure and GFR in the face of marked peripheral vasodilatation. Inhibition of the RAAS may precipitate hypotension and a deterioration of renal function.

- Assess effective circulating volume. While excess total body water is present, it usually extravasates intra-abdominally or in peripheral tissue, and patients are still intravascularly deplete.

12. **How is volume expansion used in the treatment of type 1 HRS?**
Albumin not only improves the effective arterial blood volume, but it may also reduce systemic arterial vasodilatation by binding systemic vasodilators. The recommended dose is 20 to 40 g of albumin per day in combination with vasoconstrictors (see later), after the initial dose of 1 g/kg of body weight on the first day. Albumin alone appears to be ineffective in the treatment of HRS.

The peritoneovenous (PV) shunt drains ascitic fluid into the internal jugular vein, thus achieving sustained central volume expansion. It has failed to demonstrate any survival advantage in HRS and is therefore no longer used because of significant complications, such as coagulopathy, postoperative sepsis, and shunt occlusion. Furthermore, PV shunts are no longer in production; thus many surgeons lack the technical expertise to insert a PV shunt.

Linas SL, Schaefer JW, Moore EE, et al. Peritoneovenous shunt in the management of hepatorenal syndrome. *Kidney Int* 1986;30:736–740.

Martin-Llahi M, Pepin MN, Guevara M, et al. Randomized comparative study of terlipressin and albumin vs albumin alone in patients with cirrhosis and hepatorenal syndrome. [Abstract] *J Hepatol* 2007;46:S36.

Moskovitz M. The peritoneovenous shunt: Expectations and reality. *Am J Gastroenterol* 1990;85:917–929.

Wong F. The role of albumin in the management of chronic liver disease. *Nat Clin Pract Gastroenterol Hepatol* 2007;4:43–51.

13. **How are renal vasodilators used in the treatment of type 1 HRS?**
There is no proven efficacy for renal vasodilators such as low-dose dopamine, prostaglandin E1 analogues such as misoprostol, or endothelin receptor antagonists.

Angeli P, Volpin R, Gerunda G, et al. Reversal of type 1 hepatorenal syndrome with the administration of midodrine and octreotide. *Hepatology* 1999;29:1690–1697.

Gines A, Salmeron JM, Gines P, et al. Oral misoprostol or intravenous prostaglandin E2 do not improve renal function in patients with cirrhosis and ascites with hyponatremia or renal failure. *J Hepatol* 1993;17:220–226.

Wong F, Moore K, Dingemanse J, Jalan R. Lack of renal improvement with non-selective endothelin antagonism with tezosentan in type 2 hepatorenal syndrome. *Hepatology* 2008;47:160–168.

14. **How are systemic vasoconstrictors used in the treatment of type 1 HRS?**
See Table 8-1. By reducing the extent of systemic vasodilatation, these medications lead to a rise in the systemic arterial blood pressure, which in turn improves the renal perfusion pressure. In addition, the resultant improvement in the effective arterial blood volume will reduce vasoconstrictor levels, leading to reduced renal vasoconstriction, with overall improvement in glomerular filtration.

Isolated case reports have suggested the use of *N*-acetylcysteine (NAC) in combination with systemic vasoconstrictors or endothelin-receptor antagonists. This is based on a small case study of 12 patients with HRS who showed an improvement in serum creatinine after intravenous infusion of NAC, but it is not standard clinical practice at this time.

Holt S, Goodier D, Marley R, et al. Improvement in renal function in hepatorenal syndrome with *N*-acetylcysteine. *Lancet* 1999;353:294–295.

Izzedine H, Kheder-Elfekih R, Deray G. Endothelin-receptor antagonist/N-acetylcysteine combination in type 1 hepatorenal syndrome. *J Hepatol* 2009;50:1055–1056.

Sen S, Mookerjee RP, Jalan R. Terlipressin-induced vasoconstriction reversed with *N*-acetylcysteine: A case for combined use in hepatorenal syndrome? *Gastroenterology* 2002;123:2160–2161.

TABLE 8-1.   PHARMACOLOGIC TREATMENT OF HRS

Medication	Mechanism	Dosage	Comments
Midodrine	Alpha agonist ↑ blood pressure ↑ renal perfusion pressure	Start with 5 mg tid and titrate to maintain a mean arterial pressure >70 mm Hg	Used in combination with octreotide
Octreotide	Long-acting analogue of somatostatin ↓ splanchnic vasodilatation	Continuous intravenous infusion of 25 μg stat followed by 25 μg/hour; or 100 μg tid subcutaneously	Used in combination with midodrine
Vasopressin	V1 receptor agonist Vasoconstriction of systemic and splanchnic circulations		Not commonly used because of ischemic side effects
Terlipressin	Vasopressin analogue	0.5–2 mg q4-6h IV	Less ischemic side effects Improves, but does not normalize, renal function
Norepinephrine	Alpha, beta-adrenergic agonist Systemic vasoconstriction	0.5–3 mg/hr	Pilot study Reversal of HRS No significant ischemic side effects

15. **How is transjugular intrahepatic portosystemic stent shunt used in the treatment of type 1 HRS?**
TIPS is a prosthesis that bridges a branch of the portal vein with a branch of the hepatic vein. It is effective in reducing portal pressure. In addition, it returns a significant part of the splanchnic vascular volume into the systemic circulation, decreasing the activity of various vasoconstrictor systems.

To date, there are no controlled studies assessing the efficacy of TIPS for the management of HRS. An improvement in renal function has been observed, but this improvement falls short of normalization of the GFR. However, in one study where vasoconstrictor therapy was followed by TIPS insertion, TIPS was able to normalize renal function over the course of 12 months. The overall survival rate was 50%.

Guevara M, Gines P, Bandi JC, et al. Transjugular intrahepatic portosystemic shunt in hepatorenal syndrome: Effects on renal function and vasoactive systems. *Hepatology* 1998;28:416–422.

Wong F, Pantea L, Sniderman K. The use of midodrine, octreotide and transjugular intrahepatic portosystemic stent shunt in the treatment of cirrhotic patients with ascites and renal dysfunction including hepatorenal syndrome. *Hepatology* 2004;40:55–64.

16. **How is extracorporeal albumin dialysis used in the treatment of type 1 HRS?**
Albumin dialysis removes albumin-bound substances, such as cytokines and bile acids, which are also systemic vasodilators. Albumin dialysis can filter out creatinine and artificially reduces the serum creatinine without changing the GFR. Clinicians can be lured into a false sense of improvement when there is no recovery of renal function. There are not enough data to accept it as standard of care.

17. **How is liver transplantation used in the treatment of type 1 HRS?**
Transplantation corrects liver dysfunction and eliminates portal hypertension. Renal function improves in many patients after transplantation, but up to 40% of patients can remain dependent on dialysis.
    Liver transplantation is the treatment of choice for type-1 and type-2 HRS. Reversal of HRS by pharmacologic treatment (e.g., midodrine and octreotide, terlipressin) or TIPS increases survival and the probability of receiving definitive treatment (i.e., liver transplantation).

    Marik PE, Wood K, Starzl TE. The course of type 1 hepato-renal syndrome post liver transplantation. *Nephrol Dial Transplant* 2006;21:478–482.

KEY POINTS: HEPATORENAL SYNDROME

1. Sepsis (especially spontaneous bacterial peritonitis), overdiuresis, large-volume paracentesis (≥5 liters) without intravascular volume replacement in patients with refractory ascites, and gastrointestinal bleeding are well-known precipitants of type 1 HRS.

2. In hospitalized patients with cirrhosis, prerenal azotemia is the most common cause of acute renal failure, followed by acute tubular necrosis, hepatorenal syndrome, and postrenal failure.

3. Liver transplantation is the treatment of choice for type 1 and type 2 HRS.

4. Pharmacologic treatment (e.g., midodrine and octreotide, terlipressin) or TIPS increase survival in order to increase the probability of receiving definitive treatment (i.e., liver transplantation).

18. **Should dialysis be used for the treatment of HRS?**
Intermittent hemodialysis has been used as a short-term bridge to liver transplantation. However, there is no evidence that it increases long-term survival without transplantation.

    Witzke O, Baumann M, Patschan D, et al. Which patients benefit from hemodialysis therapy in hepatorenal syndrome? *J Gastroenterol Hepatol* 2004;19(12):1369–1373.

19. **What is the prognosis of HRS?**
If left untreated, the median survival of type 1 hepatorenal syndrome is 2 weeks, whereas that of type 2 HRS is 50% at 6 months.

    Alessandria C, Ozdogan O, Guevara M, et al. MELD score and clinical type predict prognosis in hepatorenal syndrome: Relevance to liver transplantation. *Hepatology* 2005;41:1282–1289.

20. **Are there any scenarios in which HRS can be prevented?**
    - **Alcoholic hepatitis:** Pentoxifylline is a nonselective phosphodiesterase inhibitor. In one study, its use was associated with a 40% reduction in mortality, thought to be secondary to a 65% reduction in the occurrence of HRS. Patients in this study were quite ill, with jaundice and a Maddrey discriminant factor ≥32.
    - **Spontaneous bacterial peritonitis (SBP):** One third of patients with SBP will develop renal impairment despite appropriate antibiotic therapy. Patients who receive albumin in addition to antibiotics have been shown to have a lower incidence of renal impairment and death compared to those treated with antibiotics alone. Patients in this study

received intravenous albumin at a dose of 1.5 g/kg body weight on day 1, then 1 g/kg body weight on day 3.

- Although antibiotics alone have not been shown to directly reduce the incidence of HRS, primary prophylaxis of SBP with norfloxacin reduces the incidence of SBP, which is itself a risk factor for HRS.
- **Large-volume paracentesis:** Removal of large (≥ 5 liters) amounts of ascites may precipitate postparacentesis circulatory dysfunction, which can induce renal failure in up to 20% of patients. Giving albumin at a dose of 8 g/L of ascitic fluid removed has been shown to reduce the incidence of renal failure but not mortality.

Akriviadis E, Botla R, Briggs W, et al. Pentoxifylline improves short-term survival in severe acute alcoholic hepatitis: A double-blind, placebo-controlled trial. *Gastroenterology* 2000;119:1637–1648.

Fernandez J, Navasa M, Planas R, et al. Primary prophylaxis of spontaneous bacterial peritonitis delays hepatorenal syndrome and improves survival in cirrhosis. *Gastroenterology* 2007;133:818–824.

Follo A, Llovet JM, Navasa M, et al. Renal impairment after spontaneous bacterial peritonitis in cirrhosis: Incidence, clinical course, predictive factors and prognosis. *Hepatology* 1994;20:1495–1501.

Gines P, Tito L, Arroyo V, et al. Randomized comparative study of therapeutic paracentesis with and without intravenous albumin in cirrhosis. *Gastroenterology* 1988;94:1493–1502.

Sort P, Navasa M, Arroyo V et al. Effect of intravenous albumin on renal impairment and mortality in patients with cirrhosis and spontaneous bacterial peritonitis. *N Engl J Med* 1999;341:403–409.

CHAPTER 9

CARDIORENAL SYNDROME

Claudio Ronco, MD, and Edgar V. Lerma, MD

1. **What is cardiorenal syndrome?**

   Cardiorenal syndrome (CRS) is referred to as a group of "disorders of the heart and kidneys, whereby acute or chronic dysfunction in one organ may induce acute or chronic dysfunction in the other."

   As of now, this disease entity has been receiving much attention because of the multitude of recent publications of so-called epidemiologic observational studies highlighting this rather complex interrelationship between increased cardiovascular morbidity and mortality associated with progressive kidney dysfunction and congestive heart failure (CHF).

   Although the exact pathophysiologic mechanisms have yet to be defined, it can be surmised that the chronology of events begin and end with dysfunction of either the heart or kidney (Table 9-1 and Fig. 9-1). Five subtypes were identified and defined as follows:

   - **Type 1 CRS** reflects an abrupt worsening of cardiac function (e.g., acute cardiogenic shock or decompensated CHF) leading to acute kidney injury (AKI).
   - **Type 2 CRS** describes chronic abnormalities in cardiac function (e.g., chronic CHF) causing progressive and permanent chronic kidney disease (CKD).
   - **Type 3 CRS** consists of an abrupt worsening of kidney function (e.g., acute kidney ischemia or glomerulonephritis) causing acute cardiac disorder (e.g., heart failure, arrhythmia, ischemia).
   - **Type 4 CRS** describes a state of chronic kidney disease (e.g., chronic glomerular disease) contributing to decreased cardiac function, cardiac hypertrophy, and/or increased risk of adverse cardiovascular events.
   - **Type 5 CRS** reflects a systemic condition (e.g., diabetes mellitus, sepsis) causing both cardiac and kidney dysfunction.

2. **Discuss the epidemiology of the various types of CRS.**

   In patients with heart failure, evidence of kidney dysfunction (i.e., elevated serum creatinine) is considered to be one of the "independent" risk factors for all-cause mortality and poor outcome, directly correlating with increased hospitalization rates and duration of stay and death. When compared to the left ventricular ejection fraction (LVEF) and NYHA Functional class, the baseline kidney function (GFR, or glomerular filtration rate), appears to be an even stronger predictor of mortality in such patients.

   Thirty percent of patients admitted for acute decompensated heart failure (ADHF) who were included in the Acute Decompensated Heart Failure National Registry (ADHERE) had significant kidney dysfunction, with 21% having serum creatinine of at least 2 mg/dL and 9% having serum creatinine of at least 3 mg/dL.

   - **Acute cardiorenal syndrome (type 1):** In the United States, more than 1 million hospital admissions every year result from acute heart failure (AHF) or acute decompensated chronic heart failure (ADHF), and these patients are predisposed to developing AKI. Patients with impaired LVEF seem to be more prone to severe AKI compared to those with preserved LVEF, and the severity of left ventricular dysfunction correlates with the severity of AKI. In cardiogenic shock, more than 70% of patients can develop AKI. Furthermore, renal dysfunction in turn worsens the AHF and is associated with higher mortality.

Syndromes	Acute Cardiorenal (Type 1)	Chronic Cardiorenal (Type 2)	Acute Renocardiac (Type 3)	Chronic Reno-Cardiac (Type 4)	Secondary CRS (Type 5)
Organ failure sequence					
Definition	Acute worsening of heart function leading to kidney injury and/or dysfunction	Chronic abnormalities in heart function leading to kidney disease or dysfunction	Acute worsening of kidney function leading to heart injury and/or dysfunction	Chronic kidney disease leading to heart injury, disease, and/or dysfunction	Systemic conditions leading to simultaneous injury and/or dysfunction of heart and kidney
Primary events	Acute decompensated heart failure (ADHF) Acute coronary syndrome (ACS) Cardiogenic shock	Chronic heart disease (LV remodeling and dysfunction, diastolic dysfunction, chronic abnormalities in cardiac function, cardiomyopathy)	Acute kidney injury (AKI)	Chronic kidney disease (CKD)	Systemic disease (sepsis, amyloidosis, etc.)
Criteria for primary events	ESC, AHA/ACC	ESC, AHA/ACC	RIFLE - AKIN	KDOQI	Disease-specific criteria
Secondary events	Acute kidney injury (AKI)	Chronic kidney disease	ADHF, ACS, arrythmias, shock	Chronic heart disease (LV remodeling and dysfunction, diastolic dysfunction, abnormalities in cardiac function), ADHF, ACS	ADHF, ACS, AKI, CHD, CKD
Criteria for secondary events	RIFLE - AKIN	KDOQI	ESC, AHA/ACC	ESC, AHA/ACC	ESC, AHA/ACC, RIFLE / AKIN, ESC, AHA/ACC, KDOQI
Cardiac biomarkers	Troponin, BNP, MPO	BNP, CRP	BNP, CRP	CRP	CRP, procalcitonin
Renal biomarkers	Serum cystatine, creatinine, NGAL, urinary KIM-1, IL-18, NGAL, NAG	Creatinine, cystatic C, urea, uric acid, CRP Decreased GFR	Serum cystatine, creatinine, NGAL, urinary KIM-1, IL-18, NGAL, NAG	Creatinine, cystatic C, urea, uric acid CRP, decreased GFR	Creatinine, NGAL, IL-18, KIM-1, NAG
Prevention strategies	Key issue: ADHF and ACS are most common scenarios What is the inciting event? Is the inciting event common to cardiac and renal decompensation? What is the role of iodinated contrast and cardiac surgery associated AKI in the pathogenesis? If understood, if inciting event is attenuated/eliminated, can CR syndrome avoided?	Key issue: common pathophysiology (neurohumeral, inflammatory, oxidative injury) Will reduction of the decline in cardiac function impact the incidence or progression of CKD be lessened? What is the impact of subclinical acute (ischemia) on chronic disease worsen both systems? If a common pathophysiologic mechanism is attenuated, can both organ systems benefit?	Key issue: Na and volume overload If Na and volume overload is avoided, will cardiac decompensation be eliminated? If early bidirectional signaling can be understood, can new preventive targets be developed?	Key issues: cardiac and renal fibrosis, LVH, vascular stiffness, chronic Na and volume overload Will reduction of the decline in renal function, impact the incidence or progression of CVD be lessened? What is the role of chronic uremia, anemia, and changes in Ca, P, bone, and PTH on the cardiovascular system?	Key issue: potential systemic factors that negatively impact function of both organs Will reduction/elimination of key factor(s) (immune, inflammatory, oxidative stress, thrombosis) prevent both cardiac and renal decline? Can both organ systems be protected in the setting of a simultaneous insult?
Management strategies	Specific—depends on precipitating factors General supportive—oxygenate, relieve pain and pulmonary congestion, treat arrhythmias appropriately, differentiate left from right heart failure, treat low cardiac output or congestion according to ESC guidelines,* avoid nephrotoxins, monitor kidney function	Treat CHF according to ESC guidelines,* exclude precipitating pre-renal AKI factors (hypovolemia and/or hypotension), adjust therapy accordingly and avoid nephrotoxins, whilst monitoring renal function and electrolytes	Follow ESC guidelines for acute CHF.* Specific management may depend on underlying etiology, may need to exclude renovascular disease and consider early renal support, if diuretic resistant	Follow KDOQI guidelines for CKD management, exclude precipitating causes (cardiac tamponade). Treat heart failure according to ESC guidelines,* consider early renal replacement support.	Specific—according to etiology General—see CRS management* * as advised by ESC guidelines 2008

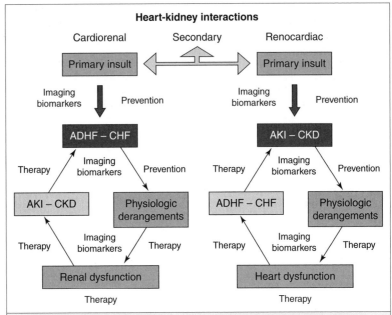

Figure 9-1. In cardiorenal syndromes, there are two important aspects: The first is the sequence of organ involvement and the second is the bidirectionality of signaling leading to a vicious cycle. Another important aspect is the time frame in which the derangements occur (chronic or acute). In all cases, there are moments in which prevention is possible; in others mitigation of the insult is potentially feasible; and in others, therapeutic strategies must be implemented. At different times, a crucial role is played by imaging techniques and biomarkers, enabling the clinician to make an early diagnosis, establish illness severity, and potentially predict outcomes. This flowchart describes a series of conditions indicating that patients may move from one type to another of cardiorenal syndromes. (From Ronco C, McCullough P, Anker SD, et al. Cardio-renal syndromes: Report from the consensus conference of the Acute Dialysis Quality Initiative. *Eur Heart J* 2010;31:703–711, 2010, by permission of the European Society of Cardiology.)

- **Chronic cardiorenal syndrome (type 2):** Patients with chronic heart failure are prone to worsening renal function, which results in prolonged hospitalization and adverse clinical outcomes. About 45% of patients with CHF and impaired LVEF have a decrease in estimated GFR (eGFR). However, even a small decrease of GFR in patients with CHF appear to confer a significantly increased risk of hospitalization and mortality.
- **Acute renocardiac syndrome (type 3):** AKI has been identified in 9% of in-hospital patients and in more than 35% of intensive care unit (ICU) patients who are critically ill. It is difficult to evaluate the epidemiology of type 3 CRS because very few studies have specifically reported the temporal occurrence of acute cardiovascular events following AKI. Incorporation of cardiovascular events as outcomes is needed to better understand and characterize the epidemiology of type 3 CRS and factors associated with those at-risk or those susceptible for acute cardiac dysfunction in AKI.
- **Chronic renocardiac syndrome (type 4):** Patients with CKD, particularly those receiving renal replacement therapies (RRT), are at risk for developing cardiovascular (CV) complications, such as coronary artery disease and hypertension. More than 50% of death in stage 5 CKD cohorts are attributed to CAD and its associated complications. The 2-year mortality rate following myocardial infarction in patients with stage 5 CKD is 50%, but in comparison, the 10-year mortality rate postmyocardial infarction for the general population without CKD is only 25%. Less severe forms of CKD also appear to be associated with

significantly higher CV risk. In patients with stages 3 through 5 CKD, the leading cause of death is CV disease, with >40% of mortality related to a CV event. It is well-established that individuals with CKD have a 10- to 20-fold increased risk for cardiac death compared to age-matched and gender-matched controls without CKD.

- **Secondary cardiorenal syndromes (type 5):** Usually seen in those with multiple organ failure (MOF), one classical example is sepsis. Severe sepsis occurs in about 30% of all patients in ICU, whereas severe AKI occurs in 6% of these patients. AKI has been associated with a more than two-fold increase in the risk of death, as compared to those without AKI. Moreover, for those with AKI requiring some form of RRT, the mortality rate can be as high as 60%.

3. What are some of the novel biomarkers of acute kidney injury?
   - **Neutrophil gelatinase-associated lipocalin (NGAL):** A 25 kDa protein belonging to the lipocalin superfamily, NGAL is one of the earliest kidney markers of ischemic or nephrotoxic injury first described in animal models and is detected in the blood and urine of humans soon after AKI. In a recent study, a single measurement of urinary NGAL was able to differentiate those with subsequent AKI, with a sensitivity and specificity of 90% and 99%, respectively. NGAL could be used as an earlier marker of impending WRF during the treatment of ADHF.
   - **Cystatin C:** This is a cysteine protease inhibitor that appears to be a better predictor (unaffected by age, gender, muscle mass, or race) of glomerular function than serum creatinine in patients with CKD. It is freely filtered by the glomerulus, reabsorbed completely by the proximal convoluted tubule, and not secreted in the urine. In AKI, urinary excretion of cystatin C has been shown to predict the requirement for RRT earlier than creatinine.
   - **Kidney injury molecule-1 (KIM-1):** A transmembrane protein, this protein is detectable in the urine after ischemic or nephrotoxic insults to proximal tubular cells, where it is markedly overexpressed. Urinary KIM-1 seems to be highly specific for ischemic AKI and not for prerenal azotemia, CKD, or contrast-induced nephropathy. In one study, it was demonstrated to be useful in distinguishing ischemic AKI from prerenal AKI and CKD and also a predictor of renal replacement therapy and mortality in AKI.
   - **N-acetyl-β-(D)glucosaminidase:** A lysosomal brush border enzyme found predominantly in proximal tubular cells, N-acetyl-β-(D)glucosaminidase has been shown to function as a marker of kidney injury, reflecting particularly the degree of tubular damage. It is not only found in elevated urinary concentrations in AKI and CKD, but also in patients with diabetes, essential hypertension, and heart failure (HF).
   - **Interleukin-18 (IL-18):** A proinflammatory cytokine detected in the urine after acute ischemic proximal tubular damage, IL-18 displays good sensitivity and specificity for ischemic AKI with an area under the curve >90%, with increased levels 48 hours prior to increases in serum creatinine. Urinary NGAL and IL-18 have been studied as joint biomarkers for delayed graft function following kidney transplantation.

   Of the biomarkers presented, NGAL (urine and plasma) and cystatin C are most likely to be integrated into clinical practice in the near future. Clinical trials will be needed to see if earlier identification of AKI and the use of specific treatment algorithms based on these markers will improve prognosis.

   Other novel biomarkers that are currently under investigation include glutathione-s-transferase (GST), glutamyl transpeptidase (GT), sodium hydrogen exchanger (NHE), liver fatty acid binding protein (L-FABP), aprotinin, IL-6, IL-10, matrix metalloproteinase 9 (MMP-9), alpha 1 microglobulin, and others.

4. What are some of the known biomarkers of cardiorenal syndrome?
   The **natriuretic peptides**, B-type natriuretic peptide (BNP) and its precursor N-terminal-proBNP (NT-proBNP), have been considered not only as tools for the diagnosis of heart failure, but also as "independent" predictors of mortality. However, the relationship among BNP, kidney function, and severity of HF has been less than precise.

In fact, patients with CKD have been demonstrated to have elevated baseline levels of both BNP and NT-proBNP, even in the absence of HF. This has been attributed primarily to significantly decreased renal elimination of the peptides. Another postulated contributory factor is that of increased myocardial stress secondary to hypertension, subclinical ischemia, cardiac hypertrophy, or myocardial fibrosis.

Cardiac **troponins,** namely cTnT (troponin T) and cTnI (troponin I), have been time-honored markers of myocardial necrosis. Similar to the natriuretic peptides, increased levels of troponins in patients with CKD (including those receiving renal replacement therapy or dialysis) have been attributed to reduced renal elimination. It is for this reason that their utility in establishing the diagnosis of acute coronary syndrome (ACS) remains questionable. What is known, however, is that increased levels of troponins correlate positively with mortality in patients with CKD.

Other biomarkers currently under investigation include asymmetric dimethylarginine, plasminogen activator inhibitor type 1, homocysteine, C-reactive protein (CRP), and serum amyloid A protein, all of which correlate with outcome in patients with CKD.

5. **What is bioimpedance vector analysis (BIVA), and what is its significance in CRS?**
   Bioimpedance vector analysis (BIVA) is performed by the placement of bipolar electrodes at the wrist and ankle. Data then are graphically displayed such that volume status can be more accurately quantified. BIVA is able to provide indices of general cellular health, which has known significant prognostic implications, and total body volume.

   Information obtained via BIVA may be used in combination with NGAL and BNP to guide fluid management strategies. In this way, patients will be kept within the narrow window of adequate hydration while preventing worsening of both kidney and heart function.

6. **What imaging studies can be used in CRS?**
   Imaging techniques provide important complementary information with respect to the laboratory biomarkers in CRS.

   In patients known or suspected to have CRS, it is of utmost importance that the use of iodinated contrast media for imaging studies be avoided at all causes unless absolutely necessary. The presence or absence of coronary disease should be established by other means such as stress echo or stress myocardial perfusion (SPECT/PET) in patients with CRS.

   Even the use of magnetic resonance imaging studies are now limited since the realization that gadolinium contrast can potentially cause "nephrogenic systemic fibrosis," especially in those with underlying CKD.

   Future investigations should focus on molecular imaging techniques (MRI and MRS, PET, etc.) and search for in vivo specific markers for diagnosis and severity evaluation of the different types of CRS.

   Less invasive imaging techniques to quantify renal blood flow need to be developed. Similarly, data obtained thereafter can then be viewed as complementary with the known cardiac and renal biomarkers (see earlier) and most importantly guide ongoing therapy designed to optimize renal blood flow and ultimately preserve kidney function.

7. **What is the goal of management strategies for CRS?**
   The primary goal in the treatment of these patients with underlying kidney–heart dysfunction is to decrease CV morbidity and mortality.

8. **What are the current recommended management strategies for atherosclerotic heart disease?**
   - **Control of blood pressure:** The use of renin-angiotensin-aldosterone (RAAS) blockers combined with diuretics to achieve a systolic blood pressure <130 mm Hg is the mainstay of treatment. It must be recognized that with more advanced stages of kidney disease, blood pressure goals may be more difficult to achieve. The use of β-blockers also deserves

mention because of their known cardioprotective benefits (e.g., decreased rates of hospitalization, decreased rates of sudden death, and improvement in LV function).

- **Reduction of proteinuria:** This can also be achieved by RAAS blockade therapy, discussed earlier. Dual combination therapy (ACE-I + ARB, ARB + spironolactone, ARB + eplerenone, etc.) has been increasingly used for this purpose. The JNC VII recommends a target blood pressure <125/75 for patients with proteinuria >1 g/day. One has to be cautious of the risk of "hyperkalemia" with such combination RAAS blockade therapies, especially on top of underlying CKD.
- **Control of dyslipidemias:** The most common pattern of dyslipidemia seen in patients with CKD includes decreased HDL-C, increased triglyceride (TG), and increased LDL-C. Current goals of therapy are as follows: total cholesterol <200 mg/dL, LDL-C <100 mg/dL, and HDL-C >40 mg/dL. Treatment regimens consist of lifestyle modification combined with the use of nicotinic acid and fibrates. This is the primary regimen because it addresses the typical features of increased TG and low HDL-C. For elevated LDL-C, statins are the agents of choice. The combination of such medications has been demonstrated to cause nontraumatic rhabdomyolysis/myoglobinuric kidney failure, with those with underlying CKD at highest risk.
- **Antiplatelet therapy:** Aspirin 81 mg/day or clopidogrel 75 mg/day, are the platelet inhibitors of choice.
- **Control of the vitamin D-calcium-phosphorus metabolism:** Active vitamin D drugs are recommended if vitamin D levels are <30 mg/mL.

9. **What are the current recommended management strategies for cardiomyopathy?**
   - **Diuretics:** These are the mainstays of therapy for fluid overload in patients with ADHF. Whereas thiazide diuretics are the initially preferred agents of this class, they are only efficacious with GFR >30 mL/min/1.73 m^2. Below that, loop diuretics are the preferred agents. Combination diuretics have been used to achieve more effective diuresis in those who may have some degree of "diuretic resistance." At times, a continuous infusion of a long-acting loop diuretic (e.g., furosemide, bumetanide) may be necessary. Some recommend the addition of salt-poor albumin to the IV infusion. Caution should be exercised to avoid hypokalemia and its attendant complications (e.g., cardiac arrhythmias, ileus, hypotension).
   - **Vasodilators:** The use of nitrates has been advocated to immediately reduce central venous and ventricular filling pressures (pulmonary congestion), leading to decreased myocardial oxygen consumption, and systemic vascular resistance, leading to improved cardiac output. Of interest, nesiritide is another known vasodilator with additional diuretic properties, albeit mild. When given in low doses (i.e., 0.0025–0.005 µg/kg/mL), it can be particularly useful in those with underlying hypotension. It is hoped that the Acute Study of Clinical Effectiveness of Nesiritide in Decompensated Heart Failure (ASCEND-HF) trial will provide information regarding outcomes, with the use of nesiritide in the setting of CRS.
   - **Continuous renal replacement therapy (CRRT):** Continuous renal replacement therapy is a novel alternative to pharmacologic diuresis in patients with CRS. When compared with diuretics, CRRT led to a significantly greater fluid and weight reduction, as demonstrated in the Ultrafiltration Versus Intravenous Diuretics for Patients Hospitalized for Acute Decompensated Heart Failure (UNLOAD) study. Although there was also a significant decrease in the rates of hospitalization and rehospitalization (with CRRT), the benefit on morbidity and mortality (in terms of kidney function and clinical outcomes) remain elusive to this date.
   - **Inotropes:** The use of dopamine and milrinone has not been shown to improve survival in these patients.
   - **Vasopressin (ADH, or antidiuretic hormone) antagonists:** In patients with HF, vasopressin antagonists have been shown to modify the renal response to water retention, leading to a significant weight loss (increase urine output and serum sodium) within the first 24 hours of administration. There was, however, no significant change in long-term outcomes (e.g., LV remodeling or recovery of kidney function).

- **Adenosine antagonists:** In CKD, there is impaired glomerular filtration; release of adenosine leads to vasoconstriction of afferent arterioles. Adenosine antagonists have been shown to promote an increased renal blood flow and increased excretion of sodium. Combining such agents with loop diuretics has been shown to enhance diuresis while preserving kidney function. However, the Prophylaxis of Thromboembolism in Critical Care Trial (PROTECT) failed to show any benefit of such agents in patients with ADHF.
- **β-blockers:** These are recommended in patients with CKD and HF. They have been demonstrated to slow the progression of LV disease, recurrent myocardial infarction, and sudden cardiac death.
- **Erythropoietin stimulating agents (ESAs):** See Question 10.

KEY POINTS: CARDIORENAL SYNDROME

1. Cardiorenal syndromes are characterized by significant heart–kidney interactions that share similarities in pathophysiology.

2. Patients with impaired left ventricular ejection fraction (LVEF) seem to be more prone to severe acute kidney injury (AKI) compared with those with preserved LVEF, and the severity of left ventricular dysfunction correlates with the severity of AKI.

3. It is well established that individuals with chronic kidney disease (CKD) have a 10- to 20-fold increased risk for cardiac death compared with age-matched and gender-matched controls without CKD.

4. Patients with CKD have higher levels of B-type natriuretic peptide (BNP) and NT-proBNP than age- and gender-matched subjects without reduced renal function, even in the absence of clinical congestive heart failure.

5. The most important preventive approach in patients with *de novo* heart failure call for blood pressure control, use of drugs that block the renin-angiotensin-aldosterone system, beta-adrenergic blockers, coronary artery disease risk factor modification, and compliance with dietary and drug treatments.

10. **What is the relationship between anemia and CRS?**
    Anemia is commonly seen in patients with CHF and has been associated with increased morbidity and mortality, increased hospitalization rates, and progression of renal failure. In the Organized Program To Initiate Lifesaving Treatment in Hospitalized Patients with Heart Failure (OPTIMIZE-HF) registry, 51% of patients with HF had hemoglobin levels <12 g/dL, whereas 25% had levels ranging between 5 and 10.7 g/dL. However, at present, it remains unclear whether anemia plays a causative role in worsening CHF.
    There are two mechanisms by which anemia occurs in CRS:
    1. In patients with CKD, there is decreased production of erythropoietin by the kidneys. CHF is characterized by significantly reduced cardiac output, leading to decreased perfusion of the kidneys, thence hypoxic injury to the tubules.
    2. Excessive cytokine production (e.g., TNF-α, and IL-6) in CHF can cause not only a reduction in erythropoietin production by the kidneys, but also decreased responsiveness of the bone marrow to erythropoietin. In particular, IL-6 causes release of "hepcidin" from the liver. Hepcidin is believed to interfere with the absorption of iron from the gut and also causes a condition called "functional iron deficiency" (i.e., decreased delivery of iron to the bone marrow, even in the presence of normal iron stores) secondary to trapping of iron within macrophages and hepatocytes.

       In the FAIR-HF (Ferric Carboxymaltose in Patients with Heart Failure) study, administration of iron intravenously to patients with CHF resulted in an improvement in NYHA class and in renal function. It has been suggested that on the cellular level, iron may have additional direct positive effects on mitochondrial function (i.e., increased oxygen utilization and adenosine triphosphate production).

A recent review (Ngo et al.) showed that treatment with erythropoietin-stimulating agents (ESA) was associated with decreased rates of hospitalizations secondary to HF, decreased all-cause mortality, decreased BNP, and improved LV ejection fraction.

The only guidelines in existence at the present time pertain to the use of ESAs in patients with CKD, with the goal hemoglobin level between 10 and 12 g/dL. Whether such guidelines will be applicable to patients with CHF will hopefully be answered by the Reduction of Events with Darbepoetin alfa in Heart Failure (RED-HF) study, due by 2011.

BIBLIOGRAPHY

1. Adams KF Jr, Fonarow GC, Emerman CL, et al.; for the ADHERE Scientific Advisory Committee and Investigators. Characteristics and outcomes of patients hospitalized for heart failure in the United States: Rationale, design, and preliminary observations from the first 100,000 cases in the acute decompensated heart failure National registry (ADHERE). *Am Heart J.* 2005;149:209–216.

2. Anker SD, Comin Colet J, Fillipatos G, et al. Ferric carboxymaltose in patients with heart failure and iron deficiency. *New Engl J Med* 2009;361:2436–2448.

3. Delanaye P, Lambermont P, Chapelle JP, et al. Plasmatic cystatin C for the estimation of glomerular filtration rate in intensive care units. *Intens Care Med* 2004;30:980–983.

4. Forman DE, Butler J, Wang Y, et al. Incidence, predictors at admission, and impact of worsening renal function among patients hospitalized with heart failure. *J Am Coll Cardiol* 2004;43:61–67.

5. Gheorghiade M, Konstam MA, Burnett JC Jr, et al. Short-term clinical effects of tolvaptan, an oral vasopressin antagonist, in patients hospitalized for heart failure: The EVEREST Clinical Status Trials. *JAMA* 2007;297:1332–1343.

6. Gottlieb SS, Brater DC. Thomas I, et al. BG9719 (CVT-124), an A1 adenosine receptor antagonist, protects against the decline in renal function observed with diuretic therapy. *Circulation* 2002;105:1348–1353.

7. Han WK, Bailly V, Abichandani R, et al. Kidney injury molecule-1 (KIM-1): A novel biomarker for human renal proximal tubule injury. *Kidney Int* 2002;62:237–244.

8. Hillege HL, Girbes AR, de Kam PJ, et al. Renal function, neurohormonal activation, and survival in patients with chronic heart failure. *Circulation* 2000;102:203–210.

9. Liangos O, Perlanayagam MC, Vaidya VS, et al. Urinary N-acetyl-beta-(D)-glucosaminidase activity and kidney injury molecule-1 level are associated with adverse outcomes in acute renal failure. *J Am Soc Nephrol* 2007;18:904–912.

10. McMurray JJV, Anand IS, Diaz R, et al. Design of the reduction of events with darbepoetin alfa in Heart failure (RED-HF): A Phase III, anemia correction morbidity-mortality trial. *Eur J Heart Failure* 2009;11:795–801.

11. Meyer B, Huelsmann M, Wexberg P, et al. N-terminal pro-B-type natriuretic peptide is an independent predictor of outcome in an unselected cohort of critically ill patients. *Crit Care Med* 2007;35:2268–2273.

12. Ngo K, Kotecha D, Walters JA, et al. Erythropoiesis stimulating agents for anemia in chronic heart failure patients. *Cochrane Database Syst Rev* 2010;20(1):CD 007613.

13. Poniatowski B, Malyszko J, Bachorzewska-Gajewska H, et al. Serum neutrophil gelatinase-associated lipocalin as a marker of renal function in patients with chronic heart failure and coronary artery disease. *Kidney Blood Press Res* 2009;32:77–80.

14. Ronco C, McCullough P, Anker SD, et al. Cardio-renal syndromes: Report from the consensus conference of the Acute Dialysis Quality Initiative. *Eur Heart J* 2010;31(6):703–711.

15. Ronco C, Cruz D. Biomarkers in cardiorenal syndrome (Rassegna). *Ligand Assay* 2009;14(4):340–349.

16. Ronco C, Haapio M, House AA, et al. Cardiorenal syndrome. *J Am Coll Cardiol* 2008;52(19):1527–1539.

17. Villa P, Jimenez M, Soriano MC, et al. Serum cystatin C concentration as a marker of acute renal dysfunction in critically ill patients. *Crit Care* 2005;9:R139–R143.

18. Weatherley BD, Cotter G, Dittrich HC, et al; PROTECT Steering Committee, Investigators, and Coordinators. Design and rationale of the PROTECT study: A placebo-controlled randomized study of the selective A1 adenosine receptor antagonist rolofylline for patients hospitalized with acute decompensated heart failure and volume overload to assess treatment effect on congestion and renal function. *J Card Fail* 2010;16:25–35.

19. Yancy CW, Singh A. Potential applications of outpatient nesiritide infusions in patients with advanced heart failure and concomitant renal insufficiency (from the Follow-Up serial Infusions of Nesiritide [FUSION I] trial). *Am J Cardiol* 2006;98:226–229.

20. Young JB, Abraham WT, Albert NM, et al; for the OPTIMIZE-HF Investigators and Coordinators. Relation of low hemoglobin and anemia to morbidity and mortality in patients hospitalized with heart failure (insight from OPTIMIZE-HF registry). *Am J Cardiol* 2008;101:223–230.

CHAPTER 10

MEDICATIONS

Mark A. Perazella, MD

1. **What are the classic renal syndromes associated with nonsteroidal anti-inflammatory drugs (NSAIDs)?**

The NSAIDs are well described to cause a number of clinical renal syndromes, many of which are related to the decrease in renal prostaglandin (PG) production by these drugs. Others are idiosyncratic. Included are the following: (1) acute kidney injury (AKI), (2) hyponatremia, (3) hyperkalemia/type 4 renal tubular acidosis (RTA), (4) hypertension, (5) edema/congestive heart failure, (6) acute interstitial nephritis, and (7) minimal change/membranous nephropathy and acute papillary necrosis.

2. **Aside from potential gastrointestinal benefits, what renal benefits are associated with the selective cyclo-oxygenase-2 (COX-2) inhibitors?**

The selective COX-2 inhibitors were initially hoped (and in some cases predicted) to provide analgesia with minimal or no nephrotoxicity. However, it became rapidly apparent that these drugs caused the same clinical renal syndromes described with traditional NSAIDs (see Question 1). In some cases, they appeared to be associated with more hypertension and adverse cardiovascular effects. This was particularly true for rofecoxib, which was subsequently voluntarily withdrawn from the market. The latter effects of these drugs were speculated to be a result of inhibition of vasodilatory PGs (vasoconstriction) without inhibiting platelet thromboxanes (intact platelet function). In regard to the safety of other NSAIDs, neither sulindac nor nabumetone are "renal safe" when used at usual analgesic doses. Sulindac was promoted as more renal safe based on its property as a prodrug (sulfoxide), which is converted to active drug (sulfide) by the liver and back to sulfoxide and sulfone in the kidney, where it is excreted. However, like other NSAIDs, it causes renal dysfunction in at-risk patients, probably as a result of the effect of sulfide inhibition of PGs prior to conversion to inactive drug. Nabumetone, which is a slightly more selective COX-2 inhibitor, suffers from the same adverse renal effects of the more selective COX-2 inhibitors. Tramadol, a centrally acting analgesic, is safe in patients with underlying kidney disease but must be dose adjusted for level of kidney function.

3. **What are clinical scenarios where angiotensin-converting enzyme (ACE) inhibitors and angiotensin-receptor blockers (ARBs) are likely to cause acute kidney injury?**

Any clinical circumstance where renal perfusion is impaired will be associated with a decline in glomerular filtration rate (GFR) and AKI by induction of efferent arteriolar vasodilatation through blockade of angiotensin II production or receptor binding. Included are the following: (1) disease states associated with hypotension; (2) decreased true (e.g., diuretics, diarrhea, vomiting) or effective (e.g., congestive heart failure, cirrhosis, nephrotic syndrome) circulating blood volume; (3) critical renal artery stenosis; and (4) treatment with certain medications such as NSAIDs, calcineurin inhibitors, and vasoconstrictors. The typical clinical scenario is that the GFR continues to decline with ACE inhibitor/ARB therapy and does not stabilize until drug withdrawal or correction of the underlying disease process.

4. **What are the major adverse renal effects of the ACE inhibitors and ARBs?**
ACE inhibitors and ARBs are associated with AKI and hyperkalemia/type 4 RTA. These adverse effects result from inhibition of angiotensin II production by ACE inhibitors or competitive antagonism of the angiotensin II receptor by ARBs. This results in loss of angiotensin II-induced efferent arteriolar tone and a drop in glomerular filtration fraction and GFR. Hyperkalemia/type 4 RTA occurs from reduced adrenal aldosterone synthesis from decreased angiotensin II production/receptor binding. Rare cases of acute interstitial nephritis have been described with the ACE inhibitors.

5. **What are risk factors for the development of acute phosphate nephropathy?**
Exposure to a phosphate-containing purgative for colonoscopy has been associated with the development of both acute and chronic kidney disease (CKD). This entity has been called acute phosphate nephropathy (APN). As with other forms of drug-induced kidney disease, not all patients develop the complications with exposure. Review of the published literature suggests that the following factors increase risk for development of APN, especially when more than one factor is present: age >60 years, female gender, GFR <60 mL/min, hypertension, ACE inhibitor/ARB use, and diuretic use. It is notable that two thirds of patients who developed APN had three or more of these risk factors.

6. **What are the histopathologic lesions associated with acute phosphate nephropathy?**
The hallmark of APN is abundant tubular and less prominent interstitial calcium phosphate deposits. With adequate biopsy samples, greater than 30 calcifications are typically encountered and sometimes greater than 100 calcifications may be seen. The calcifications form basophilic rounded concretions, are mainly confined to distal tubules and the collecting duct, and are more prominent in the renal cortex than medulla. The calcifications do not polarize and have a strong histochemical reaction with the von Kossa stain, indicating that they are composed of calcium phosphate. Other findings include acute tubular degenerative changes and interstitial edema with early lesions. However, biopsies performed more than 3 weeks following oral sodium phosphate (OSP) exposure exhibit evidence of chronicity in the form of tubular atrophy and interstitial fibrosis. A pattern of renal injury described as acute and chronic tubulointerstitial nephropathy may be present and is reminiscent of changes seen in patients with nonresolving acute tubular necrosis. Mild to moderate interstitial inflammation is also often seen. Vascular disease is a frequent finding, correlating with the high incidence of hypertension and older patient age.

7. **What are the adverse renal effects of atazanavir?**
The protease inhibitor atazanavir has been noted to cause three renal lesions. The most common is nephrolithiasis, in which the stones are composed primarily of atazanavir. Along the same lines, AKI has been associated with atazanavir from crystal deposition in the distal renal tubules. Finally, several cases of acute interstitial nephritis have been described with atazanavir.

8. **What are the major adverse effects of gadolinium-based contrast in patients with underlying kidney disease?**
In 2006 a sentinel observation was made when Grobner described gadolinium-based contrast (GBC) as the trigger for nephrogenic systemic fibrosis (NSF). Since that time, most cases of NSF have been linked to GBC exposure and several groups have shown the presence of gadolinium within tissues of patients with NSF. Patients with advanced underlying kidney disease who are exposed to linear-based chelates (vs. macrocyclic chelates) are most at risk. The GBC most often described is gadodiamide (nonionic linear chelate) followed by gadopentetate (ionic linear chelate). The macrocyclic chelate-based agents have rarely been described and none have been noted in the published literature. The other GBC-associated lesion that occurs in patients with underlying kidney disease is AKI. However, this is uncommon and much less than AKI that follows iodinated radiocontrast. When AKI develops,

it is often in patients with advanced kidney disease (GFR <30 mL/min) who are exposed to high GBC doses, often with intra-arterial administration.

9. **What renal lesions are the bisphosphonates pamidronate and zoledronate described to cause?**
The bisphosphonates have been described to cause a couple of renal lesions. High-dose pamidronate causes a collapsing focal and segmental glomerulosclerosis (FSGS) and minimal change lesion, along with some tubular injury. In contrast, high-dose zoledronate causes a pure tubular injury pattern with severe acute tubular necrosis. It is thought that these two agents target the epithelial cells: visceral epithelial cells with pamidronate and tubular epithelial cells with zoledronate.

10. **What are the renal lesions associated with antiangiogenesis therapy such as bevacizumab, sorafenib, and sunitinib?**
Drugs that target the angiogenesis pathway—in this case, vascular endothelial growth factor (VEGF)—have added significant benefit to treatment of certain malignancies. However, as is common with new drugs, a number of renal lesions have been described. The two most common are hypertension and proteinuria. These lesions appear to be the result of VEGF deficiency. In the systemic vasculature, VEGF is required to maintain vasodilatation, primarily through the nitric oxide pathway. Hypertension results when the anti-angiogenesis drugs disturb this process. Proteinuria occurs from the loss of VEGF effect to maintain healthy glomerular endothelial cell function and nephrin expression in the podocytes. Ultimately, microvascular injury is not repaired and thrombotic microangiopathy, the most common renal lesion, develops. Other forms of glomerular disease have been noted (membranoproliferative GN, focal segmental glomerulosclerosis, cryoglobulinemic GN, and immune complex GN), all demonstrating some form of glomerular endothelial cell injury. Rare cases of acute interstitial nephritis have also been described with sorafenib and sunitinib.

11. **What are the clinical renal syndromes associated with proton pump inhibitors?**
The proton pump inhibitors (PPIs) were first released into clinical practice in 1989, with omeprazole the initial agent. Since then, numerous cases of acute interstitial nephritis have been reported for omeprazole. Of note, all classes of PPIs have been noted to cause acute interstitial nephritis. Other less common adverse renal effects include hyponatremia, likely the result of the syndrome of inappropriate antidiuretic hormone (SIADH) production. All of the PPIs, except rabeprazole, are metabolized predominantly by hepatic CYP450 enzymes, in particular CYP3A4 and CYP2C19. In contrast, rabeprazole has predominantly nonenzymatic pathways for its metabolism, which allows it to be used safely with other agents that compete for the CYP pathway, such as cyclosporine. The CYP450 enzymatic pathway of metabolism of PPIs has broad implications for excessive drug concentrations when these agents are used concurrently with calcineurin inhibitors, which also use the CYP3A4 pathway for metabolism. This is particularly a concern in patients with mutations in the CYP2C19 enzyme gene, as metabolism with CYP3A4 becomes important for appropriate calcineurin inhibitor metabolism. In this circumstance, treatment with a PPI (except rabeprazole) in transplant patients is likely to cause calcineurin toxicity because of high levels. Finally, although PPIs inhibit the H^+/K^+-ATPase pump, they have not been associated with clinically important renal tubular acidosis.

12. **How does cisplatin cause acute kidney injury and proximal tubular injury?**
Cisplatin is a classic chemotherapy drug that causes kidney injury, which ultimately limits its very effective tumor killing. The drug is a platinum-based agent whose nephrotoxicity is thought to be related in part to the chloride in the *cis* position. Cisplatin gains entry into tubular cells via uptake by the organic cation transport (OCT-2) system on the basolateral membrane of proximal tubular cells. Once within the cell cytoplasm, it has multiple effects that cause cellular injury. Cellular apoptosis/necrosis develops as a result of endoplasmic reticulum–induced stress, mitochondrial injury pathways, and a death receptor pathway.

Also, normal cell-cycle regulation is disrupted by cisplatin, leading to tubular apoptosis and kidney injury. Cisplatin-induced DNA damage activates p53, which through various intracellular signals promotes cell apoptosis. In addition, cisplatin cause formation of reactive oxygen species and oxidative stress by depleting and inactivating glutathione and other related antioxidants. Finally, cisplatin induces both inflammation (triggers tumor necrosis factor-alpha) and vascular injury, which further promotes kidney injury. In addition to AKI, cisplatin causes proximal tubulopathy, salt wasting, loss of urinary-concentrating ability, and magnesium wasting. Other compounds in the class of chemotherapeutic agents (carboplatin, oxaliplatin, and nedaplatin) are less nephrotoxic than cisplatin but still maintain some nephrotoxicity when used in high doses.

13. **What is the mode of renal excretion of tenofovir, and how is it related to the drug's nephrotoxicity?**
Tenofovir, an acyclic nucleotide analogue that effectively treats HIV infection, is now recognized as a cause of a couple of renal lesions. The most common adverse kidney effects are AKI and Fanconi syndrome; nephrogenic diabetes insipidus occurs less commonly. The proximal tubule is the target of tenofovir and the ultimate cause of AKI and Fanconi syndrome. Renal excretion of tenofovir occurs by the following pathway. Tenofovir is delivered to the proximal tubule via the basolateral circulation whereupon it is then transported into the intracellular space via the human organic anion transporter (hOAT). Once inside the cell, it is shuttled through the intracellular space and subsequently secreted into the urinary space via efflux transporters such as multidrug-resistant protein-2 (MRP-2). Competition by endogenous substance or other drugs for the MRP-2 efflux transporter can impair tenofovir excretion and lead to higher intracellular concentrations. Additionally, a single nucleotide polymorphism of the MRP-2 gene, which causes a loss-of-function mutation, has been described to increase risk for Fanconi syndrome in patients with HIV treated with tenofovir. Mitochondrial injury is the major cause of the proximal tubulopathy associated with high intracellular tenofovir concentrations.

14. **How do intravenous immune globulin and intravenous hydroxyethyl starch cause AKI?**
Intravenous immune globulin (IVIG) is used for a variety of indications. Some of the IVIG preparations are stabilized with sucrose (vs. maltose and glucose), which can cause kidney injury in the form of "osmotic nephropathy." Similarly, hydroxyethyl starch (HES), which is used as a plasma expander, causes an osmotic nephropathy–type of renal lesion. In fact, large prospective sepsis trials comparing HES to other plasma expanders demonstrate an association of HES use with AKI and increased dialysis requirement. The underlying pathomechanism is thought to be the following: Sucrose and HES (small molecular weight particles) are both filtered by the glomerulus and then endocytosed by proximal tubular cells. Once inside the cells, they are transported to lysosomes where they are unable to be degraded. The cells become swollen with enlarged lysosomes containing these substances. Swollen cells can occlude tubular lumens and cause tubular obstruction with increased tubular pressure that exceeds the glomerular filtration pressure. Also, as the cells are injured, they detach from the basement membrane and are released into the tubular lumens. In general, only patients with underlying risk factors such as CKD and other renal impairment are at risk of developing osmotic nephropathy.

15. **What renal lesion does the weight loss drug orlistat cause in at-risk patients?**
Orlistat is a weight loss drug that is available both by prescription and over the counter. It promotes weight loss by inducing fat malabsorption by inhibiting gastric and pancreatic lipase. Several cases of AKI associated with high-dose orlistat use in patients with underlying risk factors (CKD, volume depletion, etc.) have been described. Renal biopsy in these patients demonstrated intratubular calcium oxalate crystal deposition. In one case, discontinuation of orlistat was associated with renal recovery, and renal biopsy noted clearing of calcium oxalate

crystals. Orlistat therapy in these cases can be considered similar to enteric hyperoxaluria that occurs with intestinal bypass procedures or small bowel resection in Crohn's disease and other malabsorption syndromes (pancreatic insufficiency). Malabsorption allows bowel fats to bind (soap out) calcium, which allows free intestinal oxalate (normally bound to calcium) to be reabsorbed in the colon, which is "leaky" to oxalate from bile salt injury.

16. **How are aristolochic acid nephropathy and Balkan nephropathy similar?**
Aristolochic acid nephropathy (Chinese herb nephropathy) is a chronic tubulointerstitial lesion that develops in patients who are exposed to the substance aristolochic acid. The disease was first described in Belgium in patients taking a slimming regimen, where these patients were noted to develop chronic kidney disease, often progressing to dialysis requirement. Uroepithelial cancers were also described in these patients. Investigation and analysis of the common link in these patients, herbal slimming regimens, allowed identification of the culprit substance, aristolochic acid (AA). *Aristolochia fanghi,* the source of AA, was used in place of the innocuous herb (*Stephania tetrandra)* in the herbal slimming regimen. Work in humans and animals identified the mechanism of tubulointerstitial injury and malignancy. Aristolochic acid is metabolized by the CYP450 enzyme to intermediates that form DNA adducts that cause DNA alkylation. For many years, the cause of endemic Balkan nephropathy remained a puzzle, with a leading trigger considered to be a food contaminant or some other environmental exposure. Because of the similarity of the histopathologic lesions (chronic tubulointerstitial nephritis) between Balkan nephropathy and aristolochic acid nephropathy, search for evidence to support AA as the cause of Balkan nephropathy was undertaken. It appears that AA may in fact be the causative agent because Baltic families were unintentionally consuming *Aristolochia clematitis,* which grew as weeds in their wheat fields. This plant species was poisoning people who consumed bread contaminated with aristolochic acid.

17. **What is the renal lesion associated with high doses of the herbal energy supplement ephedra?**
Ephedra was used in numerous "energy" and weight loss supplements sold in health food stores. Multiple reports of ephedra-containing kidney stones have been published. Patients who developed this adverse renal effect were ingesting very large amounts of ephedra. Because ephedra has been removed from most "energy" supplements, it has become a rare renal complication.

18. **What renal lesions are described with the baby formula adulterant melamine?**
A recent example of adulteration of food products was seen worldwide. To falsely elevate protein content of baby formula to meet standards, melamine was added to the formula. Contamination came to light when infants were developing kidney failure and kidney stones. The common link in these children was melamine-contaminated formula. The renal lesions seen with melamine include nephrolithiasis with melamine-containing stones and AKI, probably related to direct tubular toxicity and/or melamine intratubular crystal deposition (demonstrated in animals). Hematuria and proteinuria have also been noted in affected neonates. Stones can be diagnosed with renal ultrasonography.

19. **What is the adverse renal effect of topiramate, and what is the underlying pathomechanism?**
Topiramate is an antiseizure drug that is also used to treat/prevent migraine headaches. However, the adverse renal effect of nephrolithiasis was noted at a higher than expected rate in patients treated with this medication, raising the possibility of a drug-related complication. It was shown that topiramate is able to block carbonic anhydrase activity and cause a type 2 RTA. This type of RTA is associated with alkalinization of the urine and formation of calcium phosphate stones, which is the type of stone found in patients receiving topiramate.

KEY POINTS: MEDICATIONS

1. More than two thirds of patients that developed acute phosphate nephropathy had three or more of the following risk factors: 1) Age >60 years, 2) female gender, 3) GFR <60 mL/min, 4) hypertension, 5) ACE inhibitor/ARB use, and 6) diuretic use.

2. Hypertension and proteinuria are the most common renal adverse effects of the anti-angiogenesis inhibitors (bevacizumab, sorafenib, sunitinib), which target the vascular endothelial growth factor (VEGF) signaling pathway.

3. The proton pump inhibitors (PPIs) are associated primarily with acute interstitial nephritis, however, less common adverse renal effects include hyponatremia, impaired calcineurin inhibitor metabolism and hypomagnesemia.

4. The weight loss drug orlistat may rarely cause acute kidney injury and nephrolithiasis through its effect to cause intestinal malabsorption and enteric hyperoxaluria.

5. The anti-seizure and migraine drug topiramate is a carbonic anhydrase inhibitor that is associated with proximal renal tubular acidosis and calcium phosphate stone formation.

20. **What are risk factors for ciprofloxacin-associated crystal nephropathy?**
The most well-known renal complication of ciprofloxacin is acute interstitial nephritis. However, another cause of AKI associated with ciprofloxacin use has been described. Crystalluria commonly occurs following administration of ciprofloxacin to experimental animals. The drug is insoluble at neutral or alkaline pH and crystallizes in alkaline urine. In humans, ciprofloxacin causes crystalluria when the urine pH is greater than 7.3, especially with higher drug doses. Ciprofloxacin has been noted to cause clinically important crystal-induced AKI within 2 days to 2 weeks of ingestion of oral ciprofloxacin. Age >70 years was present in all but one patient, whereas ACE-I therapy was prescribed in two patients. Urinalysis revealed crystals of varying shapes, which were composed of ciprofloxacin salt. Renal biopsy in three cases revealed needle-shaped birefringent crystals within the tubules without evidence of acute or chronic interstitial nephritis. Renal function returned to baseline on withdrawal of ciprofloxacin. The ciprofloxacin crystals showed a wide array of appearances including needles, sheaves, stars, fans, butterflies, and other unusual shapes. All crystals had a lamellar structure, with sizes ranging from 30×5 μm to 360×237 μm, and were strongly birefringent under polarizing light. Ciprofloxacin-induced intrarenal crystal deposition should be considered as a possible cause of AKI in elderly patients, those with impaired kidney function, those who are volume depleted, and those with a urine pH higher than 6.0. Examination of the urine sediment following drug exposure will facilitate diagnosis, potentially obviating the need for a kidney biopsy. To prevent AKI and crystalluria, ciprofloxacin should be dose adjusted for level of GFR, the patient should be volume replete, and alkalinization of the urine should be avoided.

21. **What is the risk of lactic acidosis with metformin therapy in patients with acute or chronic kidney disease?**
Metformin is an effective and generally well-tolerated oral glucose-lowering agent. However, rarely it can be associated with lactic acidosis in patients who have predisposing factors. The greatest risk factor is impaired kidney function, with risk most significant as the GFR declines to less than 30 mL/min. Both acute and chronic liver disease are also contraindications. Acute illnesses (sepsis, myocardial infarction, major surgery, etc.) that are likely to lower GFR are also settings where metformin should be discontinued and certainly not initiated. Metformin-associated lactic acidosis is reversible with drug discontinuation and improvement of kidney function, but it has been associated with fatalities. In cases of overdose, hemodialysis should be undertaken to remove metformin and correct the underlying acidosis.

BIBLIOGRAPHY

1. Brewster UC, Perazella MA. Proton pump inhibitors and the kidney: Critical review. *Clin Nephrol* 2007;68:65–72.
2. Gambaro G, Perazella MA. Adverse renal effects of anti-inflammatory agents: Evaluation of selective and nonselective cyclooxygenase inhibitors. *J Intern Med* 2003;253:643–652.
3. Grobner T. Gadolinium—a specific trigger for the development of nephrogenic fibrosing dermopathy and nephrogenic systemic fibrosis? *Nephrol Dial Transplant* 2006;21(4):1104-1108.
4. Gurevich F, Perazella MA. Renal effects of anti-angiogenesis therapy: Update for the internist. *Am J Med* 2009;122:322–328.
5. Markowitz GD, Perazella MA. Drug-induced renal failure: A focus on tubulointerstitial disease. *Clin Chimica Acta* 2005;351:31–47.
6. Markowitz GS, Perazella MA. Acute phosphate nephropathy. *Kidney Int* 2009;76(10):1027–1034.
7. Perazella MA. Current status of gadolinium toxicity in patients with kidney disease. *Clin J Am Soc Nephrol* 2009;4(2):461–469.
8. Perazella MA. Renal vulnerability to drug toxicity. *Clin J Am Soc Nephrol* 2009;4:1275–1283.
9. Perazella MA, Markowitz GS. Bisphosphonate nephrotoxicity. *Kidney Int* 2008;74(11):1385–1393.
10. Yarlagadda S, Perazella MA. Drug-induced crystal nephropathy: An update. *Expert Opin Drug Safety* 2008;7(2):147–158.

CHAPTER 11

SEPSIS AND ACUTE KIDNEY INJURY

Mitchell H. Rosner, MD, and Uta Erdbruegger, MD

1. **How is septic acute kidney injury defined?**

   Septic acute kidney injury (AKI) is characterized by the simultaneous presence of the RIFLE (risk, injury, failure, loss, and end stage) criteria for AKI (change in blood creatinine or glomerular filtration rate [GFR] from baseline and decreased urine flow rates over time) and the consensus criteria for sepsis (symptoms of the systemic inflammatory response syndrome and signs of organ hypoperfusion or dysfunction). Nonseptic-related causes of AKI (e.g., nephrotoxic drugs or rhabdomyolysis) should be ruled out. However, there is no standardized method for distinguishing septic AKI from nonseptic AKI, and in many cases the cause of AKI may be multifactorial and thus difficult to attribute to sepsis.

2. **What are the key epidemiologic aspects of AKI in the setting of sepsis?**

   Several recent studies have looked at the incidence of sepsis in patients admitted to an intensive care unit (ICU). These studies reveal that a range of 8.2% to 35.3% of all patients admitted to an ICU have a diagnosis of sepsis. Recently, a large study in the United States demonstrated an 8.7% annual increase in the incidence of a primary sepsis diagnosis.

   Although the etiology of AKI in patients who are critically ill is likely often multifactorial, sepsis has consistently been found to be an important contributing factor. Several studies have shown that approximately 40% to 50% of patients with AKI on presentation to an ICU have concomitant sepsis and that approximately 11% to 64% of patients who are critically ill with a diagnosis of severe sepsis or septic shock have concomitant AKI.

3. **Does the degree of sepsis determine the incidence and severity of AKI?**

   In contrast to AKI, sepsis syndrome has benefited from the development of a consensus-driven standardized definition for greater than 15 years. The diagnosis of sepsis syndrome begins with fulfilling criteria for the systemic inflammatory response syndrome (SIRS), characterized by abnormalities in temperature, heart rate, respiratory rate, or white blood cell count. The presence of suspected or confirmed infection plus the concomitant occurrence of two out of four SIRS criteria define the diagnosis of sepsis syndrome. This syndrome is then classified according to severity based on the presence of organ dysfunction (severe sepsis) and/or lack of response to initial fluid resuscitation (septic shock).

   There is a stepwise increase in the severity of AKI in patients who are critically ill when they are stratified by the severity of sepsis. For instance, in one study, the incidence of AKI, defined by the AKIN (Acute Kidney Injury Network) criteria, increased markedly when stratified by sepsis severity: 4.2% for sepsis, 22.7% for severe sepsis, and 52.8% for septic shock, respectively. Furthermore, as patients progress from sepsis to severe sepsis to septic shock, the incidence of AKI that requires dialysis increases from 24% to 39% to 89%, respectively.

4. **What is the timing of AKI resulting from sepsis?**

   It has been observed that the development of AKI in sepsis is predominately evident at the time of ICU admission or develops early in the illness course. In a multicenter study of patients who are critically ill presenting with septic shock, investigators found 64% had evidence of AKI, defined by the RIFLE criteria, within 24 hours of onset of shock.

5. **When should physiologic derangements in sepsis be corrected?**

It has been shown that timely intervention, also called "early goal-directed therapy," in treatment of severe sepsis and septic shock improves outcome. Rivers et al. showed that besides improvement of hemodynamic factors, the acid–base status was improved in patients who received early goal-directed therapy in the first 6 hours after admission to the emergency room (ER). This "golden hour" for sepsis resuscitation is also well established for other conditions such as stroke, acute coronary syndrome, or trauma. Regarding timing of intervention, another study demonstrated that patients who have been admitted to the ICU during morning rounds have higher severity of illness and mortality rates. These patients were more often transfers from the ER or the same hospital ward ("nocturnal disease worsening transfers"). The majority of patients admitted during nonround times were from the recovery or operating rooms. The authors speculate that under-recognition of patient's critical illness during rounds (e.g., seeing patients from one bed to the other and not from the sickest patient to the least sick) might have caused this outcome. Nevertheless, the patients admitted during rounds have been sicker and had more complex conditions.

Rivers E, Nguyen B, Havstad S, et al. Early goal-directed therapy in the treatment of severe sepsis and septic shock. *N Engl J Med* 2001;345:1368–1377.

Afessa B, Gajic O, Morales IJ, et al. Association between ICU admission during morning rounds and mortality. *Chest* 2009;136:1489–1495.

6. **Is lactate clearance better than central venous oxygen saturation as a goal for early sepsis therapy?**

Central venous oxygen saturation is one of the parameters used to guide early goal-directed therapy. Per protocol, IV fluids are given initially to improve central venous pressures. Vasoactive agents are administered as a second step to increase the mean arterial pressures. Central venous oxygen saturation ($ScvO_2$) is a third parameter used to improve tissue oxygenation. If the $ScvO_2$ is <70%, red blood cells are transfused. Lactate clearance, a marker of anaerobic glycolysis in hypoxic tissue, was recently compared to $ScvO_2$ as a marker for total body oxygen metabolism. There was no difference found in mortality for patients with severe sepsis and septic shock resuscitated with a protocol using lactate clearance. Monitoring $ScvO_2$ or lactate clearance to assess response to early goal-directed therapy seems to be equally acceptable.

Jones AE, Shapiro NI, Trzeciak S, et al. Lactate clearance vs central venous oxygen saturation as goals of early sepsis therapy: A randomized clinical trial. *JAMA* 2010;303(8):739–749.

7. **What are the demographic characteristics of AKI resulting from sepsis?**

Observational data have found septic AKI occurs more commonly among elderly patients and females when compared with nonseptic AKI. Patients with septic AKI are also more likely to have a higher burden of pre-existing comorbid disease when compared with patients with nonseptic AKI. In particular, patients with septic AKI have a higher prevalence of congestive heart failure, chronic obstructive pulmonary disease, chronic kidney disease, liver disease, diabetes mellitus, active malignancy, and immune system compromise. Investigators have also found that positive blood cultures were associated with a significantly higher likelihood for developing AKI (37% vs. 29%).

Patients with septic AKI have been shown across a range of observational studies to have higher rates of oliguria, despite having received more fluid therapy and/or diuretic therapy when compared with patients with nonseptic AKI or those with sepsis only. Consequently, these patients are more likely to accumulate fluid and develop a positive fluid balance early in their clinical course. Recent data have accumulated to suggest significant fluid accumulation is associated with worse clinical outcome in patients who are critically ill with AKI.

8. **What are the hemodynamic factors that play a role in the development of septic AKI?**
   - **Old concept:** Normally, GFR is maintained by preglomerular arteriolar dilatation and postglomerular arteriolar constriction preserving glomerular perfusion and filtration pressure (a process termed autoregulation). In systemic hypoperfusion, such as that occurs during sepsis, arteriolar and venular constriction and stimulation of cardiac function occur to return systemic blood pressure and cardiac output toward normal. Vasoconstriction occurs primarily in the renal, splanchnic, and musculocutaneous circulations, resulting in the relative preservation of blood flow to the heart and brain. Thus, systemic vasoconstriction leads to renal hypoperfusion and reversible loss of GFR, which is initially without histopathologic injury to the kidney (prerenal failure). But hypoperfusion, if severe enough or prolonged in duration, can evolve to acute tubular injury (acute tubular necrosis) and irreversible loss of GFR.
   - **New concept:** In septic AKI, high cardiac output leads to preserved or increased renal blood flow (hyperaemia), according to recent data in animals and humans. It is possible that this concept describes the actual pathophysiology more accurately, but this still remains to be proven. When the afferent arterioles dilate and efferent arterioles dilate even more, renal blood flow increases but the pressure in the glomerulus will decrease, resulting in a decrease in GFR.
   In contrast, low cardiac output can occur in mixed septic and cardiogenic shock, leading to low renal blood flow following the old pathophysiologic concept.

9. **What are the nonhemodynamic factors that occur in sepsis that can lead to AKI?**
   - Inflammatory mediators (cytokines, vasoactive substances, arachidonate metabolites) are released during sepsis and may play a biological role. The role of tumor necrosis factor (TNF) in kidney injury seems predominant from a large body of experimental evidence.
   - Apoptosis (programmed cell death) occurs in response to immune-mediated cell injury. In contrast, tubular necrosis caused by ischemia also happens in sepsis. There is now good evidence to show that human renal tubular cells die by apoptosis and necrosis in experimental models of acute ischemic and toxic renal injury.
   - Endothelial cell dysfunction may also lead to ischemia.
   - Activation of coagulation pathways may impair renal microcirculatory blood flow.

10. **What are the histopathologic findings associated with AKI resulting from sepsis?**
    There is no consistent or typical renal histopathologic pattern. In part, this is a result of a lack of data because kidney biopsies are not typically performed in these patients who are critically ill. Acute tubular necrosis may be seen in some cases.

11. **What are the urinary findings in AKI resulting from sepsis?**
    The urinary findings are highly variable in this setting. Studies have shown either a high or low fractional excretion of sodium or urea and either high or low urinary osmolalities. This wide range of findings likely reflects the timing of the urine studies in relation to the amount of irreversible injury versus hemodynamic factors (i.e., the fractional excretion of sodium may be initially low when the mechanism of AKI results from vasoconstriction but may be elevated in the setting of tubular injury).

    The most common findings on urine microscopic examination are granular ("muddy brown") casts that represent shedding and degradation of tubular cells. However, the absence of these casts does not exclude the diagnosis of AKI.

12. **What is the mortality rate in septic AKI?**

Patients with septic AKI have a mortality rate of approximately 70% compared to 20% for patients with severe sepsis or 49% for patients with septic shock in the absence of AKI. In addition, septic AKI is an independent predictor of hospital death. Furthermore, the development of AKI is associated with a doubling in the length of ICU stays.

KEY POINTS: SEPSIS AND ACUTE KIDNEY INJURY

1. Several recent studies have shown that approximately 40% to 50% of patients with AKI on presentation to an intensive care unit have concomitant sepsis and that approximately 11% to 64% of patients who are critically ill with a diagnosis of severe sepsis or septic shock have concomitant acute kidney injury (AKI).

2. AKI resulting from sepsis occurs early in the course of the disease. Of patients presenting with septic shock, investigators found 64% had evidence of AKI, defined by the RIFLE criteria, within 24 hours of onset of shock.

3. Physiologic derangements resulting from sepsis need to be corrected as early as possible utilizing goal-directed therapy.

4. Patients with septic AKI have a mortality rate of approximately 70% compared to 20% for patients with severe sepsis or 49% for patients with septic shock in the absence of AKI.

13. **What are the clinical factors in patients with septic AKI associated with worse outcomes?**
    - Older age
    - Higher acuity of disease
    - Greater burden of illness
    - Longer stays in ICU and hospital
    - AKI severity as defined by the RIFLE criteria
    - Recently, it has been shown that a delay in initiation of appropriate antimicrobial therapy in patients who are critically ill with septic shock is an independent predictor of both AKI and poor outcomes

14. **What is the therapy of AKI resulting from sepsis?**

Currently, there are no specific therapies for either prevention or treatment of septic AKI. However, it is critically important that appropriate and timely supportive care be delivered. This includes the following:
    - Rapid fluid resuscitation to ensure adequate blood pressure and organ perfusion
    - Appropriate use of vasopressors to ensure adequate blood pressure and organ perfusion
    - Timely administration of antimicrobials
    - Avoidance of nephrotoxic exposures such as intravenous contrast or nonsteroidal anti-inflammatory drugs
    - Timely initiation of dialysis in patients with oliguria, positive fluid balance, and signs of irreversible kidney injury

    Novel therapies that target specific pathogenic pathways are being actively studied in animal models and offer promise for future human use.

15. **Is there a role for low-dose dopamine in the treatment or prevention of AKI resulting from sepsis?**

For much of the last four decades, low-dose dopamine has been considered the drug of choice to treat and prevent renal failure in the ICU. The multifactorial etiology of renal failure in the ICU and the presence of coexisting multisystem organ dysfunction make the design and execution of clinical trials to study this problem difficult. However, in the past decade, several meta-analyses and one large randomized trial have all shown a lack of benefit of low-dose dopamine in improving renal function. There are multiple reasons for this lack of efficacy. Although dopamine does cause a diuretic effect, it does very little to improve mortality, creatinine clearance, or the incidence of dialysis. Evidence is also growing of its adverse effects on the immune, endocrine, and respiratory systems. It may also potentially increase mortality in sepsis and thus has no role in the prevention or treatment of AKI.

16. **In patients who develop AKI from sepsis, what is the rate of recovery of renal function?**

Recovery of kidney function is increasingly recognized as an important determinant of morbidity with long-term health resource implications. Data have suggested that renal recovery and independence from dialysis may be greater in septic compared with nonseptic AKI. In the BEST Kidney study (a large multicenter study of patients with AKI), in survivors to hospital discharge with normal baseline kidney function, 5.7% of septic AKI compared with 7.8% of nonseptic AKI were dialysis dependent. However, in patients with pre-existing chronic kidney disease, recovery to dialysis independence trended lower in septic compared with nonseptic AKI (16.7% vs. 24.7%, p = 0.28). Recently, another study found 95.7% of patients with septic AKI had complete renal function recovery occurring on average 10.1 ± 8 days after hospital discharge.

BIBLIOGRAPHY

1. Afessa B, Gajic O, Morales IJ, et al. Association between ICU admission during morning rounds and mortality. *Chest* 2009;136:1489–1495.

2. Bagshaw SM, Uchino S, Bellomo R, et al. Septic acute kidney injury in critically ill patients: Clinical characteristics and outcomes. *Clin J Am Soc Nephrol* 2007;2:431–439.

3. Hoste EA, Lameire NH, Vanholder RC, et al. Acute renal failure in patients with sepsis in a surgical ICU: Predictive factors, incidence, comorbidity, and outcome. *J Am Soc Nephrol* 2003;14:1022–1030.

4. Jones AE, Shapiro NI, Trzeciak S, et al. Lactate clearance vs central venous oxygen saturation as goals of early sepsis therapy: A randomized clinical trial. *JAMA* 2010;303(8): 739–749.

5. Langenberg C, Bagshaw SM, May CN, et al. The histopathology of septic acute kidney injury: A systematic review. *Crit Care* 2008;12:2.

6. Lopes JA, Jorge S, Resina C, et al. Acute kidney injury in patients with sepsis: A contemporary analysis. *Int J Infect Dis* 2009;13:176–181.

7. Marshall JC, Vincent JL, Fink MP, et al. Measures, markers, and mediators: Toward a staging system for clinical sepsis. A report of the Fifth Toronto Sepsis Roundtable, Toronto, Ontario, Canada, October 25–26, 2000. *Crit Care Med* 2003;31:1560–1567.

8. Rivers E, Nguyen B, Havstad S, et al. Early goal-directed therapy in the treatment of severe sepsis and septic shock. *N Engl J Med* 2001;345:1368–1377.

9. Zaccaria R, Ronco C. Pathogenensis of acute kidney injury during sepsis. *Curr Drug Targets* 2009;10:1179–1183.

CHAPTER 12

RHABDOMYOLYSIS

Scott D. Bieber, DO, and J. Ashley Jefferson, MD

1. **What is rhabdomyolysis?**

   Rhabdomyolysis is a condition characterized by muscle injury leading to myocyte necrosis with the subsequent release of toxic intracellular contents into the circulation. The term is usually applied when acute kidney injury (AKI) results from the muscle injury, but note that AKI does not always occur, even following severe muscle injury.

2. **What are the mechanisms by which rhabdomyolysis causes acute kidney injury?**

   Rhabdomyolysis causes acute kidney injury through a combination of renal vasoconstriction, direct oxidant injury, and tubular obstruction.

   - **Renal vasoconstriction:** Effective circulatory volume decreases as fluid moves from the intravascular space into the interstitial space of damaged muscle tissue. This leads to activation of neurohormonal systems such as the renin-angiotensin-aldosterone system (RAAS) and sympathetic nervous system. Vasoconstrictor mediators including endothelin-1, thromboxane-A2, tumor necrosis factor-α, and F2-isoprostanes are also upregulated. The binding of nitric oxide to myoglobin may limit the availability of this vasodilator and further contribute to vasoconstriction. The net result is early, but prolonged vasoconstriction, which may manifest clinically as oliguria with a low urine sodium concentration prior to progression to acute tubular injury.

   - **Oxidant injury:** Free iron released from myoglobin may lead to the formation of oxygen free radicals as ferrous iron is converted to ferric iron (Fenton reaction). Myoglobin itself has been found to be directly toxic to tubular cells by causing lipid peroxidation of tubular cellular membranes.

   - **Tubular obstruction:** Under normal conditions, small amounts of myoglobin are filtered, then endocytosed and metabolized by proximal tubular cells. When myoglobin levels in the tubules exceed the absorptive capacity of the proximal tubular cells, myoglobin may complex with Tamm-Horsfall protein (THP) in the distal nephron to form casts leading to intratubular obstruction. An acidic environment (urine pH <6.5) favors the formation of these complexes.

3. **What are some of the causes of muscle injury in rhabdomyolysis?**

   - **Trauma:** Crush injuries (motor vehicle accidents, earthquakes)
   - **Vascular occlusion:** Thrombosis, embolism, vessel clamping during surgery
   - **Muscular strain:** Exercise induced, seizures, delirium tremens, tetanus, status asthmaticus
   - **Toxins/drugs:** Alcohol, HMG-CoA reductase inhibitors, barbiturates, corticosteroids, colchicine, fibrates, isoniazid, zidovudine, amphetamines, ecstasy, opiates, cocaine, neuroleptic malignant syndrome
   - **Infection:** Influenza A/B, toxic shock syndrome, human immunodeficiency virus, Epstein-Barr virus, tetanus, malaria, legionella, polio, coxsackievirus, *Streptococcus, Staphylococcus, Clostridium*
   - **Inherited disorders of metabolism:** Carnitine palmitoyl transferase II deficiency, phosphofructokinase deficiency, myophosphorylase deficiency (McArdle), coenzyme Q10 deficiency, myoadenylate deaminase deficiency

- **Electrolyte disorders:** Hypokalemia, hypophosphatemia, hypocalcemia
- **Autoimmune:** Polymyositis, dermatomyositis
- **Other:** Hyperthermia, hypothermia, electrical injury

4. **What are some of the common examples of rhabdomyolysis?**

Rhabdomyolysis may be caused by a wide range of conditions (see Question 3). Trauma or direct muscle injury is the most common cause and is important to consider in any patient who presents with multiple injuries/trauma.

Alcohol intoxication is associated with rhabdomyolysis from multiple mechanisms. Alcohol itself is directly toxic to myocytes (and also proximal tubular cells). Alcoholics are often depleted of phosphorus, magnesium, and potassium. Hypokalemia may contribute to muscle injury through disturbances in the function of the sodium potassium ATPase pump, but hypokalemia also impairs the ability of muscle arterioles to vasodilate, promoting ischemic muscle injury. Hypomagnesemia can worsen concurrent hypokalemia. Phosphorus deficiency may result from poor diet, the use of phosphorus-binding medications for gastrointestinal upset, and urinary phosphorus wasting. Phosphorus is critical for the production of adenosine triphosphate (ATP) and multiple cellular enzymes and is an important component of the lipid bilayer of cell membranes. Furthermore, alcohol intoxication leading to altered mental status may result in compressive injuries to muscle in individuals who are found down and motionless for a prolonged period.

HMG-CoA reductase inhibitors (statins) have been associated with myositis and, in rare cases, AKI. It has been suggested that statins cause muscle cell damage by interfering with coenzyme Q and the electron transport chain, leading to problems with ATP generation. Statin-induced myositis can occur within days of starting the drug but has been described years later. Muscle pain is a common reason to discontinue statin use.

Exercise-induced muscle injury may lead to rhabdomyolysis and AKI. It is believed that muscle injury during strenuous exercise is secondary to thermal injury to the muscle cells combined with ATP depletion. Hypokalemia may also play a role. High temperature and humidity conditions put athletes at increased risk for exercise-induced rhabdomyolysis. Inherited disorders of muscle metabolism may be present in subjects with recurrent episodes of exercise-induced rhabdomyolysis.

5. **Why do some people develop recurrent episodes of rhabdomyolysis?**

Recurrent episodes of rhabdomyolysis should raise a red flag in the clinician's mind. Behavioral issues should be explored in patients with recurrent rhabdomyolysis. Often recurrent episodes of rhabdomyolysis are linked to alcohol and substance abuse. Toxicology screening can be useful to identify drug or alcohol ingestions as a cause of recurrent muscle injury. The man with alcoholism who is frequently presenting for medical attention with altered mental status and renal failure is one example. The marathon runner who is abusing diuretics or laxatives is another example. In the latter setting, the combination of strenuous exercise with concurrent diuretic- or laxative-induced hypokalemia can lead to muscle injury.

Less frequently, patients with recurrent episodes of rhabdomyolysis have an underlying inherited disorder of cell metabolism. Some of the common genetic conditions that are associated with rhabdomyolysis are listed in Question 3. These disorders affect cellular energetics as a result of abnormalities in carbohydrate or lipid metabolism. Usually patients with inherited metabolic myopathies present in childhood, but adult presentation also occurs. The most common inherited disorder causing rhabdomyolysis is carnitine palmitoyltransferase (CPT) deficiency. Often these inherited disorders of metabolism present with a concurrent precipitating factor such as strenuous exercise or infection.

6. **Do the creatine kinase or myoglobin levels help with the diagnosis of rhabdomyolysis?**

Creatine kinase (CK) or creatine phosphokinase (CPK) is an enzyme that is present in all striated muscle. The main role of CK is to catalyze the formation of phosphocreatine from creatine. Muscle tissue has a high need for energy in the form of ATP. Phosphocreatine in muscle serves as a store for high-energy phosphates, which can be donated to ADP when extra ATP is needed. CK levels are the most sensitive marker of muscle injury. Normal CK levels can go as high as 400 U/L. In muscle injury, CK levels tend to rise in the first 12 hours and peak in 1 to 3 days, with levels remaining elevated for up to 5 days after resolution of the muscle injury. CK levels correlate with the amount of muscle injury and may correlate with the risk of acute kidney injury. The risk of developing acute kidney injury is usually low when the CK level is below 15,000 U/L. Persons who develop acute kidney injury with CK levels below 15,000 often have coexisting conditions predisposing to development of acute kidney injury, such as sepsis or hypotension.

Myoglobin is another marker of muscle injury. Myoglobin levels rise rapidly (within 3 hours) and serum levels peak prior to serum CK levels. Myoglobin has a short half-life of 2 to 3 hours and is rapidly excreted by the kidneys. Rapid and unpredictable metabolism makes serum myoglobin a less useful marker of muscle injury than CK and is rarely used in assessing the risk of acute kidney injury. Urinary myoglobin has been proposed as a marker for AKI in rhabdomyolysis when concentrations of urine myoglobin are above 20 mg/L, but this is rarely used clinically.

7. **What are the clinical features of rhabdomyolysis?**
The clinical features of rhabdomyolysis are variable depending on the underlying cause and extent of the muscle injury. Patients usually complain of myalgias and may have associated muscle weakness. Blood pressure in rhabdomyolysis is often maintained even in the setting of large amounts of fluid loss secondary to vasoconstriction, in part because of the sequestration of nitric oxide by free myoglobin. Affected muscles may be tender, sometimes with marked stiffness and swelling. The large muscles of the leg and lower back are most commonly involved. Sometimes muscle swelling within a myofascial compartment may compress blood vessels and limit local blood supply, leading to further muscle ischemia. This is known as compartment syndrome and often requires surgical intervention (fasciotomy) to prevent ongoing ischemic muscle damage. Measurement of intramuscular pressures can be used to help guide decisions regarding the need for surgical intervention. Compartment pressures greater than 30 mm Hg are usually associated with muscle ischemia. Fasciotomy should be performed emergently if intramuscular pressures are greater than 50 mm Hg or remain above 30 mm Hg for 6 hours. In severe rhabdomyolysis, the patient is typically oliguric and may demonstrate the classic "tea-colored" urine secondary to myoglobinuria. Muddy-brown casts typical of acute tubular necrosis are commonly seen. A low urine sodium concentration secondary to vasoconstriction may be seen at early stages. Note that occasionally rhabdomyolysis may be asymptomatic and may only be detected on routine laboratory testing. Fortunately, with resolution of the underlying muscle injury, the renal function typically recovers.

8. **What laboratory abnormalities are commonly seen in patients with rhabdomyolysis?**
Common laboratory findings in rhabdomyolysis include an increase in muscle enzyme levels (e.g., creatinine kinase), hyperkalemia, hypocalcemia, hyperphosphatemia, hyperuricemia, and an anion gap acidosis. Potassium and phosphorus are released from damaged muscle cells into the circulation as muscle cells are lysed. If muscle injury is coupled with acute kidney injury, the excretion of potassium and phosphorus by the kidneys is impaired, contributing to higher serum levels. These electrolyte abnormalities are almost universally present in clinically significant cases of muscle injury and rhabdomyolysis. In cases of rhabdomyolysis without elevations of potassium and phosphorus, one should consider underlying hypokalemia or hypophosphatemia as an underlying factor mediating the muscle injury.

Calcium levels in rhabdomyolysis are typically decreased. In the early stages of muscle injury calcium precipitates in the injured muscle and occasionally massive heterotrophic calcification occurs. High phosphorus levels directly decrease calcium levels by binding free calcium, but hyperphosphatemia also inhibits 1-α hydroxylase, the enzyme that catalyzes the conversion of 25-hydroxycholecalciferol to 1,25-dihydroxycholecalciferol, the active form of vitamin D. There may also be decreased bone responsiveness to parathyroid hormone, impairing the body's ability to correct hypocalcemia.

An anion gap metabolic acidosis is commonly seen from the combination of anaerobic respiration in hypoxic muscles producing a lactic acidosis and the accumulation of organic acids from acute kidney injury. The acidosis may cause a shift of potassium from the intracellular compartment, exacerbating hyperkalemia. Elevated uric acid levels are a direct result of the release of purine nucleosides from degrading muscle cells. Adenosine and guanine from DNA and RNA are converted to uric acid by xanthine oxidase. It should be noted that a low urine pH promotes the formation of tubular myoglobin casts and uric acid crystals, both of which can lead to tubular obstruction in the development of acute kidney injury.

9. **What is the differential diagnosis in a patient with reddish-brown urine? How does the urinalysis help you in the diagnosis of rhabdomyolysis?**
The differential diagnosis for red–brown urine is broad. Most cases involve the presence of heme pigment in the urine or foods and drugs that alter the color of the urine. Some of the more common causes of red–brown urine are as follows:

- **Heme pigment:** Gross hematuria, hemoglobin, myoglobin, bile pigments, porphyria
- **Foods:** Beets, rhubarb, food coloring, fava beans, blackberries
- **Drugs:** Rifampin, phenolphthalein, vitamin B_{12}, phenytoin, deferoxamine, doxorubicin, chloroquine, ibuprofen, methyldopa, levodopa, metronidazole, nitrofurantoin, iron sorbitol

In rhabdomyolysis, a discrepancy between the urinalysis (dipstick) and the urine microscopy can indicate pigmenturia. The urinalysis does not identify whether or not there is blood in the urine; it simply identifies the presence of heme pigments (myoglobin or hemoglobin). Microscopy can be used to identify the presence of cells in the urine. The urine sediment can be separated from supernatant after spinning the urine sample in a centrifuge. In rhabdomyolysis, the urine supernatant will remain red–brown. A red sediment with clear supernatant implies the presence of red blood cells in the urine (hematuria), which can be confirmed by microscopy. When foods or drugs alone are causing the discoloration of the urine, the urine dipstick and microscopy should be negative for blood.

10. **How do we prevent kidney injury in patients with rhabdomyolysis?**
It should be noted that the treatment of rhabdomyolysis should be specific to the patient and take into consideration the underlying mechanism that is leading to muscular damage. Reversal of the underlying cause of muscle injury is of paramount importance.

Volume resuscitation is the key in the initial therapy. This is especially true in patients with crush syndrome and trauma. Crush syndrome occurs when compression of a limb or torso leads to rhabdomyolysis and subsequently renal dysfunction or even multiple organ failure. Not infrequently, crush syndrome is associated with sepsis syndrome, acute respiratory distress syndrome, disseminated intravascular coagulation, bleeding, arrhythmias, and electrolyte disturbances. Ideally, patients with crush syndrome should be started on intravenous fluids prior to extraction or relief of the compressive injury. Severe muscle injuries also may be present that require surgical intervention, such as amputation or fasciotomy for compartment syndrome.

The amount of fluid that is administered should be tailored to the patient and take into account the underlying etiology of muscle injury. In traumatic crush injury cases, 1 to 2 L of isotonic saline should be given as a bolus prior to extrication. Patients with traumatic muscle injury may require 10 to 15 L per day of fluid resuscitation. In comparison, it would be inadvisable to administer large amounts of fluid to an elderly patient with heart failure and statin-related rhabdomyolysis. Solutions containing potassium or lactate (lactated ringers) should be avoided.

11. **Should sodium bicarbonate or mannitol be given to prevent kidney injury in rhabdomyolysis?**

Tubular obstruction by myoglobin-THP casts, direct oxidant injury by myoglobin, and free iron lead to acute tubular injury in rhabdomyolysis. Alkalinization of the urine in animal models has been shown to increase the solubility of myoglobin-THP complex and inhibit reduction-oxidation cycling of myoglobin and lipid peroxidation. Therefore, alkali therapy has been proposed to have a role in prevention of tubular injury. Lowering the serum pH may also reduce potassium levels by shifting potassium back into cells. Some advocate alternating administration of normal saline with 5% dextrose containing 100 mmol bicarbonate (D5W with 2 amps of $NaHCO_3$) for fluid resuscitation in rhabdomyolysis, aiming for a urine pH greater than 6.5. The disadvantage of this therapy is that alkalinization has the potential to lower serum ionized calcium levels (not total calcium) in patients who are already hypocalcemic as a result of enhanced binding to albumin. Randomized controlled trials to support the use of bicarbonate in the treatment of rhabdomyolysis are currently lacking. Retrospective studies have shown that bicarbonate administration does not improve outcomes with regard to renal failure, need for dialysis, or mortality in most patients, although there may be benefit in the subgroup with severe rhabdomyolysis (CK level >30,000 U/L).

Mannitol is an osmotic diuretic that can increase urinary flow, flushing toxic agents such as myoglobin through the tubules. It also facilitates the osmotic shift of water out of cells, supporting the extracellular volume and decreasing compartment effects. Mannitol is also a weak free-radical scavenger. Unfortunately, mannitol can potentially worsen acute kidney injury by causing osmotic nephrosis and can accumulate if the urine output falls and is now rarely used.

The term "forced alkaline diuresis" has been used to describe the combination of intravenous fluids, bicarbonate therapy for urinary alkalinization, and diuretics to increase urinary flow. Although this therapy has shown some success in retrospective studies, there currently are little data available to recommend this approach. Notably, diuretic therapy should be limited to patients who have been resuscitated and are volume replete.

12. **How should electrolyte abnormalities be managed in rhabdomyolysis?**

Hyperkalemia is a frequent laboratory finding in rhabdomyolysis. Elevated serum potassium levels are a direct consequence of potassium release from injured myocytes. The hyperkalemia seen in rhabdomyolysis can develop rapidly and may be life threatening if the muscle injury is marked. In crush syndrome or traumatic injuries, serum potassium levels can also rise rapidly after perfusion is restored to muscle tissues via fluid resuscitation or fasciotomy. In nontraumatic rhabdomyolysis, hyperkalemia is less pronounced. Acute kidney injury also impairs potassium clearance. Hyperkalemia in rhabdomyolysis should be managed in a similar fashion to hyperkalemia from other causes (see Chapter 77). It should be noted that patients who receive dialysis for hyperkalemia may have a post dialysis "rebound" elevation in their potassium levels. Potassium levels may need to be monitored very closely.

Serum calcium levels drop, as described earlier. Replacing the calcium may only exacerbate muscle calcium deposition and can lead to rebound hypercalcemia as the calcium leaves myocytes during the recovery period. Indications for calcium replacement include symptomatic hypocalcemia (e.g., seizures, tetany), ionized serum calcium <0.8 mmol/L and severe hyperkalemia (> .0 mmol/L) with electrocardiogram changes. High phosphorus levels in rhabdomyolysis are difficult to manage and usually do not respond to oral PO_4 binder medications. As muscle injury resolves and kidney injury improves, hyperphosphatemia usually will resolve on its own. Acute hyperphosphatemia is rarely of clinical significance; however, in severe cases of hyperphosphatemia dialysis can be considered to correct serum phosphorus levels.

13. **When is renal replacement therapy indicated in the treatment of rhabdomyolysis?**

Indications for renal replacement therapy or dialysis in acute kidney injury from rhabdomyolysis are similar to acute kidney injury and renal failure from any other cause.

Life-threatening hyperkalemia, refractory acidosis, and volume overload are standard indications for renal replacement therapy in rhabdomyolysis. Clearance of myoglobin using conventional intermittent hemodialysis or continuous therapies such as continuous venovenous hemofiltration (CVVH), continuous venovenous hemodiafiltration (CVVHDF), or slow extended daily dialysis (SLED) is low and currently does not have a role in prevention of acute kidney injury in rhabdomyolysis. Plasmapheresis has not been shown to be effective in myoglobin clearance either. Super-high-flux dialyzers have increased myoglobin clearance; however, their role in the treatment or prevention of acute kidney injury remains unclear.

KEY POINTS: RHABDOMYOLYSIS

1. Early and vigorous volume resuscitation of patients with rhabdomyolysis (even prior to extrication in crush syndrome) is the key to preventing acute kidney injury.

2. Serum creatine kinase levels correlate with the degree of muscle injury and help predict the risk of acute kidney injury (rare if <15,000 U/L)

3. Blood pressure in rhabdomyolysis is often maintained, even in the setting of large amounts of fluid loss secondary to vasoconstriction, in part because of nitric oxide sequestration by free myoglobin.

4. Life-threatening hyperkalemia may be prominent as a result of the lysis of muscle cells and release of intracellular potassium.

BIBLIOGRAPHY

1. Bosch X, Poch E, Grau JM. Rhabdomyolysis and acute kidney injury. *N Engl J Med* 2009;361:62–72.

2. Holt SG, Moore KP. Pathogenesis and treatment of renal dysfunction in rhabdomyolysis. *Intens Care Med* 2001;27:803–811.

3. Huerta-Alardin AL, Varon J, Marik PE. Bench-to-bedside review: Rhabdomyolysis—An overview for clinicians. *Crit Care* 2005;9:158–169.

4. Vanholder R, Sever MS, Erek E, et al. Rhabdomyolysis. *J Am Soc Nephrol* 2000;11:1553–1561.

CHAPTER 13

TUMOR LYSIS SYNDROME

Scott D. Bieber, DO, and J. Ashley Jefferson, MD

1. **What is tumor lysis syndrome?**

   Tumor lysis syndrome (TLS) is a condition in which the necrosis of large numbers of tumor cells causes the release of toxic amounts of intracellular contents into the circulation resulting in acute hyperuricemia, electrolyte abnormalities (hyperkalemia, hyperphosphatemia, hypocalcemia), and acute kidney injury (AKI).

2. **What causes TLS?**

   TLS is usually caused by the administration of chemotherapeutic agents to patients with cancer resulting in rapid cell necrosis. Common agents implicated include cisplatin, etoposide, fludarabine, cytosine arabinoside, methotrexate, paclitaxel, rituximab, and corticosteroids. Radiation therapy rarely may cause TLS. Occasionally, spontaneous TLS may arise, especially in rapidly growing tumors that outgrow their blood supply.

3. **What are the risk factors for the development of TLS?**

   TLS typically occurs following the chemotherapeutic treatment of hematologic malignancies—in particular, Burkitt's lymphoma and acute B-cell lymphoblastic leukemia. TLS has only rarely been described following the treatment of solid organ tumors. Specific risk factors for the development of TLS include the following:

   Host-related factors:
   - Volume depletion
   - Pre-existing renal disease
   - Hyponatremia (in solid organ tumors only)

   Disease-related factors:
   - Large tumor burden or "bulky" disease
   - High tumor cell proliferation rate
   - Lactate dehydrogenase (LDH) levels >1500 IU (or twice the upper limit of normal)
   - Uric acid level >8.0 mg/dL
   - Extensive bone marrow involvement
   - Highly chemosensitive or radiosensitive tumors

4. **What laboratory findings are associated with TLS?**

   Electrolyte balance is often profoundly disturbed in TLS. Similar to the electrolyte abnormalities seen in patients with rhabdomyolysis, laboratory analysis in TLS typically reveals hyperkalemia, hyperphosphatemia, hypocalcemia, hyperuricemia, and elevated LDH levels. In TLS the uric acid and LDH levels are often elevated to a much greater degree. Potassium, a predominantly intracellular cation, is released into the extracellular space as tumor cell membranes are damaged. Malignant cells are often intensely metabolically active with large amounts of adenosine triphosphate (ATP) and can contain up to four times the amount of phosphorus found in normal cells. If AKI develops, decreased renal clearance of phosphorus and potassium can further elevate serum levels. Hypocalcemia develops in tumor lysis as calcium complexes with the phosphorus that is released from lysed cells forming calcium–phosphorus complexes in tissues and lowering the serum calcium level.

Hyperuricemia develops in TLS as purine nucleic acids are released from cells that are often rich in nucleic acid material as a result of their high turnover rates. Purines are subsequently metabolized into hypoxanthine, xanthine, and uric acid, which raises the level of uric acid in the blood (described later). Levels of LDH are often increased in TLS as this enzyme is also released from lysed cells into the serum. The pretreatment LDH level is considered a risk factor because it is a marker of a greater tumor burden.

5. **What are the expected findings on urinalysis in a patient with TLS?**
Urinalysis in a patient with acute TLS may reveal uric acid crystals or amorphous urates. Calcium–phosphate crystals can also be seen. It should be noted that lack of crystalluria does not rule out TLS. When AKI develops, there will typically be evidence of tubular injury or acute tubular necrosis, manifested by the presence of renal tubular epithelial cells and granular or muddy-brown casts.

6. **What is the mechanism of uric acid formation?**
As illustrated in Figure 13-1, purines from nucleic acids (DNA, RNA) are broken down into xanthine and hypoxanthine. Xanthine oxidase catalyzes the conversion to uric acid, which is a less soluble compound, especially in acidic urine. In other species, urate oxidase catalyzes the conversion of uric acid to the much more soluble allantoin, which is more readily excreted by the kidney. In humans and higher primates, a missense mutation in the gene encoding urate oxidase occurred some time in early hominid evolution, and the nitrogenous waste is excreted as uric acid.

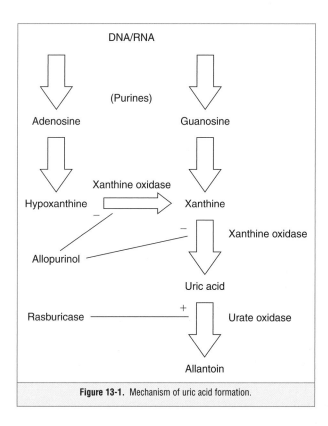

Figure 13-1. Mechanism of uric acid formation.

7. **How does TLS cause AKI?**

The primary mechanism of AKI in TLS is a crystal-induced nephropathy. When tumor cells undergo lysis, large amounts of nucleic acids from DNA and RNA are acutely released into the circulation. The purines (adenosine and guanine) are metabolized into xanthine and hypoxanthine, and subsequently, xanthine oxidase converts these into uric acid. The resultant high uric acid levels may precipitate in joints as acute gout. Glomerular filtration results in high concentrations of uric acid in tubular fluid and the consequent precipitation of uric acid crystals. Factors that enhance uric acid crystallization include volume depletion (nausea and vomiting, diarrhea, poor sodium intake) and low urinary pH (from metabolic acidosis). The intratubular uric acid crystals may lead to direct tubular obstruction but may also cause tubular injury with stimulation of a profound inflammatory response. There is also some evidence that soluble uric acid may act as a renal vasoconstrictor, exacerbating renal hypoperfusion.

It should be recognized that AKI secondary to TLS may not solely be a result of uric acid. Other intracellular components may also be toxic to renal tubular cells. In particular, hyperphosphatemia may enhance the intratubular precipitation of calcium–phosphate crystals and lead to nephrocalcinosis. This is especially relevant in the setting of overzealous alkalinization of the urine as the precipitation of calcium–phosphate stones is promoted in the presence of alkaline urine.

8. **Is there any way to prevent TLS in patients at high risk?**

- **Hydration:** The amount of hydration that a patient requires should be based on a clinical evaluation of the volume status of the patient and should take into account any underlying comorbidities that exist. Vigorous hydration is ideal but should be avoided in patients with impaired cardiac function or those already showing clinical signs of volume excess. In general, patients should receive at least 2 L/m^2/day with a goal urine output of greater than 100 mL/hour, ideally beginning 24 hours prior to the administration of chemotherapy. The increased hydration will increase tubular urine flow, enhancing uric acid and phosphate excretion and decreasing intratubular concentrations. Lactated Ringer's and other potassium-containing solutions should be avoided.
- **Alkalinization:** In the presence of acidic urine, uric acid can precipitate. By contrast, in more alkaline environments, uric acid is converted to urate salts, which are more soluble. In theory, administration of bicarbonate would increase the solubility of uric acid and diminish crystal-induced injury. Maximal uric acid solubility occurs at a urine pH >7.0. However, it should be noted that calcium–phosphate crystals precipitate readily in more alkaline environments and that xanthine and hypoxanthine crystals also precipitate at a higher urine pH. Thus, the role of alkalinization in tumor lysis syndrome is controversial and is not routinely used.
- **Allopurinol:** Allopurinol and its metabolite oxypurinol are competitive inhibitors of xanthine oxidase. Xanthine oxidase is an enzyme found predominantly in the liver, which converts xanthine and hypoxanthine into uric acid. By blocking xanthine oxidase, one can decrease the production of uric acid. The recommended prophylactic dose of allopurinol is 100 mg/m^2 three times daily with a maximum dose of 800 mg/day. It should be noted that allopurinol will not decrease the amount of uric acid already present; it will only prevent new generation of uric acid. For this reason it should be started 48 to 72 hours prior to the initiation of chemotherapy.
- **Rasburicase:** One can also decrease uric acid levels by converting uric acid to allantoin. Allantoin is 5 to 10 times more soluble than uric acid and is easily excreted by the kidneys. Rasburicase is a recombinant urate oxidase enzyme that converts uric acid to allantoin, replacing the deficient enzyme in humans. The dose recommended for prophylaxis is 0.2 mg/kg/day administered over 30 minutes and should be given at least 4 hours prior to chemotherapy and continued for 3 to 5 days following initiation of chemotherapy as needed. No dosage adjustment is necessary for impaired renal

function. Rasburicase will lower the serum uric acid levels dramatically within 24 hours, and clinical studies have shown it to be highly effective in both the prevention and treatment of TLS.

KEY POINTS: TUMOR LYSIS SYNDROME

1. Tumor lysis syndrome typically occurs following chemotherapy in the treatment of acute hematologic malignancies with a large tumor burden.

2. Both rhabdomyolysis and tumor lysis syndrome can cause profound electrolyte abnormalities (hyperkalemia, hyperphosphatemia, hypocalcemia, and hyperuricemia) as a result of the release of intracellular constituents.

3. Rasburicase, a recombinant uric oxidase, rapidly lowers uric acid levels and, although expensive, is an effective therapy in the prevention and treatment of acute kidney injury associated with tumor lysis syndrome.

9. **When should a patient get prophylaxis for TLS?**
Clinical judgment should be used to categorize patients as either low risk or high risk. Risk assessment should take into account the whole patient, keeping in mind the presence or absence of underlying renal compromise, the type of malignancy, the tumor burden, and the cytotoxic therapy that is going to be used. In general, patients at high risk have one or more of the risk factors described previously. Patients at low risk should receive intravenous hydration and allopurinol. Patients at high risk for TLS may receive intravenous hydration and rasburicase. Allopurinol and rasburicase are typically not given together because allopurinol will block xanthine oxidase, decreasing the substrate for rasburicase.

10. **How should the electrolyte abnormalities be managed in TLS?**
Hyperkalemia is a frequent laboratory abnormality in TLS as a consequence of potassium release from lysed tumor cells. If the amount of tumor lysis is massive, hyperkalemia can be life threatening. Associated oliguria or anuria can worsen clearance of potassium as urine flow drops off. Hyperkalemia in tumor lysis should be managed in a similar fashion as hyperkalemia that is attributable to other causes (see Chapter 77).
In the absence of symptoms, it is not necessary to treat hypocalcemia in TLS. Worrisome clinical signs of symptomatic hypocalcemia include paresthesias, cramping, tetany, seizures, and a prolonged QT interval on electrocardiogram. Symptomatic hypocalcemia is rare in TLS. That being said, if symptoms are present, they should prompt calcium replacement. Electrocardiogram changes such as a prolonged PR interval, widened QRS complex, or peaked T waves in the setting of hyperkalemia would also be an indication for calcium therapy. Hyperphosphatemia in tumor lysis syndrome can be managed similarly to elevated phosphorus from other causes. If severe, aluminum hydroxide (600 mg/5 mL) at a starting dose of 30 mL three to four times daily, orally or via nasogastric tube, can be given. Unfortunately, phosphate binders are of limited value because they only bind gastrointestinal phosphorus. Hypocalcemia often resolves quickly after resolution of hyperphosphatemia.

11. **Once a patient has developed TLS, is there any therapy available to help protect the kidneys?**
Treatment of the metabolic sequelae of tumor lysis by increasing urinary flow with intravenous hydration and lowering uric acid with rasburicase is the key to preventing AKI in TLS. Dialysis may be necessary to reverse the metabolic derangements in TLS and can have some renal protective effects through removal of uric acid and phosphorus.

12. **What is the role for renal replacement therapy in the treatment and/or prevention of TLS?**

In general, indications for dialysis in patients with AKI secondary to TLS are similar to indications for dialysis in AKI from other causes. Indications include life-threatening hyperkalemia, volume overload refractory to diuretics, uremic pericarditis, or severe uremic encephalopathy. Dialysis has the added benefit of being able to clear uric acid and phosphorus from the extracellular space, which may help prevent further kidney damage. If rasburicase is not available, early hemodialysis for uric acid clearance should be considered and has been shown to increase urine output in oliguric AKI as the uric level falls below 10 mg/dL. Clearance rates of uric acid with hemodialysis (70–145 mL/min) are much greater than peritoneal dialysis (6–10 mL/min) and it is the renal replacement therapy of choice.

BIBLIOGRAPHY

1. Conger JD. Acute uric acid nephropathy. *Med Clin N Am* 1990;74(4):859–871.

2. Davidson MB, Thakkar S, Hix JK, et al. Pathophysiology, clinical consequences, and treatment of tumor lysis syndrome. *Am J Med* 2004;116:546–554.

3. Hochberg J, Cairo MS. Tumor lysis syndrome: Current perspective. *Hematologica* 2008;93(1):9–13.

4. Tosi P, Barosi G, Lazzaro C, et al. Consensus conference on the management of tumor lysis syndrome. *Haematologica* 2008;93:1877–1885.

CONTRAST-INDUCED NEPHROPATHY

Ami M. Patel, MD, and Michael R. Rudnick, MD

CHAPTER 14

1. **What is contrast-induced nephropathy (CIN), and how does it occur?**
   Iodinated contrast media can lead to a usually reversible form of acute renal injury that occurs soon after intravenous or intra-arterial administration of contrast. CIN does not occur with oral delivery of contrast media because it is not absorbed through the gut. Contrast media causes acute kidney injury (AKI) through two major mechanisms: renal vasoconstriction and direct tubular epithelial toxicity. After contrast administration, there is a transient increase in renal blood flow followed by a prolonged period of reduced flow resulting in renal ischemia. Contrast media stimulate release of vasoconstrictive mediators such as endothelin while blocking the release of vasodilatory ones such as prostaglandins and nitric oxide. The renal medulla, which is poorly oxygenated in normal condition, is susceptible to reduced oxygen delivery. Higher osmolar contrast can increase the work of active transporters in the medulla in response to the osmotic diuresis, which thereby reduces the oxygen tension further. This ischemic injury generates reactive oxygen species, which causes renal damage. Furthermore, contrast agents are directly toxic to renal epithelial cells, causing proximal tubular vacuolization, interstitial inflammation, and cellular necrosis.

2. **What is the typical clinical presentation of CIN? What is the differential diagnosis for renal failure following cardiac catheterization?**
   The differential diagnoses of renal failure following cardiac catheterization include ischemic acute tubular necrosis, cardiorenal syndrome, and renal atheroemboli/cholesterol emboli syndrome. The presence of diffuse atherosclerosis predisposes a patient to renal atheroemboli, which is characterized by renal failure that usually occurs days to weeks after the procedure with little or no recovery of renal function. Other distinguishing features are the presence of embolic lesions (as on the toes and fingers), livedo reticularis, transient eosinophilia, hypocomplementemia, vague abdominal pain (due to small vessel ischemic disease), and Hollenhorst plaques (cholesterol emboli to retinal vessels).

3. **What are the risk factors for the development of CIN?**
   The main predisposing factor is pre-existing kidney disease with serum creatinine ≥ 1.5 mg/dL or estimated glomerular filtration rate below 60 mL/min/1.73 m^2. Because contrast media are eliminated renally, clearance of contrast is significantly reduced in renal disease, increasing the risk for CIN. The presence of diabetes further enhances this risk; however, diabetes itself without renal disease has not been associated with CIN. Any amount of contrast can cause CIN, but high doses of contrast, defined as higher than 140 mL, are associated with increased risk. Other important risk factors include advanced age, proteinuria, hypotension, volume depletion, congestive heart failure, nonsteroidal anti-inflammatory drugs (NSAIDs), and multiple myeloma.

4. **What prophylactic measures are recommended?**
   Volume expansion and removal of nephrotoxins, including NSAIDs, are the principal prophylactic measures to reduce the risk for CIN. The theoretic rationale behind volume expansion is that it should decrease the activity of the renin-angiotensin system, reduce the levels of vasoconstrictive mediators, and dilute the contrast media. Another prophylactic treatment is *N*-acetylcysteine (also known as Mucomyst), which can be used for its

antioxidative properties by increasing intracellular glutathione levels; thus, it is believed to decrease the production of reactive oxygen species. However, there are debatable results about the effectiveness of *N*-acetylcysteine because the drug undergoes significant first-pass metabolism when delivered orally. Nevertheless, *N*-acetylcysteine is considered safe and inexpensive, and we recommend prescribing *N*-acetylcysteine 1200 mg twice daily with two doses before and two doses after contrast administration.

KEY POINTS: CONTAST-INDUCED NEPHROPATHY

1. Contrast media cause acute kidney injury through two major mechanisms: renal vasoconstriction and direct tubular epithelial toxicity.

2. In most cases, contrast-induced nephropathy (CIN) is characterized by an elevation of creatinine within 24 to 48 hours following exposure, reaching a peak within 3 to 5 days, followed by a return to baseline within 7 to 10 days. Typically, the urinalysis is characterized by coarse granular casts and renal tubular epithelial cells along with a high specific gravity and fractional excretion of sodium <1%.

3. The main predisposing factor for CIN is preexisting kidney disease with serum creatinine ≥1.5 mg/dL or estimated glomerular filtration rate <60 mL/min/1.73 m^2. Other risk factors include diabetes, high contrast load, advanced age, proteinuria, hypotension, volume depletion, congestive heart failure, nonsteroidal anti-inflammatory drug (NSAID) use, and multiple myeloma.

4. Volume expansion and removal of nephrotoxins including NSAIDs are the principal prophylactic measures to reduce the risk for CIN. Although studies have shown conflicting outcomes in regards to whether isotonic bicarbonate is superior to isotonic saline, we suggest using isotonic sodium bicarbonate unless there is a coexisting metabolic alkalosis.

5. Another prophylactic treatment is *N*-acetylcysteine (also known as Mucomyst), which can be used for its antioxidative properties. Although there are debatable results about its effectiveness, *N*-acetylcysteine is generally recommended because it is safe and inexpensive.

5. **What kind of hydration is recommended?**
Isotonic sodium bicarbonate has recently been recommended over isotonic saline. The basis for this suggestion is that the generation of reactive oxygen species is pH dependent, and systemic alkalinization is believed to decrease the level of reactive oxygen species, thereby decreasing the risk of CIN. However, several studies have shown conflicting outcomes in regards to whether isotonic bicarbonate is superior to isotonic saline. If there is no contraindication such as coexisting metabolic alkalosis, we suggest using isotonic bicarbonate 3 mL/kg for 1 hour precontrast and 1 mL/kg/hour for 6 hours postcontrast.

6. **What other therapies are available to reduce CIN risk and how effective are they?**
Several classes of pharmacologic agents have been reported to have effects on CIN prevention including theophylline and diuretics. Theophylline has been examined as a prophylactic treatment for CIN because of its effect on renal vasodilation through nonselective blockage of adenosine receptor; however, it is not generally recommended because of its potential drug-related toxicity when administered intravenously (such as ventricular arrhythmias, seizures, and shock). Likewise, mannitol and furosemide were hypothesized to decrease CIN by promoting renal vasodilation along with increasing diuresis, which then resulted in less contact time between the contrast and tubular epithelium. However, a prospective randomized

trial demonstrated that saline alone was as effective or superior than saline with mannitol or furosemide, and in fact diuretics may enhance renal toxicity. Other therapies that are considered ineffective include dopamine, atrial natriuretic peptide, fenoldopam, and endothelin receptor antagonist.

7. **Does hemodialysis prevent CIN?**
   The use of hemodialysis or hemofiltration for the prevention of CIN is currently a controversial issue. Although dialysis can remove a majority of the contrast media, a recent meta-analysis has failed to show that periprocedural dialysis decreases the risk for CIN. One explanation for this finding is that there is an immediate hemodynamic change in the renal vasculature within seconds of contrast administration, and subsequent histopathologic changes occur within 15 minutes. It is unfeasible to arrange for dialysis within 30 minutes of contrast delivery, and there is significant associated risk involved with dialysis, such as catheter placement. Therefore, we do not generally recommend dialysis as a prophylactic treatment against CIN.

8. **Is there any benefit to discontinuing angiotensin-converting enzyme inhibitors/angiotensin receptor blockers (ACE-I/ARBs) prior to contrast exposure?**
   There are two opposing theories concerning the renal effects of ACE-I/ARBs in the setting of contrast administration. First, ACE-I/ARBs increase the risk of CIN because these drugs are associated with decreasing the glomerular filtration rate and thus often raising the serum creatinine. The second theory is that ACE-I/ARBs are protective against CIN by counteracting the afferent arteriolar vasoconstriction and the subsequent medullary ischemia precipitated with contrast. The current literature in regards to the value of withdrawing or giving ACE-I/ARBs prior to contrast exposure is inconclusive. Some research studies have indicated that there is a benefit for holding these drugs, whereas others showed no difference in outcome. Furthermore, a few studies exhibit that ACE-I/ARBs are protective against CIN. Many of these studies are flawed with retrospective data, presence of confounders, poor study design, and/or small heterogeneous study group. In a recent randomized controlled trial, discontinuing ACE-I/ARBs 24 hours prior to contrast administration did not reduce the incidence of CIN. Thus, we do not recommend holding these drugs, especially if they are critical for blood pressure control, unless there are issues with hyperkalemia and hypotension.

9. **Is there a role for statin therapy in preventing contrast nephropathy?**
   Statins were recently shown to possess pleiotropic effects including antioxidant and anti-inflammatory properties. Because reactive oxygen species are involved in the pathogenesis of CIN, statins were assumed to reduce the risk for CIN by scavenging oxygen-free radicals and stabilizing the endothelium. However, in recent randomized controlled trials, short-term high-dose statin therapy has failed to decrease the occurrence of CIN.

10. **What different types of iodinated contrast are available? Is there one contrast agent that is more nephrotoxic than others?**
    Clinical studies have suggested that the osmolality of contrast might have an impact on the development of CIN. Iodinated contrast media are either ionic or nonionic, and they are further classified by their osmolality. The first-generation contrast media were considered as high-osmolal agents with typical osmolar range of 1500 to 1800 mOsm/kg (whereas human plasma is 290 mOsm/kg) and were also ionic. In the 1980s, the second-generation contrast media replaced first-generation contrast because they were shown to be less nephrotoxic. They were known as low-osmolal agents with an osmolality around 600 to 700 mOsm/kg. The newest class or third generation of contrast media are referred to as iso-osmolol agents, such as iodixanol, with a typical osmolality around 290 mOsm/kg. The initial hypothesis was that iso-osmolal agents were less nephrotoxic than low-osmolal because of the lower osmolality; however, recent randomized control trials failed to show superiority of iso-osmolal agents over several specific low-osmolal agents (iopamidol, ioversol, and iopromide) in CIN prevention. Iso-osmolal agents can be more viscous, causing increased red blood cell aggregation and

decreased renal blood flow, offsetting any reduction in medullary hypoxia from the decreased osmolarity. However, there are varying renal toxicities associated with individual agents. The current recommendation by experts is to preferentially use specific (see above) low-osmolal or iso-osmolal agents rather than high-osmolal agents in patients at high risk.

11. **What is the treatment of CIN? Does CIN increase mortality?**
CIN is considered the third most common cause of renal failure in hospitalized patients, and there is no cure once CIN has occurred. The treatment is largely supportive, including withdrawal of concomitant nephrotoxins, treatment of hypotension, and initiation of dialysis if necessary. Those who develop CIN have a higher mortality risk, with the greatest risk in those who require dialysis. The in-hospital morality rates reported by McCullough et al. was 1.1% mortality with no CIN, 7.1% in nephropathy alone, and 35.7% for those with nephropathy requiring dialysis. Thus, CIN is associated with significant increase in morbidity and mortality, and for those patients at high risk for CIN, the risk and benefit of an iodinated contrast study should be assessed carefully. However, it is difficult to prove a causal relationship because the same risk factors that raise the risk of CIN are also associated with increased morbidity and mortality.

McCullough PA, Wolyn R, Rocher LL, Levin RN, et al. Acute renal failure after coronary intervention: Incidence, risk factors, and relationship to mortality. *Am J Med* 1997;103:368–375.

12. **What is gadolinium, and what risks are associated with it?**
Gadolinium is a lanthanide metal with paramagnetic properties, making it a suitable contrast agent. Initially gadolinium was assumed to be a safe alternative to iodinated contrast, but it can cause both AKI and nephrogenic systemic fibrosis (NSF). Subsequently, it has been demonstrated that gadolinium can also cause AKI, although it remains unclear if the risk is similar to iodinated contrast. As with iodinated contrast, impaired renal function decreases the clearance of gadolinium, increasing the risk for nephrotoxicity and NSF. NSF is a severe fibrosing disorder of the skin and systemic organs that can be debilitating and fatal. The majority of cases of NSF occur in patients with end-stage renal disease who were receiving dialysis, whereas a minority were associated with stage 5 chronic kidney disease and AKI. No cases have been reported with stage 1 to 3 chronic kidney disease, and only a few cases have occurred in stage 4 kidney disease. Experts recommend the following measures to reduce the risk of NSF: using a macrocyclic ionic chelate-based gadolinium rather than linear nonionic type, administering the lowest dosage possible, avoiding repeated exposures, and considering hemodialysis postexposure in patients at high risk. No current evidence supports the use of hemodialysis for the prevention of NSF, but in our opinion dialysis should be performed because there is increased clearance of gadolinium with dialysis.

BIBLIOGRAPHY

1. Brar SS, Hiremath S, Dangas G, et al. Sodium bicarbonate for the prevention of contrast induced-acute kidney injury: A systematic review and meta-analysis. *Clin J Am Soc Nephrol* 2009;4(10):1584–1592.

2. Cruz DN, Perazella MA, Bellomo R, et al. Extracorporeal blood purification therapies for prevention of radiocontrast-induced nephropathy: A systematic review. *Am J Kidney Dis* 2006;48(3):361–371.

3. Jefferson JA, Schrier RW. Pathophysiology and etiology of acute renal failure. In: Feehaly J, Floege J, Johnson R (eds.). *Comprehensive Clinical Nephrology*, 3rd ed. Philadelphia: Mosby Elsevier, 2007, pp. 755–770.

4. Jo S, Koo B, Park J, et al. Prevention of radiocontrast medium-induced nephropathy using short-term high-dose simvastatin in patients with renal insufficiency undergoing coronary angiography (PROMISS) trial—A randomized controlled study. *Am Heart J* 2008;155:499e1–499e8.

5. Katzberg RW, Haller C. Contrast-induced nephrotoxicity: Clinical landscape. *Kidney Int* 2006;69:S3–S7.

6. Kiski D, Stepper W, Brand E, et al. Impact of renin-angiotensin-aldosterone blockade by angiotensin-converting enzyme inhibitors or AT-1 blockers on frequency of contrast medium-induced nephropathy: A post-hoc analysis from the Dialysis-versus-Diuresis (DVD) trial. *Nephrol Dial Transplant* 2010;25:759–764.

7. Lameire N, Van Biesen W, Vanholder R. Epidemiology, clinical evaluation, and prevention of acute renal failure. In: Feehaly J, Floege J, Johnson R (eds.). *Comprehensive Clinical Nephrology*, 3rd ed. Philadelphia: Mosby Elsevier, 2007, pp. 771–785.

8. Maioli M, Toso A, Leoncini M, et al. Sodium bicarbonate versus saline for the prevention of contrast-induced nephropathy in patients with renal dysfunction undergoing coronary angiography or intervention. *J Am Coll Cardiol* 2008;52:599–604.

9. Majumdar SR, Kjellstrand CM, Tymchak WJ, et al. Forced euvolemic diuresis with mannitol and furosemide for prevention of contrast-induced nephropathy in patients with CKD undergoing coronary angiography: A randomized controlled trial. *Am J Kidney Dis* 2009;54:602–609.

10. McCullough PA, Wolyn R, Rocher LL, et al. Acute renal failure after coronary intervention: incidence, risk factors, and relationship to mortality. *Am J Med* 1997;103:368–375.

11. Meier P, Ko DT, Tamura A, et al. Sodium bicarbonate-based hydration prevents contrast-induced nephropathy: A meta-analysis. *BMC Med* 2009;7:23.

12. Navaneethan SD, Singh S, Appasamy S, et al. Sodium bicarbonate therapy for prevention of contrast-induced nephropathy: A systematic review and meta-analysis. *Am J Kidney Dis* 2009;53:617–627.

13. Perazella MA. Current status of gadolinium toxicity in patients with kidney disease. *Clin J Am Soc Nephrol* 2009;4:461–469.

14. Persson PB, Tepel M. Contrast medium-induced nephropathy: The pathophysiology. *Kidney Int* 2006;69:S8–S10.

15. Rosenstock JL, Bruno R, Kim JK, et al. The effect of withdrawal of ACE inhibitors or angiotensin receptor blockers prior to coronary angiography on the incidence of contrast-induced nephropathy. *Int Urol Nephrol* 2008;40:749–755.

16. Rudnick M, Feldman H. Contrast-induced nephropathy: What are the true clinical consequences? *Clin J Am Soc Nephrol* 2008;3:263–272.

17. Rudnick MR, Kesselheim A, Goldfarb S. Contrast-induced nephropathy: How it develops, how to prevent it. *Cleve Clin J Med* 2006;73:75–87.

18. Solomon R. Preventing contrast-induced nephropathy: Problems, challenges and future directions. *BMC Med* 2009;7:24.

19. Sterling KA, Tehrani T, Rudnick MR. Clinical significance and preventive strategies for contrast-induced nephropathy. *Curr Opin Nephrol Hypertens* 2008;17:616–623.

20. Tepel M, Zidek W. *N*-Acetylcysteine in nephrology; contrast nephropathy and beyond. *Curr Opin Nephrol* 2004;13:649–654.

21. Toso A, Maioli M, Leoncini M, et al. Usefulness of atorvastatin (80 mg) in prevention of contrast-induced nephropathy in patients with chronic renal disease. *Am J Cardiol* 2010;105:288–292.

22. Trivedi H, Daram S, Szabo A, et al. High-dose *N*-acetylcysteine for the prevention of contrast-induced nephropathy. *Am J Med* 2009;122:874e9–874e15.

23. Wu S, Shah S, Sterling K, et al. Prevention of contrast-induced nephropathy. *US Nephrol* 2009;4:35–38.

CHAPTER 15

ACUTE GLOMERULONEPHRITIS AND RAPIDLY PROGRESSIVE GLOMERULONEPHRITIS

John R. Sedor, MD

1. **What is the syndrome of acute glomerulonephritis?**

   Acute glomerulonephritis is an acute kidney injury (AKI) syndrome characterized by the sudden onset of edema and new-onset or worsening hypertension. Urinalysis demonstrates an active sediment, including significant proteinuria (usually >30 mg/dL or 1+ on a semiquantitative scale), hematuria, and red cell casts. Patients with acute glomerulonephritis often are azotemic (i.e., they have elevated serum blood urea nitrogen and creatinine concentrations) and occasionally develop severe renal failure requiring dialysis. Acute glomerulonephritis can be a primary kidney disease, usually classified on the basis of renal histopathology, or can result from a number of systemic diseases. Although this chapter focuses on primary acute glomerulonephritis, the diagnostic and therapeutic approaches for renal-limited and systemic diseases are similar. The reader is referred to the Sections on primary and secondary glomerular disorders for more information.

2. **What are the major causes of acute glomerulonephritis? What approach should be used to develop an appropriate differential diagnosis?**

   Table 15-1 presents major causes of acute glomerulonephritis and uses serum complement levels as a tool to focus the differential diagnosis. Measuring serum complement levels (C3, C4) and/or activity (CH50) is a somewhat arbitrary choice of initial tests but provides a practical approach to diagnosis and management of the patient with presumptive glomerulonephritis.

   The history and physical examination can provide clues to the diagnosis of acute glomerulonephritis. Focusing on presence of skin lesions and concurrent disease in other organ systems can help determine if the cause of the acute glomerulonephritis syndrome is a result of renal-limited or systemic diseases. A focused laboratory examination, including serologic studies, directed by the findings in the patient's history and physical examination, can also be useful in establishing a diagnosis. Hematuria with dysmorphic red blood cells and red cell casts are usually detected on urinalysis. Moderate proteinuria, usually in the non-nephrotic range, is typical. Nephrotic-range proteinuria occurs in <30% of patients. Mild to severe azotemia is universally present. A renal biopsy is often indicated to establish or confirm the clinical diagnosis and direct treatment. The extent of acute inflammation and fibrosis present in the biopsy can provide important data on prognosis and can be used to project responsiveness to therapy.

3. **What are dysmorphic red cells?**

   Phase-contrast morphology can be used to characterize urinary erythrocyte morphology. Glomerular bleeding, a characteristic of glomerulonephritis, causes red cells in the urine to have a nonuniform morphology with irregular outlines and small blebs projecting from their surfaces (i.e., the red cells are "dysmorphic"). Red cells in the urine from nonglomerular bleeding in the urinary tract are uniform in shape and similar in appearance to red cells in the circulation. Urine can be analyzed by the clinical laboratory for the presence of dysmorphic red cells. The sensitivity, specificity, and predicative values for this test are limited, and results need to be interpreted in context of other clinical and diagnostic data.

TABLE 15-1.   CAUSES OF ACUTE GLOMERULONEPHRITIS (SEROLOGIC AND OTHER TESTS THAT PROVIDE DIAGNOSTIC CLUES)

	Low Serum Complement Level	Normal Serum Complement Level
Systemic diseases	Systemic lupus erythematosus (ANA, anti-DNA antibodies) Cryoglobulinemia (cryoglobulins) Henoch-Schönlein purpura Subacute bacterial endocarditis (positive blood cultures) "Shunt" nephritis (positive blood cultures)	Microscopic polyangiitis (ANCA) Wegener's granulomatosis (ANCA) Goodpasture syndrome (anti-GBM Ab) Hypersensitivity vasculitis Visceral abscess (positive blood cultures)
Primary renal diseases	Acute postinfectious glomerulo-nephritis (antistreptococcal Ab) Membranoproliferative glomerulonephritis Type I (C4Nef, C3Nef, NFt) Type II (C3Nef) Type III (NFt)	IgG-IgA nephropathy Idiopathic RPGN Type I: Anti-GBM disease (anti-GBM Ab) Type II: Immune complex/immune deposit disease Type III: Pauci-immune (ANCA)

Adapted from Waldman M, Schelling JR, Chung-Park M, et al. Immune-mediated and other glomerular diseases. In: Alpern RJ, Hebert SC (eds.). The Kidney Physiology and Pathophysiology, 4th ed. San Diego: Academic Press, 2008, p. 2400.

4. **Define the syndrome of rapidly progressive glomerulonephritis (RPGN).**
   Patients with RPGN have evidence of glomerular disease (proteinuria, hematuria, and red cell casts) accompanied by rapid loss of renal function over days to weeks. If untreated, RPGN often results in renal failure. The pathologic hallmark of RPGN is the presence of crescents on kidney biopsy, and RPGN is also described as crescentic nephritis (see later for further discussion). Fortunately, the disorders associated with this syndrome are rare, so that RPGN makes up only 2% to 4% of all cases of glomerulonephritis.

5. **What are crescents in renal biopsies?**
   Crescent formation is a nonspecific response to severe injury of the glomerular capillary wall. As a result, fibrin leaks into Bowman's space, causing parietal epithelial cells to proliferate and mononuclear phagocytes to migrate into the glomerular tuft from the circulation. Large crescents can compress glomerular capillaries and impair filtration. Although crescent formation can resolve, some inflammatory chemotactic signals recruit fibroblasts into Bowman's space, which ultimately can cause both the crescents and glomeruli to scar. Extensive scarring results in end-stage renal disease.

6. **Do crescentic nephritis and RPGN describe the same syndrome?**
   Although the terms crescentic nephritis and RPGN are used interchangeably, these diagnoses are not synonymous. RPGN describes a *clinical* syndrome of rapid loss of renal function over days to weeks in patients with evidence of glomerulonephritis. In contrast, crescentic nephritis is a *histopathologic* description of kidney biopsy specimens that demonstrate the presence of crescents in more than 50% of glomeruli. Biopsies of patients with RPGN very commonly

reveal crescentic nephritis. However, RPGN can occur in the absence of crescentic nephritis, and extensive glomerular crescent formation rarely is identified in kidney biopsy specimens from patients without the clinical syndrome of RPGN.

7. **How is primary RPGN classified?**
   RPGN can occur as a primary disorder in the absence of other glomerular or systemic diseases and is classified pathologically into three types using immunofluorescence microscopy to describe the presence or absence of immune deposits and the character of their distribution within the glomerular basement membrane (Tables 15-1 and 15-2). Type I RPGN is characterized by linear deposition of antibodies directed against type IV collagen, a matrix protein that is a constituent of the glomerular basement membrane (GBM). These antibodies are commonly referred to as anti-GBM antibodies (discussed later). Type I RPGN comprises approximately 20% of patients with primary RPGN without pulmonary hemorrhage. A granular or discrete pattern of immune complex deposition is detected in renal biopsies from an additional 30% of patients (type II RPGN). The remaining patients have type III RPGN, and no immune deposits ("pauci-immune") are detectable in glomeruli using immunofluorescence microscopy.

8. **What diseases are associated with RPGN ("secondary RPGN")?**
   RPGN can complicate the clinical course of some primary glomerular diseases such as immunoglobulin A (IgA) nephropathy, membranous nephropathy, membranoproliferative

---

TABLE 15-2.   CLASSIFICATION OF RPGN

PRIMARY
Type I: Anti-GBM antibody disease (Goodpasture disease)
Type II: Granular glomerular immune complex association
Type III: Pauci-immune glomerulonephritis

SECONDARY TO SYSTEMIC DISEASE
Superimposed on a primary glomerular disease
Postinfectious
   Poststreptococcal and postviral glomerulonephritis
   Visceral abscess
Vasculities:
   Small Vessel (Pauci-Immune):
      Microscopic polyangiitis
      Wegener's granulomatosis
      Churg-Strauss syndrome
   Small Vessel (Immune Complex):
      Systemic lupus erythematosus
      Henoch-Schönlein purpura
      Cryoglobulinemia
   Medium Vessel:
      Polyarteritis nodosa (rare)
   Goodpasture syndrome
   Carcinoma
   Medication-associated:
      Allopurinol
      Penicillamine

glomerulonephritis, and hereditary nephritis (Alport syndrome). In addition, RPGN is associated with infectious and multisystem diseases including systemic lupus erythematosus, cryoglobulinemia, and systemic vasculitides. Table 15-2 summarizes the renal-limited and systemic causes of RPGN.

9. **Aside from urinalysis, which other laboratory tests are useful in determining the etiology of acute glomerulonephritis?**
   Certain serologic studies or other laboratory tests may be useful in narrowing the differential diagnosis, but ordering these labs should be guided by the patient's history and clinical presentation. Complement levels (C3, C4) are usually normal in most patients with either primary RPGN or RPGN associated with systemic disease (Table 15-1). However, patients with underlying systemic lupus erythematosus often have depressed circulating C3 and C4 levels. In almost all patients, an antinuclear antibody level is a useful screen for lupus or other connective tissue diseases. Identification of circulating anti-GBM antibodies and antineutrophil cytoplasmic antibody (ANCA) can be useful in establishing a diagnosis in patients who present with RPGN. Patients who are ANCA positive frequently have a primary small vessel vasculitis, although disease may be limited to the kidney. The patient's clinical presentation also determines the predictive value of ANCA testing. For example, the predictive value of a positive ANCA test is low in a patient who presents with hematuria, proteinuria, and a normal creatinine than in a patient with similar urinalysis findings in the presence of azotemia. Laboratory testing to identify infections with *streptococcus,* hepatitis, or HIV or causes of autoimmune diseases in addition to lupus and ANCA vasculitis may be indicated.

10. **What are anti-GBM antibodies?**
    Anti-GBM antibodies are targeted toward the NC1 domain of the α3 chain of type IV collagen, which is a component of the GBM. Formation of the type IV collagen network in normal GBM sequesters these epitopes from the immune system, preventing tolerance during fetal development. Anti-GBM–associated disease probably occurs after the kidney is injured in some manner that exposes these regions of the collagen molecule, which is not recognized as "self" and generates an immune response. Anti-GBM antibodies are found in approximately 90% to 95% of patients with Goodpasture disease. On kidney biopsy, they form linear deposits of immunoglobulin along basement membranes detected by immunofluorescence.

11. **Are Goodpasture syndrome and anti-GBM glomerulonephritis (Goodpasture disease) the same?**
    No. Although both disease entities result from circulating anti-GBM antibodies, **Goodpasture syndrome** describes a systemic disease with a clinical constellation of pulmonary hemorrhage, circulating anti-GBM antibodies, and glomerulonephritis. Anti-GBM glomerulonephritis, or **Goodpasture disease,** is kidney-limited and describes a proliferative glomerulonephritis, which results from deposition of anti-GBM antibodies. Anti-GBM antibodies are the same in patients with Goodpasture syndrome and Goodpasture disease. Because alveolar basement membrane contains the epitope of type IV collagen that is recognized by anti-GBM antibodies, the variable presence of pulmonary disease seems to reflect whether alveolar basement membrane is accessible to the circulating anti-GBM antibodies. Alveolar injury from infections, smoking, toxins, or other underlying lung disease may predispose the lungs to deposition of anti-GBM antibodies.

12. **What are antineutrophil cytoplasmic antibodies?**
    Renal biopsies from patients with type III RPGN have no immune deposits, but type III RPGN usually results from small-vessel vasculitides associated with circulating ANCA. The ANCA-associated small vessel vasculitides are Wegener's granulomatosis, microscopic polyangiitis (systemic and renal-limited), and Churg-Strauss syndrome. These are often systemic diseases but can be limited to the kidney. ANCA are directed against neutrophil proteinase 3 (PR3) and myeloperoxidase (MPO). Screening for ANCA uses an indirect immunofluorescence examination of normal neutrophils, which, if positive, demonstrates a

staining pattern characteristic of the target antigen (cytoplasmic for ANCA against PR3 [C-ANCA] and perinuclear for anti-MPO ANCA [P-ANCA]). The P-ANCA screening test has low specificity because other antineutrophil antibodies give a similar pattern by indirect immunofluorescence. A screening test positive for either C-ANCA or P-ANCA needs confirmation with an antigen-specific technique.

13. **What is the treatment for acute glomerulonephritis?**
The treatment for acute glomerulonephritis is primarily supportive: diuretics to reduce the edema and antihypertensive drugs to reduce elevated blood pressure. Anti-inflammatory therapy with corticosteroids, cytotoxic agents, and other classes of immunosuppressive agents are used for some etiologies of acute glomerulonephritis. Therapeutic approaches for acute glomerulonephritis from systemic lupus nephritis and the pauci-immune vasculitides have been most extensively studied, and reasonable evidence from multicenter trials is available to guide treatment for these diseases. Treatment strategies used for other etiologies of acute glomerulonephritis are often based on observational studies of small numbers of patients. Approaches to therapy in children and adults with the same etiology of acute glomerulonephritis are not always identical.

14. **What are the treatment options for patients with RPGN?**
RPGN needs to be treated aggressively and early in its course to reduce the likelihood of end-stage renal failure. Glucocorticoid and immunosuppressive regimens are the mainstay of RPGN treatment. The benefit of these agents is particularly great in patients with ANCA-associated vasculitis. The most common complications of therapy are infections. Hemorrhagic cystitis, a complication of cyclophosphamide therapy, occurs less commonly with use of aggressive intravenous saline infusions to promote excretion of metabolites toxic to bladder epithelial cells. In addition, 2-mercaptoethanesulfonate (MESNA), an agent that binds and sequesters the metabolite responsible for injury to the uroepithelia, often is given concomitantly with cyclophosphamide. Malignancies, especially bladder cancers and leukemias, can occur decades after treatment of Wegener's granulomatosis with cyclophosphamide.

15. **Should treatment for RPGN be initiated prior to definitive diagnosis?**
Yes. Data obtained in experimental animal models of acute glomerulonephritis/crescentic nephritis show that fibrosis begins within days after disease initiation. Because patients usually present with evidence of active renal inflammation and often are azotemic, significant renal scarring has likely occurred by the time patients receive medical attention. Starting treatment should be viewed as urgent.

16. **What is appropriate empiric therapy for patients with acute glomerulonephritis or RPGN?**
Renal biopsy should be performed expeditiously and appropriate laboratory studies should be sent when the patient presents. While waiting for these results, initiation of steroid therapy, the mainstay inductive anti-inflammatory therapy for most acute inflammatory glomerular diseases, is reasonable. Toxicities from high-dose steroid therapy are minimal and manageable during this short "window" between patient presentation and obtaining diagnostic test results. Initiation of cytotoxic or other immunosuppressive treatments, which consolidate treatment response to steroids, or plasma exchange should wait until definitive diagnosis is established. Analysis of clinical trials outcomes for some glomerular diseases suggests that benefit from cytotoxic drugs occurs well after disease onset, and most experts feel use of these agents can be delayed until diagnosis is established. Dosing for cyclophosphamide must be adjusted in the patient with renal insufficiency to avoid leukopenia.

17. **Is there any role for plasma exchange in the therapy for RPGN?**
Plasma exchange is thought to remove circulating pathogenic autoantibodies from the circulation. Trials evaluating efficacy of plasma exchange for all causes of RPGN have been small. However, plasma exchange is a safe procedure in experienced centers and may be an appropriate therapeutic

modality for subsets of patients with RPGN, in view of the high risk of renal failure with this syndrome. The European Vasculitis Study Group published a randomized trial that demonstrated that adjunctive plasma exchange improved renal outcomes in patients with severe renal failure (serum creatinine >2.3 mg/dL) and active ANCA vasculitis. In addition, prompt initiation of plasma exchange and aggressive immunosuppression with corticosteroids and cyclophosphamide can be lifesaving in patients with ANCA vasculitis and diffuse alveolar hemorrhage. Patients who are dialysis dependent with ANCA vasculitis can respond to treatment (see question 18).

Plasma exchange and immunosuppressive therapy are standard treatments for patients with anti-GBM antibody disease. Most evidence supporting use of plasma exchange in anti-GBM–associated diseases is from case reports, although one small, randomized, controlled trial demonstrated a nonsignificant trend toward improved outcome in patients treated with plasma exchange. Patients who are dialysis dependent with anti-GBM disease are unlikely to respond to aggressive treatment, and the potential benefit of treatment does not outweigh risk in these individuals (see question 18).

KEY POINTS: ACUTE GLOMERULONEPHRITIS AND RAPIDLY PROGRESSIVE GLOMERULONEPHRITIS

1. Acute glomerulonephritis is an acute kidney injury syndrome characterized by the sudden onset of edema, new onset or worsening hypertension, and the presence of an active urinary sediment.

2. Rapidly progressive glomerulonephritis is a clinical syndrome characterized by rapid loss of renal function that often results in end-stage renal disease.

3. If you think a patient has RPGN, early diagnosis and initiation of therapy is vital because early intervention is associated with better outcomes.

4. Steroid treatment can be initiated prior to establishing a definitive diagnosis.

5. Plasma exchange improves outcomes in patients with active renal vasculitis and severe renal failure.

18. **What is the prognosis of RPGN?**
Prognosis and response to treatment in patients with anti-GBM antibody or Goodpasture disease have not been studied in large trials. Data from a number of small case series with similar, but not identical, treatment strategies suggest that patient survivals are high (70%–90%). Overall, only 40% of patients remain off dialysis at 1 year after presentation. However, patients who do not require dialysis and who are treated with immunosuppression and plasma exchange have 1-year renal survivals of approximately 70% to 75%, even if renal failure is severe. In contrast, renal survival is poor in patients with anti-GBM antibody–associated disease, who require dialysis within 72 hours of presentation. Aggressive therapy with immunosuppressive drugs and plasma exchange may not be appropriate in this subgroup of anti-GBM antibody patients, unless significant acute tubular necrosis, in addition to crescentic nephritis, is demonstrated on renal biopsy. Clinical, laboratory, and pathologic parameters do not have predictive value for renal outcome to be used in an individual patient.

Although data on patients with kidney-limited, ANCA-positive RPGN are limited, treatment responses have been reported recently in several cohorts of patients with ANCA-associated necrotizing glomerulonephritis and either Wegener's granulomatosis or microscopic polyangiitis. Many patients (approximately 75%) achieve remission after induction therapy, but only 40% to 50% remain in long-term remission after 4 to 10 years. Serum creatinine at presentation is the strongest predictor of renal survival in patients who are ANCA positive. In contrast to patients with anti-GBM glomerulonephritis, patients with ANCA-associated glomerulonephritis can respond to therapy even if they have already required initiation of dialysis.

BIBLIOGRAPHY

1. Dooley MA, Falk RJ. Human clinical trials in lupus nephritis. *Semin Nephrol* 2007;27:115–127.

2. Hudson BG, Tryggvason K, Sundaramoorthy M, et al. Alport's syndrome, Goodpasture's syndrome, and type IV collagen. *N Engl J Med* 2003;348:2543–2456.

3. Jayne DRW, Gaskin G, Rasmussen N, et al. Randomized trial of plasma exchange or high-dosage methylprednisolone as adjunctive therapy for severe renal vasculitis. *J Am Soc Nephrol* 2007;18:2180–2188.

4. Klemmer PJ, Chalermskulrat W, Reif MS, et al. Plasmapheresis therapy for diffuse alveolar hemorrhage in patients with small-vessel vasculitis. *Am J Kidney Dis* 2003;42:1149–1153.

5. Levy JB, Turner AN, Rees AJ, et al. Long-term outcome of anti-glomerular basement membrane antibody disease treated with plasma exchange and immunosuppression. *Ann Intern Med* 2001;134:1033–1042.

6. Madaio MP, Harrington JT. The diagnosis of glomerular diseases: Acute glomerulonephritis and the nephrotic syndrome. *Arch Intern Med* 2001;161:25–34.

7. Savige J, Davies D, Falk RJ, et al. Antineutrophil cytoplasmic antibodies and associated diseases: A review of the clinical and laboratory features. *Kidney Int* 2000;57:846–862.

8. Salant DJ. Intravenous methylprednisolone or plasma exchange for adjunctive therapy of severe renal vasculitis? *Nat Clin Pract Nephrol* 2008;4:14–15.

9. Waldman M, Schelling JR, Chung-Park M, et al. Immune-mediated and other glomerular diseases. In: Alpern RJ, Hebert SC (eds.). *The Kidney Physiology and Pathophysiology*, 4th ed. San Diego: Academic Press, 2008, pp. 2399–2445.

NEPHROTIC SYNDROME

Howard Trachtman, MD

CHAPTER 16

1. What is nephrotic syndrome?

Nephrotic syndrome is one of the most rigidly defined entities in clinical medicine. Specifically, it comprises four distinct elements: edema, massive proteinuria, hypoalbuminemia, and hypercholesterolemia. A hypercoagulable state is an optional fifth feature, especially in adults who have a 10-fold higher risk of thromboembolic complications compared to pediatric patients. The hypercoagulable state in the nephrotic syndrome is the result of many factors including urinary loss of antithrombin III, increased platelet aggregation, and endothelial dysfunction. It is important to note that reduced glomerular filtration rate (GFR) or azotemia is not a defining feature of the nephrotic syndrome in any age group.

2. How does one make the diagnosis of the nephrotic syndrome?

The diagnosis is made in a patient with edema and in whom there is massive proteinuria (i.e., a urine protein:creatinine ratio greater than 2 [mg:mg] in a first morning sample). Quantitation of urine protein excretion is mandatory to confirm the diagnosis of new-onset nephrotic syndrome. However, subsequent monitoring can be accomplished using qualitative dipstick urine testing. It is important to exclude cirrhosis, congestive heart failure, or gastrointestinal disease (protein-losing enteropathy or malabsorption) before conclusively attributing edema to a renal cause.

3. What are the causes of nephrotic syndrome?

The cause of primary nephrotic syndrome is generally unknown. Nephrotic syndrome is classified into primary (or idiopathic) and secondary causes. There are four principal primary etiologies of nephrotic syndrome: minimal change nephrotic syndrome (MCNS), focal segmental glomerulosclerosis (FSGS), membranous nephropathy (MN), and membranoproliferative glomerulonephritis (MPGN) (Table 16-1). Variants of MCNS are characterized by subtle changes in mesangial cell hypercellularity or deposition of specific immunoglobulins such as immunoglobulin M (IgM). However, the clinical significance of these entities is unclear. In MCNS, an immune-mediated mechanism has been proposed based on the association of the disease with atopy, various malignancies, and the response to immunosuppressive medications. In addition, a variety of permeability factors including vascular endothelial growth factor (VEGF) and interleukin-8 (IL-8), presumably derived from immunoeffector cells, has been linked to proteinuria.

Genetic mutations (see later) are increasingly recognized as the cause of primary FSGS.

The pathogenesis of idiopathic membranous nephropathy may be linked to the development of antibodies to M-type phospholipase A2 receptor.

Types I and III MPGN are immune-complex disorders, whereas type II disease is associated with abnormal regulation of the alternative pathway of complement.

In adults, IgA nephropathy, fibrillary, and immunotactoid glomerulonephritis can present with nephrotic syndrome.

The secondary causes of nephrotic syndrome include postinfectious glomerulonephritis, systemic lupus erythematosus, Henoch-Schönlein purpura, medications, infections (e.g., hepatitis B, HIV) malignancies (Hodgkin's lymphoma), amyloidosis, and diabetes. This

TABLE 16-1. COMMON GLOMERULAR DISEASES PRESENTING AS NEPHROTIC SYNDROME IN ADULTS

Disease	Associations	Serologic Tests Helpful in Diagnosis
Minimal change disease	Allergy, atopy, NSAIDs, Hodgkin's lymphoma	None
Focal segmental glomerulonephritis	African Americans HIV infection Heroin	— HIV antibody —
Membranous nephropathy	Drugs: gold, penicillamine, NSAIDs Infections: hepatitis B, C; malaria Lupus nephritis Malignancy: breast, lung, gastrointestinal tract	— Hepatitis B surface antigen, anti-HCV antibody Anti-DNA antibody —
Membranoproliferative glomerulonephritis (type I)	C4 nephritic factor	C3 ↓, C4 ↓
Membranoproliferative glomerulonephritis (type II)	C3 nephritic factor	C3 ↓, C4 normal
Cryoglobulinemic MPGN	Hepatitis C	Anti-HCV antibody, rheumatoid factor, C3 ↓, C4 ↓, CH_{50} ↓
Amyloid	Myeloma Rheumatoid arthritis, bronchiectasis, Crohn's disease (and other chronic inflammatory conditions), familial Mediterranean fever	Serum protein electrophoresis, urine immunoelectrophoresis —
Diabetic nephropathy	Other diabetic microangiopathy	None

NSAIDs = nonsteroidal anti-inflammatory drugs; HCV = hepatitis C virus; = MPGN = membranoproliferative glomerulonephritis.
From Johnson RJ, Feehally J. *Comprehensive Clinical Nephrology*, 2nd ed. Philadelphia: Mosby, 2003.

chapter will focus on primary nephrotic syndrome as a group because the secondary causes are detailed in specific chapters for each entity.

4. **Is there a genetic contribution to nephrotic syndrome?**
In nearly 30% to 40% of cases of primary FSGS, genetic mutations in podocyte proteins have been identified. The most commonly affected protein is podocin, detected in up to 20% of sporadic and familial cases. Other proteins linked to FSGS include α-actinin-4, CD2AP, Wilms' tumor-1 (WT-1), phospholipase C epsilon1 (PLICE1), TRPC6, and the formin gene INF2. Defects in the nephrin gene are associated with congenital nephrotic syndrome and disease in the first year of life. Currently, the role of genetic testing in patients with new-onset nephrotic

syndrome that is resistant to corticosteroids is subject to ongoing debate. Patients with nephrotic syndrome who have a genetic basis for the disease may have a lower response rate to immunosuppressive therapy but may also have a lower risk of recurrent disease following transplantation.

5. **What is the incidence and prevalence of nephrotic syndrome? Has it changed in recent years?**
The incidence of nephrotic syndrome is approximately two to four new cases per 100,000 population per year. This overall figure has been fairly steady and is applicable around the world and in all ethnic groups. There may be a difference in the incidence of specific types of primary nephrotic syndrome with a rising incidence of FSGS in African American compared to white patients. Nephrotic syndrome represents a prevalent cause of end-stage renal disease (ESRD) in children and adults. The prevalence of nephrotic syndrome as a cause of chronic kidney disease will vary from country to country depending on the practice patterns for disease detection and treatment. Nonetheless, primary nephrotic syndrome is an uncommon illness and qualifies for designation as a rare disease.

6. **What is the clinical presentation of patients with nephrotic syndrome?**
The most common presenting complaint for patients with nephrotic syndrome is edema. It usually involves the lower extremities in adults, whereas children may have a greater propensity to periorbital edema and ascites because of their increased physical activity. The edema is symmetric and painless.

7. **Are there extrarenal manifestations of nephrotic syndrome?**
Less common presentations include peritonitis, which can occur before implementation of immunosuppressive therapy, and thromboembolic events. The latter complaint is much more common in adults. In addition, patients with unremitting nephrotic syndrome and persistent hypercholesterolemia are at risk of premature atherosclerosis and cardiovascular disease.

8. **What is the natural history of nephrotic syndrome?**
The natural history of the primary nephrotic syndrome depends on the underlying cause. Patients with MCNS have an excellent long-term prognosis. Most patients are responsive to therapy and, although it may follow a relapsing course, eventually most patients outgrow the disease without any permanent renal injury. However, some children with MCNS continue to have relapsing disease well into adulthood. Nearly half of patients with primary FSGS will progress to ESRD over 5 to 10 years of follow-up, and 25% to 30% of these patients may experience recurrent disease in a kidney transplant. Similarly, nearly 50% of patients with MPGN will progress to ESRD over 10 to 15 years of follow-up, and 20% to 25% of these patients may experience recurrent disease in a kidney transplant. The long-term course of membranous nephropathy is more variable. Approximately one third will go into remission, another third have persistent proteinuria with stable kidney function, and the remaining patients will experience a steady decline in kidney function.

9. **Are there any patient groups at special risk of developing nephrotic syndrome or adverse long-term outcomes?**
Primary nephrotic syndrome occurs in all racial ethnic groups. It affects boys more commonly than girls; however, the outcomes are similar, irrespective of the patient's gender.

10. **What is the appropriate workup for patients with nephrotic syndrome?**
Patients with primary nephrotic syndrome require quantitation of urine protein excretion to demonstrate nephrotic-range proteinuria. This can be accomplished by measuring the protein:creatinine ratio in the first morning urine specimen, with a value >2 mg:mg indicative

of nephrotic syndrome. Alternatively, a 24-hour urine collection can be performed, and a level of protein in excess of 1 g/m^2 per 24 hours is diagnostic of nephrotic syndrome. A complete metabolic profile is obtained to demonstrate hypoalbuminemia and hypercholesterolemia. The blood urea nitrogen and creatinine are generally normal. The total serum calcium level is low secondary to hypoalbuminemia. The serum sodium concentration may be low if there is water reabsorption in excess of sodium. Artifactual hyponatremia secondary to hyperlipidemia is no longer a concern with the widespread use of ion-selective electrodes in clinical chemistry analyzers. The C3 level is measured in all patients to exclude MPGN. A complete blood count is part of the routine evaluation, although it usually has little information value about the cause of nephrotic syndrome.

11. **Are there any unique laboratory tests that are relevant to patients with nephrotic syndrome?**
    Ancillary studies such as antistreptolysin O (ASLO), antinuclear antibody, and double-stranded DNA titers are obtained if there are clinical features suggestive of a secondary cause of nephrotic syndrome. Under these circumstances, measurement of C3 level can be used to guide the need for further serologic studies. Testing for other secondary causes of nephrotic syndrome, such as HIV infection or hepatitis B and C, should be guided by the clinical scenario or specific findings in the kidney biopsy. A complement protein profile and assays for C3 nephritic factor are performed in children and adults with MPGN. Measurement of antibodies to M-type phospholipase A(2) receptor (PLA(2)R) may be useful in the diagnosis of idiopathic membranous nephropathy. Venography is often performed routinely in adults with new-onset primary nephrotic syndrome to detect renal vein thrombosis, especially in patients with membranous nephropathy.

12. **What is the role of a kidney biopsy in the assessment of patients with nephrotic syndrome?**
    A kidney biopsy is necessary to definitely distinguish between the four causes of primary nephrotic syndrome. There are differences in the application of renal biopsy in pediatric and adult patients. In children, criteria for performing a kidney biopsy prior to treatment include age younger than 6 months, onset in adolescence, a low C3 level, or any unusual clinical feature. Otherwise, most pediatric nephrologists defer a kidney biopsy in a patient with new-onset nephrotic syndrome until after completion of a course of steroids and verification of resistance to this treatment. The underlying rationale for this approach is the high frequency of MCNS in children with new-onset nephrotic syndrome. Moreover, a standard course of steroids will not modify the underlying renal histopathology if there is a lesion other than MCNS. Thus, a kidney biopsy is not an urgent procedure under these circumstances. Patients with nephrotic syndrome who require a biopsy but who have a relative contraindication to the procedure such as a solitary kidney or a bleeding diathesis may need to have the procedure done under more controlled conditions (i.e., as an operative procedure or under direct visualization). In contrast, in adults with nephrotic syndrome, because of the more diverse pathology and the reduced tolerance to corticosteroids, a renal biopsy is often done prior to initiation of any therapy. The tissue sample should be processed for light microscopy, immunofluorescence, and electron microscopy to establish the diagnosis. Special stains for glomerular proteins such as synaptopodin and dystroglycan may help discriminate among the causes of primary nephrotic syndrome.

13. **What is the first-line treatment for nephrotic syndrome?**
    Corticosteroids are generally considered the first agent to be tried to reduce proteinuria in all patients with nephrotic syndrome, unless there is a clinical contraindication to their use. The dose and duration of therapy is highly contingent on the age of the patient, and the likelihood of response varies from greater than 90% in children with MCNS to less than 20% in patients with FSGS.

KEY POINTS: NEPHROTIC SYNDROME

1. The nephrotic syndrome comprises four distinct elements: edema, massive proteinuria, hypoalbuminemia, and hypercholesterolemia, with an optional fifth feature, a hypercoagulable state.

2. Nephrotic syndrome is classified into primary (or idiopathic) and secondary causes, with four principal primary etiologies: minimal change nephrotic syndrome (MCNS), focal segmental glomerulosclerosis (FSGS), membranous nephropathy (MN), and membranoproliferative glomerulonephritis (MPGN).

3. A kidney biopsy is necessary to definitely distinguish between the four causes of primary nephrotic syndrome or confirm a secondary cause.

4. The natural history of the primary nephrotic syndrome depends on the underlying cause. Thus, patients with MCNS have an excellent long-term prognosis in contrast to those with primary FSGS, in whom nearly 50% will progress to ESRD over 5 to 10 years of follow-up, and 25% to 30% of these patients may experience recurrent disease in a kidney transplant.

5. Corticosteroids are generally considered the first agent tried to reduce proteinuria in all patients with nephrotic syndrome, unless there is a clinical contraindication to their use.

14. **What are the second-line therapies for nephrotic syndrome?**
The choice of therapy in patients with steroid-resistant nephrotic syndrome is a highly contentious topic because of a lack of sufficiently powered clinical trials. Alternative therapies are applied in MCNS in children who are suffering intolerable side effects from steroids. These patients respond well to mycophenolate mofetil, cyclophosphamide, or calcineurin inhibitors. Cyclosporine is the only agent that has been proven to be superior to placebo in patients with FSGS. In those with membranous nephropathy, combined therapy with steroids and an alkylating agent may be effective in patients at high risk of progressive deterioration in kidney function. In those with MPGN, a regimen involving steroids, antiplatelet drugs, and an alkylating agent has been utilized with uncertain efficacy.

15. **What is appropriate supportive care for patients with nephrotic syndrome?**
Patients who have edema from nephrotic syndrome require dietary sodium restriction and judicious use of diuretics. These agents are often needed in combination (site of action in the loop of Henle and distal tubule), and careful monitoring for hyponatremia, hypokalemia, and metabolic alkalosis is mandatory. Angiotensin-converting enzyme inhibitors and angiotensin receptor blockers can be used to lower blood pressure and reduce urinary protein excretion. Hypercholesterolemia can be treated with an HMG-CoA reductase inhibitor—namely, a statin. Immunization against *S. pneumoniae* should be administered to prevent bacterial infections such as peritonitis. In select cases, prophylactic antibiotics may be necessary. Careful surveillance for thromboembolic complications and administration of anticoagulants may be needed in adult patients.

16. **What is the role of kidney transplantation in the treatment of patients with nephrotic syndrome?**
Kidney transplantation is a viable option in all patients with nephrotic syndrome who progress to ESRD. However, there is a substantial risk of recurrent disease that is in the range of 20% to 40% for patients with FSGS and MPGN. Thus, patients who have lost more than one kidney allograft to recurrent glomerular disease are often considered ineligible for subsequent transplant procedures.

17. Are there novel therapies for nephrotic syndrome that are under development?
Rituximab, a monoclonal antibody to CD20 on B cells, is being tested in the full array of causes of nephrotic syndrome. Strategies to prevent renal fibrosis using thiazolidinediones (rosiglitazone) and monoclonal antitumor necrosis factor antibodies (adalimumab) are under evaluation to protect the kidney in resistant forms of nephrotic syndrome.

BIBLIOGRAPHY

1. Barisoni L, Schnaper HW, Kopp JB. Advances in the biology and genetics of the podocytopathies: Implications for diagnosis and therapy. *Arch Pathol Lab Med* 2009;133:201–216.

2. Beck LH Jr, Bonegio RG, Lambeau G, et al. M-type phospholipase A2 receptor as a target antigen in idiopathic membranous nephropathy. *N Engl J Med* 2009;361:11–21.

3. Chesney RW. The changing face of childhood nephrotic syndrome. *Kidney Int* 2004;66:1294–1302.

4. Fakhouri F, Bocqueret N, Taupin P, et al. Children with steroid-sensitive nephrotic syndrome come of age: Long-term outcome. *J Pediatr* 2005;147:202–207.

5. Giannico G, Yang H, Neilson EG, et al. Dystroglycan in the diagnosis of FSGS. *Clin J Am Soc Nephrol* 2009;4:1747–1753.

6. Hlatky M. Is renal biopsy necessary in adults with nephrotic syndrome? *Lancet* 1982;310:1264–1268.

7. Knebelmann B, Broyer M, Grunfeld JP, et al. Steroid-sensitive nephrotic syndrome: From childhood to adulthood. *Am J Kidney Dis* 2003;41:550–557.

8. Orth SR, Ritz E. The nephrotic syndrome. *N Engl J Med* 1998;338:1202–1211.

9. Ruth EM, Landolt MA, Neuhaus TJ, et al. Health-related quality of life and psychosocial adjustment in steroid-sensitive nephrotic syndrome. *J Pediatr* 2004;145:778–783.

10. Stadermann MB, Lilien MR, van de Kar NCAJ, et al. Is biopsy required prior to cyclophosphamide in steroid-sensitive nephrotic syndrome? *Clin Nephrol* 2003;60:315–317.

OBSTRUCTIVE UROPATHY

Mathew D. Sorensen, MD, and Marshall L. Stoller, MD

CHAPTER 17

1. What is obstructive uropathy?

Obstructive uropathy is structural or functional interference with normal urine flow anywhere along the urinary tract.

2. What is obstructive nephropathy?

Long-standing obstructive uropathy may ultimately lead to renal damage. Obstructive nephropathy typically involves dilation of the collecting system and tubules with progressive ischemia of the cells of the renal tubules leading to atrophy and interstitial fibrosis.

3. What are the most common causes of obstructive uropathy?

The causes of obstructive uropathy vary with age and gender. In older men, benign prostatic hypertrophy and prostate cancer are the most common causes. In young men and women, nephrolithiasis is the most common cause. In children obstruction is most often a result of congenital obstructions such as ureteropelvic junction obstruction and posterior urethral valves in newborn boys. Obstruction is common in pregnancy, although it is rarely clinically significant. This is hypothesized to result from hormonal changes (progesterone) and mechanical extrinsic compression from the uterus.

4. What is a normal and abnormal postvoid residual?

Normal patients should have the ability to void at least 80% of their bladder volume with a postvoid residual of less than 50 cc. With bladder outlet obstruction or poor bladder contractility, however, the efficiency of bladder emptying may decrease and residual urine may increase. An elevated postvoid residual is associated with increased risk of infection and can lead to bladder decompensation.

5. Is pain always present in obstructive uropathy?

The pain in urinary tract obstruction is a result of distention of the collecting system. If obstruction and distention occur acutely, then pain can be excruciating. However, if obstruction is slowly progressive, then the process can be painless.

6. What happens to the ureteral physiology proximal to an obstructing ureteral stone?

There is progressive dilation of the ureter with an increase in intraluminal resting pressure. This results in a decrease in the difference between the ureteral contractile pressure and the ureteral resting pressure. As the ureter dilates, there is ineffective coaptation of the ureteral walls resulting in ineffective peristalsis. With prolonged obstruction, peristalsis decreases such that urine transport depends entirely on hydrostatic forces from the kidney.

7. What happens to ureteral peristalsis with ureteral obstruction and after obstruction is relieved?

Ureteral peristalsis is triggered by calcium-dependent pacemaker cells in ureteral smooth muscle. With obstruction, ureteral peristalsis increases in amplitude and frequency. Peristalsis decreases with chronic obstruction and may cease entirely with concurrent infection. Immediately after the obstruction is relieved, peristalsis slowly normalizes.

8. **What are the contributors to the glomerular filtration rate?**
Glomerular filtration rate (GFR) is determined by glomerular capillary pressure (P_{GC}) as the primary driving force for GFR. This is inhibited by the hydrostatic pressure within the tubule (P_T) and the oncotic pressure in the glomerulus (π_{GC}). GFR is also dependent on the permeability of the glomerular basement membrane (Kf):

$$GFR = Kf(P_{GC} - P_T - \pi_{GC})$$

9. **What effect do changes to the afferent and efferent arterioles have on GFR?**
The afferent arteriole is primarily mediated by the presence (or inhibition) of prostacyclin and prostaglandins, which exert a vasodilatory effect, causing increased renal blood flow and increased GFR. The efferent arteriole is primarily mediated by angiotensin II and with vasoconstriction there is an increase in GFR.

10. **What happens to GFR and renal blood flow with acute urinary obstruction?**
Single-nephron GFR decreases with obstruction primarily because of an increase in tubular pressure. An acute release of prostacyclin and prostaglandin E2 causes afferent arteriolar dilation and an increase in renal blood flow of up to 40% in an attempt to maintain GFR.

11. **What happens to GFR and renal blood flow with prolonged urinary obstruction?**
With prolonged obstruction the efferent arteriole constricts as a result of increased angiotensin II levels. This further contributes to increase GFR but results in increased vascular resistance and ultimately a decrease in renal blood flow. Ultimate recovery of function is based on the degree and duration of obstruction and the patient age and baseline renal function. Animal studies and human case reports describe some potential recovery of renal function as long as 6 to 8 weeks after complete obstruction, but longer periods of obstruction are associated with diminished return of GFR.

12. **How are unilateral ureteral obstruction and bilateral ureteral obstruction similar?**
Both unilateral and bilateral ureteral obstruction are marked by a decrease in GFR resulting from an increase in intratubular pressure. Compensatory afferent arteriolar dilation and an increase in renal blood flow occur. With prolonged obstruction there is an increase in renin release and activation of the renin-angiotensin-aldosterone system.

13. **How are unilateral ureteral obstruction and bilateral ureteral obstruction different?**
In unilateral ureteral obstruction the renin release from the obstructed kidney causes a compensatory increase in renal blood flow and GFR in the contralateral kidney. Overall there is little change to total GFR, urine output, electrolyte levels, or serum creatinine. In bilateral ureteral obstruction there is no compensation by the contralateral kidney. Thus there can be dramatic decreases in GFR and urine output with electrolyte abnormalities, creatinine elevation, and fluid retention as a result of release of atrial natriuretic peptide.

14. **What are the contributors to the hypertension seen in bilateral ureteral obstruction?**
Hypertension is initially a result of elevated renin levels and later of fluid retention.

15. **What electrolyte abnormalities are seen in obstructive uropathy?**
Obstructive uropathy is often associated with hyperkalemia and metabolic acidosis resulting from defects in the excretion of potassium and hydrogen in the distal convoluted tubules from relative resistance to aldosterone.

16. **What is the most common complication of obstructive uropathy?**
Urinary tract infection is the most common complication of urinary tract obstruction and results from stasis of urine. Elimination of infection is difficult until the obstruction is relieved.

KEY POINTS: OBSTRUCTIVE UROPATHY

1. Long-standing urinary tract obstruction can lead to renal damage.

2. Acute urinary obstruction is often associated with pain, whereas chronic urinary obstruction may be asymptomatic.

3. Ultimate recovery of renal function after obstruction is based on the degree and duration of obstruction and the patient age and baseline renal function.

4. Hypertension from bilateral urinary obstruction is initially a result of the release of renin and later a result of retention of fluid.

5. Diuresis after obstruction may result from a physiologic excretion of water and urea but can become pathologic. Patients should have electrolytes checked and replaced regularly with free access to oral fluids. If necessary, the type and amount of intravenous fluids should be determined by serum and urinary electrolyte levels.

6. Infection is the most common complication of urinary tract obstruction and is a result of stasis of urine.

---

17. **What is postobstructive diuresis?**

After obstruction is relieved, a physiologic diuresis occurs with the excretion of excess total body water and an osmotic diuresis mainly from urea. This process can persist with a pathologic diuresis because of decreased expression of aquaporin channels in the collecting duct, excessive presence of atrial natriuretic peptide, and concentrating defect from dysfunction of the corticomedullary gradient. Excess volume replacement, especially with isotonic solutions containing glucose or saline, may cause the diuresis to persist. Patients should have electrolytes checked and replaced regularly with free access to oral fluids. If intravenous fluids are required, their type and amount should be determined by serum and urinary electrolyte levels.

18. **What is the role of renal ultrasound in diagnosing obstruction?**

Ultrasound is a noninvasive diagnostic test. In obstruction there is typically dilation of the ureter or collecting system. In a dehydrated state or in early acute obstruction (first 1–3 days) dilation may be absent. An intrarenal pelvis may limit dilation of the renal pelvis, whereas an extrarenal pelvis may dramatically expand with obstruction. Chronic obstruction may limit the visibility of echo-rich fat in the plane of Gil Vernet. Ultrasonography is operator dependent and requires clinical correlation.

19. **What is the role of computed tomography in diagnosing obstruction?**

Computed tomography (CT) allows the clinician to visualize the entire urinary collecting system. The preliminary noncontrast phase may identify urinary stones. All stones are visible on noncontrast CT, with the exception of stones associated with protease inhibitors in the treatment of HIV, and the Hounsfield units may help determine stone composition. The acute nephrogram phase after contrast administration provides information about renal arterial inflow. The contrast portion of the scan may identify extrinsic sources of obstruction such as retroperitoneal lymphadenopathy or pelvic malignancy. Delayed images after contrast administration may reveal ureteral filling defects from ureteral urothelial cell carcinoma or ureteral stricture. CT scans are associated with ionizing radiation, and repeated imaging should be limited if possible.

20. **When is retrograde pyelography indicated in diagnosing obstruction?**

When other imaging studies are equivocal or in patients with renal insufficiency or contrast dye allergies, retrograde pyelography may be necessary. Retrograde pyelography provides excellent delineation of urothelial-filling defects and can give a road map to the clinician to better direct therapy. Collection of urinary cytology is possible during retrograde pyelography. This route also allows for intervention at the same setting such as with a ureteral stent.

21. **What is a nuclear medicine renogram?**

A renogram is a nuclear medicine evaluation of the kidneys after administration of a radiotracer. The examination provides functional information regarding perfusion of the kidneys and their ability to uptake and excrete the tracer. After the administration of a diuretic, the study may demonstrate delayed washout consistent with urinary obstruction. Several radiotracers are available including DMSA, MAG-3, and DTPA.

BIBLIOGRAPHY

1. Campbell MF, Wein AJ, Kavoussi LR. *Campbell-Walsh Urology*, 9th ed., Philadelphia: W.B. Saunders, 2007, 4 v. (xlii, 3945, cxv p.).

2. Harris RH, Yarger WE. Renal function after release of unilateral ureteral obstruction in rats. *Am J Physiol* 1974;227:806–815.

3. Kerr WS. Effect of complete ureteral obstruction for one week on kidney function. *J Appl Physiol* 1954;6:762–772.

4. Kim SW, Lee JU, Park JW, et al. Increased expression of atrial natriuretic peptide in the kidney of rats with bilateral ureteral obstruction. *Kidney Int* 2001;59:1274–1282.

5. Klahr S, Morrissey J. Obstructive nephropathy and renal fibrosis. *Am J Physiol* 2002;283:F861–F875.

6. Rokaw MD, Sarac E, Lechman E, et al. Chronic regulation of transepithelial Na+ transport by the rate of apical Na+ entry. *Am J Physiol* 1996;270:C600–C607.

7. Schlossberg SM, Vaughan ED Jr. The mechanism of unilateral post-obstructive diuresis. *J Urol* 1984;131:534–536.

8. Vaughan ED, Gillenwater JY. Recovery following complete chronic unilateral ureteral occlusion: Functional, radiographic, and pathologic alterations. *J Urol* 1971;106:27–35.

CHAPTER 18

NEPHROLITHIASIS

John R. Asplin, MD

1. **How common are kidney stones?**

   In industrialized countries, approximately 12% of men and 7% of women will form at least one kidney stone in their life and the prevalence of nephrolithiasis is increasing. Historically, men were much more likely to form kidney stones than women, but recent data show the prevalence in women is approaching that of men. After presenting with their initial stone, about 50% of patients will have a second stone within 8 years. Some patients will have multiple recurrent stones, with the most severe patients forming new stones every few weeks.

2. **What are kidney stone made of?**

   Approximately 80% of kidney stones are predominantly calcium salts. Calcium oxalate is the major component in 85% to 90% of calcium stones, the rest being calcium phosphate, in the form of apatite or brushite. It is common for small amounts of apatite to be found in calcium oxalate stones. About 10% of stones are uric acid and 5% to 10% are struvite (magnesium ammonium phosphate). Cystine accounts for about 1% of all stones. Stones may be a single pure substance or may be a mix of crystal types, such as calcium oxalate and uric acid.

3. **What is the best radiologic test to diagnose kidney stones?**

   Computed tomography (CT) scan without intravenous or oral contrast is the preferred radiologic study for patients presenting with renal colic. Advantages of CT scans include much greater sensitivity for small stones, no intravenous contrast, ability to detect uric acid stones (which are radiolucent on standard x-rays), and the potential to diagnose other causes of flank/abdominal pain if no stones are found. The main drawback with CT scans is the radiation dose. If a patient requires serial radiologic evaluation, a KUB (kidneys, ureters, and bladder) x-ray is preferred but only if the stone of interest can be adequately visualized.

   Ultrasound can identify hydronephrosis and document stones, but it is not as sensitive or specific as CT. Ultrasound is clearly the preferred imaging method in pregnant women, and many clinicians prefer to use it in children to avoid excessive radiation.

4. **Do all patients with renal colic require urologic intervention to remove the stone?**

   Most patients with renal colic will pass the stone without surgical intervention. Stones <5 mm will pass without intervention 80% to 90% of the time; stones >6 mm pass only 25% of the time. Pharmaceuticals can be used to promote stone passage, such as the alpha blocker tamsulosin or calcium channel blockers, which act as ureteral muscle relaxants. Corticosteroids may be added to the muscle relaxants to reduce swelling and inflammation. In addition to medical expulsive therapy, hydration and pain control are key components in the management of renal colic. Indications for emergent removal of a ureteral stone include fever, intractable pain, persistent nausea and vomiting, obstruction of a unilateral kidney, or a stone deemed unlikely to pass because of its size.

5. **What is extracorporeal shock-wave lithotripsy?**

   Extracorporeal shock-wave lithotripsy (ESWL) is a noninvasive method to remove urolithiasis in the renal pelvis or in the ureter. Shock waves are conducted through water to the patient's flank. The shock waves are focused on the stone, pulverizing it into multiple small pieces. ESWL is an outpatient procedure that requires only mild anesthesia. Disadvantages include the requirement for the patient to pass the fragments, which may cause renal colic, and the potential for some stone fragments to remain in the kidney, particularly stones in the lower pole of the kidney. Some stones, such as cystine and brushite, are resistant to fracture by ESWL.

6. **Is open surgery still used for kidney stones?**
   Open surgery has been replaced by percutaneous nephrolithotomy (PCNL) and ureteroscopy. PCNL is performed by placing a nephroscope through the patient's flank into the renal pelvis. Stones can be directly visualized and fragmented, and fragments are removed through the scope. PCNL most often is used for large stones (>2 cm), stones in a lower pole of the kidney, or stones that have been resistant to ESWL. Ureteroscopy is used for stones in the ureter and some stones in the renal pelvis. The ureteroscope is introduced through the urethra, into the bladder, and then the ureter. Stones may be removed using a basket or may be destroyed using a laser. The choice of surgical approach depends on the type of stone, location of the stone, and expertise of the urologist.

7. **Is it worthwhile having kidney stone composition analyzed?**
   Whenever stone material is available, crystallographic analysis should be performed. Although 70% of stones will be composed of calcium oxalate, it is the finding of noncalcium stones that provides the most benefit. Struvite and cystine stones are uncommon but serious stone diseases; their diagnosis via stone analysis leads to specific and intensive therapy. Uric acid stones are always treated with alkalinization. Crystallization of medications such as indinavir, guaifenesin, and triamterene in the urinary tract can lead to stones, which can only be diagnosed by the analysis of stone material. Of note, patients may have kept stones they had passed previously; such stones can be analyzed because they do not decompose with time.

8. **If an initial stone has been analyzed, do subsequent stones need to be analyzed?**
   Yes. Analysis of stones as they recur may reveal that stone composition has changed, which could require revision of the stone prevention protocol. In fact, a change in stone type may be a result of preventive therapy, such as calcium phosphate stones forming as a result of excessive alkalinization in a patient with cystinuria.

9. **How much of a workup should a patient with a single kidney stone have?**
   When adults present with their initial stone episode, they should have a limited workup to identify the more serious issues related to nephrolithiasis. Serum chemistries will reveal hypokalemia and/or acidosis that would indicate distal renal tubular acidosis (RTA), hypercalcemia to identify patients who should be evaluated for hyperparathyroidism, and serum creatinine to estimate kidney function. Stone analysis should always be performed. Urinalysis and/or urine culture should be done to identify infection and microscopy for stone-related crystals. Radiographic evaluation should be performed to quantify stone burden. A patient with only one symptomatic stone should not be considered a single stone former if multiple stones are seen on CT scan or x-ray.

10. **Who should have 24-hour urine chemistries measured as part of their evaluation?**
    Adults with recurrent stone disease should have 24-hour urine chemistries measured. Some adults with a single stone event will require full evaluation as dictated by their career, such as airline pilots. In addition, all children with kidney stones should have urine chemistries performed because they have a higher likelihood of having a severe inherited form of nephrolithiasis such as cystinuria or primary hyperoxaluria.

11. **What chemistries should be ordered on a 24-hour urine collection?**
Urine chemistries should include calcium, oxalate, uric acid, and phosphorus because all are common components of kidney stones. Urine volume is a key factor because all patients should try to maintain a urine volume of at least 2.5 liters/day. Citrate forms a complex with calcium in the urine; thus low urine citrate is a commonly found risk factor for calcium stone formation. pH should be measured in a 24-hour urine sample; low pH is a risk factor for uric acid stones, and high pH is a risk factor for calcium phosphate stones. Creatinine should be measured in all timed urine specimens to ensure that the urine specimen was collected properly (14–20 mg creatinine/kg body weight in women, 18–25 mg/kg in men).

12. **Is a random urine pH an adequate replacement for a 24-hour urine pH?**
A random urine pH should not be used to assess stone risk because pH is too variable for a single measurement to provide meaningful information. Urine pH in a normal subject varies from 5.0 to 7.0 depending on diet and time of day. A 24-hour sample gives the time-averaged urine pH; normal range is 5.7 to 6.3 for a 24-hour collection.

13. **Is a single 24-hour urine collection adequate when evaluating a patient with nephrolithiasis?**
Urine chemistries vary much more than serum chemistries because urine excretions are dependent on lifestyle, diet, and each patient's particular physiology. As such, it is wise to perform at least two 24-hour urine collections during the initial evaluation. Optimally, one collection would be on a weekend and the other on a weekday to assess both the home and work environment because diet, fluid intake, and levels of exertion can vary tremendously.

14. **Are crystals seen during urine microscopy helpful in the diagnosis of stone disease?**
Cystine crystals and struvite crystals are always abnormal and diagnostic of an underlying disorder (Fig. 18-1). Cystine crystals are only present in people with cystinuria, an uncommon genetic disorder in which cystine is not reabsorbed normally by the kidney. Struvite crystals only form in humans when there is urinary infection with bacteria that possess urease activity. Uric acid and calcium crystals may be more frequent in the urine of stone formers, but they are not diagnostic of disease because they also may be found in healthy people. One situation in which the finding of calcium or uric acid crystals may be helpful is in patients with renal colic without a documented stone, where transient bursts of crystalluria may be causing symptoms.

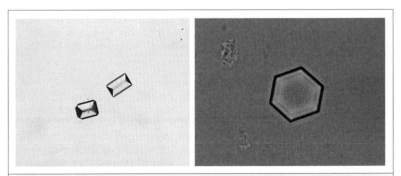

Figure 18-1. Struvite crystals (*left panel*) are rectangular prisms with the appearance of coffin lids. Cystine crystals (*right panel*) are hexagonal plates.

KEY POINTS: FEATURES OF CYSTINURIA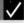

1. Cystinuria is a stone disease that follows an autosomal recessive pattern.
2. Reduced proximal tubule reabsorption of cystine and dibasic amino acids is present.
3. Hexagonal crystals may be seen in the urine.
4. First presentation is usually in childhood.
5. The mainstays of therapy are very high fluid intake, alkalinization of the urine, and use of thiol-binding drugs such as tiopronin or D-penicillamine.

15. Is it really true that drinking water prevents kidney stones?
Creating dilute urine will reduce the concentration of lithogenic substances and thus the driving force for crystallization. A prospective randomized trial proved the effectiveness of high fluid intake; the urine volume in the treated group averaged 2.5 liters/day, providing a reasonable goal for patients with nephrolithiasis. Generally, it is better to prescribe a specified urine flow rather than an absolute amount of fluid intake because patients' fluid needs vary. Although physicians usually recommend water as the preferred fluid, other beverages seem to provide equal benefit. The unique exception is grapefruit juice; daily ingestion was shown to increase the risk of kidney stones. The mechanism of this peculiar association is not known.

16. Why do uric acid stones form?
Urate is an end product of purine metabolism. Urate solubility is pH dependent; as urine pH falls below 5.5, uric acid becomes the predominant form of urate. Uric acid is poorly soluble such that even at normal rates of urate excretion, uric acid can crystallize when urine pH is low. In fact, the majority of patients with uric acid stones do not overexcrete uric acid, but rather have an abnormally low urine pH as the cause of stone formation. Low urine pH may be the result of high dietary intake of animal protein, chronic kidney disease, metabolic syndrome, or gastrointestinal (GI) alkali loss as may be seen with chronic diarrhea.

17. How does metabolic syndrome lead to kidney stones?
Metabolic syndrome is a constellation of abnormalities (hypertension, glucose intolerance, dyslipidemia, increased waist size) associated with an increased risk of cardiovascular disease. Recent studies also have shown an increased risk of uric acid stone formation. Patients with metabolic syndrome have a lower urine pH because they excrete more of their daily net acid production as titratable acid and less as ammonia, with the net effect being a lower urine pH. The lower ammonia production by the proximal tubule results from insulin resistance because insulin is a stimulus for ammonia production. As might be expected, patients with diabetes appear to develop uric acid stones more frequently than patients who do not have diabetes.

18. What is the best treatment for uric acid stones?
Lowering dietary intake of animal protein will reduce the dietary acid load, raising urine pH. Because most dietary purine comes from animal tissue, lowering animal protein intake will lower uric acid excretion. The mainstay of therapy to prevent uric acid stone formation is to raise urine pH with alkali. Potassium citrate is generally preferred. If a patient cannot tolerate potassium salts because of GI side effects or hyperkalemia, then sodium alkali may be used. The goal of therapy is a 24-hour urine pH of 6.0 to 6.5; raising urine pH to higher levels will not provide additional benefit. Allopurinol is a second-line drug for uric acid stones, used when the patient also has gout or when the patient is unable to take sufficient alkali to raise urine pH higher than 6.0. Allopurinol should be used in diseases with massive urate overproduction such as Lesch-Nyhan syndrome.

19. **What is idiopathic hypercalciuria?**
    Idiopathic hypercalciuria is generally defined as a urine calcium excretion higher than 300 mg/day in a man or 250 mg/day in a woman, with normal serum calcium in the absence of any systemic disorder known to affect mineral metabolism, such as sarcoidosis or primary hyperparathyroidism.

20. **How much calcium should a patient with calcium stones have in their diet?**
    For many years low-calcium diets (400 mg/day) were standard for patients with calcium stones and hypercalciuria. Although low-calcium diets clearly reduce urine calcium, there is not a clinical trial proving that low-calcium diets reduce stone formation. Epidemiologic studies challenged this approach by showing people with low-calcium diets were more likely to form kidney stones than those on a high-calcium diet. A subsequent study showed that a low-sodium, low-protein diet with normal calcium intake was more effective in preventing stones than a standard low-calcium diet. In general, patients should be encouraged to avoid calcium gluttony but should maintain a calcium intake of 1000 to 1200 mg/day.

21. **What treatments are available to prevent recurrent nephrolithiasis?**
    Treatments vary depending on the type of stone and the underlying metabolic abnormality that has caused the stone to form. Table 18-1 lists possible treatments to prevent stone recurrence.

22. **Do patients with nephrolithiasis get bone disease from renal calcium losses?**
    Multiple studies have documented reduced bone mineral density in calcium stone formers, particularly those with idiopathic hypercalciuria. Patients with hypercalciuria are likely to go into negative calcium balance when placed on a low-calcium diet. Because many patients avoid dairy

TABLE 18-1. MEDICAL THERAPY FOR RECURRENT NEPHROLITHIASIS

Stone Type	Metabolic Abnormality	Potential Treatment
Calcium oxalate (therapy for calcium phosphate stone focuses on hypercalciuria and hypocitraturia)	Hyperparathyroidism	Parathyroidectomy
	Hypercalciuria	Low-sodium, low-protein diet
		Thiazide diuretic
	Dietary hyperoxaluria	Low-oxalate, normal-calcium diet
	Enteric hyperoxaluria	Low-oxalate, low-fat diet
		Calcium supplements with meals
	Primary hyperoxaluria	Pyridoxine
		Neutral phosphate
		Potassium citrate
	Hypocitraturia	Potassium citrate
		Sodium bicarbonate if potassium salts not tolerated
	Hyperuricosuria	Low-purine diet
		Allopurinol
Uric acid	Low urine pH	Alkali salts, potassium citrate preferred
	Severe hyperuricosuria	Allopurinol
Cystine	Cystinuria	Alkali salts, potassium citrate preferred
		Tiopronin, D-penicillamine

products after a stone episode, they may be contributing to their bone loss. Higher fracture rates have been noted in stone formers. To treat bone loss, diet calcium should be 1000 to 1200 mg/day and diet sodium should be 2300 to 3000 mg/day. Thiazide diuretics can improve bone mineral level and reduce stone risk. Bisphosphonates may improve bone mineral density and perhaps reduce urine calcium, although long-term use has not been well studied in patients with nephrolithiasis.

23. **How does distal RTA cause kidney stones?**
In distal RTA stone formation is common and most stones are calcium phosphate. The systemic metabolic acidosis leads to increased proximal tubule reabsorption of citrate, lowering urine citrate excretion. Because there is less citrate available to complex calcium, there is more calcium available to combine with phosphate or oxalate. Acidosis increases renal calcium excretion, further increasing the risk of stones. Finally, the inability to acidify urine leads to a persistent alkaline urine, which increases the amount of divalent phosphate (pK = 6.8) and thus the risk of calcium phosphate crystallization. Medications such as topiramate and acetazolamide can cause kidney stones by creating an RTA by inhibiting renal carbonic anhydrase.

KEY POINTS: MEDICATIONS THAT CAN LEAD TO STONE FORMATION

1. Protease inhibitors
2. Topiramate
3. Calcium supplements
4. Triamterene
5. Guaifenesin/ephedrine

24. **Why do patients with bowel disease have a higher risk of kidney stone formation?**
Diarrheal states cause low urine flow as patients lose excess water from the GI tract and patients may restrict fluid intake to lower GI output. In addition, chronic diarrhea leads to GI bicarbonate loss with resultant metabolic acidosis. The acidosis leads to low urine pH, a risk factor for uric acid stones, and low urine citrate, a risk factor for calcium stones. These abnormalities are commonly found in patients who have colectomy, with or without ileostomy. If a patient has fat malabsorption, from Crohn's disease or small bowel surgery, he or she can develop enteric hyperoxaluria as fat malabsorption leads to increased oxalate absorption in the colon. Note that enteric hyperoxaluria does not occur in patients who have had a colectomy.

25. **Does bariatric surgery lead to kidney stones?**
Only the malabsorptive bariatric procedures, roux-en-Y gastric bypass and biliopancreatic diversion, have been linked to an increased risk of kidney stones. The purely restrictive procedures such as gastric banding are not associated with stones. Stone risk from the malabsorptive procedures is mainly a result of hyperoxaluria. The mechanism is not well studied but likely is the result of fat malabsorption leading to increased oxalate absorption resulting from increased oxalate permeability of the colon wall and binding of calcium in the gut lumen by fatty acids. Hyperoxaluria can be severe, leading to stone formation and at times loss of kidney function from oxalate nephropathy.

26. **What are infection stones?**
Infection stones are composed of struvite. Struvite stones only form in the presence of urinary infection with bacteria that possesses the enzyme urease, which converts urea to ammonium

and bicarbonate, leading to the unique condition of high urine ammonium concentration with a high urine pH. The bacteria most likely to possess urease are the *Proteus* species, although many other bacterial species may also possess urease. *Escherichia coli,* the most common urinary tract pathogen, does not possess urease. Struvite stones can grow to fill the entire renal pelvis (staghorn stones) and may lead to recurrent infection and loss of kidney infection. Treatment of struvite stones requires complete surgical removal of the stone and a prolonged course of antibiotics.

27. **Do kidney stones cause damage and lead to chronic kidney disease?**
Cystine and struvite stones have long been recognized as causing kidney damage and even loss of a kidney. These stones can form large staghorn calculi and recur frequently, which leads to kidney damage. Recently, it has been recognized that patients with kidney stones as a whole have slightly lower estimated glomerular filtration rate (eGFR) than a healthy population. Whether the chronic kidney disease (CKD) is a result of recurrent surgical procedures, lithotripsy, or intermittent obstruction during stone passage is not known.

28. **How should symptomatic stone disease be managed during pregnancy?**
Ultrasound is the radiologic procedure of choice, although it may be difficult to interpret because ureters become dilated during pregnancy, making the diagnosis of hydronephrosis difficult. If a patient has a symptomatic stone, hydration and observation to let the stone pass spontaneously are the preferred approaches. If the stone does not pass and pain persists, infection/pyelonephritis is present, or there is complete unilateral obstruction, then the stone should be removed ureteroscopically. If the stone cannot be removed, then placement of a stent may be needed to relieve the obstruction. ESWL is not recommended during pregnancy. Final surgical removal of a stone may be delayed until after delivery, if necessary. Medical evaluation for cause of the stone should be delayed until after pregnancy and nursing are over because urine calcium excretion will be markedly different than the nonpregnant state.

29. **Are magnesium salts or pyridoxine (vitamin B$_6$) effective therapies for calcium nephrolithiasis?**
Both of these agents have been proposed as ways to lower urine oxalate excretion—magnesium because it can bind dietary oxalate and lower intestinal absorption and pyridoxine because it is a cofactor for a key enzyme that can lower endogenous oxalate production. There are no controlled trials to prove that these therapies are effective in lowering urine oxalate or preventing calcium stone recurrence. However, a subset of patients with primary hyperoxaluria, an autosomal recessive disorder characterized by severe hyperoxaluria, nephrolithiasis, and CKD, may significantly lower urine oxalate excretion when treated with pyridoxine.

BIBLIOGRAPHY

1. Asplin JR. Evaluation of the kidney stone patient. *Semin Nephrol* 2008;28:99–110.
2. Asplin JR. Treatment of renal stones. In: Rosen CJ (ed.). *Primer on the Metabolic Bone Diseases and Disorders of Mineral Metabolism*, 7th ed. Washington, DC: American Society of Bone and Mineral Research, 2008, pp. 470–473.
3. Goldfarb DS. Prospects for dietary therapy of recurrent nephrolithiasis. *Adv Chronic Kidney Dis* 2009;16:21–29.
4. Mandeville JA, Nelson CP. Pediatric urolithiasis. *Curr Opin Urol* 2009;19:419–423.
5. Patel BN, Passman CM, Assimos DG. Evaluation and management of the patient with acute renal colic. In: Pearle MS, Nakada SY (eds.). *Urolithiasis: Medical and Surgical Management*, 1st ed. Essex: Informa Healthcare, 2009, pp. 68–74.
6. Patel BN, Passman CM, Fernandez A, et al. Prevalence of hyperoxaluria after bariatric surgery. *J Urol* 2009;181:161–166.
7. Sakhaee K, Maalouf NM. Metabolic syndrome and uric acid nephrolithiasis. *Semin Nephrol* 2008;28:174–180.
8. Seitz C, Liatsikos E, Porpiglia F, et al. Medical therapy to facilitate the passage of stones: What is the evidence? *Eur Urol* 2009;56:455–471.
9. Tiselius HG. New horizons in the management of patients with cystinuria. *Curr Opin Urol* 2010;20:169–173.

EPIDEMIOLOGY, ETIOLOGY, PATHOPHYSIOLOGY, AND STAGING OF CHRONIC KIDNEY DISEASE

CHAPTER 19

Meguid El Nahas, MD, PhD; B.S. Kawar, MBBS, MD; and Mohsen El Kossi, MD

1. **What is the definition of chronic kidney disease?**

   In 2002 the Kidney Disease Outcomes Quality Initiative (K/DOQI) classified chronic kidney disease (CKD) into five stages based on the level of glomerular filtration rate (GFR) and/or the presence of associated renal abnormalities: proteinuria/albuminuria, hematuria, or radiological/histological abnormalities (Table 19-1). In 2005 the classification was revised by KDIGO (Kidney Disease: Improving Global Outcomes) to include the suffix D for patients in CKD5 on dialysis and T for those with a functioning renal transplant.

   In 2008 the UK National Institute of Health and Clinical Excellence (NICE) modified the K/DOQI CKD classification by subdividing CKD stage 3 into CKD3a and 3b, which is estimated GFR (eGFR) between 59 and 45 mL/min/1.73 m^2 and 44 and 30 mL/min/1.73 m^2, respectively. The NICE CKD guidelines also stipulated that the suffix "p" is added to the stages in patients with proteinuria. This modification of the KDOQI CKD classification by NICE assumes that there is a distinction between patients with GFR <60 mL/min/1.73 m^2 and those with GFR <45 mL/min/1.73 m^2 in terms of prognosis and that the prognostic significance of proteinuria/albuminuria has to be acknowledged in the classification.

   National Kidney Foundation. K/DOQI clinical practice guidelines for chronic kidney disease: Evaluation, classification, and stratification. *Am J Kidney Dis* 2002;39(suppl 1):S1–S266.

   Early Identification and Management of Chronic Kidney Disease in Adults in Primary and Secondary Care. Available at: http://www.nice.org.uk/cg73.

2. **What are the advantages and limitations of the current CKD classification?**

   Advantages:
   - The current classification has simplified the categorization of people suffering from CKD.
   - It has considerably increased awareness of CKD among nephrologists, non-nephrologists, and the public at large. In the past, a number of people suffering from CKD were not recognized because they had serum creatinine levels within the "normal range".
   - It has allowed assessment of the impact of different levels of GFR on outcomes, including cardiovascular disease (CVD).

   Limitations:
   - It classifies people with isolated microalbuminuria (MA) as suffering from CKD, when it may merely reflect underlying vascular pathology, endothelial dysfunction, and/or atherosclerosis or chronic inflammatory conditions such as hepatitis, dermatitis, and colitis. Microalbuminuria is also associated with aging, obesity, and smoking. Microalbuminuria is often transient and reversible.
   - GFR estimated by the Cockroft-Gault and MDRD formulas tend to underestimate renal function at high levels of GFR (>60 mL/min/1.73 m^2), therefore potentially overestimating the number of people with CKD.
   - It relies on calculated GFR to categorize individuals with GFR >60 mL/min/1.73 m^2 as suffering from stage 1 or 2 CKD in spite of the imprecision of calculated GFR above 60 mL/min/1.73 m^2.

TABLE 19-1. CLASSIFICATION OF CHRONIC KIDNEY DISEASE (CKD) ACCORDING TO K/DOQI (2002) AND MODIFIED BY NICE (2008)	
CKD Stages	Definition
1	Normal or increased GFR; some evidence of kidney damage reflected by microalbuminuria, proteinuria, hematuria, as well as radiologic or histologic changes
2	Mild decrease in GFR (89-60 mL/min/1.73 m^2) with some evidence of kidney damage reflected by microalbuminuria, proteinuria, hematuria, as well as radiologic or histologic changes
3	GFR 59-30 mL/min/1.73 m^2
3a	GFR 59-45 mL/min/1.73 m^2
3b	GFR 44-30 mL/min/1.73 m^2
4	GFR 29-15 mL/min/1.73 m^2
5/ESRD	GFR <15 mL/min/1.73 m^2; when renal replacement therapy in the form of dialysis or transplantation has to be considered to sustain life

CKD = chronic kidney disease; K/DOQI = Kidney Disease Outcomes Quality Initiative; NICE = National Institute of Health and Clinical Excellence; GFR = glomerular filtration rate; ESRD = end-stage renal disease. The suffix "p" should be added to the stage in patients with proteinuria (proteinuria >0.5 g/24h).

- It does not differentiate between age-related impaired kidney function and progressive disease-induced CKD. This risks detecting a large number of elderly individuals with reduced but stable GFR and labeling them as suffering from a disease.

Glassock RJ, Winearls C. Diagnosing chronic kidney disease. *Curr Opin Nephrol Hypertens* 2010;19(2): 123–128.

3. **How common is CKD?**
The true incidence and prevalence of CKD within a community is difficult to ascertain because early to moderate CKD is usually asymptomatic. Epidemiologic studies have suggested a prevalence of CKD of around 10%, albuminuria (mostly microalbuminuria) of around 7%, and GFR <60 mL/min/1.73 m^2 of around 3% (Table 19-2). Of note, the majority of those found to be suffering from CKD in the community are older people mostly aged >55 years.

4. **What are the limitations of most CKD population screening studies?**
   - Most screening programs rely on single testing to define CKD.
   - Microalbuminuria is invariably accepted as the sole definer of CKD.
   - The majority of those screened within the community and found to have reduced GFR are elderly individuals at low risk of progression.
   - Screening programs use formulae such as the Modification of Diet in Renal Disease (MDRD) and Gault-Cokcroft (GC) equation to estimate GFR despite their known limitations and underestimation of normal kidney function.

   The limitations of current CKD definition, classification, and screening strategies may tend to overinflate the overall prevalence of significant CKD.

5. **Who should I screen for CKD?**
There is little evidence that whole-population screening for CKD either by measuring albuminuria or serum creatinine is warranted or cost effective. However, most national and

TABLE 19-2.	REPRESENTATIVE STUDIES OF THE PREVALENCE OF CKD IN COMMUNITIES	
Country	Name of the Study	CKD Prevalence (%)
USA	NHANESIII	CKD = 11, MA = 12
Netherlands	PREVEND	MA = 7
UK	NEOERICA	CKD = 11 (F), 6 (M)
Australia	AUSDIAB	CKD = 10, MA = 6
China	Beijing	CKD = 13
Japan	Takahata	MA = 14

CKD = chronic kidney disease; NHANES = National Health and Nutrition Evaluation Survey; MA = microalbuminuria; PREVEND = Prevention of Endstage Renal and Vascular Disease; NEOERICA = New Opportunities for Early Renal Intervention by Computerised Assessment; M = male; F = female; AUSDIAB = Australian Diabetes, Obesity and Lifestyle Study.

international guidelines recommend screening individuals at risk of CKD, such as those with a history of the following:

- Hypertension
- Diabetes mellitus
- Family history of CKD
- Recurrent urinary tract infections
- Systemic disease that can affect the kidneys such as vasculitis
- Excessive or prolonged use of analgesics or nonsteroidal anti-inflammatory drugs (NSAIDs)

6. **Is a low eGFR a sign of CKD in older people?**
This is a difficult question to answer and remains subject to considerable debate. It is generally accepted that the majority of individuals lose kidney function with age; it has been estimated that from the age of 40 to 50 years onward, most individuals have a reduction of GFR of around 0.5 to 0.8 mL/min/year. Some have described this loss as "physiological" whereas others have described it as "pathological". It is likely that the loss of GFR with aging is a reflection of a more generalized vascular aging process affecting the kidneys. In the absence of significant proteinuria, the renal prognosis of older individuals with CKD3 is good because very few progress to end-stage renal disease (ESRD). However, the increased CVD morbidity and mortality associated with reduced GFR or albuminuria cannot be overlooked.

Weiner DE, Tabatabai S, Tighiouart H, et al. Cardiovascular outcomes and all-cause mortality: Exploring the interaction between CKD and cardiovascular disease. *Am J Kidney Dis* 2006;48(3):392–401.

7. **How common is end-stage renal disease?**
Although the prevalence of CKD may be as high as 10% of the general population, there is little doubt that the prevalence of ESRD seldom exceeds 0.2% of the population. This discrepancy may be a result of a number of factors, including lack of progression of CKD3 in the majority of the elderly classified as such, the death of many with progressive CKD3 and 4 before reaching CKD5 (ESRD), and/or the lack of renal replacement therapy (RRT) facilities to treat patients with CKD5. The latter is particularly true in developing countries where the cost of RRT is prohibitive.

8. **Why are there such disparities in ESRD incidence and prevalence?**
Disparities in the incidence and prevalence of ESRD within and between developed countries reflect racial and ethnic diversity and their impact on the prevalence of diabetes and

hypertension in respective countries and communities (Table 19-3). Disparities within developing countries are likely to reflect availability of, and access to, RRT in low and middle-income economies. The cost of treating patients with ESRD is substantial (more than $30 billion/year in the United States) and affects provision of care. There is a clear and direct relationship between gross national product (GNP) and the availability of RRT in most countries.

9. **What is the natural history of CKD?**
The natural history of CKD depends to a large extent on the cause and stage of CKD, the presence or absence of hypertension and/or proteinuria, and the severity of the complications of CKD. In general, patients with glomerular pathology and those with diabetic nephropathy tend to progress with steadily declining kidney function, hypertension, and increasing proteinuria. Those suffering from hypertensive nephrosclerosis or chronic interstitial nephropathies tend to have much slower rates of CKD progression because GFR can remain stable for years in the absence of severe/uncontrolled hypertension, proteinuria, or persistent insults.

The majority of patients with CKD 1 and 2 are non-progressive because they have preserved renal function and either isolated albuminuria or isolated hematuria. Patients with CKD stage 3 tend to progress with declining GFR when CKD is associated with albuminuria (>1 g/24 h or protein to creatinine ratio (PCR) >100 mg/mmol). Hypertension is also a major risk factor for the progression of CKD.

In addition, CKD progression can be accelerated by intercurrent illnesses, the use of nephrotoxic agents such as NSAIDs, or episodes of superimposed acute kidney injury (AKI).

As mentioned earlier, the majority of patients with CKD1–3 do not seem to progress to CKD4–5. In fact, although the prevalence of CKD1–3 may be as high as 10%, the prevalence of CKD4–5 seldom exceeds 1%. This is likely to reflect the non-progressive nature of CKD3 in the elderly in the absence of proteinuria/albuminuria; the fact that those with declining kidney function, hypertension, and albuminuria often die from cardiovascular disease (CVD) before they reach ESRD; and the fact that many patients with CKD5 do not have access to RRT and therefore do not feature in the registries of prevalence of ESRD.

10. **What are the causes of CKD?**
There are different ways of classifying causes of CKD. One approach is to consider the pathologic sieve:
- Congenital (e.g., renal dysphasia)
- Inherited (e.g., autosomal dominant polycystic kidney disease)
- Inflammatory (e.g., primary glomerulonephritis, systemic vasculitis such as systemic lupus erythematosus)

TABLE 19-3. APPROXIMATE GLOBAL INCIDENCE AND PREVALENCE OF RENAL REPLACEMENT THERAPY

Country	Incidence (patients per million per year)	Prevalence (patients per million of population)
USA	~350	~1600
Caucasians	~280	~1200
African Americans	~1000	~5000
Japan	~280	~2000
Europe	~150	~800
Africa	30–150	0–300

- Infective (e.g., chronic pyelonephritis)
- Metabolic (e.g., diabetic nephropathy)
- Vascular (e.g., renovascular disease)
- Toxins (e.g., drugs, radiocontrast material)
- Malignancy (e.g., renal tumors, multiple myeloma)

Another approach is to consider which part of the kidney is affected:

- Glomerular diseases: glomerulonephritis, diabetic nephropathy, systemic diseases such as lupus and Wegener's granulomatosis
- Tubulointerstitial diseases: chronic pyelonephritis, drug-induced interstitial nephritis, cast nephropathy in multiple myeloma
- Vascular: diffuse atherosclerosis affecting renal arteries and intrarenal arterioles causing atherosclerotic renovascular disease (ARVD)
- Gross structural abnormalities/malformations: congenital dysplasia, autosomal dominant polycystic kidney disease (ADPKD)

The problem with these approaches is that they do not reflect the relative prevalence of these conditions. Therefore, you may wish to answer the question by listing the causes starting with the most common. In the developed world the most common causes of CKD are as follows:

- Diabetic nephropathy
- Hypertension/renovascular disease
- Glomerulonephritis
- Pyelointerstitial nephritis
- ADPKD

In the developing world glomerulonephritis remains the leading cause for CKD/ESRD. However, because of the obesity epidemic, diabetes is a rapidly growing cause of CKD in the developing world and is likely to overtake glomerulonephritis as the leading cause.

11. **What do you need to know about diabetic nephropathy?**
There is little doubt that type 2 diabetes mellitus (DM) is on the increase worldwide. The number of those suffering is predicted to double by 2030. Consequently, diabetic nephropathy is rapidly becoming one of the most common causes of CKD worldwide. It is estimated that about one third of patients with DM will have some manifestations of CKD. The disease starts with microalbuminuria (albumin excretion rate: 30–300 mg/24 h) and then progresses to overt proteinuria and even nephrotic syndrome. Increasing proteinuria is associated with declining kidney function. Diabetic nephropathy is a manifestation of the widespread microvascular disease affecting these individuals and is often associated with diabetic retinopathy. Microscopic hematuria is not an uncommon feature of diabetic nephropathy. A renal biopsy is seldom warranted in these patients because the diagnosis of diabetic nephropathy makes little doubt.

Elderly patients with type 2 DM may have a different course to that described previously because systemic hypertension, diffuse atherosclerosis, and ischemic nephropathy also contribute to the renal involvement. In the absence of significant proteinuria, hypertensive and ischemic nephropathy are more likely to prevail. Such a distinction is important because angiotensin-converting enzyme (ACE) inhibitors/angiotensin receptor blockers (ARBs) are the treatment of choice for typical/proteinuric diabetic nephropathy, although they should be used with caution and may be contraindicated in ischemic nephropathy.

12. **What are the risk factors for CKD?**
- **Age:** The majority of those labeled as suffering from CKD are older than 55 years of age.
- **Hypertension:** Long-standing and poorly controlled hypertension causes CKD.
- **Diabetes:** Up to one third of people with diabetes may have some manifestations of CKD.
- **Family history of CKD:** CKD often runs in families.
    Also, albeit of less importance:
- **Smoking:** Heavy and sustained smoking has been associated with albuminuria.
- **Hyperlipidemia:** Persistent dyslipidemia has been associated in the long term with albuminuria.

- **Obesity:** Obesity has been associated with albuminuria and glomerulosclerosis.
- **Poverty:** Poverty is also perceived as a risk factor for CKD, its progression, and ESRD.

13. **What factors affect the rate of progression of CKD?**
    - **Hypertension:** Poorly controlled hypertension is the single most important factor contributing to the progression of CKD.
    - **Proteinuria:** Heavy proteinuria (1 g/24 h) is often associated with a fast rate of GFR decline.
    - **Poorly controlled diabetes**: In diabetic nephropathy, hyperglycemia has been implicated as a contributing factor along with hypertension and proteinuria in the progression of CKD.

    Other cardiovascular factors such as smoking, dyslipidemia, and obesity may play a role but have not been consistent in epidemiologic studies.

    Exposure to nephrotoxic agents/drugs can affect the rate of progression of CKD. This includes radio-contrast material, NSAIDs, and occasionally inhibitors of the renin-angiotensin-aldosterone system (RAAS). These agents/drugs should be used with caution in older patients and those with diabetic and/or ischemic nephropathy. In the elderly, CKD progression can also be adversely affected by intercurrent illnesses and episodes of AKI.

    An acute-on-chronic exacerbation of CKD warrants thorough investigation of a reversible cause/insult. Dehydration, nephrotoxicity, and obstruction should be ruled out and corrected as soon as possible.

    Pregnancy can exacerbate CKD. This is often the case in the last trimester when hypertension and proteinuria tend to increase, leading in some to pre-eclampsia. Subsequently, renal function can be adversely affected. In pregnant patients with CKD, close monitoring of hypertension and proteinuria is warranted with tight blood pressure (BP) control throughout. ACE inhibitors and ARBs should be avoided in pregnancy and statins should be discontinued. There is no contraindication to pregnancy in CKD1 and 2. The outcome of pregnancy in women with mild renal functional impairment, normal BP, and absent or minimal proteinuria is excellent for mother and fetus. Women suffering from CKD3 should be warned that the risks associated with a pregnancy on the fetus and their kidney function is inversely proportional to the level of GFR. A recent study showed accelerated GFR loss after delivery in a group of women with GFR <40 mL/min/1.73 m^2 and proteinuria >1 g/day. This would imply that women with CKD3b are at increased risk. In fact, more than 70% of women with a serum creatinine >2.5 mg/dL will experience preterm delivery and 40% will develop pre-eclampsia. Pregnancy seldom occurs in stages 4 and 5 and is contraindicated.

    Maynard SE, Thadani R. Pregnancy and the kidney. *J Am Soc Nephrol* 2009;20:14–22.

14. **How should the patient with CKD be approached?**
    History and examination should guide investigations. This could be used as a general guide.
    All patients should have the following:
    - Serum electrolytes, urea, and creatinine
    - Complete blood count and hematinics
    - Bone biochemistry and parathyroid hormone to assess CKD complications
    - Myeloma screen, especially in the elderly
    - Ultrasound scan to rule out structural abnormalities/obstruction; size of kidney and cortical thickness indicate the chronicity of the condition

    Patients with urinary abnormalities (hematuria/proteinuria) should have the following:
    - Autoantibodies, e.g., ANCA, anti-GBM, anti-dsDNA antibodies
    - Serum complement level
    - Serum protein electrophoresis
    - Virology screening for viruses such as hepatitis B and C virus and, when indicated, HIV
    In patients with preserved renal parenchyma on renal ultrasound (good cortical thickness), a kidney biopsy should be performed if there is no obvious cause.

15. **How should kidney function be measured?**

In the past, assessment of overall kidney function relied on the measurement of serum creatinine. Unfortunately, serum creatinine levels can be raised but remain within the normal range, thus misleading physicians to believe that the patient's kidney function is normal. More recently, a calculated GFR derived from the serum creatinine value has been used to estimate glomerular filtration rate. A number of formulas are used to calculate GFR; the most common is the Modification of Diet in Renal Disease (MDRD) abbreviated formula:

$$\text{GFR (mL/min/1.73 m}^2) = 186 \times (PCR)^{-1.154} \times (age)^{-0.203} \times (0.742 \text{ if female}) \times (1.210 \text{ if African American})$$

16. **What are the limitations of the MDRD formula-based eGFR calculation?**
   - The derived estimation of GFR is inaccurate at high levels of GFR (>60 mL/min).
   - The formula underestimates GFR at levels >50 to 60 mL/min.
   - The formula overestimates GFR in CKD stage 5.
   - The formula has not been validated in people with diabetes.
   - The formula has not been validated in individuals who are obese.
   - The formula has not been validated in elderly individuals with muscle wasting.
   - The formula has not been fully validated in non-African American ethnic minorities.

   New and alternative formulas are constantly being put forward. Also, calculation of kidney function and GFR based on the measurement of another endogenous substances filtered by the glomeruli, namely cystatin C, has been advocated by some. Combining creatinine and cystatin measurements and GFR derivation has also been proposed. Most forms of calculated GFR remain inferior to measured GFR by means of inulin,[51] Cr-EDTA, or iohexol/iothalamate clearance but have the advantage of being noninvasive and easy to calculate and disseminate.

17. **How should proteinuria be measured?**
   - Urine dipstick: semiquantitative.
   - 24-hour urine collection: cumbersome, often inaccurate or incomplete
   - Spot urine PCR: more convenient; most useful for monitoring of proteinuria.
   - Spot urine albumin to creatinine ratio (ACR): as above but more specific to albumin; does not measure tubular proteins or light chains; therefore, a better indicator of glomerular disease.

   For PCR and ACR, a first morning void is most reliable. Both measurements are only reliable in the chronic "steady state" of metabolism setting where creatinine excretion is constant.

18. **How does CKD present?**
   - Incidental finding of urine abnormalities or raised creatinine (e.g., routine medicals or investigation of other medical conditions)
   - Finding on routine screening of high-risk groups (e.g., patients with diabetes or hypertension)
   - Symptomatic: symptoms of renal disease are rare.
     - Uremic symptoms are nonspecific (e.g., lethargy and suppressed appetite). They only occur in advanced CKD, usually stage 4.
     - Symptoms related to a systemic inflammatory disease with renal involvement (e.g., Wegner's granulomatosis, lupus).
     - CKD secondary to symptomatic urologic disease (e.g., obstructive symptoms)
     - Symptomatic proteinuria: only occurs when proteinuria is in the nephrotic range

19. **What are the manifestations of CKD?**
   - Asymptomatic urine abnormalities: proteinuria and hematuria
   - Reduced GFR
   - Hypertension
   - Nephrotic syndrome
   - Nephritic syndrome

20. **What are the features of the nephrotic syndrome?**
    - Proteinuria >3.5 g/24 h
    - Edema
    - Hypoalbuminemia
    - Hyperlipidaemia
    - Hypercoagulability

21. **What is the nephritic syndrome?**
    This is less well defined than the nephrotic syndrome and is usually referred to in the acute rather than the chronic setting. It refers to the presence of "nephritis" and includes an active urinary sediment (proteinuria <3.5 g/24 h or "subnephrotic"), hypertension, and reduced GFR.

22. **What are the complications of CKD?**
    The major complications of CKD are as follows:
    - Cardiovascular disease
      - Hypertension
      - Congestive heart failure (CHF)
      - Vascular calcifications and accelerated atherosclerosis
      - Major adverse cardiovascular events (MACE), coronary artery disease, strokes, *peripheral vascular disease*
    - Anemia
    - Mineral and bone disorder
    - Malnutrition

23. **What do patients with CKD die from?**
    The high death rate of patients with CKD is directly related to the adverse cardiovascular impact of CKD. The CVD mortality of CKD is directly related to the CKD stage with up to a 10- to 100-fold increase in CVD mortality in patients with CKD5. It accounts for 50% of deaths in this patient group. The high CVD morbidity and mortality associated with CKD results from the presence of conventional risk factors such as hypertension and dyslipidemia but also renal-specific risk factors such as anemia and abnormalities of the calcium-phosphorus-PTH-vitamin D axis.
    Weiner DE, Tabatabai S, Tighiouart H, et al. Cardiovascular outcomes and all-cause mortality: Exploring the interaction between CKD and cardiovascular disease. *Am J Kidney Dis* 2006;48(3):392–401.

24. **Why do patients with CKD have such a high incidence of CVD?**
    The causes of CVD in CKD are multiple. They consist of the occurrence in CKD of conventional risk factors associated with CVD such as family history of CVD, hypertension, diabetes, and dyslipidemia. Also, many patients with CKD smoke, thus increasing their CVD risk.

    Patients with CKD also have nonconventional CVD risk factors associated with renal insufficiency, including uremia, anemia, abnormalities of the calcium-phosphorus-PTH-vitamin D axis, chronic inflammation, raised serum homocysteine levels, and increased blood oxidant capacity. These various factors combine to increase the CVD morbidity and mortality in CKD.

25. **What is cause of anemia in CKD?**
    The causes of anemia in CKD are multiple:
    - Reduced erythropoietin production
    - Resistance to erythropoietin
    - Iron deficiency

    Also, but of less importance:
    - Folate deficiency
    - Hyperparathyroidism
    - Excessive oxidant stress

26. **What are the mineral and bone disorders (MBD) associated with CKD?**
From CKD stage 3, the ability of the kidneys to appropriately excrete a phosphate load is diminished, leading to hyperphosphatemia. The conversion of 25(OH)D to 1,25(OH)D$_2$ is also impaired, reducing intestinal calcium absorption. Both eventually lead to secondary hyperparathyroidism. There is evidence also of downregulation of vitamin D receptors and resistance to the actions of PTH.

These abnormalities are associated with decreased bone mineral density (renal osteodystrophy), vascular calcifications, and increased CVD morbidity and mortality. The range of renal osteodystrophy spans from low bone turnover and adynamic bone disease to high bone turnover associated with raised PTH levels and osteitis fibrosa.

27. **Why are patients with uremia malnourished?**
Undernutrition and malnutrition are common in patients suffering from ESRD. This stems from a number of factors, prominent among which are the following:
- Decreased food consumption
  - Decreased intake; loss of appetite
  - Decreased absorption
- Hypercatabolism
  - Resistance to anabolic hormones such as insulin and growth hormone
  - Increased catabolic hormones such as catecholamines and glucagon
  - Metabolic acidosis
  - Cytokines release and complement activation during haemodialysis
- Chronic inflammation: malnutrition-inflammation-atherosclerosis (MIA) syndrome
- Diet restriction: e.g., low phosphate diet may lead to protein malnourishment

28. **How should I manage a patient with CKD?**
The two cornerstones of the management of patients with CKD are prevention of CKD progression and management of CKD complications.

29. **Can I prevent the progression of CKD?**
Many years ago, it was thought that the majority of patients with CKD progressed relentlessly to ESRD. Today it is acknowledged that this is not the case because many patients with CKD do not progress and some even regress as their kidney function improves. In general, progression is associated with poorly controlled hypertension (>130/80 mm Hg) and heavy proteinuria (>1 g/24 h).

To slow or prevent progression, we need to do the following:
- Optimize BP control (BP <130/80 mm Hg)
- Reduce proteinuria (<1 g/24 h)
- Use ACE inhibitors and ARBs as appropriate to control BP and reduce proteinuria; this is particularly relevant in diabetic nephropathy and proteinuric CKD.
Key clinical trials include REIN for nondiabetic proteinuric CKD, RENAAL for type 2 diabetic nephropathy, and IDNT for type 2 diabetic nephropathy.

Also, the control of other potential progression cofactors such as dyslipidemia and smoking may have additional benefit. Avoidance of nephrotoxic agents such as NSAIDs is also essential to prevent the decline in kidney function in susceptible individuals. Caution should be exerted with ACE inhibitors or ARBs used in the elderly because they can cause a significant and progressive reduction in kidney function.

30. **How can I minimize and treat cardiovascular CKD complications?**
The most important complication that we should aim to minimize is CVD. Clearly, early intervention is recommended with optimization of BP control, correction of anemia, improvement of the Ca-Pi-PTH-vitamin D axis abnormalities, and treatment of dyslipidemia. Patients with CKD should be advised to stop smoking. Unfortunately, most interventions started late in the course of CKD failed to show an impact on the high mortality rate.

A key clinical trial on lipid lowering is AURORA, 4D.

KEY POINTS: CHRONIC KIDNEY DISEASE

1. Chronic kidney disease (CKD) is common—it is estimated that CKD may affect up to 10% of the population. Most of those affected are older than 55 years of age.

2. Diabetes and hypertension are the most common causes of CKD.

3. CKD may be preventable through lifestyle modification that would have an impact on the incidence of diabetes and hypertension.

4. CKD is treatable, with slowing of its progression by optimization of blood pressure control.

5. CKD increases cardiovascular morbidity and mortality.

6. Most patients with CKD die from cardiovascular disease before reaching end-stage renal disease.

---

31. **How can I minimize and treat anemia in CKD?**
    The management of anemia in CKD consists of correction of any deficiency, including that of iron. In CKD stages 4 and 5/ESRD, the correction of iron deficiency relies on parenteral administration of iron supplements because oral administration is hampered by poor absorption.

    If anemia persists after correction of iron deficiency and repletion of iron stores, then the patient should be treated with regular parenteral administration of an erythropoiesis stimulating agent (ESA). Causes of ESA resistance include uremia (underdialysis), DM, hyperparathyroidism, chronic infections, chronic inflammation, malignancy and myelofibrosis.

    Target Hb levels are around 11 to 12.5 g/dL, according to most guidelines and best renal practice. Higher target levels failed to improve outcomes and were associated in a number of clinical trials with increased mortality.

    Key clinical trials include CREATE, CHOIR, and TREAT.

32. **How can I minimize and treat bone and mineral disturbances in CKD?**
    Treatment aims at correcting hyperphosphatemia and secondary hyperparathyroidism. To reduce hyperphosphatemia, we recommend dietary phosphate restriction while avoiding protein deficiency. Also, we use gut phosphate binders whether calcium based or calcium free. Correction of vitamin D deficiency is also important either with the active metabolite calcitriol or precursors that need the liver for activation as alfacalcidol. It is extremely rare to find refractory cases of hyperparathyroidism in CKD cases before initiation of renal replacement therapy. Severe and refractory hyperparathyroidism on dialysis is treated by either the oral administration of calcimimetics and/or parathyroidectomy.

33. **How can I minimize and treat malnutrition in CKD?**
    Prevention of malnutrition in ESRD involves avoiding exacerbating intervention such as low-protein or low-calorie diets in CKD stage 5, optimization of dialysis, increased protein (>1.2 g/kg/day) and caloric (>35 kcal/kg/day) intake, control of metabolic acidosis, correction of underlying infections or inflammatory processes, and correction of anemia. Attempts have been undertaken at stimulation of anabolism with recombinant human growth hormone or IGF-1.

34. **When should I refer my patient with CKD to a nephrologist?**
    The UK CKD and NICE guidelines give clear guidance as to referral of patients to nephrologists and tertiary centers:
    - All patients with CKD stage 5 should be immediately referred.
    - All patients with CKD stage 4 should be referred unless RRT by dialysis is not considered an option.
    - CKD 4 and 5 should be referred for optimal preparation for RRT. Late referral was found to increase risk in CKD4 and 5.

- Patients with CKD3b should be referred. This is primarily to assess the potential of slowing progression and minimizing complications.
- The following patients are often referred for further investigations and often a renal biopsy:
    - Patients with CKD3a and declining GFR
    - Patients with CKD3a and significant proteinuria (>1 g/24 h)
    - Patients with CKD 1 and 2 with significant proteinuria (>1 g/24 h)
    - Patients with CKD1 and 2 with hematuria and proteinuria (>0.5 g/24 h)
- Patients with CKD1 and 2 and isolated hematuria should be investigated urologically but do not require nephrologic referral
- Patients with CKD1, 2, and 3 and stable renal function should be referred unless they have hematuria, proteinuria, or declining kidney function

35. **How is a renal replacement therapy option chosen?**
    Most patients reaching a GFR should be considered for renal replacement therapy unless futile. Treatment options include dialysis, hemo or peritoneal dialysis, and transplantation. Clearly transplantation is the preferred option, although it depends on the availability of a kidney donor. Patients unsuitable for RRT have been offered medical management. In one study overall patient survival from the time of first-known CKD 5 was 21 months. Patients known to a nephrologist before reaching CKD 5 survived longer than those presenting with CKD 5. Serum albumin >35 g/L was associated with greater survival, but other biochemical parameters, comorbidity grade, and age did not predict survival. In another study of patients who were not dialysis treated, the Stoke Comorbidity Score (SCG), a validated scoring system for the survival of patients on RRT was an independent prognostic factor in predicting survival. In those patients who chose not to dialyze, SCG provides a potentially useful indication of expected prognosis (6).

    Wong CF, McCarthy M, Howse ML, et al. Factors affecting survival in advanced chronic kidney disease patients who choose not to receive dialysis. *Ren Fail* 2007;29(6):653–659.

CHAPTER 20

ANEMIA IN CHRONIC KIDNEY DISEASE

Jay B. Wish, MD

1. **What causes anemia in patients with renal disease?**
   The anemia of chronic kidney disease (CKD) is primarily caused by deficiency of erythropoietin. The kidneys are the major source of erythropoietin and, as renal function declines, production of erythropoietin declines proportionately. As a result, there tends to be a linear relationship between hemoglobin (Hb) level and glomerular filtration rate (GFR) in patients with CKD, although a wide range of Hb may be observed for any degree of renal disease.

   A number of other factors tend to decrease red cell life span from the normal of 120 days to approximately 70 to 80 days in patients with CKD. These include red cell trauma as a result of microvascular disease from diabetes or hypertension, blood loss from the hemodialysis (HD) procedure, an increased incidence of gastrointestinal bleeding from peptic ulcer disease and angiodysplasia of the bowel, and increased oxidative stress leading to shortened red cell survival.

2. **How does one evaluate anemia in a patient with CKD?**
   Erythropoietin deficiency is a diagnosis of exclusion, and determination of erythropoietin levels in patients with CKD is generally not indicated. The routine evaluation of such patients should include measurement of red blood cell (RBC) indices, reticulocyte count, transferrin saturation, and serum ferritin and a test for occult blood in the stool. If these tests reveal no easily correctable cause of anemia, such as gastrointestinal bleeding or iron deficiency, it can be presumed that the anemia results primarily from erythropoietin deficiency.

3. **How are the tests of iron status in patients with CKD interpreted?**
   The two most commonly used tests of iron status are transferrin saturation and serum ferritin. Transferrin saturation is computed by dividing the serum iron level by the total iron-binding capacity. The total iron-binding capacity correlates with circulating transferrin, which is the major iron-binding protein in plasma. Transferrin saturation correlates with the amount of iron available for erythropoiesis because only circulating iron is available to the bone marrow for incorporation into newly synthesized red blood cells. The serum ferritin level correlates with storage iron located primarily in the reticuloendothelial system. Interpretation of serum ferritin levels is confounded by the fact that ferritin will rise as an acute-phase reactant in the setting of acute or chronic inflammation. In patients with CKD, a serum ferritin level less than 100 ng/mL correlates with a deficiency in storage iron; such patients will almost invariably respond to supplemental iron therapy. Patients with a transferrin saturation of less than 20% have decreased iron delivery to the erythroid marrow, but supplemental iron may or may not correct this problem, depending on whether storage iron can effectively be released to the transferrin carrier protein.

   The reticulocyte hemoglobin content (cHr) measures the amount of hemoglobin in the youngest red blood cells and is a useful marker of current iron availability to the bone marrow. The cHr test is available on some hematology analyzers that perform complete blood counts. A cHr value of <29 pg correlates with functional iron deficiency.

4. **What is functional iron deficiency?**

Functional iron deficiency is a phenomenon that occurs in patients treated with pharmacologic doses of erythropoiesis-stimulating agents (ESAs) when the bone marrow is stimulated to produce red blood cells faster than the transferrin carrier protein can deliver adequate iron substrate. In such patients, the transferrin saturation tends to be low or low-normal, whereas the serum ferritin level may be normal or even high. The operative definition of functional iron deficiency is based on a response to intravenous iron supplementation characterized by either an increase in hemoglobin or a decrease in ESA requirements to achieve the same Hb. Studies have demonstrated that functional iron deficiency is common in patients with end-stage renal disease who are treated with ESAs and that intravenous iron supplementation will decrease ESA requirements by approximately 20% to 25%. Because of the risk of fatal anaphylactic reactions, iron dextran has fallen out of favor as an intravenous iron supplement and has been replaced by sodium ferric gluconate, iron sucrose, and ferumoxytol.

5. **Why are oral iron supplements often ineffective in treating the iron deficiency in patients receiving chronic hemodialysis?**

Oral iron absorption tends to be inversely proportional to serum ferritin levels. In patients with a serum ferritin of 100 ng/mL or higher, oral iron absorption is approximately 1% to 2% of the administered load. A patient taking ferrous sulfate, 325 mg three times daily, will consume 200 mg of elemental iron, of which 2 to 4 mg will be absorbed daily. The iron requirements in patients with anemia undergoing hemodialysis are often enormous. Increasing the Hb from 8 g/dL to 11 g/dL in a 70-kg patient requires the incorporation of 600 mg of elemental iron into the newly synthesized red blood cells. In addition, the estimated daily iron losses in hemodialysis patients are approximately 4 to 7 mg. Thus, the 2 to 4 mg of oral iron absorbed daily would barely keep pace with ongoing iron losses, let alone repair the accumulated iron deficit. Compounding this problem is the phenomenon of functional iron deficiency, which often results in the need for high levels of storage iron to facilitate release of iron to transferrin and delivery of that iron to the erythroid marrow. As a result, most patients undergoing hemodialysis and receiving ESAs require intravenous iron supplements.

6. **How are ESAs administered?**

Human recombinant erythropoietin (epoetin) is a polypeptide hormone that, like insulin, must be given parenterally through a subcutaneous or intravenous route. A number of studies have demonstrated that subcutaneously administered epoetin, because of its slower absorption and longer half-life, is more effective than a comparable dose administered intravenously. Several studies have demonstrated a 20% to 30% reduction in the epoetin dose required to achieve the same Hb when patients are switched from the intravenous to the subcutaneous route of administration.

For patients receiving epoetin intravenously on HD, the recommended starting dose is 50 units/kg of body weight three times weekly, with the dose titrated at monthly intervals depending on the hemoglobin response. For patients receiving epoetin therapy subcutaneously, the recommended starting dose is 30 units/kg administered three times weekly (as is typically done in HD facilities) or 100 units/kg/week administered weekly or biweekly (which is typical for predialysis and peritoneal dialysis patients). Again, the dose would be titrated at monthly intervals depending on the Hb response. **Darbepoetin alfa,** an analogue of human erythropoietin with two extra carbohydrate side chains, has a longer duration of action when compared with both native and recombinant hormone. The recommended starting dose for darbepoetin alfa is 0.45 μg/kg administered weekly or 0.75 μg/kg administered biweekly in dialysis and patients with CKD for both intravenous and subcutaneous administration, with subsequent titration based on the hemoglobin concentration. Success with longer dosing intervals for both epoetin and darbepoetin has been reported.

7. **What is the target hemoglobin for patients with CKD receiving ESA therapy?**
   The practice guidelines prepared by the National Kidney Foundation's Kidney Disease Outcomes Quality Initiative (NKF-KDOQI) recommend a target Hb of 11 to 12 g/dL and avoiding Hb >13 g/dL in patients with CKD (dialysis and predialysis) with anemia and being treated with ESAs. This is supported by a number of studies, mostly observational, that demonstrate this Hb is associated with improved functional and cognitive status, improved quality of life, regression of left ventricular hypertrophy, and decreased morbidity and mortality when compared with patients with CKD and lower Hb levels. The U.S. Food and Drug Administration (FDA) has recommended a target Hb of 10 to 12 g/dL in patients with anemia and CKD treated with ESA. A number of randomized prospective trials of ESA treatment for such patients have failed to confirm the benefits of higher, as opposed to lower, Hb levels suggested by observational data. The Normal Hematocrit Cardiovascular Trial, published in 1998, demonstrated a tendency toward more cardiovascular events among patients undergoing HD and receiving epoetin who were randomized to a target hematocrit to 42% versus 30%. Three additional studies comparing high versus low Hb targets for ESA therapy in patients with nondialysis CKD are summarized in Table 20-1.

   Retrospective analyses of the Normal Hematocrit Cardiovascular Trial and Correction of Hemoglobin and Outcomes in Renal Insufficiency (CHOIR) by the FDA and the CHOIR investigators suggest that the risk of adverse outcomes in these trials is correlated with the ESA dose received rather than the Hb level achieved. A similar pattern is observed in the Trial to Reduce Cardiovascular Events with Aranesp Therapy (TREAT) study. In other words, a patient who achieves an Hb of 13 g/dL using a low dose of ESA is at lower risk than a patient who requires a large dose of ESA to increase the Hb level from 9 to 11 g/dL.

TABLE 20-1. LARGE RANDOMIZED STUDIES IN PATIENTS WITH ANEMIA AND CKD NOT RECEIVING DIALYSIS			
	CHOIR	**CREATE**	**TREAT**
Location	United States	Europe	International
ESA	Epoetin alfa	Epoetin beta	Darbepoetin alfa
Number of patients	1432	603	4038, type 2 diabetics
High Hb target g/dL	13.5	13–15	13
Low Hb target g/dL	11.3	10.5–11.5	9
Cardiovascular endpoints	Higher in high Hb group	No difference	No difference except higher stroke in high Hb group
Progression of CKD	No difference	More in high Hb group	No difference
Cancer deaths	Not noted	Not noted	Higher in high Hb group among patients with prior cancer
Quality of life	No difference	Better in high Hb group	No difference except less fatigue in high Hb group

CKD = chronic kidney disease; CHOIR = Correction of Hemoglobin and Outcomes in Renal Insufficiency; CREATE = Cardiovascular Risk Reduction of Early Anemia Treatment with Epoetin Beta; TREAT = Trial to Reduce Cardiovascular Events with Aranesp Therapy; ESA = erythrocyte-stimulating agent; Hb = hemoglobin.

KEY POINTS: ANEMIA

1. The anemia of chronic kidney disease (CKD) is primarily caused by deficiency of erythropoietin.

2. Many patients with CKD not receiving hemodialysis and most patients receiving hemodialysis are iron deficient and require iron supplementation.

3. The FDA has determined that the target hemoglobin (Hb) level for patients with anemia receiving erythropoiesis-stimulating agents (ESAs) is 10 to 12 g/dL, but this has become a matter of some controversy.

4. Randomized controlled studies consistently demonstrate that normalizing the Hb level of patients with CKD with ESAs is associated with poorer outcomes than a Hb target in the 9.0 to 11.5 g/dL range.

8. **Are ESAs toxic?**

Since their approval for the treatment of CKD-associated anemia in 1989, ESAs have been considered by many patients and physicians to be a therapeutic miracle. ESAs are administered to more than 95% of patients receiving dialysis in the United States. Like any other pharmacologic agent, ESAs have risks that must be weighed against their benefits. The most compelling benefits of ESA therapy are improvement in quality of life and transfusion avoidance. These are most dramatic in patients receiving dialysis whose historical Hb in the pre-ESA era was 7 to 8 g/dL. None of the randomized clinical trials of ESA therapy has ever shown a mortality benefit, and the three large trials in patients with CKD who are not receiving dialysis summarized in Table 20-1 suggest that caution must be used when treating patients with ESAs to minimize the risk of adverse cardiovascular outcomes. Based on retrospective rather than intention-to treat analyses, it is suspected that high ESA doses (rather than high Hb levels) accelerate cardiovascular disease. The increased number of cancer deaths noted in the high Hb arm of the TREAT study, coupled with data from the oncology literature demonstrating increased tumor progression or recurrence among patients treated with ESAs, suggests that ESAs should be used with caution in patients with CKD with existing malignancies. The recommendation is that ESA treatment and dosing should be individualized in the patient with CKD to weigh benefit versus risk and that very high doses of ESAs should be avoided.

9. **What are EPO mimetics?**

A number of pharmaceutical agents are under development that are not derivatives of human recombinant erythropoietin and have been shown to increase Hb levels in anemic subjects with and without kidney disease. The first category consists of agents that are based on synthetic polypeptides with strong affinity for the human EPO receptor but that have no homology to the human EPO molecule. These polypeptides are pegylated and administered parenterally (subcutaneously or intravenously) and have a duration of action that is significantly longer than the currently available ESAs. Peginesatide (Hematide) is one such agent in late clinical trials. It is effective when administered once monthly and has been shown to be effective in patients who develop pure red cell aplasia (PRCA) as the result of formation of antibodies against agents derived from human recombinant erythropoietin. The second category of EPO mimetics consists of modifications of the human recombinant erythropoietin molecule. A number of these agents are currently in use in countries other than the United States, but their introduction into the U.S. market has been delayed until 2014 by patent infringement issues. These include a pegylated form of EPO (Micera) and a gene-activated EPO (Dynepo). Like peginesatide, Micera has been show to be effective when administered once monthly. The third category of EPO mimetics are agents that potentiate the activity of hypoxia-inducible factor (HIF), the substance in the kidney and other tissues that senses decreased delivery of oxygen (from hypoxemia or anemia) and stimulates the production of EPO. In the absence of hypoxia, HIF is rapidly degraded by an enzyme, prolyl hydroxylase (HIF-PH). A number of agents are under development that inhibit HIF-PH, thereby increasing HIF and endogenous EPO activity. These agents are orally active and, interestingly, effective even in patients with end-stage renal disease (ESRD), suggesting that significant EPO production can be induced in nonrenal tissues. Finally, there are a number of "biosimilar" (the term used for "generic" biopharmaceutcal agents) ESAs in use outside the United States. These agents have been associated with a relatively high incidence of PRCA as a result of subtle differences in manufacturing and packaging, which may make them more immunogenic than the agents currently available in the United States, where the incidence of PRCA is extremely low.

10. **What is the role of carnitine?**
Carnitine is an essential intracellular substance that is responsible for the transport of fatty acids into the mitochondria for oxidation. Carnitine is synthesized in the liver and kidneys, and many patients with ESRD have low levels of carnitine in the blood. It has been proposed that carnitine deficiency in patients with ESRD may contribute to anemia and ESA resistance and that L-carnitine supplementation improves red blood cell survival through enhanced RBC membrane stability. Although Medicare has paid for intravenous (IV) L-carnitine supplements in patients undergoing dialysis and requiring high doses of ESAs, the results of clinical trials for this indication have been less than compelling, using small numbers of patients and providing conflicting results. Based on a review of this evidence, the NKF-KDOQI guidelines do not advocate the use of IV L-carnitine for the treatment of ESA-resistant anemia in patients ESRD, but there are some authors who consider a 6-month trial of IV L-carnitine reasonable in this setting if no other cause for the ESA-resistance can be identified.

11. **Are there special considerations for patients with CKD and sickle cell disease?**
There are no evidence-based guidelines regarding whether the anemia of patients with CKD and sickle cell disease should be treated differently from other patients with anemia and CKD. As a result of ongoing red blood cell destruction, patients with sickle cell disease have lower Hb levels and higher ESA requirements than their anemic CKD counterparts. Concerns regarding toxicity of high-dose ESAs may lead to placing a ceiling on the ESA dose administered to such patients (300 units of epoetin/kgBW/week in patients with CKD not undergoing hemodialysis and 450 units of epoetin/kgBW/week in patients receiving hemodialysis has been suggested as such a ceiling). Furthermore, patients with sickle cell disease may become more symptomatic at higher Hb levels, so a target Hb range lower than 10 to 12 g/dL may be appropriate. Transfusions are more often required in patients with sickle cell disease than in other patients with anemia and CKD, so attention must be paid to the potential for iron overload and sensitization for future renal transplantation. As in all patients, ESA and transfusion therapy in patients with sickle cell disease should carefully weigh risk versus benefit.

12. **What is the role of transfusions in the treatment of CKD-associated anemia?**
RBC transfusion therapy for the anemia of CKD in the pre-ESA era was associated with the transmission of bloodborne infections, iron overload, and sensitization for future renal transplantation. Despite the newly emerging controversies regarding the risk versus benefits of ESA therapy, there is no dispute that ESAs decrease RBC transfusion requirements and far fewer patients receiving ESAs require RBC transfusions than patients not receiving ESAs. Nonetheless, RBC transfusions are occasionally required in patients with anemia and CKD despite the use of ESA and iron therapy, especially in the setting of acute blood loss. Because RBC transfusions still carry the risk of sensitization for future renal transplantation, they should be used judiciously in patients with CKD, especially those who are transplant candidates. There is no single Hb or Hb range that is considered a trigger for RBC transfusions, and the NKF-KDOQI anemia guidelines emphasize that the Hb target/trigger for transfusion is not the same as the Hb

target range for ESA therapy. The decision to transfuse a patient with anemia and CKD should weigh the Hb level, symptoms, comorbidities such as coronary artery disease, cause of anemia, and whether the anemia can be treated effectively with alternate therapies. A patient with a critically low Hb level who is a Jehovah's Witness and declines transfusions may require higher ESA doses than those typically used. The use of blood substitutes may also be considered in this setting.

BIBLIOGRAPHY

1. Aranesp (darbepoetin alfa) for injection [prescribing information]. Thousand Oaks, CA: Amgen Inc, 2007. Available at: http://www.aranesp.com/pdf/aranesp_pi.pdfprescribing_information.jsp. Accessed Jan. 15, 2011.

2. Besarab A, Bolton WK, Browne JK, et al. The effects of normal as compared with low hematocrit values in patients with cardiac disease who are receiving hemodialysis and epoetin. *N Engl J Med* 1998;339(9):584–590.

3. Brewster UC. Intravenous iron therapy in end-stage renal disease. *Semin Dial* 2006;19(4):285–290.

4. Drueke TB, Locatelli F, Clyne N, et al. CREATE Investigators. Normalization of hemoglobin level in patients with chronic kidney disease and anemia. *N Engl J Med* 2006;355(20):2071–2084.

5. Hedayati SS. Dialysis-related carnitine disorder. *Semin Dial* 2006;19(4):323–328.

6. Kimel M, Leidy NK, Mannix S, et al. Does epoetin alfa improve health-related quality of life in chronically ill patients with anemia? Summary of trials of cancer, HIV/AIDS, and chronic kidney disease. *Value Health* 2008;11(1):57–75.

7. Ling B, Walczyk M, Agarwal A, et al. Darbepoetin alfa administered once monthly maintains hemoglobin concentrations in patients with chronic kidney disease. *Clin Nephrol* 2005;63(5):327–334.

8. Macdougall IC, Ashenden M. Current and upcoming erythropoiesis-stimulating agents, iron products, and other novel anemia medications. *Adv Chronic Kidney Dis* 2009;16(2):11–130.

9. National Kidney Foundation. *KDOQI Clinical Practice Guidelines and Clinical Practice Recommendations for Anemia in Chronic Kidney Disease.* Available at: www.kidney.org/PROFESSIONALS/kdoqi/guidelines_anemia/guide2.htm#cpr11 Accessed Jan. 15, 2011.

10. Pfeffer, M, Burdmann, E, Chen, C, et al. A trial of darbepoetin alfa in type 2 diabetes and chronic kidney disease. *N Engl J Med* 2009;361(21):2019–2032.

11. Procrit (epoetin alfa) for injection [prescribing information]. Thousand Oaks, CA: Amgen Inc. Distributed by Ortho Biotech Products, LP: Raritan, NJ, 2007. Available at: http://www.procrit.com/sites/default/files/shared/OBI/PI/ProcritBooklet.pdf#page=1. Accessed Jan 15, 2011.

12. Provenzano R, Bhaduri S, Singh AK, PROMPT Study Group. Extended epoetin alfa dosing as maintenance treatment for the anemia of chronic kidney disease: The PROMPT study. *Clin Nephrol* 2005;64(2):113–123.

13. Regidor DL, Kopple JD, Kovesdy CP, et al. Associations between changes in hemoglobin and administered erythropoiesis-stimulating agent and survival in hemodialysis patients. *J Am Soc Nephrol* 2006;17(4):1181–1191.

14. Szczech LA, Burnhart HXS, Inrig JK, et al. Secondary analysis of the CHOIR trial epoetin-a dose and achieved hemoglobin outcomes. *Kidney Int* 2008;74:791–798.

15. Singh AK, Szczech L, Tang KL, et al, CHOIR Investigators. Correction of anemia with epoetin alfa in chronic kidney disease. *N Engl J Med* 2006;355(20):2085–2098.

16. Spinowitz BS, Kausz AT, Baptista J, et al. Ferumoxytol for treating iron deficiency anemia in CKD. *J Am Soc Nephrol* 2008;19:1599–1605.

CHAPTER 21

RENAL OSTEODYSTROPHY

Stuart M. Sprague, DO

1. **What is chronic kidney disease-mineral and bone disorder?**
   Chronic kidney disease-mineral and bone disorder (CKD-MBD) is a systemic disorder of mineral and bone metabolism resulting from CKD that may be manifested by either one or a combination of the following:
   - Laboratory abnormalities associated with disturbed mineral metabolism including calcium, phosphorus, parathyroid hormone (PTH), or vitamin D metabolism
   - Bone disease defined as renal osteodystrophy including abnormalities in bone turnover, mineralization, volume, linear growth, or strength
   - Calcification of extraskeletal tissue, which would include vascular or other soft tissue calcification

2. **How do we define renal bone diseases?**
   Renal osteodystrophy (ROD) is the term used to describe the bone lesions associated with CKD-MBD. ROD is an alteration of bone morphology in patients with CKD. It is one measure of the skeletal component of the systemic disorder of CKD-MBD that is quantifiable by bone histomorphometry. It is defined by three key histologic descriptors—bone turnover, mineralization, and volume (TMV system)—with any combination of each of the descriptors possible in a given specimen. The TMV classification scheme provides a clinically relevant description of the underlying bone pathology.

3. **Name the factors contributing to sustained increases in PTH secretion, parathyroid hyperplasia, and ultimately high-turnover bone disease.**
   The factors responsible for secondary hyperparathyroidism associated with CKD include hyperphosphatemia from diminished renal phosphorus excretion, hypocalcemia, impaired renal production of active 1,25-dihydroxyvitamin D, alterations in the control of PTH gene transcription, and skeletal resistance to the calcemic action of PTH. Fibroblastic growth factor 23 (FGF23) may indirectly promote hyperparathyroidism as it further inhibits production of 1,25-dihydroxyvitamin D.

4. **Describe the bone lesion associated with hyperparathyroidism.**
   The primary histologic bone lesion associated with moderate to severe hyperparathyroidism is a high-turnover lesion, which has been referred to as osteitis fibrosa cystic. Clinically it is associated with nonspecific bone pain, proximal myopathy. The serum-intact PTH level is usually higher than 350 to 500 pg/mL. Radiologic features are subperiosteal resorption, Brown tumors, and a mottled and granular salt-and-pepper appearance to the skull. The histologic features include bone resorption and formation with increased numbers of osteoclasts and osteoblasts, increased tetracycline uptake with increased of woven bone, and peritrabecular fibrosis. There may or may not be increased osteoid.

5. **How is high-turnover bone disease treated?**
   Treatment of this disorder entails prevention and correction of the factors leading to secondary hyperparathyroidism. This includes phosphorus control (dietary restriction, phosphate binders, adequate dialysis); prevention of hypocalcemia (oral calcium supplements,

correction of vitamin D deficiency, dialysis); and suppression of PTH production and secretion with the use of vitamin D receptor activators (VDRA), including calcitriol, paricalcitol, and doxercalciferol, and/or the use of calcimimetics (cinacalcet) (Table 21-1). In severe cases, parathyroidectomy may be required; however, bone biopsy should be considered prior to proceeding with parathyroidectomy.

6. **What are the disorders associated with low-turnover bone disease?**
   Low-turnover or adynamic bone disease is defined by the presence of low or absent bone formation as determined by decreased tetracycline uptake into bone, in conjunction with a paucity of bone-forming osteoblasts and bone-resorbing osteoclasts. It may also be associated with a defect in mineralization, resulting in the histologic lesion referred to as

TABLE 21-1.   IMPACT AND CHALLENGES WITH VITAMIN D TO TREAT SHPT IN PATIENTS WITH CKD

Vitamin D Compound	Biologic and Clinical Impact	Challenges
Ergocalciferol (D_2) Cholecalciferol (D_3)	Effective in repleting 25-D and 1,25-D in patients with early-stage CKD and adequate kidney function	Requires activation in the liver to generate 25-D Requires activation in the kidney to generate active 1,25-D Provides only partial suppression of PTH in patients with later-stage CKD
Calcitriol	Biologically active VDR agonist Effectively suppresses SHPT Reduces abnormal high bone turnover	Hypercalcemia, hypercalciuria, and hyperphosphatemia evident at high doses
Doxercalciferol	Suppresses SHPT similar to or better than calcitriol Noted reduction in serum bone-specific alkaline phosphatase and osteocalcin	Requires activation in liver to generate active 1,25-D Induces significant elevation of serum P, elevating need for phosphate binder use
Alphacalcidol	Suppresses SHPT similar to or better than calcitriol	Requires activation in kidney to generate active 1,25-D Induces significant elevation of serum P, elevating need for phosphate binder use
Paricalcitol	Biologically active VDR agonist Effectively suppresses SHPT Noted reduction in serum bone-specific alkaline phosphatase and osteocalcin	Minimal elevation in Ca, P, and Ca $\times$ P product, requiring Ca and P monitoring

SHPT, secondary hyperparathyroidism; CKD = chronic kidney disease; 25-D = 25-hydroxyvitamin; 1,25-D = 1,25-dihydroxyvitamin D; PTH = parathyroid hormone; VDR = vitamin D receptor; P = phosphorus; Ca = calcium.

osteomalacia. Clinically it may be manifested by nonspecific bone pain and fractures. PTH concentrations are relatively low (less than 100–200 pg/mL) and hypercalcemia is a common feature. There may be a tendency for increased extraskeletal calcification. Low turnover is characterized histologically by absence of cellular (osteoblast and osteoclast) activity, osteoid formation, and endosteal fibrosis. It appears that this is essentially a disorder of decreased bone formation, accompanied by a secondary decrease in bone mineralization. Although low turnover disease is common in the absence of aluminum, it was initially described as a result of aluminum toxicity. Aluminum bone disease is diagnosed by special staining, which demonstrates the presence of aluminum deposits at the mineralization front. The major risk factors for low turnover bone disease include diabetes, aging, and malnutrition. The other causes of low bone formation in CKD are multifactorial and include such remedial causes as vitamin D deficiency, high serum phosphate, metabolic acidosis, elevated circulating cytokine levels (interleukin [IL]-I, tumor necrosis factor [TNF]), and low estrogen and testosterone levels. Normal or mildly elevated serum PTH concentrations have been associated as a cause of adynamic bone when in fact what is meant is that there is a resistance to the bone stimulatory effect of PTH in CKD. Parathyroid hormone receptor downregulation is one potential mechanism to explain the bone resistance effect to PTH resulting, in part, from persistently elevated PTH.

7. **What is osteomalacia?**
Osteomalacia is characterized by an excess of unmineralized osteoid, manifested as wide osteoid seams and a markedly decreased mineralization rate. The presence of increased unmineralized osteoid per se does not necessarily indicate a mineralizing defect because increased quantities of osteoid appear in conditions associated with high rates of bone formation when mineralization lags behind the increased synthesis of matrix. Other features of osteomalacia include the absence of cell activity and the absence of endosteal fibrosis; there is normal or decreased osteoid volume and decreased mineralization. Frequently, aluminum disease is associated with osteomalacia. Serum PTH is, in general, normal or low, and hypercalcemia is common. Looser zones or pseudofractures are radiologic characteristics.

8. **What is mixed uremic osteodystrophy?**
Mixed uremic osteodystrophy (MUO) is the term that has been used to describe bone biopsies that have features of secondary hyperparathyroidism together with evidence of a mineralization defect. There is extensive osteoclastic and osteoblastic activity and increased endosteal peritrabecular fibrosis coupled with more osteoid than expected, and tetracycline labeling uncovers a concomitant mineralization defect. Unfortunately, mixed uremic osteodystrophy, in particular, and high- and low-turnover bone disease have been inconsistent and poorly defined. Thus, it is best to describe bone histology or renal osteodystrophy according to the TMV system as defined as part of CKD-MBD.

9. **What is calcific uremic arteriolopathy?**
Calcific uremic arteriolopathy (CUA, or calciphylaxis) is a rare but life-threatening syndrome characteristically occurring in individuals with ESRD but has been described in patients with normal kidney renal function and calcium/phosphate metabolism. CUA generally presents as excruciatingly painful eschars on the lower limbs but may affect other sites, including the abdominal wall, breasts, and penis, but rarely the face or upper extremities. The syndrome typically begins with dysesthesia, followed by the development of erythema resembling livedo reticularis, and progression to frank ulceration. There may be palpable deposits of calcium subcutaneously. The lesions are intensely painful and the surrounding tissue may be pruritic. The lesions have been proposed to occur at sites of adipose tissue where diminished blood flow contributes to hypoxia. Major risk factors appear to be female gender, diabetes mellitus, obesity, malnutrition, elevated serum phosphate, and the use or warfarin. The underlying pathology is of vascular calcification. Initially assumed to be a passive event caused by

deranged calcium and phosphate metabolism, this calcification is fundamentally an actively regulated process. Elevated phosphate levels have been regarded as one of the most important factors in initiating CUA, with persistent hyperphosphatemia and hypercalcemia promoting further vascular mineralization. Defects in a number of inhibitors of calcification including matrix GLA protein and fetuin have also been identified as playing a causative role. Most patients with CUA die from complications associated with wound infections. Therapy should be focused on wound management and controlling serum phosphate levels. Parathyroidectomy is controversial and is generally not recommended. Aggressive dialysis, nutrition, and noncalcium-containing phosphate binders are the mainstay of therapy. Some studies have demonstrated anecdotal response to sodium thiosulfate. It is unclear if calcimimetics or bisphosphonates are beneficial.

10. **How should treatment be approached for patients with CKD stages 3–4?**
The earliest manifestations of CKD-MBD in the evolution of CKD are phosphate retention, decreases in calcitriol, then increases in PTH, and finally (in late stage 4, early stage 5 disease) hyperphosphatemia and eventually hypocalcemia. Most patients are also calcidiol (25-hydroxy vitamin D) deficient. Thus, the approach to therapy should be aimed at reversing or preventing these perturbations in mineral metabolism. Unfortunately, adequate studies demonstrating benefit to various therapies are lacking; thus recommendations have been based on expert opinion and clinical judgment. A reasonable approach would be to prevent phosphate retention either through moderate phosphate restriction or the introduction of phosphate binders (Table 21-2). To date, the use of phosphate binders has not been approved in CKD stages 3 and 4, nor are there adequate studies demonstrating that the use of phosphate binders results in improved patient outcome. It is also reasonable to correct the calcidiol deficiency by replacing nutritional vitamin D, either with cholecalciferol (1200–2000 units/day) or ergocalciferol (50,000 units once monthly to once weekly). If PTH levels remain elevated after some degree of phosphate control and correction of calcidiol deficiency, then it would be reasonable to use a VDRA—calcitriol, paricalcitol, or doxercalciferol. There does not appear to be a role for calcimimetics in CKD stages 3 and 4. Although the National Kidney Foundation's Kidney Disease Outcomes Quality Initiative (K/DOQI) and Kidney Disease: Improving Global Outcomes (K/DIGO) have suggested therapeutic targets for PTH concentrations, unfortunately there are insufficient data to support those targets and patients should be treated upon clinical judgment (Table 21-3).

11. **How should treatment be approached for patients with CKD stage 5?**
Patients with stage 5 disease who have not been previously treated generally present with hyperphosphatemia, hyperparathyroidism, and very low calcitriol concentrations and may have low, normal, or elevated serum calcium. Furthermore, most of these patients are also calcidiol deficient. Therapy should definitely be focused to control serum phosphate to at least 5.5 mg/dL, if not to normal values by the use of adequate dialysis, dietary phosphate restriction, and phosphate binders. The use of calcium-containing binders (calcium carbonate or calcium acetate) should be limited to less than 1500 mg of calcium a day. If patients have evidence of vascular calcifications, calcium-containing binders should be avoided. The noncalcium-containing binders that could be used include either sevelamer or lanthanum. Both of these agents appear to be effective in treating hyperphosphatemia with few side effects or long-term risk. However, the dose for sevelamer generally requires three to four times the number of pills than that required for lanthanum with comparable phosphate control. If patients have extremely elevated serum phosphorus, a short course of aluminum-containing phosphate binder may be considered; however, its use should be avoided because of the risk of aluminum toxicity. Hyperparathyroidism and calcitriol deficiency could be addressed with the use of VDRAs. Calcitriol is effective but carries a greater risk of causing hypercalcemia and/or hyperphosphatemia, whereas paricalcitol appears to have the lowest risk for hypercalcemia and hyperphosphatemia. Doxercalciferol, a prohormone, is also

TABLE 21-2. CHARACTERISTICS OF COMMONLY USED PHOSPHATE BINDERS

Phosphate Binder	Benefits	Hazards	Bone Biopsy Findings
Aluminum	Potent and effective Useful for short term in severe hyperphosphatemia	Dementia Low-turnover bone disease/osteomalacia Anemia Should not be used as maintenance therapy	Accumulation of unmineralized matrix Wide osteoid seams Absence of osteoblasts
Calcium salt based	Effective Inexpensive Treats hypocalcemia Antacid properties useful for reflux and peptic ulcer disease	High calcium load Hypercalcemia Development of adynamic bone disease Extraosseous/vascular calcifications	Lack of osteoid accumulation Absence of bone formation or resorption
Sevelamer chloride	Effective No systemic absorption Lowers level of low-density lipoprotein cholesterol Lower risk of hypercalcemia Reduces aortic and coronary calcification versus calcium salts Lower risk of adynamic bone disease versus calcium salts	Expensive Metabolic acidosis Binds bile acids Not effective in acidic environment Gastrointestinal symptoms such as diarrhea High pill burden	Unknown
Sevelamer carbonate	Effective No metabolic acidosis	Expensive Limited postmarketing experience Unclear if has same side effects of Sevelamer HCl	Does not appear to cause low bone turnover
Lanthanum carbonate	Potent and effective over wide pH range Lack of hypercalcemia No evidence of increased risk of low bone turnover disease Potential reduced pill burden	Expensive Systemic absorption with minimal body tissue accumulation (no clinical consequence to date)	1 year increases in markers of bone turnover—improved activation frequency and bone formation rate/bone surface 2 year increases in overall bone volume

TABLE 21–3. COMPARISON OF K/DOQI WITH K/DIGO MINERAL GUIDELINES

	K/DIGO	K/DOQI
Monitoring of Ca, phos, PTH	Starting at CKD stage 3 CKD stage 5 Ca and phos monthly PTH quarterly Include alkaline phosphatase: high or low levels may predict bone turnover	Same, no comment on alkaline phosphatase
Goal calcium	Normal range CKD stages 3–5	Same, weighted to lower end of normal range (8.4–9.5 mg/dL)
Goal phosphorus	Normal range stages 3–5	Range 2.7–4.6 mg/dL stages 3–4, 3.0–5.5 mg/dL for stage 5
Goal PTH	Evaluate patients with PTH above upper limits of normal for correctable factors: low phos/ca, low vitamin D. Treat based on trends to achieve PTH between 2 and 9 times the upper limit of normal	Target ranges: CKD3 35–70 pg/mL CKD4 70–110 pg/mL CKD5 150–300 pg/mL
Bone biopsy	Reasonable in various settings and prior to bisphosphonate therapy in CKD-MBD	Should be considered

K/DOQI = Kidney Disease Outcomes Quality Initiative; K/DIGO = Kidney Disease: Improving Global Outcomes; ca = calcium; phos = phosphorus; PTH = parathyroid hormone; CKD = chronic kidney disease; CKD-MBD = chronic kidney disease-mineral and bone disorder.

effective at reducing PTH but may have a higher incidence of hypercalcemia and/or hyperphosphatemia than paricalcitol. Only one study has directly compared VDRAs in patients receiving dialysis, and that was between calcitriol and paricalcitol. The calcimimetic cinacalcet is also effective in lowering PTH concentrations and lowering both serum calcium and phosphate concentrations. Although it has been shown to be effective when used in the absence of VDRA therapy, it is most commonly used as an adjunct to VDRA therapy, when the PTH remains elevated or to assist in controlling hyperphosphatemia or if hypercalcemia develops with therapy.

There has been some controversy as to the optimal PTH concentration to achieve in patients with stage 5 CKD. K/DIGO has expanded the K/DOQI range (150–300 pg/mL) to two to nine times the upper limit of normal for the particular PTH assay being used. The problem is that it has not clearly been defined as to what PTH values are consistently associated with normal bone histology. Furthermore, it has been noted that there are great discrepancies between various PTH assays. Thus, a reasonable approach is to manage patients with only one PTH assay, to follow trends in PTH levels (as suggested by K/DIGO), and to use appropriate clinical judgment in managing PTH levels. Whether it is reasonable to correct the calcidiol deficiency by replacing nutritional vitamin D with cholecalciferol or ergocalciferol remains open for debate.

KEY POINTS: RENAL OSTEODYSTROPHY

1. Chronic kidney disease-mineral and bone disorder (CKD-MBD) is a systemic disorder of mineral and bone metabolism resulting from CKD that may be manifested by either one or a combination of the following: laboratory abnormalities associated with disturbed mineral metabolism including calcium, phosphorus, parathyroid hormone (PTH), or vitamin D metabolism; bone disease, defined as renal osteodystrophy, including abnormalities in bone turnover, mineralization, volume, linear growth, or strength; and/or calcification of extraskeletal tissue, which would include vascular or other soft tissue calcification.

2. The earliest manifestations of CKD-MBD in the evolution of CKD are phosphate retention, decreases in calcitriol, then increases in PTH, and finally (in late stage 4, early stage 5 disease) hyperphosphatemia and eventually hypocalcemia. Most patients are also calcidiol (25-hydroxy vitamin D) deficient. Thus the approach to therapy should be aimed at reversing or preventing these perturbations in mineral metabolism.

3. In stage 5 CKD, therapy should definitely be focused to control serum phosphate to at least 5.5 mg/dL, if not to normal values by the use of adequate dialysis, dietary phosphate restriction, and phosphate binders. The use of calcium-containing binders (calcium carbonate or calcium acetate) should be limited to less than 1500 mg of calcium a day. If patients have evidence of vascular calcifications, calcium-containing binders should be avoided. The noncalcium-containing binders that could be used include either sevelamer or lanthanum. Both of these agents appear to be effective in treating hyperphosphatemia with few side effects or long-term risk. However, the dose for sevelamer generally requires three to four times the number of pills than that required for lanthanum with comparable phosphate control.

4. Treatment of hyperparathyroidism in stage 5 CKD should be addressed with the use of vitamin D receptor activators (VDRAs) and calcimimetics. Although cinacalcet has been shown to be effective when used in the absence of VDRA therapy, it is most commonly used as an adjunct to VDRA therapy, when the PTH remains elevated or to assist in controlling hyperphosphatemia or if hypercalcemia develops with therapy.

5. There has been some controversy as to the optimal PTH concentration to achieve in patients with stage 5 CKD. Kidney Disease: Improving Global Outcomes (K/DIGO) has expanded the Kidney Disease Outcomes Quality Initiative (K/DOQI) range (150–300 pg/mL) to two to nine times the upper limit of normal for the particular PTH assay being used. The problem is that it has not clearly been defined as to what PTH values are consistently associated with normal bone histology. Furthermore, it has been noted that there are great discrepancies between various PTH assays. Thus, a reasonable approach is to manage patients with only one PTH assay, to follow trends in PTH levels (as suggested by K/DIGO), and to use appropriate clinical judgment in managing PTH levels.

12. **Is there a role for parathyroidectomy?**
    Ideally, parathyroidectomy should be avoided with the initiation of early therapy to prevent development of severe hyperparathyroidism with monoclonal nodular transformation of the parathyroid gland. As the parathyroid glands develop monoclonal nodularity, there is loss of both the calcium-sensing receptor (CaR) and the vitamin D receptor (VDR). Thus, as the glands develop large nodules they are no longer responsive to normal physiologic control, which is a poor prognostic sign. An attempt should be made to treat patients with severe hyperparathyroidism with high-dose VDRAs and cinacalcet; however, if severe hyperparathyroidism persists and patients develop hypercalcemia and hyperphosphatemia, a parathyroidectomy may be required. There is much controversy as to the best approach for parathyroidectomy, whether a subtotal parathyroidectomy should be performed or a total

parathyroidectomy with reimplantation of part of a gland into either the forearm or the sternocleidomastoid muscle. The problem of reimplantation is that frequently the implanted tissue becomes fibrotic and does not function or the patient (rarely) could develop parathyroidomatosis, in which microscopic cells produce high levels of PTH. If parathyroidectomy is to be performed, I generally recommend using an experienced parathyroid surgeon who would perform a partial parathyroidectomy, trying to selectively remove the nodular tissue, while leaving behind normal-appearing gland. The procedures should be performed utilizing intraoperative PTH measurements. Recent studies have suggested improved survival in dialysis patients following parathyroidectomy.

13. **What are the biochemical changes in mineral metabolism following kidney transplantation?**
Significant changes in mineral metabolism are observed following transplantation. PTH concentrations decrease significantly during the first 3 months but typically stabilize at elevated values after 1 year. It is common for PTH values to range from one to two times the upper limit of normal. Serum calcium tends to increase after transplant and then stabilize at the higher end of the normal range within 2 months. A small percentage of patients will have persistent hypercalcemia. Serum phosphorus generally decreases rapidly to within or below normal levels after surgery, and hypophosphatemia, if present, generally resolves within 2 to 4 months. However, a small group of patients will have persistent hypophosphatemia. Low levels of calcitriol typically do not normalize until almost 18 months after transplantation. If patients have persistent hypercalcemia with hyperparathyroidism, the practice is to wait at least 1 year prior to considering a parathyroidectomy. Lately, it has become relatively common practice to treat patients with hypercalcemia and hyperparathyroidism with cinacalcet; however, data demonstrating a long-term benefit of this practice presently are lacking.

14. **What bone lesion is typical after kidney transplantation?**
Fractures are very common following kidney transplantation associated with bone loss in the first 1 to 2 years. The use of corticosteroids for immunosuppression is considered to be the major contributor. However, other factors such as persistent hyperparathyroidism, vitamin D deficiency, persistent and/or progressive CKD, and hypophosphatemia are contributing factors. Therapy should be focused on identifying the underlying metabolic disorder and appropriately managing it.

BIBLIOGRAPHY

1. Andress DL. Adynamic bone in patients with chronic kidney disease. *Kidney Int* 2008;73:1345–1354.

2. Andress DL, Coyne DW, Kalantar-Zadeh K, et al. Management of secondary hyperparathyroidism in stages 3 and 4 chronic kidney disease. *Endocrine Pract* 2008;14:1–10.

3. Gal-Moscovici A, Sprague SM. Role of bone biopsy in stages 3 to 4 chronic kidney disease. *Clin J Am Soc Nephrol* 2008;3:S170–174.

4. Moe SM, Drüeke T, Cunningham J, et al. Definition, evaluation, and classification of renal osteodystrophy: A position statement from Kidney Disease: Improving Global Outcomes (KDIGO). *Kidney Int* 2006;69:1945–1953.

5. Rogers NM, Teubner DJO, Coates PTH. Calcific uremic arteriolopathy: Advances in pathogenesis and treatment. *Semin Dial* 2007;20:150–157.

6. Sprague SM, Belozeroff V, Danese M, et al. Abnormal bone and mineral metabolism in kidney transplant patients—A review. *Am J Nephrol* 2008;28:246–253.

7. Sprague SM, Coyne D. Control of secondary hyperparathyroidism by vitamin D receptor activators in chronic kidney disease. *Clin J Am Soc Nephrol* 2010;5:512–518.

CHAPTER 22

CARDIOVASCULAR DISEASE IN CHRONIC KIDNEY DISEASE

Anuja Pradip Shah, MD, and Rajnish Mehrotra, MBBS, MD

1. **What is the relationship between decreased glomerular filtration rate and cardiovascular disease?**

   Patients with chronic kidney disease (CKD) have a substantial increase in risk for death from cardiovascular disease. Even small decreases in renal function, as measured by estimated glomerular filtration, are associated with this higher risk and it increases progressively as renal function declines. Patients with chronic kidney disease are substantially more likely to die from heart disease than progress to dialysis. In patients with end-stage renal disease, the risk for death is 10- to 100-fold higher than for age- and gender-matched individuals without kidney disease. Conversely, in patients with known heart disease (like coronary artery disease or heart failure), as the severity of renal disease increases, the patient outcome worsens.

2. **What is the relationship between albuminuria/proteinuria and cardiovascular disease?**

   The presence of albuminuria is also associated with a higher risk of death from cardiovascular disease. This risk begins even when the amount of urine albumin is not enough to meet the criteria for the diagnosis of microalbuminuria. As the amount of urine albumin increases, so does the risk for death from heart disease; the risk is higher in individuals with microalbuminuria and even higher among those with overt proteinuria.

3. **Why is the risk for cardiovascular disease increased in chronic kidney disease?**

   Both traditional and nontraditional risk factors are important contributors to cardiovascular disease. Diabetes mellitus and hypertension are the two most common causes of CKD—and both are also known cardiovascular risk factors. Moreover, diseases such as hypertension are more severe in the setting of chronic kidney disease. However, traditional risk factors are insufficient to explain the high cardiovascular risk seen with CKD. A large number of nontraditional risk factors have been identified—systemic inflammation, high serum phosphorus, oxidative stress, among others. At this time, however, it remains unclear whether any of the nontraditional risk factors can be modified to reduce the risk of heart disease.

4. **What types of cardiovascular disease are seen in patients with chronic kidney disease?**

   There are two major overlapping categories of cardiovascular disease associated with CKD: disorders of cardiovascular perfusion, which includes atherosclerotic cardiovascular disease, and disorders of cardiac function, such as congestive heart failure and left ventricular hypertrophy. Disorders of vascular perfusion include coronary artery disease, cerebrovascular disease, peripheral vascular disease, and renovascular disease.

5. **Are there other forms of vascular disease seen in patients with chronic kidney disease?**

   Vascular calcification is a frequent manifestation of vascular disease in CKD—it can occur either in the tunica intima or tunica media of the blood vessels. Calcified blood vessels can often be seen on plain x-rays in patients with chronic kidney disease, particularly among the elderly or those being treated with dialysis. The greater the severity of vascular calcification, the greater the risk of death. Patients with chronic kidney disease develop vascular calcification for many reasons; increase in serum phosphorus is considered to be an important contributor and this may be a potentially modifiable risk factor. Hence, management of elevated phosphorus levels may reduce risk for heart disease; however, this approach remains unproven.

6. **What are the clinical manifestations of cardiovascular disease in CKD?**
Manifestations of cardiovascular disease include angina pectoris, myocardial infarction, congestive heart failure, stroke, peripheral vascular disease, arrhythmias, and sudden death. In advanced CKD, cardiovascular disease is often manifested by left ventricular hypertrophy, diastolic dysfunction, and heart failure. The left ventricular hypertrophy may be accompanied by left ventricular remodeling and fibrosis, and these changes, with or without coronary artery disease, in addition to electrolyte shifts and volume expansion may contribute to the high incidence of sudden cardiac death in this population. Indeed, sudden cardiac death is the most common cause of death in patients undergoing dialysis.

The clinical manifestations of acute coronary syndrome are also atypical in patients with chronic kidney disease and the electrocardiographic findings are often obscured by the presence of left ventricular hypertrophy.

7. **What should be the goal blood pressure for the treatment of hypertension in patients with chronic kidney disease?**
Aggressive control of blood pressure has been shown to slow the rate of decline in renal function and progression to end-stage renal disease in both diabetics and nondiabetics with chronic kidney disease. In contrast, there is no convincing evidence that aggressive lowering of blood pressure reduces the cardiovascular morbidity and mortality in ESRD. In light of the benefits in retarding progression of CKD, the target blood pressure should be <140/90; a lower goal may be appropriate for those with proteinuric renal diseases.

8. **Does reduction in proteinuria decrease cardiovascular risk?**
As proteinuria amount increases, so does the cardiovascular risk. Reduction in urine protein excretion is associated with slowing of progression to end-stage renal disease. However, whether reduction in proteinuria will reduce cardiovascular risk is unclear at this time. Nevertheless, given the benefit of slowing rate of decline of glomerular filtration rate, attempts should be made to reduce urine protein excretion to at least <1.0 g/day.

There are two broad strategies for reducing urine protein excretion: therapies specific to the underlying disease (as for glomerular diseases) or nonspecific therapies. Angiotensin-converting enzyme inhibitors or angiotensin-receptor blockers are the most effective nonspecific antiproteinuric therapies and should be the first-line antihypertensive therapies as long as there are no contraindications for their use.

9. **What is the role of lipid management in CKD?**
The greater the amount of urine protein excretion, the worse the abnormalities in lipid panel. Patients with proteinuria generally have elevated total cholesterol and low-density lipoprotein cholesterol and low levels of high-density lipoprotein cholesterol. Patients with diabetes may have, in addition, elevated triglyceride levels.

Lipid-lowering therapies are as effective in lowering cholesterol levels in patients with chronic kidney disease as in the general population. No dosage adjustments are required for statins, bile-acid sequestrants, niacin, or ezetimibe. Fibrates do require a dosage adjustment for renal function. The magnitude of effect of these drugs on reducing cardiovascular disease, however, may not be as large as is seen in the general population. Three large randomized controlled trials have been unable to show any significant reduction in all-cause or cardiovascular events in patients undergoing dialysis. Secondary analyses of the data from participants with CKD enrolled in large primary and secondary prevention clinical trials, however, do show some benefit in reducing cardiovascular events. Some other clinical trials are currently under way.

10. **What is the relationship between anemia and its management to the cardiovascular mortality in chronic kidney disease?**
Anemia is a cardinal manifestation of CKD, and it generally is apparent when the estimated glomerular filtration rate is <30 mL/min/1.73 m². Observational studies have shown that as anemia increases in severity, the risk of death also increases. However, several randomized controlled trials have failed to demonstrate a reduction in mortality risk with erythropoietin therapy, the cornerstone of anemia management in patients with chronic kidney disease. In fact, some of these studies have shown a higher risk for stroke and/or death when the treatment was targeted to achieve a hemoglobin of 13 g/dL. Hence, erythropoietin therapy should not be started unless the hemoglobin level decreases to between 9.0 and 10.0 g/dL and care should be exercised to prevent it from increasing to higher than 12.0 g/dL.

11. **Can serum troponin be used in the diagnosis of myocardial infarction in patients with kidney disease?**
The use of biomarkers for the diagnosis of myocardial infarction in patients with CKD can be problematic. Serum troponin has been found to be elevated in patients with chronic kidney disease who have no clinical suspicion of acute myocardial injury. It is not absolutely clear why this is the case. This may have to do with subclinical myocardial ischemia or decreased clearance of troponin degradation products because of kidney disease.
    Baseline elevations in troponin are associated with increased risk of cardiovascular death in these patients. Troponin I is a more specific marker of infarction that troponin T in these patients. Even so, whether or not an elevation in serum troponin in a given patient indicates acute myocardial injury, it is necessary to take into account the patient's clinical presentation and change in the blood levels of troponin over time. For example, a rising troponin level in a patient who presents with typical chest pain would be consistent with the diagnosis of acute myocardial infarction. However, small and unchanging elevations in an otherwise asymptomatic patient would portend a poor long-term prognosis but are unlikely to be of any immediate import.

12. **Are there special considerations for treatment of myocardial infarction in chronic kidney disease?**
Patients with CKD who present with acute myocardial infarction generally do not do as well as those without kidney disease. Furthermore, patients with CKD do not do as well after percutaneous coronary intervention, with or without stenting, or after coronary artery bypass grafting. The risk–benefit ratio of all these procedures should be carefully considered and a decision should be made on a case-by-case basis.
    The treatment of an acute myocardial infarction with percutaneous coronary intervention also involves a risk for acute kidney injury that may be secondary to contrast-induced nephropathy or cholesterol emboli. Patients at increased risk of contrast-induced nephropathy are those with a serum creatinine ≥1.5 mg/dL or an estimated glomerular filtration rate <60 mL/min/1.73 m², patients with diabetes mellitus, those treated with biguanides, and the elderly.

13. **What are the clinical manifestations of cholesterol emboli?**
Patients will have progressive and often irreversible loss of renal function after an intra-arterial procedure (over days and weeks), which often does not improve. Livedo reticularis, low complement levels, peripheral and or urinary eosinophilia, and physical findings of distal emboli (in the digits or retina) may be seen.

14. **How reliable is the measurement of serum brain natriuretic peptide in patients with chronic kidney disease?**
Like serum troponin, serum levels of brain natriuretic peptide are elevated in patients with chronic kidney disease; in many cases, marked elevations are noted. The magnitude of increase in serum brain natriuretic peptide depends on the degree of left ventricular hypertrophy and/or left ventricular systolic dysfunction. It is unclear if serum brain natriuretic

peptide can be used to diagnose circulatory congestion in patients with CKD or to serially monitor response to diuretics or ultrafiltration with dialysis. A fair bit of caution should be exercised before ordering and/or interpreting brain natriuretic peptide levels in patients with advanced chronic kidney disease or those treated with dialysis.

KEY POINTS: CARDIOVASCULAR DISEASE

1. Even small changes in renal function—either a decrease in glomerular filtration rate or an increase in urine albumin excretion—are associated with a higher risk of death from cardiovascular causes.

2. Both traditional and nontraditional cardiovascular risk factors are more common and often severe in patients with chronic kidney disease and account for the high risk for heart disease.

3. Serum levels of biomarkers, like troponin and brain natriuretic peptide, are sometimes increased in patients with chronic kidney disease; their diagnostic value depends on the clinical setting and change over time.

15. **Is there an increased risk of stroke from atrial fibrillation in CKD?**
Atrial fibrillation causes an increased risk of thromboembolic stroke in patients with CKD. The U.S. Renal Data System reported an annual incidence of 15.1% in patients receiving hemodialysis compared with 9.6% in patients with other stages of CKD and 2.6% in a control cohort without CKD. The 2-year mortality rates after stroke in these subgroups were 74%, 55%, and 28%, respectively.

Oral anticoagulation, which is the treatment of choice to prevent these complications, also increases risk of bleeding, which is magnified in patients undergoing hemodialysis. Hence, careful monitoring of the degree of anticoagulation is necessary in these patients.

BIBLIOGRAPHY

1. Abboud H, Henrich WL. Clinical practice. Stage IV chronic kidney disease. *N Engl J Med* 2010;362(1):56–65.
2. Dukipatti R, Adler SA, Mehrotra R. Cardiovascular implications of chronic kidney disease in older adults. *Drugs Aging* 2008;25(3):241–253.
3. Fellström BC, Jardine AG, Schmieder RE, et al. Rosuvastatin and cardiovascular events in patients undergoing hemodialysis. *N Engl J Med* 2009;360:1395–1407.
4. Go AS, Chertow GM, Fan D, et al. Chronic kidney disease and the risks of death, cardiovascular events, and hospitalization. *N Engl J Med* 2004;351:1296–1305.
5. Kanderian AS, Francis GS. Cardiac troponin and chronic kidney disease. *Kidney Int* 2006;69(7):1112–1114.
6. National Kidney Foundation. K/DOQI clinical practice guidelines for chronic kidney disease: Evaluation, classification and stratification. *Am J Kidney Dis* 2002;39(Suppl 1):S1–S266.
7. Pfeffer MA, Burdmann EA, Chen C-Y, et al. A trial of darbepoetin alfa in type 2 diabetes and chronic kidney disease. *N Engl J Med* 2009;361:2019–2032.
8. Pun PH, Smarz TR, Honeycutt EF, et al. Chronic kidney disease is associated with increased risk of sudden cardiac death among patients with coronary artery disease. *Kidney Int* 2009;76:652–658.
9. Reinecke H, Brand E, Mesters R, et al. Dilemmas in the management of atrial fibrillation in chronic kidney disease. *J Am Soc Nephrol* 2009;20(4):705–711.
10. Rucker D, Tonelli M. Cardiovascular risk and management in chronic kidney disease. *Nat Rev Nephrol* 2009;5:287–296.

CHAPTER 23

HYPERLIPIDEMIA

Christoph Wanner, MD, and Christiane Drechsler, MD, PhD

1. **What is the typical lipid profile in patients with chronic kidney disease?**

   Hyperlipidemia or dyslipidemia in patients with chronic kidney disease (CKD) and no nephrotic syndrome can be characterized by high triglyceride levels and low high-density lipoprotein (HDL) concentrations, whereas total and low-density lipoprotein (LDL) cholesterol levels are normal or even low. Patients with proteinuria and those receiving peritoneal dialysis have higher levels of LDL cholesterol than do patients without proteinuria or those receiving hemodialysis. Although the lipid abnormalities captured by routine laboratory measurements may not be impressive, more sophisticated research analyses reveal profound disturbances in lipid metabolism. One example is a shift in the size distribution of LDL to increased content of small, dense LDL, which can undergo oxidation during prolonged circulation.

   Prinsen BH, de Sain-van der Velden MG, de Koning EJ, et al. Hypertriglyceridemia in patients with chronic renal failure: Possible mechanisms. *Kidney Int Suppl* 2003;S121–S124.

   Ritz E, Wanner C. Lipid abnormalities and cardiovascular risk in renal disease. *J Am Soc Nephrol* 2008;19:1065–1070.

2. **What causes hyperlipidemia or dyslipidemia in patients with chronic kidney disease?**

   Mainly as a result of decreased catabolism, the concentration of triglyceride-rich lipoproteins (very-low-density lipoprotein [VLDL], intermediate-density lipoprotein [IDL]) is increased, in particular in the postprandial phase. Lipolysis of the highly atherogenic VLDL and chylomicron (CM) remnants is impaired partly as a result of the decreased lipoprotein lipase (LPL) on the vascular endothelium and partly as a result of increased levels of the major LPL inhibitory apolipoprotein apo CIII. Increased levels of small, dense LDL result from increased triglyceride concentration, which via the action of cholesterol ester transfer protein (CETP) and hepatic lipase (HL) are involved in the formation of small, dense LDL.

   Functional deficiencies in lecithin:cholesterol acyltransferase (LCAT) and LPL activity affect HDL maturation, and disorders in processes favoring HDL maturation are associated with a greater abundance of large, mature HDL affecting serum levels. The formation of these HDL particles is mediated by LCAT—resulting in the esterification of cholesterol—and by LPL.

   In addition, elevated levels of Lp(a) have been found in CKD. Lp(a) is an LDL-like particle that has an additional protein, apolipoprotein(a), and constitutes an important independent risk factor for atherosclerosis.

   Cressman MD, Heyka RJ, Paganini EP, et al. Lipoprotein(a) is an independent risk factor for cardiovascular disease in hemodialysis patients. *Circulation* 1992;86:475–482.

   Frischmann ME, Kronenberg F, Trenkwalder E, et al. In vivo turnover study demonstrates diminished clearance of lipoprotein(a) in hemodialysis patients. *Kidney Int* 2007;71:1036–1043.

   Kaysen GA. New insights into lipid metabolism in chronic kidney disease: What are the practical implications? *Blood Purif* 2009;27:86–91.

   Kronenberg F, Konig P, Neyer U, et al. Multicenter study of lipoprotein(a) and apolipoprotein(a) phenotypes in patients with end-stage renal disease treated by hemodialysis or continuous ambulatory peritoneal dialysis. *J Am Soc Nephrol* 1995;6:110–120.

   Levine DM, Gordon BR. Lipoprotein(a) levels in patients receiving renal replacement therapy: Methodologic issues and clinical implications. *Am J Kidney Dis* 1995;26:162–169.

   Longenecker JC, Klag MJ, Marcovina SM, et al. High lipoprotein(a) levels and small apolipoprotein(a) size prospectively predict cardiovascular events in dialysis patients. *J Am Soc Nephrol* 2005;16:1794–1802.

3. **What impact does proteinuria have on dyslipidemia?**

Abnormal lipid metabolism is most prominent in the nephrotic syndrome. Studies have shown that about half of the patients with nephrotic syndrome (proteinuria >3 g/day) had total cholesterol concentrations higher than 300 mg/dL, and 80% of the patients had LDL cholesterol levels higher than 130 mg/dL. Many patients also have elevated levels of triglycerides, and high-density lipoproteins are distributed abnormally (increased HDL_3 fraction and decreased HDL_2 fraction). Hyperlipidemia in the nephrotic syndrome results from increased hepatic synthesis and decreased catabolism of lipoproteins. Increased triglyceride-rich lipoprotein concentration, VLDL and IDL primarily, results from decreased clearance, partly because of reduced LPL activity. Lipoprotein lipase is necessary for normal lipolysis. In addition, both LDL and Lp(a) synthesis are increased, whereby evidence exists that LDL synthesis may be augmented through a mechanism bypassing its normal precursor VLDL. Finally, because of decreased activity of LCAT in proteinuric renal disease, the number of spherical HDL particles is decreased. These particles are important carriers for several cofactors (apoCII) affecting LPL activity and VLDL levels.

de Sain-van der Velden MG, Reijngoud DJ, Kaysen GA, et al. Evidence for increased synthesis of lipoprotein(a) in the nephrotic syndrome. *J Am Soc Nephrol* 1998;9:1474–1481.

de Sain-van der Velden MG, Kaysen GA, Barrett HA, et al. Increased VLDL in nephrotic patients results from a decreased catabolism while increased LDL results from increased synthesis. *Kidney Int* 1998;53:994–1001.

Kaysen GA, de Sain-van der Velden MG. New insights into lipid metabolism in the nephrotic syndrome. *Kidney Int Suppl* 1999;71:S18–S21.

Kronenberg F, Lingenhel A, Lhotta K, et al. Lipoprotein(a)- and low-density lipoprotein-derived cholesterol in nephrotic syndrome: Impact on lipid-lowering therapy? *Kidney Int* 2004;66:348–354.

Radhakrishnan J, Appel AS, Valeri A, et al. The nephrotic syndrome, lipids, and risk factors for cardiovascular disease. *Am J Kidney Dis* 1993;22:135–142.

Weiner DE, Sarnak MJ. Managing dyslipidemia in chronic kidney disease. *J Gen Intern Med* 2004;19: 1045–1052.

4. **What impact does dialysis have on dyslipidemia?**

The lipid abnormalities in CKD stages 2–4 as characterized by an increase in plasma triglycerides, VLDL and IDL, along with a reduction in HDL cholesterol, generally also apply for patients undergoing dialysis. Dyslipidemia becomes more pronounced as kidney failure advances to CKD stage 5 requiring dialysis.

Hemodialysis and peritoneal dialysis appear to have different effects on uremic dyslipidemia. Patients undergoing peritoneal dialysis show higher cholesterol, triglyceride, LDL, and Lp(a) levels than patients receiving maintenance hemodialysis. Possible reasons may be a considerable loss of protein (7–14 g/day) into the peritoneal dialysate and the absorption of glucose (150–200 g/day) from the dialysis fluid. This leads to an increase in the pool size of triglycerides and apoB100 in the VLDL fraction of patients undergoing peritoneal dialysis.

Attman PO, Samuelsson OG, Moberly J, et al. Apolipoprotein B-containing lipoproteins in renal failure: The relation to mode of dialysis. *Kidney Int* 1999;55:1536–1542.

Deighan CJ, Caslake MJ, McConnell M, et al. Atherogenic lipoprotein phenotype in end-stage renal failure: Origin and extent of small dense low-density lipoprotein formation. *Am J Kidney Dis* 2000;35:852–862.

5. **How to evaluate dyslipidemia in a patient with chronic kidney disease?**

In daily clinical routine a complete lipid profile consisting of total cholesterol, LDL cholesterol, HDL cholesterol, and triglyceride level should be obtained and repeated in yearly intervals or at every visit when a change in lipid-lowering medication has occurred.

European best practice guidelines for hemodialysis (part 1). Section VII. Vascular disease and risk factors. *Nephrol Dial Transplant* 2002;17(Suppl 7):88–109.

National Kidney Foundation. K/DOQI Clinical Practice Guidelines for management of dyslipidemias in patients with kidney disease. *Am J Kidney Dis* 2003;41(4Suppl 3):I–IV, S1–S91.

National Kidney Foundation. K/DOQI Clinical Practice Guidelines and Clinical Practice Recommendations for diabetes and chronic kidney disease. *Am J Kidney Dis* 2007;49(Suppl 2):S88–S95.

6. **Is hyperlipidemia of chronic kidney disease origin atherogenic?**

Lipid abnormalities, which are common in patients with kidney disease, have been suggested to play a major role in cardiac and vascular disease, although multiple other causes are apparent. A log linear relationship among blood total and LDL cholesterol levels, triglyceride levels, and cardiovascular risk has never convincingly been established in patients with CKD, mainly stage 5. In fact, a number of studies have even found that low (not high) serum total cholesterol was associated with increased mortality. U- and J-shaped curves have been described for the relationship between serum cholesterol and mortality. This probably reflects the influence of malnutrition and chronic inflammation, resulting in the phenomenon known as reverse causation. Concomitant illnesses are associated with an increased risk of death; when they then induce a decrease in cholesterol synthesis, the result may be an artifactually negative association between cholesterol and mortality. Supporting this hypothesis, hypercholesterolemia was shown to be an independent risk factor for cardiovascular and all-cause mortality in patients undergoing dialysis without, but not in those with, evidence of malnutrition or inflammation.

Although lipid profiles differ between patients receiving peritoneal dialysis and those receiving hemodialysis, abnormalities in lipid metabolism qualitatively have similarities regarding the pathogenesis of atherosclerosis and endothelial dysfunction in these groups. Therefore, it is tempting to propose a general need for treatment of lipid disorders in this patient group. However, caution is required on translating observational findings into possible therapeutic treatments. Extrapolation of data from the general population may not meet the special disease pattern of patients with kidney disease.

Despite cardiovascular deaths being a major cause of mortality in patients who receive dialysis, the proportion of myocardial infarctions in cardiac deaths is much lower in patients with chronic kidney disease as compared to the general population. Only 25% of the cardiac deaths in patients receiving hemodialysis can be attributed to myocardial infarctions, whereas the majority of events constitute sudden cardiac deaths. Although sudden cardiac death may to some extent also result from infarctions and arrhythmias, other reasons such as structural heart diseases presumably play an important role. Whether these may be modifiable with cholesterol-lowering treatment is unlikely. Therefore, it is obvious that the classical guidelines cannot generally be applied to patients with renal disease. In particular, treatment indications may differ according to the severity of chronic kidney disease.

Habib AN, Baird BC, Leypoldt JK, et al. The association of lipid levels with mortality in patients on chronic peritoneal dialysis. *Nephrol Dial Transplant* 2006;21:2881–2892.

Iseki K, Yamazato M, Tozawa M, et al. Hypocholesterolemia is a significant predictor of death in a cohort of chronic hemodialysis patients. *Kidney Int* 2002;61:1887–1893.

Kilpatrick RD, McAllister CJ, Kovesdy CP, et al. Association between serum lipids and survival in hemodialysis patients and impact of race. *J Am Soc Nephrol* 2007;18:293–303.

Kovesdy CP, Anderson JE, Kalantar-Zadeh K. Inverse association between lipid levels and mortality in men with chronic kidney disease who are not yet on dialysis: Effects of case mix and the malnutrition-inflammation-cachexia syndrome. *J Am Soc Nephrol* 2007;18:304–311.

Liu Y, Coresh J, Eustace JA, et al. Association between cholesterol level and mortality in dialysis patients: Role of inflammation and malnutrition. *JAMA* 2004;291:451–459.

7. **Does dyslipidemia cause progression of renal disease?**

Animal experiments have suggested that hyperlipidemia may also enhance the rate of progressive glomerular injury, possibly by promoting an intraglomerular equivalent of atherosclerosis. Dyslipidemia, partly explained by its association with proteinuria, predicts progressive loss of kidney function. This was seen particularly in early stages of diabetic nephropathy. Elevated levels of triglycerides seem to contribute to the progression of albuminuria, diabetic nephropathy, and retinopathy. They were furthermore associated with a higher risk of end-stage renal disease requiring renal replacement therapy. In addition, higher levels of HDL were found to be protective of albuminuria in type 1 diabetes.

Cusick M, Chew EY, Hoogwerf B, et al. Risk factors for renal replacement therapy in the Early Treatment Diabetic Retinopathy Study (ETDRS), Early Treatment Diabetic Retinopathy Study Report No. 26. *Kidney Int* 2004;66:1173–1179.

Earle KA, Harry D, Zitouni K. Circulating cholesterol as a modulator of risk for renal injury in patients with type 2 diabetes. *Diabetes Res Clin Pract* 2008;79:68–73.

Ficociello LH, Perkins BA, Silva KH, et al. Determinants of progression from microalbuminuria to proteinuria in patients who have type 1 diabetes and are treated with angiotensin-converting enzyme inhibitors. *Clin J Am Soc Nephrol* 2007;2:461–469.

Hadjadj S, Duly-Bouhanick B, Bekherraz A, et al. Serum triglycerides are a predictive factor for the development and the progression of renal and retinal complications in patients with type 1 diabetes. *Diabetes Metab* 2004;30:43–51.

Misra A, Kumar S, Kishore VN, et al. The role of lipids in the development of diabetic microvascular complications: Implications for therapy. *Am J Cardiovasc Drugs* 2003;3:325–338.

Molitch ME, Rupp D, Carnethon M. Higher levels of HDL cholesterol are associated with a decreased likelihood of albuminuria in patients with long-standing type 1 diabetes. *Diabetes Care* 2006;29:78–82.

Ozsoy RC, van der Steeg WA, Kastelein JJ, et al. Dyslipidaemia as predictor of progressive renal failure and the impact of treatment with atorvastatin. *Nephrol Dial Transplant* 2007;22:1578–1586.

8. **Who should be treated with a statin, and why do the current treatment recommendations distinguish between stages of CKD?**
Observational data provide indirect evidence that patients with CKD stages 2 and 3 may benefit from a lipid-lowering intervention. Based on many post hoc analyses of past statin trials on subcohorts of patients with early CKD, data are sufficiently suggestive to justify the administration of statins in these patients.

Few data are available addressing the effect of lipid-lowering medication on outcome in patients at CKD stage 4. These patients represent a population with advanced kidney failure, where all-cause mortality markedly increases and the pattern of cardiac and vascular disease may change, compared to CKD stages 2 and 3. Novel information is provided by the SHARP trial, which assessed the effects of lipid lowering in 9438 patients with CKD, of whom 2197 patients were in stage 3, 2628 patients in stage 4, and 1237 were in stage 5 CKD (not dialysis dependent). The SHARP trial provides evidence that patients with CKD not on dialysis clearly benefit from statin treatment.

Finally, the 4D and AURORA studies did not provide a rationale to start statin treatment in patients receiving hemodialysis. Treatment aiming at primary prevention in the absence of signs and symptoms of coronary heart disease presumably comes too late once the patient has advanced to end-stage renal disease. In the SHARP trial, no significant heterogeneity between non-dialysis and dialysis patients was noticed, indicating a benefit of statin treatment in all patients including those on dialysis.

Ritz E, Wanner C. Lipid abnormalities and cardiovascular risk in renal disease. *J Am Soc Nephrol* 2008;19:1065–1070.

Sharp Collaborative Group. Study of Heart and Renal Protection (SHARP) randomized trial to assess the effects of lowering low-density lipoprotein cholesterol among 9438 patients with chronic kidney disease. *Am Heart J* 2010;160(5):785-794.e10.

9. **Should patients with proteinuria or the nephrotic syndrome be treated with a statin?**
There is no reason to assume that high LDL cholesterol is not toxic to the vascular wall of patients with proteinuria. Patients with persistent nephrotic syndrome and hyperlipidemia are at increased risk for atherosclerotic disease, particularly if other risk factors are present. Thus, it appears reasonable that lowering lipid levels may both protect against systemic atherosclerosis and slow the progression of the underlying kidney disease. Studies have shown that statins can efficiently lower total and LDL cholesterol concentrations by 20% to 45% and to a lesser extent triglyceride levels in patients with nephrotic syndrome. Despite the lack of studies using "hard" endpoints, statins are suggested as the treatment of choice for persistent hyperlipidemia in the nephrotic syndrome. Other lipid-lowering medication such as nicotinic acid/laropiprant, fibric acid, or bile-acid sequestrants are difficult to install and have higher side effects.

Brown CD, Azrolan N, Thomas L, et al. Reduction of lipoprotein(a) following treatment with lovastatin in patients with unremitting nephrotic syndrome. *Am J Kidney Dis* 1995;26:170–177.

Massy ZA, Ma JZ, Louis TA, et al. Lipid-lowering therapy in patients with renal disease. *Kidney Int* 1995;48:188–198.

Ordonez JD, Hiatt RA, Killebrew EJ, et al. The increased risk of coronary heart disease associated with nephrotic syndrome. *Kidney Int* 1993;44:638–642.

Rabelink AJ, Hene RJ, Erkelens DW, et al. Effects of simvastatin and cholestyramine on lipoprotein profile in hyperlipidaemia of nephrotic syndrome. *Lancet* 1988;2:1335–1338.

Thomas ME, Harris KP, Ramaswamy C, et al. Simvastatin therapy for hypercholesterolemic patients with nephrotic syndrome or significant proteinuria. *Kidney Int* 1993;44:1124–1129.

Wheeler DC, Bernard DB. Lipid abnormalities in the nephrotic syndrome: Causes, consequences, and treatment. *Am J Kidney Dis* 1994;23:331–346.

10. **Should patients in CKD stages 2–3 receive statin treatment?**

The effects of a lipid-lowering therapy on cardiovascular, cerebrovascular, and renal endpoints were investigated in a subgroup analysis of the *Pravastatin Pooling Project,* including 12,333 patients with mild CKD (stage 2) and 4491 patients with moderate CKD (stage 3). Pravastatin 40 mg/day resulted in a significant 23% relative risk reduction in the combined endpoint of nonfatal myocardial infarction, cardiac death, and percutaneous or surgical revascularizations in patients with moderate CKD. A similar effect was seen in patients with mild CKD, among whom even total mortality was reduced. The achieved relative risk reduction corresponds to the effect, which would have been expected in the general population without kidney disease. The corresponding absolute risk reduction was—as a result of the higher event rate—even more than twice as high compared to patients with normal kidney function (6.3% versus 2.9%). Further post hoc analysis of endpoint trials with different statins confirm these results (Anglo-Scandinavian Cardiac Outcomes Trial [ASCOT], Heart Protection Study [HPS], Treat to New Targets [TNT], the MEGA trial, the Alliance study, the CARE study). Finally, the SHARP study was a randomized controlled trial designed to assess the effect of lipid lowering in 9438 patients with CKD. The primary outcome was major atherosclerotic events, comprising coronary death, myocardial infarction, non-hemorrhagic stroke, and any revascularization. The SHARP trial included 67 patients with stage 2 and 2197 patients with stage 3 CKD. Treatment with simvastatin 20mg and ezetimibe 10mg reduced the risk of major atherosclerotic events by 17% (risk ratio 0.83, 95% CI 0.74-0.94; $p < 0.01$) in the whole study group. Similar reductions were achieved in all subgroups studied, suggesting a clear benefit of statin treatment in early CKD.

Furthermore, there are data suggesting that statins may also slow the rate of decline in kidney function and lower urinary protein excretion. One subanalysis within the GREACE study showed that in untreated patients with coronary heart disease, dyslipidemia, and normal baseline creatinine, the glomerular filtration rate (GFR) decreased over a period of 3 years. Treatment with a statin could prevent this decline and lead to a significant improvement in kidney function. Similar data were reported from the TNT and the CARE study. Results from the randomized controlled SHARP trial, however, showed no significant effect of lipid lowering treatment on renal outcomes, suggesting no substantial effect on kidney disease progression.

Although data also exist for fibrates suggesting beneficial effects on the rate of progression of renal disease and cardiovascular risk, these drugs have been considered with caution in patients with CKD stages 3 and lower as a result of active metabolite accumulation and occasionally rhabdomyolysis. In stages 1 and 2 CKD fenofibrate is a good option to treat atherogenic dyslipidemia (triglycerides >200 mg/dL, low HDL cholesterol) and residual risk.

Athyros VG, Mikhailidis DP, Papageorgiou AA, et al. The effect of statins versus untreated dyslipidaemia on renal function in patients with coronary heart disease. A subgroup analysis of the Greek atorvastatin and coronary heart disease evaluation (GREACE) study. *J Clin Pathol* 2004;57:728–734.

MRC/BHF Heart Protection Study of cholesterol lowering with simvastatin in 20,536 high-risk individuals: A randomised placebo-controlled trial. *Lancet* 2002;360:7–22.

Nagai T, Tomizawa T, Nakajima K, et al. Effect of bezafibrate or pravastatin on serum lipid levels and albuminuria in NIDDM patients. *J Atheroscler Thromb* 2000;7:91–96.

Sever PS, Dahlof B, Poulter NR, et al. Prevention of coronary and stroke events with atorvastatin in hypertensive patients who have average or lower-than-average cholesterol concentrations, in the Anglo-Scandinavian Cardiac Outcomes Trial—Lipid Lowering Arm (ASCOT-LLA): A multicentre randomised controlled trial. *Lancet* 2003;361:1149–1158.

Sharp Collaborative Group. Study of Heart and Renal Protection (SHARP) randomized trial to assess the effects of lowering low-density lipoprotein cholesterol among 9438 patients with chronic kidney disease. *Am Heart J* 2010;160(5):785-794.e10.

Shepherd J, Kastelein JJ, Bittner V, et al. Effect of intensive lipid lowering with atorvastatin on renal function in patients with coronary heart disease: The Treating to New Targets (TNT) study. *Clin J Am Soc Nephrol* 2007;2:1131–1139.

Shepherd J, Kastelein JJ, Bittner V, et al. Intensive lipid lowering with atorvastatin in patients with coronary heart disease and chronic kidney disease: The TNT (Treating to New Targets) study. *J Am Coll Cardiol* 2008;51:1448–1454.

Tonelli M, Collins D, Robins S, et al. Gemfibrozil for secondary prevention of cardiovascular events in mild to moderate chronic renal insufficiency. *Kidney Int* 2004;66:1123–1130.

Tonelli M, Isles C, Curhan GC, et al. Effect of pravastatin on cardiovascular events in people with chronic kidney disease. *Circulation* 2004;110:1557–1563.

Tonelli M, Moye L, Sacks FM, et al. Effect of pravastatin on loss of renal function in people with moderate chronic renal insufficiency and cardiovascular disease. *J Am Soc Nephrol* 2003;14:1605–1613.

11. ## Should patients in CKD stages 4–5 undergoing dialysis receive statin treatment?

Patients with more advanced CKD (stage 4) were either absent in the aforementioned subgroup analyses (exclusion criteria in the studies), or their numbers were too small to be analyzed. Evidence is now being provided by the Study of Heart and Renal Protection (SHARP), which is a large-scale randomized controlled trial comparing the use of simvastatin and ezetimibe to placebo in 9438 patients in CKD stage 3 or 4 and undergoing dialysis. The SHARP trial included 2628 patients with CKD stage 4. The treatment with simvastatin 20mg and ezetimibe 10mg resulted in a reduction of LDL-C by 32 mg/dl. The primary endpoint of major atherosclerotic events was reduced by 17% (risk ratio 0.83, 95% CI 0.74-0.94; p<0.01) in the whole study group. Similar reductions were achieved in all subgroups studied.

In dialysis patients, two prospective, randomized controlled trials with atorvastatin and rosuvastatin had been conducted in a total of 4000 patients. The 4D study (The German Diabetes and Dialysis Study) evaluated the effect of 20 mg of atorvastatin/day versus placebo in 1255 patients receiving hemodialysis with type 2 diabetes mellitus during 4 years of follow-up. Although atorvastatin effectively lowered LDL cholesterol by 42%, the composite primary cardiovascular endpoint, consisting of death from cardiac causes, nonfatal myocardial infarction, and stroke, was only reduced by 8%, which was not statistically significant (RR 0.92, 95%CI 0.77–1.10, $p = 0.37$). The 4D study was followed by AURORA: A study to evaluate the Use of Rosuvastatin in subjects On Regular Dialysis: an Assessment of survival and cardiovascular events. In this trial, 2776 patients receiving hemodialysis were assigned to receive rosuvastatin 10 mg daily or placebo and were followed for a median of 3.8 years. Despite the mean reduction in LDL cholesterol of 43%, the combined primary endpoint of death from cardiovascular causes, nonfatal myocardial infarction, or nonfatal stroke could not be reduced (HR 0.96, 95%CI 0.84–1.11, $p = 0.59$). It remained unclear whether these data can be generalized to patients receiving peritoneal dialysis, patients with very high LDL cholesterol, and patients younger than 50 years of age without diabetes. The SHARP study included 3056 patients on dialysis, both hemodialysis and peritoneal dialysis patients, of whom 21% had diabetes mellitus. The mean age was 58.9 ± 11.8 years, and 27% of the patients were younger than 50 years of age. In the overall study group of non-dialysis and dialysis patients, the primary endpoint was significantly reduced by 17% (risk ratio 0.83, 95% CI 0.74-0.94; p<0.01). No significant heterogeneity between non-dialysis and dialysis patients was noticed, indicating a benefit of statin treatment in all patients including those on dialysis. Although the 4D and AURORA studies did not provide a rationale to start statin treatment in patients receiving hemodialysis, it has been suggested that patients who are already taking statins when entering chronic dialysis should continue taking the medication.

Baigent C, Landray M. Study of Heart and Renal Protection (SHARP). *Kidney Int Suppl* 2003;S207–S210.

Fellström BC, Jardine AG, Schmieder RE, et al. Rosuvastatin and cardiovascular events in patients undergoing hemodialysis. *N Engl J Med* 2009;360:1395–1407.

Sharp Collaborative Group. Study of Heart and Renal Protection (SHARP) randomized trial to assess the effects of lowering low-density lipoprotein cholesterol among 9438 patients with chronic kidney disease. *Am Heart J* 2010;160(5):785-794.e10.

Wanner C, Krane V, Marz W, et al. Atorvastatin in patients with type 2 diabetes mellitus undergoing hemodialysis. *N Engl J Med* 2005;353:238–248.

KEY POINTS: HYPERLIPIDEMIA

1. The characteristic lipid profile of patients with chronic kidney disease consists of high triglycerides and low high-density lipoprotein cholesterol concentrations, whereas total and low-density lipoprotein cholesterol are normal or even low.

2. The pattern of cardiac and vascular disease changes during progression of kidney disease, as do the cardiovascular risk factors.

3. Post hoc analyses of statin trials support the administration of statins in patients with early stages of chronic kidney disease (CKD stage 1–3).

4. Patients with advanced chronic kidney disease do not benefit to the same extent from lipid-lowering therapy as do patients with early stages of CKD.

12. **Should adjunctive treatment be administered under certain conditions?**
 Nutritional interventions and physical activity: These play an important role as lipid-lowering treatments in the general population. They presumably have similar importance in patients with chronic kidney disease in early stages 1–3. In stage 4, reduction in nutrient intake without sufficient physical activity may lead to a catabolic state with reduction of muscle mass. Therefore, nutritional interventions should not generally be applied to patients in advanced stages of CKD, but they should be carefully considered individually.

 Antiproteinuric therapy: Renin-angiotensin system blockers have antiproteinuric properties and thus result in a reduction of the albuminuria or proteinuria-induced dyslipidemia. Any intervention leading to a reduction of urinary protein excretion leads to a decline in 10% to 20% of plasma levels of total and LDL cholesterol and Lp(a).

Keilani T, Schlueter WA, Levin ML, et al. Improvement of lipid abnormalities associated with proteinuria using fosinopril, an angiotensin-converting enzyme inhibitor. *Ann Intern Med* 1993;118:246–254.

NUTRITION AND MALNUTRITION

Csaba P. Kovesdy, MD, and Kamyar Kalantar-Zadeh, MD, PhD

1. **How is nutritional status examined, and how is malnutrition determined in patients with chronic kidney disease?**

   There is no single way to assess nutritional status, which is a consequence of a complex interplay of nutrient intake and catabolism, with significant effect modification by comorbid conditions, especially inflammatory conditions. A recent expert panel has recommended the use of the term "protein-energy wasting" (PEW) to describe states of undernutrition that could result from a complex interplay of decreased nutrient intake and/or increased catabolism. PEW can be measured in clinical practice using five different criteria: (1) biochemical measures (serum albumin, prealbumin, transferrin, and cholesterol); (2) measures of body mass (body mass index [BMI], unintentional weight loss, and total body fat); (3) measures of muscle mass (total muscle mass, mid-arm muscle circumference, and creatinine appearance); (4) measures of dietary intake (dietary protein and energy intake); and (5) integrative nutritional scoring systems (subjective global assessment of nutrition and malnutrition-inflammation score). In addition to these readily available measures of PEW, a series of other markers have also been proposed, which could have applicability as research tools; these include measures of appetite, food intake and energy expenditure, other measures of body mass and composition (such as dual-energy x-ray absorptiometry, bioimpedance, near-infrared interactance or computed tomography/magnetic resonance imaging of muscle mass, among others), and laboratory measures (such as growth hormone levels, C-reactive protein, interleukin-1 [IL-1], IL-6, tumor necrosis factor-alpha [TNF-α], serum amyloid-A, or peripheral blood cell counts, among others) (Table 24-1).

   Fouque D, Kalantar-Zadeh K, Kopple J, et al. A proposed nomenclature and diagnostic criteria for protein-energy wasting in acute and chronic kidney disease. *Kidney Int* 2008;73:391–398.

2. **Why is malnutrition associated with mortality in chronic kidney disease?**

   Multiple pathophysiologic mechanisms have been invoked to explain the link between poor nutritional status and mortality in chronic kidney disease (CKD). These include derangements related to lower muscle and adipose mass and depleted circulating lipoprotein with subsequent unopposed effect of circulating endotoxin in activating the proinflammatory processes; gastrointestinal, hematopoietic, and immune dysfunctions leading to higher infectious events; complications related to deficiencies involving multiple micronutrients with antioxidative properties leading to oxidative stress and endothelial dysfunction; and inadequate circulating gelsolin to oppose deleterious effects of circulating actin including platelet activation leading to increased thromboembolic events. The maladaptive activation of the inflammatory and oxidative cascade can potentiate the effects of low nutrient intake by increasing catabolism. In addition to such pathophysiologic mechanisms involved in the higher mortality seen with protein-energy wasting, novel factors such as proinflammatory high-density lipoprotein, myeloperoxidase, and pentraxin may also play important roles. Because the links between PEW and mortality have been established almost exclusively in epidemiologic and observational studies, there is currently no convincing evidence that PEW is indeed the main cause of the observed poorer clinical outcomes. Such causality needs to be verified in randomized controlled

TABLE 24-1. CRITERIA FOR THE CLINICAL DIAGNOSIS OF PROTEIN-ENERGY WASTING IN PATIENTS WITH KIDNEY DISEASE

Serum Chemistry and Other Laboratory Markers
Serum albumin <3.8 g/dL (Bromcresol Green)
Serum prealbumin (transthyretin) <30 mg/dL
Serum cholesterol <100 mg/dL
Serum biochemistry: transferrin, urea, triglyceride, bicarbonate
Hormones: leptin, ghrelin, growth hormones
Inflammatory markers: CRP, IL-6, TNF-α, IL-1, SAA
Peripheral blood cell count: lymphocyte count or percentage

Body Mass and Composition
BMI <22 kg/m^2 (<65 years) <23 kg/m^2 (>65 years)
Unintentional weight loss over time: 5% over 3 months or 10% over 6 months
Total body fat percentage: <10%
Weight-based measures: weight-for-height
Total body nitrogen
Total body potassium
Energy-beam–based methods: DEXA, BIA, NIR
Underwater weighing and air displacement weighing
14 K Dalton fragment of actomyosin
Micro arrays
Muscle fiber size
Relative proportions of muscle fiber types
Muscle alkaline soluble protein
CT and/or MRI of muscle mass

Muscle Mass
Muscle wasting: reduced muscle mass 5% over 3 months or 10% over 6 months
Reduced midarm muscle circumference area (>10% of reduction in relation to 50th percentile of reference population)
Urinary creatinine appearance

Dietary Intake
Unintentional low dietary protein intake: <0.80 g/kg/day for at least 2 months for patients undergoing dialysis or <0.6 g/kg/day for patients in CKD stages 2–5

Appetite, Food Intake, and Energy Expenditure
Appetite assessment questionnaires
Population-based dietary assessments: food frequency questionnaires
Measuring energy expenditure by indirect or direct calorimetry

Nutritional Scoring Systems
SGA and its modifications
Malnutrition-Inflammation Score

CRP = C-reactive protein; IL = interleukin; TNF-α = tumor necrosis factor alpha; SAA = serum amyloid A; BMI = body mass index; DEXA = dual-energy x-ray absorptiometry; BIA = bioelectrical impedance analysis; NIR = near infrared interactance; CT = computed tomography; MRI = magnetic resonance imaging; CKD = chronic kidney disease; SGA = subjective global assessment of nutritional status.

trials of nutritional interventions, even though the association is strong, robust, and consistent.

Kovesdy CP, Kalantar-Zadeh K. Why is protein-energy wasting associated with mortality in chronic kidney disease? *Semin Nephrol* 2009;29:3–14.

3. **What is the significance of obesity in patients with chronic kidney disease?**
   Obesity has reached epidemic proportions in the general population and has been linked to increased morbidity and mortality. Several epidemiologic studies have suggested a link between obesity and higher risk of developing CKD. The link between obesity and adverse outcomes in the general population is evident from epidemiologic studies showing a linear increase in mortality associated with higher body mass index (BMI), especially higher than 30 kg/m^2. Similar epidemiologic studies in patients with moderate to advanced CKD, however, have shown a reversal of this risk factor pattern, with a linear *decrease* in mortality in those with higher BMI; patients with BMI levels reaching morbid obesity have shown the best survival, questioning the validity of the obesity paradigm in this patient population. Similar reversals in risk factor patterns, also known as "obesity paradox" or "reverse epidemiology," have emerged in other patient populations characterized by chronic disease states and a high burden of comorbid conditions (such as those with advanced chronic obstructive pulmonary disease, congestive heart failure, malignancies, or HIV) and in patients with advanced age. The common thread in the populations displaying this phenomenon of reverse epidemiology is their extremely high short-term mortality rate, which probably explains the mechanism whereby obesity appears protective within short time periods; in such patients the mechanisms responsible for the long-term deleterious effects seen in the general population (metabolic syndrome/insulin resistance/atherosclerosis) are likely overshadowed by the beneficial effects of higher overall nutritional reserves.

Hsu CY, McCulloch CE, Iribarren C, et al. Body mass index and risk for end-stage renal disease. *Ann Intern Med* 2006;144:21–28.

Kalantar-Zadeh K, Kopple JD. Obesity paradox in patients on maintenance dialysis. *Contrib Nephrol* 2006;151:57–69.

Kovesdy CP, Anderson JE, Kalantar-Zadeh K. Paradoxical association between body mass index and mortality in men with CKD not yet on dialysis. *Am J Kidney Dis* 2007;49:581–591.

4. **Can manipulations of weight improve outcomes in patients with CKD?**
   Interventions aimed at alleviating obesity are advocated in the general population as a means to prevent long-term deleterious consequences. Such interventions are based on robust evidence linking obesity to adverse outcomes. Because descriptive studies in patients undergoing chronic dialysis suggest that obesity may confer a survival benefit rather than a risk, it may be less likely that interventions validated in the general population can be extrapolated to patients receiving dialysis without critical appraisal of the consequences. There is currently no evidence from clinical trials that would have tested the risks versus benefits of weight reduction interventions in patients receiving dialysis. As a result of the marked discrepancy between epidemiologic studies of obesity in the general population and in patients receiving dialysis, any weight loss–based intervention in the latter group would have to proceed with utmost care taken to assure that no harm is done as a result of worsened nutritional status. There also has to be openness about the possibility that gain in dry (edema-free) weight could in fact be beneficial in this patient population because the complex homeostatic changes occurring in the process of increasing lean body mass and even adiposity may entail short-term benefits.

   Weight-reduction strategies bring up even more complex questions in patients with nondialysis-dependent CKD. Some, but not all, observational studies in this patient population have also indicated a salutary association between higher BMI and lower mortality, but at the same time obesity has also been linked to more severe loss of kidney function, and restriction of dietary protein intake may be beneficial in retarding progressive loss of kidney function. As a result of such complex interplays, weight loss–based interventions could have benefits on kidney function in these patients, but any attempt to induce weight loss through limiting nutrient intake in patients with nondialysis-dependent CKD has to be coordinated by trained personnel to assure no deleterious effects on broader nutritional status and consequently on survival.

Hsu CY, McCulloch CE, Iribarren C, et al. Body mass index and risk for end-stage renal disease. *Ann Intern Med* 2006;144:21–28.

Kovesdy CP, Anderson JE, Kalantar-Zadeh K. Paradoxical association between body mass index and mortality in men with CKD not yet on dialysis. *Am J Kidney Dis* 2007;49:581–591.

5. **What is the effect of cholesterol-lowering interventions in patients with CKD?**
   Blood lipid (cholesterol) level is one of the biochemical markers linked to nutritional status and used to define PEW in CKD. However, in the general population lowering blood cholesterol is the cornerstone of secondary cardiovascular prevention. Given the extremely high cardiovascular morbidity and mortality observed in the CKD population, it appeared seemingly reasonable to use cholesterol-lowering therapies in particular in patients undergoing dialysis, especially because such pharmacologic interventions are not only anti-inflammatory, but they also typically do not cause an overall worsening of protein-energy wasting and are thus devoid of a potentially significant problem caused by other nutritional interventions. One issue that appeared to contradict the cholesterol-cardiovascular disease paradigm in the CKD population was the almost unanimous findings of epidemiologic studies in both dialysis and nondialysis-dependent patients with CKD, which suggested that high cholesterol was not associated with higher mortality but may in fact be protective; this is also referred to as the "lipid paradox" and is another component of the "reverse epidemiology" phenomenon. Because of the resultant uncertainty, two large randomized controlled trials were designed to test the hypothesis that lowering blood cholesterol by statin therapy can decrease cardiovascular event rates and mortality in patients undergoing chronic dialysis. Both of these studies yielded negative results, corroborating the findings of epidemiologic studies and again suggesting that the classical Framingham risk factor patterns cannot be automatically translated to patients with kidney disease. A third study, which also enrolled patients with non-dialysis dependent CKD (besides patients receiving dialysis), has been completed, and indicated a small but significant decrease in cardiovascular events (but not in mortality) in patients treated with a combination of simvastatin and ezetimibe. Further details about this study should become available upon its publication.

Baigent C, Landry M. Study of Heart and Renal Protection (SHARP). *Kidney Int Suppl* 2003;S207–S210.

Fellstrom BC, Jardine AG, Schmieder RE, et al. Rosuvastatin and cardiovascular events in patients undergoing hemodialysis. *N Engl J Med* 2009;360:1395–1407.

Kovesdy CP, Kalantar-Zadeh K. Lipids in aging and chronic illness: Impact on survival. *Arch Med Sci* 2007;3:S74–S80.

Wanner C, Krane V, Marz W, et al. Atorvastatin in patients with type 2 diabetes mellitus undergoing hemodialysis. *N Engl J Med* 2005;353:238–248.

6. **What types of nutritional interventions are available in patients with CKD?**
   Compared to the general population, nutritional interventions in patients with CKD and especially those undergoing maintenance dialysis therapy are more complex. The most basic intervention is dietary counseling, the goals of which are aimed, on the one hand, to provide the necessary amount of energy, protein, and other nutrients and, on the other hand, to avoid biochemical imbalances that are the result of the lack of kidney function. These two goals of dietary intervention are often in conflict with each other (e.g., adequate amounts of protein in the diet will result in an obligatory intake of potassium and phosphorus and could lead to hyperkalemia and/or hyperphosphatemia). Dietary counseling is even more complex in patients with nondialysis-dependent CKD, in whom protein restriction of 0.6 to 0.75 g/kg/day has been suggested as an intervention to retard progression of kidney disease but in whom restrictions of this magnitude may result in unintended worsening in their nutritional status. Other nutritional factors that need to be addressed when providing dietary counseling to patients with CKD receiving dialysis are urinary protein losses in patients with nephrotic syndrome, peritoneal protein losses in patients on peritoneal dialysis, and amino acid losses in the dialysate of patients on hemodialysis. Because of this complexity, dietary advice should be provided by trained nutritionists to assure the adequacy of the nutritional value of any

TABLE 24-2. NUTRITIONAL SUPPORT AND THERAPY
Oral or Enteral Interventions
■ Meals during dialysis treatment
■ Intense/tailored protein energy
■ Oral nutritional supplements
■ Tube feeding
Parenteral Interventions
■ IDPN
■ TPN
Pharmacologic Interventions
■ Appetite stimulators
■ Antidepressant
■ Anti-inflammatory and/or antioxidative
■ Anabolic and/or muscle enhancing drug

imposed restricted diets. As a result of the complex medical conditions that are common in CKD, nutritional interventions often extend far beyond dietary counseling in these patients.

Nutritional interventions for patients with CKD who are malnourished can be classified into three groups of oral/enteral, parenteral, and pharmacologic (Table 24-2). Meals during hemodialysis are routine in many countries but not in the United States, although recent studies have popularized the concept of oral dietary supplements in dialysis clinics. Artificial nutrition through feeding tubes, gastrostomy tubes, or parenteral nutrition (which is sometimes applied in the context of hemodialysis, called intradialytic parenteral nutrition) can be applied in certain conditions, usually over short periods. Other interventions include pharmacologic measures to improve appetite, such as appetite stimulators (megestrol acetate), or to improve biochemical measures of protein-energy wasting, such as the use of anabolic hormones. Megestrol acetate is a synthetic derivate of progesterone that has been used as an appetite stimulant but that also inhibits the activity of proinflammatory cytokines such as IL-1, IL-6, and TNF-α. In patients receiving hemodialysis megestrol acetate was found to improve appetite, increase energy and protein intake, increase dry weight, and improve quality of life. Its application is not without risk, however, because it can induce side effects such as headaches, dizziness, confusion, diarrhea, hyperglycemia, thromboembolic phenomena, breakthrough uterine bleeding, peripheral edema, hypertension, adrenal suppression, and adrenal insufficiency. Anabolic steroids have been tested in small clinical trials, but their clinical use remains uncommon because their risks and benefits have not been adequately characterized yet. Among patients undergoing dialysis, the goal of nutritional interventions is to maintain serum albumin at higher than 4.0 g/dL, and this may be achieved by maintaining oral supplements of 1 to 2 servings per day including upon pill intake in lieu of water (Fig. 24-1). A low serum albumin level is by far the strongest predictor of mortality in patients with CKD.

Boccanfuso JA, Hutton M, McAllister B. The effects of megestrol acetate on nutritional parameters in a dialysis population. *J Ren Nutr* 2000;10:36–43.

Bossola M, Muscaritoli M, Tazza L, et al. Malnutrition in hemodialysis patients: What therapy? *Am J Kidney Dis* 2005;46:371–386.

Burrowes JD, Bluestone PA, Wang J, et al. The effects of moderate doses of megestrol acetate on nutritional status and body composition in a hemodialysis patient. *J Ren Nutr* 1999;9:89–94.

Johansen KL, Mulligan K, Schambelan M, Anabolic effects of nandrolone decanoate in patients receiving dialysis: A randomized controlled trial. *JAMA* 1999;281:1275–1281.

Kalantar-Zadeh K, Kilpatrick RD, Kuwae N, et al. Revisiting mortality predictability of serum albumin in the dialysis population: time dependency, longitudinal changes and population-attributable fraction. *Nephrol Dial Transplant* 2005;20:1880–1888.

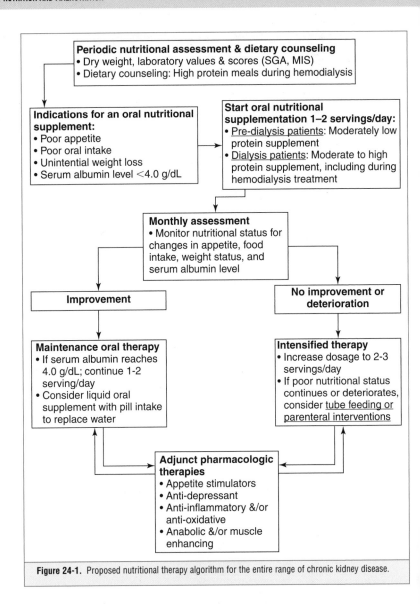

Figure 24-1. Proposed nutritional therapy algorithm for the entire range of chronic kidney disease.

Lambert CP, Sullivan DH, Evans WJ. Effects of testosterone replacement and/or resistance training on interleukin-6, tumor necrosis factor alpha, and leptin in elderly men ingesting megestrol acetate: A randomized controlled trial. *J Gerontol A Biol Sci Med Sci* 2003;58:165–170.

Mantovani G. Does megestrol acetate down-regulate interleukin-6 in patients? *Support Care Cancer* 2002;10:566–567.

Mantovani G, Maccio A, Lai P, et al. Cytokine involvement in cancer anorexia/cachexia: Role of megestrol acetate and medroxyprogesterone acetate on cytokine downregulation and improvement of clinical symptoms. *Crit Rev Oncog* 1998;9:99–106.

National Kidney Foundation. K/DOQI Clinical Practice Guidelines for Nutrition in Chronic Renal Failure. *Am J Kidney Dis* 2000;35:s1–s140.

Rammohan M, Kalantar-Zadeh K, Liang A, et al. Megestrol acetate in a moderate dose for the treatment of malnutrition-inflammation complex in maintenance dialysis patients. *J Ren Nutr* 2005;15:345–355.

Yeh SS, Wu SY, Levine DM, et al. The correlation of cytokine levels with body weight after megestrol acetate treatment in geriatric patients. *J Gerontol A Biol Sci Med Sci* 2001;56:M48–M54.

KEY POINT: NUTRITION AND MALNUTRITION

1. Protein-energy wasting is the strongest predictor of mortality in patients undergoing dialysis.

2. Obesity is associated with survival advantages in patients with chronic kidney disease.

3. Oral nutritional supplements and other nutritional interventions should maintain serum albumin at higher than 4.0 g/dL.

7. **Can nutritional interventions result in better outcomes in patients with CKD?**
Protein-energy wasting is the strongest predictor of increased mortality in patients with CKD of all stages. Based on the compelling results of epidemiologic studies it is plausible to postulate that interventions aimed at improving nutritional status could be beneficial in these patients. Unfortunately there are currently no clinical trial data to prove this concept, and because of this nutritional interventions cannot be advocated as a means to improve patient survival. Clinical trials have shown that various interventions can be successfully applied to improve biochemical measures of PEW (such as serum albumin) or to favorably change body composition, but it remains unclear if the application of such interventions (which include dietary and pharmacologic interventions) can result in better clinical outcomes. A recent study testing the effects on mortality of human growth hormone versus placebo in patients receiving dialysis was terminated as a result of inadequate enrollment, and there are currently no other similar studies to test this hypothesis.

Cano NJ, Fouque D, Roth H, et al. Intradialytic parenteral nutrition does not improve survival in malnourished hemodialysis patients: A 2-year multicenter, prospective, randomized study. *J Am Soc Nephrol* 2007;18:2583–2591.

Feldt-Rasmussen B, Lange M, Sulowicz W, et al. Growth hormone treatment during hemodialysis in a randomized trial improves nutrition, quality of life, and cardiovascular risk. *J Am Soc Nephrol* 2007;18:2161–2171.

Kopple JD, Cheung AK, Christiansen JS, et al. OPPORTUNITY: A randomized clinical trial of growth hormone on outcome in hemodialysis patients. *Clin J Am Soc Nephrol* 2008;3:1741–1751.

CHAPTER 25

MANAGEMENT OF THE PATIENT WITH PROGRESSIVE RENAL FAILURE

Lynda Anne M. Szczech, MD

1. **How do you recognize progressive renal failure?**

   Progressive renal failure is an increase in serum creatinine over time. It is, however, important to recognize that the person who goes on to have progressive renal failure may not have an abnormal creatinine in the earliest stages of their kidney disease. The person at risk for progressive renal failure may have a normal kidney function but abnormal urine with hematuria or proteinuria. Therefore, in addition to identifying patients who have increasing serum creatinine levels over time, it is also important to consider any individual who has an abnormal urine (i.e., proteinuria) with a normal serum creatinine as someone at risk for progressive renal failure.

2. **How do you monitor the rate of loss of kidney function?**

   Monitoring kidney function can be performed using serum creatinine and urinalysis. With respect to serum creatinine, the estimation of kidney function can be performed by calculating the creatinine clearance using the Cockcroft-Gault formula or the estimated glomerular filtration rate (eGFR) using either the Modification of Diet and Renal Disease (MDRD) formula or the Chronic Kidney Disease Epidemiology formula (Table 25-1).

   Although a certain degree of fluctuation in serum creatinine, creatinine clearance, or eGFR is expected related to changes in volume status, medications, and diet, creatinine values (and their respective estimates of kidney function using one of the equations in Table 25-1) should be viewed over time for a basic trend (Fig. 25-1). This is the most efficient way to judge progression.

   In addition, monitoring the amount of urine protein excretion can also provide an estimation of disease activity and progression of the kidney disease. In general, most people normally excrete <300 mg of protein per day. Any amount greater than this is considered abnormal. At approximately 3 g/day, a patient is said to have nephrotic range proteinuria correlating to a significant disease activity in the kidney. Therapy should subsequently be aimed at reducing proteinuria to attempt to slow the progression of the kidney disease. Therefore, similar to a rise in serum creatinine, a rise in urine protein excretion (or a failure to decrease urine protein excretion) can also be considered as a way to monitor kidney disease.

   Cockcroft DW, Gault MH. Prediction of creatinine clearance from serum creatinine. *Nephron* 1976;16:31–41.

   Levey AS, Green T, and Kusek JW. *J Am Soc Nephrol* 2000;11:A0828.

   Levey AS, Stevens LA, Schmid CH, et al; for the CKD-EPI Collaboration. A new equation to estimate glomerular filtration rate. *Ann Intern Med* 2009;150; 604–612.

3. **What are the parameters, diseases, and complications that are encompassed in the consideration of the management of patients with progressive renal failure?**

   See Table 25-2.

4. **What is the goal blood pressure (BP) for a person with progressive renal failure?**

   Few studies directly access differential BP goals and their effect on progression of kidney disease in general in a person with kidney disease. As per the seventh report of the Joint National Committee on Prevention, Detection, Evaluation, and Treatment of High Blood Pressure criteria, a systolic BP goal of 130 mm Hg and a diastolic goal of 80 mm Hg or below are considered

---

TABLE 25-1.   EQUATIONS TO ESTIMATE KIDNEY FUNCTION USING SERUM CREATININE

Cockcroft-Gault Formula

$$\text{Creatinine clearance (mL/min)} = \frac{(140 - age) \times Weight}{sCr \times 72} \times (0.85 \text{ if female})$$

Modification of Diet and Renal Disease Formula (Abbreviated)

Glomerular filtration rate (mL/min/1.73 m^2) = 186 × sCr$^{-1.154}$ × Age$^{-0.203}$ × (0.742 if female) × (1.210 if black)

Chronic Kidney Disease-Epidemiology:

Glomerular filtration rate = **a** × (Scr/**b**)^c × (0.993)^{Age}

a	Black	
	Female	166
	Male	163
	White/other	
	Female	144
	Male	141
b	Female	0.7
	Male	0.9
c	Female	
	Creatinine ≤0.7	$^-$0.329
	Creatinine >0.7	$^-$1.209
	Male	
	Creatinine ≤0.7	$^-$0.411
	Creatinine >0.7	$^-$1.209

Equations from Cockcroft DW, Gault MH. Prediction of creatinine clearance from serum creatinine. *Nephron* 1976;16:31–41; Levey AS, Green T, and Kusek JW, et al. *J Am Soc Nephrol* 2000;11:A0828; and Levey AS, Stevens LA, Schmid CH, et al; for the CKD-EPI Collaboration. A new equation to estimate glomerular filtration rate. *Ann Intern Med* 2009;150;604–612.

---

optimal. With the exception of the African American Study of Kidney Disease and Hypertension (AASK), few randomized controlled trials examine this question directly with the goal largely derived from observational data. In the AASK trial, African Americans with hypertension and chronic kidney disease (CKD) were randomly assigned one of two mean arterial pressure goals: 102 to 107 mm Hg or 92 mm Hg or less. Achieved BP averaged 128/78 (12/8) mm Hg in the lower BP group and 141/85 (12/7) mm Hg in the usual BP group. The mean change in GFR over the 4 years of the study did not differ significantly between arms (-2.21 versus -1.95 mL/min per 1.73 m^2 per year, in the lower and·usual BP arms, respectively; $P = 0.24$).

JNC-7. http://www.nhlbi.nih.gov/guidelines/hypertension/ accessed on December 7, 2009.

Wright JT Jr, Bakris G, Greene T, et al; for the African American Study of Kidney Disease and Hypertension Study Group. Effect of blood pressure lowering and antihypertensive drug class on progression of hypertensive kidney disease: Results from the AASK trial. *JAMA* 2002;288:2421–2431.

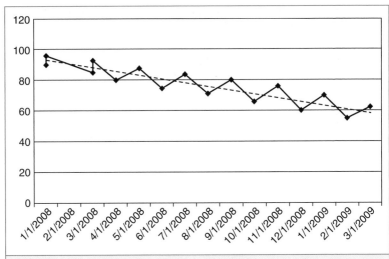

Figure 25-1. Plot of estimated glomerular filtration rate (eGFR) over time for a single patient. Points along the solid line indicate actual values, and the dotted line indicates the overall trend.

5. **What are the preferred antihypertensive medications for a patient with progressive renal failure?**

Multiple studies suggest that in a person with kidney disease, particularly one with increased urine protein excretion, an angiotensin-converting enzyme (ACE) inhibitor or angiotensin receptor blocker (ARB) is the preferred antihypertensive medication. For a patient with proteinuria, BP reduction and urine protein excretion should be goals of therapy and used to titrate doses of either of these medication classes upward. Studies of ACE inhibitors and ARBs in patients with diabetes, HIV-associated nephropathy, and multiple other glomerular diseases demonstrate a benefit toward use of these agents as antihypertensive medications in the progression of kidney disease.

Agardh CD, Garcia-Puig J, Charbonnel B, et al. Greater reduction of urinary albumin excretion in hypertensive type II diabetic patients with incipient nephropathy by lisinopril than by nifedipine. *J Hum Hypertens* 1996;10:185–192.

Brenner BM, Cooper ME, de Zeeuw D, et al. Effects of losartan on renal and cardiovascular outcomes in patients with type 2 diabetes and nephropathy. *N Engl J Med* 2001;345:861–869.

TABLE 25-2. FACTORS TO CONSIDER IN THE MANAGEMENT OF PATIENTS WITH PROGRESSIVE RENAL FAILURE	
Factors That Contribute to the Loss of Kidney Function	**Factors That Occur as a Result of a Loss of Kidney Function**
Hypertension	Anemia
Diabetes mellitus	Bone and mineral metabolism
Lipids	Lipid changes
Dietary salt and protein intake	
Proteinuria	

Burns GC, Paul SK, Toth IR, et al. Effect of angiotensin-converting enzyme inhibition in HIV-associated nephropathy. *J Am Soc Nephrol* 1997;8:1140–1146.

Chan JC, Cockram CS, Nicholls MG, et al. Comparison of enalapril and nifedipine in treating non-insulin dependent diabetes associated with hypertension: One year analysis. *BMJ* 1992;305:981–985.

De Cesaris R, Ranieri G, Andriani A, et al. Effects of benazepril and nicardipine on microalbuminuria in normotensive and hypertensive patients with diabetes. *Clin Pharmacol Ther* 1996;60:472–478.

Jafar TH, Schmid CH, Landa M, et al. Angiotensin-converting enzyme inhibitors and progression of nondiabetic renal disease. A meta-analysis of patient-level data. *Ann Intern Med* 2001;135:73–87.

Laffel LM, McGill JB, Gans DJ. The beneficial effect of angiotensin-converting enzyme inhibition with captopril on diabetic nephropathy in normotensive IDDM patients with microalbuminuria. North American Microalbuminuria Study Group. *Am J Med* 1995;99:497–504.

Maschio G, Alberti D, Janin G, et al. Effect of the angiotensin-converting-enzyme inhibitor benazepril on the progression of chronic renal insufficiency. *N Engl J Med* 1996;334:939–945.

Mathiesen ER, Hommel E, Giese J, et al. Efficacy of captopril in postponing nephropathy in normotensive insulin dependent diabetic patients with microalbuminuria. *BMJ* 1991;303:81–87.

Parving HH, Lehnert H, Brochner-Mortensen J, et al. The effect of irbesartan on the development of diabetic nephropathy in patients with type 2 diabetes. *N Engl J Med* 2001;345:870–878.

Ravid M, Lang R, Rachmani R, et al. Long-term renoprotective effect of angiotensin-converting enzyme inhibition in non-insulin-dependent diabetes mellitus. A 7-year follow-up study. *Arch Intern Med* 1996;156:286–289.

Schnack C, Hoffmann W, Hopmeier P, et al. Renal and metabolic effects of 1-year treatment with ramipril or atenolol in NIDDM patients with microalbuminuria. *Diabetologia* 1996;39:1611–1616.

Trevisan R, Tiengo A. Effect of low-dose ramipril on microalbuminuria in normotensive or mild hypertensive non-insulin-dependent diabetic patients. North-East Italy Microalbuminuria Study Group. *Am J Hypertens* 1995;8:876–883.

Viberti G, Mogensen CE, Groop LC, et al. Effect of captopril on progression to clinical proteinuria in patients with insulin-dependent diabetes mellitus and microalbuminuria. European Microalbuminuria Captopril Study Group. *JAMA* 1994;271:275–279.

Wright JT Jr, Bakris G, Greene T, et al; for the African American Study of Kidney Disease and Hypertension Study Group. Effect of blood pressure lowering and antihypertensive drug class on progression of hypertensive kidney disease: Results from the AASK trial. *JAMA* 2002;288:2421–2431.

6. **What is the goal level of blood sugar control for a person with progressive renal failure?**
   Although the goal for glucose control with respect to its effect on hard clinical outcomes is controversial and beyond the scope of the chapter, from the renal perspective glucose control close to normal range is associated with the slowest rate of progression of kidney disease. The Diabetes Control and Complications Trial (DCCT) randomly assigned approximately 1400 patients with type I diabetes to intensive therapy aimed at reaching this goal as compared to conventional therapy. Intensive therapy reduced the occurrence of microalbuminuria by 39% and albuminuria by 54%.

The Diabetes Control and Complications Trial Research Group. The effect of intensive treatment of diabetes on the development and progression of long-term complications in insulin-dependent diabetes mellitus. *N Engl J Med* 1993;329:977–986.

The Diabetes Control and Complications Trial/Epidemiology of Diabetes Interventions and Complications Research Group. Retinopathy and nephropathy in patients with type 1 diabetes four years after a trial of intensive therapy. *N Engl J Med* 2000;342:381–389.

Stratton IM, Adler AI, Neil HA, et al. Association of glycaemia with macrovascular and microvascular complications of type 2 diabetes (UKPDS 35): Prospective observational study. *BMJ* 2000;321:405–412.

UK Prospective Diabetes Study (UKPDS) Group. Intensive blood-glucose control with sulphonylureas or insulin compared with conventional treatment and risk of complications in patients with type 2 diabetes (UKPDS 33). *Lancet* 1998;352:837–853.

7. **Is hemoglobin Alc a good marker of blood sugar control in a person with progressive renal failure?**
   Although hemoglobin A1c is a sufficient marker of blood sugar control in a patient with kidney disease who does not yet require dialysis, this parameter has limited utility in patients who are receiving dialysis. Studies suggest little correlation between average blood glucose level and hemoglobin A1c as a result of nonenzymatic glycosylation of hemoglobin in the uremic serum and therefore little correlation with clinical outcomes. Although multiple other potential

markers have been studied, recent publications suggest that glycosylated albumin might be an adequate marker of blood sugar control; however, no studies have been performed to suggest that an optimal level of blood sugar control in the patient receiving dialysis effect clinical outcomes.

Peacock TP, Shihabi ZK, Bleyer AJ, et al. Comparison of glycated albumin and hemoglobin A1c levels in diabetic subjects on hemodialysis. *Kidney International* 2008;73:1062–1068.

Williams ME, Lacson E Jr, Teng M, et al. Hemodialyzed type I and type II diabetic patients in the US: Characteristics, glycemic control, and survival. *Kidney Int* 2006;70:1503–1509.

KEY POINTS: PROGRESSIVE RENAL FAILURE

1. Monitoring kidney function can be performed using serum creatinine and urinalysis.

2. Proteinuria may be considered an important surrogate outcome for disease activity in someone with progressive renal disease. In a patient with glomerular kidney disease, the level of proteinuria correlates with disease activity and potential risk for progression.

3. Although hemoglobin A1c is a sufficient marker of blood sugar control in a patient with kidney disease who does not yet require dialysis, this parameter has limited utility in patients who are receiving dialysis. Studies suggest little correlation between average blood glucose level and hemoglobin A1c as a result of nonenzymatic glycosylation of hemoglobin in the uremic serum and therefore little correlation with clinical outcomes.

8. **Does the management of lipids affect the course of patients with progressive renal failure?**
   The management of lipids in patients with renal disease is highly controversial. Although secondary analyses of clinical trials meant to evaluate the use of cholesterol-reducing medications such as statins in patients based on hard clinical outcomes suggest a similar benefit exists among people with kidney disease, dedicated studies are ongoing with respect to these outcomes and to progression of kidney disease in this population. Multiple studies both suggest and fail to suggest a benefit toward the progression of kidney disease from statins, but a recent meta-analysis suggests that the benefits may be modest. This meta-analysis included 27 studies with 39,704 participants. Overall, the change in eGFR was less in the statin recipients (1.22 mL/min per year slower, 95% CI 0.44 to 2.00). This potential benefit was statistically significant in participants with cardiovascular disease (0.93 mL/min per year slower than control subjects; 95% CI 0.10 to 1.76) but was not significant for participants with diabetic or hypertensive kidney disease or glomerulonephritis. Dedicated studies will be able to more clearly determine the benefit of statins on the course of kidney disease.

Sandhu S, Wiebe N, Fried LF, et al. Statins for improving renal outcomes: A meta-analysis. *J Am Soc Nephrol* 2006;17:2006–2016.

9. **How does diet (salt, protein, and fluids) affect the progress of kidney disease?**
   No studies directly measure the effect of various sodium diets on the progression of kidney disease. Arguably, a lower-sodium diet can frequently facilitate better BP control in patients. Given that BP is an important parameter to control in the attempt to slow the progression of chronic kidney disease, a lower-sodium diet indirectly may benefit an individual patient. On a more controversial note, early studies suggested that a lower-protein diet decreased hyperfiltration and glomerular pressure and may potentially benefit a progression of kidney disease. However, the large MDRD study failed to demonstrate a benefit to kidney disease progression among people who reduced their protein intake.

Klahr S, Levey AS, Beck GJ, et al. The effects of dietary protein restriction and blood-pressure control on the progression of renal disease. Modification of Diet in Renal Disease Study Group. *N Engl J Med* 1994;330:877–884.

10. **How should proteinuria be used as a marker and a target of disease activity in the person with progressive renal disease?**

    Proteinuria may be considered an important surrogate outcome for disease activity in someone with progressive renal disease. In a patient with glomerular kidney disease, the level of proteinuria correlates with disease activity and potential risk for progression. Therefore, therapeutic decisions aimed at lowering protein excretion should be implemented in a paradigm similar to BP management; baseline protein excretion should be estimated using a urine test such as the urine protein-to-creatinine ratio. The urine protein-to-creatinine ratio roughly approximates the amount of protein a patient excretes in a single 24-hour period. A lower value of approximately 0.3 g or less could be considered normal. A value >0.3 g is abnormal. In a patient with an abnormal level of protein excretion in their urine (e.g., 1 g, 3 g, or 5 g), therapy such as ACE inhibitors or ARBs should be initiated in an attempt to lower urine protein excretion. At an interval of approximately 3 months, the urine protein excretion should be rechecked to determine the effect of the therapy on urine protein excretion. A decrement in the urine protein-to-creatinine ratio to the lowest value possible or normal is an appropriate goal. If, after initiating the therapy, the desired urine protein-to-creatinine ratio is not reached, the medication chosen should be titrated up or another medication should be added to continue to attempt to reach the goal of the lowest urine protein-to-creatinine ratio possible.

    Gansevoort RT, Sluiter WJ, Hemmelder MH, et al. Antiproteinuric effect of blood-pressure-lowering agents: A meta-analysis of comparative trials. *Nephrol Dial Transplant* 1995;10:1963–1974.

    Jafar TH, Stark PC, Schmid CH, et al. Proteinuria as a modifiable risk factor for the progression of non-diabetic renal disease. *Kidney Int* 2001;60:1131–1140.

    Laverman GD, Navis G, Henning RH, et al. Dual renin-angiotensin system blockade at optimal doses for proteinuria. *Kidney Int* 2002;62:1020–1025.

    Maki DD, Ma JZ, Louis TA, et al. Long-term effects of antihypertensive agents on proteinuria and renal function. *Arch Intern Med* 1995;155:1073–1080.

    Schwab SJ, Christensen RL, Dougherty K, et al. Quantitation of proteinuria by the use of protein-to-creatinine ratios in single urine samples. *Arch Intern Med* 1987;147(5):943–944.

11. **When is anemia likely to occur in the person with progressive kidney disease?**

    In general, anemia becomes more frequent as kidney function declines. A person with stage III kidney disease has an approximately 5% chance of being anemic. This increases to 10% to 15% and greater than 40% in a person with stage V kidney disease who does not yet require dialysis.

    U.S. Renal Data System. *USRDS 2009 Annual Data Report.* Bethesda, MD: National Institutes of Health, National Institute of Diabetes and Digestive and Kidney Diseases, April 2009.

12. **What are the mechanisms by which anemia develops in the patient with progressive kidney disease?**

    The mechanism for anemia is likely multifactorial in the person with chronic kidney disease. An important contributor has long been felt to be decreased indigenous erythropoietin production related to decreased nephron mass; however, also contributing to anemia are factors such as iron deficiency and inflammation resulting in iron sequestration and a relative iron deficiency.

    Andrews NC, Schmidt PJ. Iron homeostasis. *Ann Rev Physiol* 2007;69:69–85.

    Fishbane S, Pollack S, Feldman HI, et al. Iron indices in chronic kidney disease in the National Health and Nutritional Examination Survey 1988–2004. *Clin J Am Soc Nephrol* 2009;4:57–61.

    McGonigle RJ, Wallin JD, Shadduck RK, et al. Erythropoietin deficiency and inhibition of erythropoiesis in renal insufficiency. *Kidney Int* 1984;25:437–444.

13. **What are the therapeutic options in the treatment of anemia in the patient with progressive kidney disease?**

    Therapies available for the patient with anemia and kidney disease include iron supplementation and erythrocytes stimulating agents (ESAs). Patients with anemia should have their iron stores checked, and those with parameters suggesting iron deficiency should have their stores repleted. Patients whose hemoglobin falls below 10 g/dL despite replete iron stores can be begun on ESAs such as epoetin-alfa or darbepoetin. Iron stores may be supplemented through oral iron supplementation. In the setting of multiple comorbidities and an increasing likelihood of inflammation, however, a cytokine such as hepcidin may prevent oral iron from being adequately bioavailable. In circumstances in which oral iron is not efficacious, particularly in someone with severe kidney disease, intravenous iron is a successful alternative.

Andrews NC, Schmidt PJ. Iron homeostasis. *Ann Rev Physiol* 2007;69:69–85.

NKF-DOQI guidelines. Available at www.kidney.org. Accessed on December 7, 2009.

Package inserts for Epogen, Darbepoetin, and Procrit. Available at www.amgen.com and www.procrit.com. Accessed on December 7, 2009.

14. **What are the treatment goals for anemia in the patient with progressive kidney disease?**

The treatment goals for anemia in a patient with progressive kidney disease are based on several clinical trials. Multiple studies suggest a quality-of-life increase in a person who has their hemoglobin elevated using therapies such as ESAs. Three clinical trials have been performed to evaluate the effect of anemia correction with ESAs on heart clinical outcomes such as death, congestive heart failure, myocardial infarction, and stroke. Two clinical trials enrolled a wide range of patients with chronic kidney disease and anemia, randomly assigning them to treatment for correction of their anemia to hemoglobin of approximately 13 versus hemoglobin of approximately 11. Although one study failed to demonstrate any benefit or harm when the two arms were compared, one study demonstrated harm in the group randomized to the higher hemoglobin. Finally, a trial randomly assigning patients to hemoglobin of approximately 13 as compared with placebo (i.e., no anemia correction) failed to demonstrate a difference in cardiovascular outcomes or mortality between the two arms. It is, however, noteworthy that this trial did demonstrate a significantly increased risk in the likelihood of stroke in the arm receiving active treatment with the ESA. Taken together, these trials support the treatment goals as put forth in the U.S. Food and Drug Administration labeling for ESAs and the National Kidney Foundation Disease Outcomes Quality Initiative guidelines of a hemoglobin level between 10 and 12 g/dL. Given these controversial results, the relative benefit to quality of life as compared to the increased risk of cardiovascular event, particularly stroke, should be considered on a case-by-case basis.

Drüeke TB, Locatelli F, Clyne N, et al; the CREATE Investigators. Normalization of hemoglobin level in patients with chronic kidney disease and anemia. *N Engl J Med* 2006;355:2071–2084.

Pfeffer MA, Burdmann EA, Chen C-Y, et al; for the TREAT Investigators. A trial of darbepoetin alfa in type 2 diabetes and chronic kidney disease. *N Engl J Med* 2009;361:2019–2032.

Singh AK, Szczech L, Tang KL, et al. Correction of anemia with epoetin alfa in chronic kidney disease. *N Engl J Med* 2006;355(20):2085–2098.

15. **What are the parameters that should be monitored in bone and mineral metabolism, and when are changes in these parameters likely to occur in the person with progressive kidney disease?**

The parameters that should be monitored in patients with progressive renal disease with respect to bone and mineral metabolism include serum calcium, serum phosphorous, and serum intact parathyroid hormone. One expected change that occurs as kidney disease progresses is initially an elevation in intact parathyroid hormone. This is a compensatory response to retention of serum phosphorous and serves to maintain serum calcium and serum phosphorous within normal ranges in the vast majority of patients until very late stages of progressive kidney disease. In that regard, monitoring of serum calcium or phosphorous alone will fail to recognize in the vast majority of patients the degree to which a bone and mineral metabolism becomes deranged as kidney function declines.

Levin A, Bakris GL, Molitch M, et al. Prevalence of abnormal serum vitamin D, PTH, calcium, and phosphorus in patients with chronic kidney disease: Results of the study to evaluate early kidney disease. *Kidney Int* 2007;71:31–38.

16. **What is the mechanism by which bone and mineral metabolism changes in the person with progressive kidney disease?**
Phosphorous that should be excreted by normal kidney function is likely the primary driver toward the derangements in bone and mineral metabolism seen in people with progressive loss of kidney function. This may trigger derangements in serum calcium through precipitation of calcium phosphate with a subsequent stimulus for increased parathyroid hormone excretion (secondary hyperparathyroidism).

17. **What are the therapeutic options in the treatment of changes in bone and mineral metabolism in the person with progressive kidney disease?**
The therapeutic options available for a person with derangements in bone and mineral metabolism include dietary counseling on decreased phosphorous intake. In the setting of hyperphosphatemia, a phosphorous binder also can be used. These binders are taken with the patient's meal and bind the phosphorous in the food that is eaten to prevent its absorption. Phosphorous binders include calcium acetate, sevelamer carbonate, and lanthanum carbonate. Additionally, to treat secondary hyperparathyroidism correction of vitamin D deficits utilizing ergocalciferol and cholecalciferol and the calcimimetic cinacalcet can serve to suppress secondary hyperparathyroidism. The relative combination of these agents should be considered on a case-by-case basis utilizing the laboratory parameters of vitamin D levels and intact parathyroid hormone levels.

Block GA, Martin KJ, de Francisco ALM, et al. Cinacalcet for secondary hyperparathyroidism in patients receiving hemodialysis. *N Engl J Med* 2004;350:1516–1525.

Chertow GM, Burke SK, Raggi P; for the Treat to Goal Working Group. Sevelamer attenuates the progression of coronary and aortic calcification in hemodialysis patients. *Kidney Int* 2002;62:245–252.

Joy MS, Finn WF; LAM-302 Study Group. Randomized, double-blind, placebo-controlled, dose-titration, phase III study assessing the efficacy and tolerability of lanthanum carbonate: a new phosphate binder for the treatment of hyperphosphatemia. *Am J Kidney Dis* 2003;42(1):96–107.

Quarles LD, Yohay DA, Carroll BA, et al. Prospective trial of pulse oral versus intravenous calcitriol treatment of hyperparathyroidism in ESRD. *Kidney Int* 1994;45:1710–1721.

Qunibi WY, Nolan CR. Treatment of hyperphosphatemia in patients with chronic kidney disease on maintenance hemodialysis: Results of the CARE study. *Kidney Int* 2004;66:SS33–SS38.

18. **What are the treatment goals for changes in bone and mineral metabolism in the patient with progressive kidney disease?**
The treatment goals for a patient with derangements in bone and mineral metabolism are focused on maintaining serum calcium, serum phosphorous, and serum parathyroid hormone levels within normal ranges.

19. **In preparation for dialysis, when and what should a patient be told to assist them in their decision regarding modality choice?**
In preparation for dialysis, patient education should begin early. Depending on the rate of progression of kidney disease, the patient may wish to understand their options very early in their disease progression; however, referral to a nephrologist and education with respect to options for renal or placement therapy should begin no later than stage IV chronic kidney disease. Options such as hemodialysis, peritoneal dialysis, and renal transplantation should each be discussed with respect to their advantages and feasibility for each individual patient.

20. **In a person interested in hemodialysis, when and what should be done to facilitate the timely placement of a functional vascular access, and why is that important?**
For a patient who is interested in hemodialysis, vascular access should be placed at such a time to attempt to have that vascular access functioning when hemodialysis should begin. In general, arterial venous fistulae require 4 to 6 months for maturation, whereas arterial venous grafts require only 2 to 3 weeks. Peritoneal dialysis requires sufficient time for not only catheter placement and healing, but also the training that will be required for the patient and

his or her family prior to the full initiation of the therapy. Having a patient's vascular access or peritoneal access ready when it is necessary to initiate renal replacement therapy is important because in the absence of this preparation an intravenous catheter will be required to initiate hemodialysis. These catheters carry with them a risk of infection that may affect survival.

21. **Can a person get a kidney transplant without having been on dialysis?**
Patients with kidney disease can receive a kidney transplant while they are undergoing dialysis or prior to the initiation of dialysis. Pre-emptive transplantation is a viable option that may provide a survival benefit over transplantation following the initiation of dialysis. In that regard, education and referral of a patient for kidney transplantation should be considered for those patients who maybe appropriate candidates even prior to the initiation of renal replacement therapy.

Mange KC, Joffe MM, Feldman HI. Effect of the use or nonuse of long-term dialysis on the subsequent survival of renal transplants from living donors. *N Engl J Med* 2001;344:726–731.

MANAGEMENT OF THE PATIENT WITH RESISTANT EDEMA

John B. Stokes, MD, and Mony Fraer, MD

CHAPTER 26

1. **How does a person adapt to diuretic administration?**
   In the initial days to weeks, the effect of loop diuretics on the extracellular fluid volume is the result of two opposing forces: sodium chloride loss during diuretic action and the postdiuretic sodium chloride retention. The first is influenced by the diuretic dose, bioavailability, dosing frequency, and half-life. Loop diuretic action is also lower when the glomerular filtration rate is low. The loss of sodium chloride induced by the diuretic is counterbalanced by several factors. A high sodium chloride diet will blunt or negate the diuretic effect. In addition, sodium absorption by nephron segments that are not blocked by the administered diuretic will increase their capacity for sodium absorption. As a consequence of contraction of the extracellular fluid volume, a neurohumoral response causes renal vasoconstriction and enhanced renal sodium reabsorption. In the proximal tubule, the sodium reabsorption is caused by angiotensin II and norepinephrine. In the distal tubule, hypertrophy is caused by a combination of high aldosterone secretion and a high rate of sodium delivery produced by the inhibition of sodium absorption in the loop of Henle. This hypertrophy of the distal nephron sodium-absorbing capacity renders patients who have received large doses of loop diuretics more sensitive to thiazide and potassium-sparing diuretics than are normal (untreated) people.

2. **What is diuretic resistance?**
   Diuretic resistance ensues when, despite a full dose of diuretic, an adequate clearance of extracellular fluid volume is not achieved. This can be defined by a set weight, by absence of peripheral edema, or by improvement in respiratory or other symptoms. Some patients require a certain degree of edema to maintain renal perfusion and general well-being.

3. **What are the causes of diuretic resistance?**
   - Noncompliance
   - Reduced absorption from the gastrointestinal tract from low bioavailability or edema (furosemide)
   - Reduced glomerular filtration rate and nephron mass
   - Competitive inhibition of tubular secretion of the diuretic (bile salts in cirrhosis)
   - Decreased renal perfusion in heart failure (as a result of the reduced cardiac output) and cirrhosis (as a result of renal vasoconstriction) leads to decreased diuretic secretion
   - Interference with diuretic secretion by other drugs (probenecid, sulfonamides, beta-lactam antibiotics, methotrexate, valproic acid, cimetidine, and some antiviral medications)
   - Drugs that enhance sodium absorption: nonsteroidal anti-inflammatory drugs (diminished synthesis of vasodilator and natriuretic prostaglandins)
   - High sodium intake
   - Inadequate diuretic dose
   - Hypoalbuminemia (see later)

4. **How should diuretic resistance be addressed?**
   The first step is to make sure that the edema is a result of inappropriate renal sodium and fluid retention rather than of lymphatic or venous obstruction or redistribution (like from the use of calcium channel blockers). The next step is to exclude noncompliance, severe blood

volume depletion, or concurrent nonsteroidal anti-inflammatory use. Noncompliance with dietary prescriptions can be determined at steady state by measuring the sodium excretion rate over 24 hours. If sodium excretion exceeds 100 to 120 mmol/day (2.5–3 g sodium) in a patient whose daily weight is stable, then excessive dietary sodium chloride intake is likely contributing to the apparent resistance to therapy. The maximum diuretic response at a given dose in stable patients is generally seen with the first dose. If the initial response is inadequate, the dose of the loop diuretic should be doubled until a response is obtained or until the ceiling dose is attained. If there is a brief diuresis, then the dose is effective but short-lived; the appropriate response is to give the same dose twice or even three times a day. If furosemide does not produce the desired effect, another loop diuretic such as bumetanide or torsemide may be more effective. Differences in kinetics, absorption, and bioavailability may allow a more favorable action for these other loop diuretics. Other strategies might include switching to intravenous administration to overcome problems associated with impaired absorption, combining different classes of diuretics, and increasing the dose of the diuretic in patients with renal impairment (inversely correlated with glomerular filtration rate).

5. **What is sequential nephron blockade?**
Concurrent use of diuretics acting on different segments of the nephron may produce an additive or synergistic response. Loop diuretics increase sodium delivery to the distal tubule, the segment of the nephron that is sensitive to thiazide diuretics; chronic use of loop diuretics also leads to hypertrophy of the distal tubule cells, increasing their ability to reabsorb sodium chloride. Blockage of sodium reabsorption at the distal tubule by coadministering a thiazide diuretic may restore diuresis in resistant states. Thiazides have a longer half-life compared to loop diuretics. This combination requires careful monitoring because an excessive diuresis can occur in which daily sodium and potassium losses can be greater than 500 meq and 200 meq, respectively. Also there is the risk of azotemia and severe volume depletion. A collecting duct diuretic added to a loop diuretic may be more effective, particularly when circulating aldosterone concentrations are increased (as in congestive heart failure and cirrhosis); this may also counteract unwanted hypokalemia or alkalosis.

6. **Is there an advantage to providing a continuous infusion of (loop) diuretics versus intravenous boluses?**
Usually used in the inpatient setting, this approach avoids periods of positive sodium balance that would otherwise occur in between diuretic doses; also, the total daily dose can be higher. The evidence is that continuous infusion produces slightly more negative sodium balance than intermittent infusion; this could make a difference for hospitalized patients. By avoiding the high-dose boluses, the toxicity is decreased. A continuous loop diuretic infusion in patients with refractory edema begins with an initial bolus. Patients who do not respond to the bolus are unlikely to respond to a continuous infusion because bolus therapy results in higher initial plasma and urinary diuretic levels. In patients who respond to the initial bolus, the infusion can be started with furosemide at a dose of 20 mg/hour and increased up to 40 mg/hour. If the diuresis is not sustained, a second bolus is given followed by a higher infusion rate of 40 mg/hour. The risk of complications is associated with infusion rates higher than 80 mg/hour.

7. **Is there a role for diuretic usage in end-stage renal disease?**
The water and sodium balance is maintained until the late stages of chronic renal disease; this seems to occur as a result of an increased level of natriuretic factors, leading to a rise in sodium and water excretion per residual nephron. In chronic renal failure, the organic acid transport system in the proximal tubule is blocked by the accumulated endogenous organic acids. Additionally, the renal blood flow is reduced and the amount of loop diuretic reaching the kidney is thus decreased. Still, intravenous and oral high-dose loop diuretics (torsemide more than furosemide) are effective in increasing fluid and sodium excretion in a dose-dependent manner; however, the decrease in interdialytic weight gain is not pronounced.

KEY POINTS: MANAGEMENT OF THE PATIENT WITH RESISTANT EDEMA

1. The most frequent causes of diuretic resistance are noncompliance (including with dietary sodium restriction) and inadequate diuretic dose (below threshold).

2. Concurrent use of diuretics acting on different segments of the nephron may produce an additive or synergistic response.

3. Other effective interventions for diuretic resistance include switching to intravenous administration (boluses or continuous infusion), increasing the dose of the diuretic in patients with renal impairment, and using a continuous intravenous infusion of a loop diuretic.

4. Loop diuretics can be used even in advanced renal failure.

8. **What is the role of hypoalbuminemia in resistant edema? Does albumin infusion increase the effects of loop diuretics?**
Hypoalbuminemia decreases loop diuretics' transport to the kidneys, increases their volume of distribution, increases their metabolism to inactive compounds, and (in the case of nephrotic syndrome) leads to increased binding of diuretic to albumin in tubular lumen. This is one of the reasons that when there is diuretic resistance, there should be attempts to decrease proteinuria. Renin-angiotensin-aldosterone system blocking agents will decrease proteinuria, enhance fluid losses, and reduce renal potassium losses. However, there is no role for concomitant furosemide and albumin infusion in patients with hypoalbuminemia from the nephrotic syndrome.

9. **What is the role of mechanical ultrafiltration in removing excessive extracellular fluid volume?**
Slow continuous ultrafiltration is a procedure that allows continuous fluid removal. It is done with a specially designed device or with a dialysis apparatus. The advantage of the smaller ultrafiltration devices is that they can be used via a peripheral vein, whereas ultrafiltration by standard dialysis can remove fluid faster but requires a central venous catheter. Most studies of mechanical ultrafiltration are in patients with diuretic-resistant decompensated heart failures. Some patients can benefit by decreased right atrial and pulmonary artery wedge pressures and improved cardiac output. In selected patients, this therapy can improve cardiac performance with minimal changes in blood pressure, heart rate, and renal function. However, its use should be reserved for the patients with heart failure who are truly refractory.

10. **What is the interpretation of an abnormally high level of brain natriuretic peptide (BNP) and NT-proBNP in the setting of decreased renal function?**
Across the ranges of chronic kidney disease, BNP and NT-proBNP have similar dependence on renal function for clearance. In patients with chronic kidney disease, their concentrations are higher and they parallel the presence and severity of heart disease and do not simply reflect a reduced clearance of these molecules. A difficult yet unsolved task is finding a cutoff point for which further assessment of cardiac function is warranted, particularly in asymptomatic patients with renal failure.

BIBLIOGRAPHY

1. Chalasani N, Gorski JC, Horlander JC, SR, et al. Effects of albumin/furosemide mixtures on responses to furosemide in hypoalbuminemic patients. *J Am Soc Nephrol* 2001;12:1010.
2. Davenport A. Ultrafiltration in diuretic-resistant volume overload in nephrotic syndrome and patients with ascites due to chronic liver disease. *Cardiology* 2001;96:190–195.
3. DeFilippi C, van Kimmenade RR, Pinto YM. Amino-terminal pro-B-type natriuretic peptide testing in renal disease. *Am J Cardiol* 2008;101(3A):82–88.
4. Dormans TP, van Meyel JJ, Gerlag PG, et al. Diuretic efficacy of high dose furosemide in severe heart failure: Bolus injection versus continuous infusion. *J Am Coll Cardiol* 1996;28:376.

5. Ellison DH. The physiologic basis of diuretic synergism: Its role in treating diuretic resistance. *Ann Intern Med* 1991;114:886–894.
6. Fliser D, Schroter M, Neubeck M, et al. Coadministration of thiazides increases the efficacy of loop diuretics even in patients with advanced renal failure. *Kidney Int* 1994;46:482–488.
7. Kindler J. Torsemide in advanced renal failure. *Cardiovasc Drugs Ther* 1993;7:75–80.
8. Kramer BK, Schweda F, Rieger GA. Diuretic treatment and diuretic resistance in heart failure. *Am J Med* 1999;106:90.
9. Oster JR, Epstein M, Smoller S. Combination therapy with thiazide-type and loop diuretic agents for resistant sodium retention. *Ann Intern Med* 1983;99:405.
10. Rudy DW, Voelker JR, Greene PK, et al. Loop diuretics for chronic renal failure: A continuous infusion is more efficacious than bolus therapy. *Ann Intern Med* 1991;115:360.
11. Salvador D, Rey N, Ramos G, Punzalan F. Continuous infusion versus bolus injection of loop diuretics in congestive heart failure. *Cochrane Database Syst Rev* 2004;1:CD003178.
12. van Meyel JJM, Smits P, Dormans T, et al. Continuous infusion of furosemide in the treatment of patients with congestive heart failure and diuretic resistance. *J Intern Med* 1994;235:329–334.
13. Wollam GL, Tarazi RC, Bravo EL, et al. Diuretic potency of combined hydrochlorothiazide and furosemide therapy in patients with azotemia. *Am J Med* 1982;72:929.

CHAPTER 27

MANAGEMENT OF THE PATIENT WITH CONGESTIVE HEART FAILURE

Jose F. Rueda, MD, and David H. Ellison, MD

1. **How common is heart failure in the United States?**

   Heart failure (HF) affects approximately 6 million Americans, with an incidence of 600,000 new cases each year. HF affects 2.3% of the population, particularly the elderly. Its annual cost is more than $33 billion. A projected future prevalence of 20% has been suggested by a few investigators who take into consideration the aging population and the epidemic of obesity, which leads to an increase incidence of diabetes, hypertension, and kidney disease. The number of deaths resulting from HF as a primary or secondary cause has increased six-fold during the past 40 years.

2. **What are the symptoms and signs of HF?**

   The diagnosis of HF is based on signs and symptoms derived from a thorough history and physical examination. The duration of symptoms and potential precipitating or exacerbating factors should be ascertained. Clinicians should determine the status of the extracellular fluid volume and the adequacy of systemic perfusion. Measurement of the ejection fraction (EF) is typically indicated.

   Patients with HF often present with symptoms of elevated left or right ventricular filling pressures, such as paroxysmal nocturnal dyspnea, orthopnea, dyspnea on exertion, or dyspnea at rest. They may also complain of fatigue or exercise intolerance or leg or abdominal swelling.

   Orthopnea has the highest sensitivity (~90%) for elevated left-sided filling pressures, although it lacks specificity. On physical examination, the presence of a third heart sound (ventricular gallop), distension of the jugular veins, pulmonary rales, and pitting edema are often present. The most specific signs of decompensated HF are elevated jugular venous pressures and S3 gallops (95% specificity).

   The Framingham HF criteria are useful to identify patients with chronic HF. The diagnosis requires the presence of two major, or one major and two minor, criteria.

Major criteria:	Minor criteria:
Paroxysmal nocturnal dyspnea	Bilateral ankle edema
Neck vein distension	Night-time cough
Rales	Dyspnea on ordinary exertion
Cardiomegaly on chest x-ray	Hepatomegaly
Pulmonary edema on chest x-ray	Pleural effusion
S3 gallop	Heart rate >120 beats/minute
Central venous pressure >16 cm H_2O	Decrease in vital capacity by one third
Hepatojugular reflux	from maximum recorded
Weight loss >4.5 kg in 5 days in response to treatment	

3. **What are the most common causes of HF?**

   The syndrome of HF can result from any disorder that affects the heart's ability to fill and/or relax or empty. HF is typically divided according to systolic function: heart failure with systolic dysfunction and heart failure with preserved systolic function (diastolic dysfunction).

HF with systolic dysfunction results from the inability of the left heart to empty appropriately, owing to decreased EF. Common causes of systolic dysfunction include the following:

- Coronary artery disease
- Nonischemic causes:
  - Hypertension
  - Valvular disease
  - Thyroid disease
  - Alcohol abuse
  - Myocarditis
  - Cardiomyopathy
  - Adult congenital heart disease

HF with preserved systolic function often results when the left ventricular relaxation is impaired, hence the elevated end diastolic pressure seen in a normal-sized chamber; it is often considered to be synonymous with diastolic dysfunction and may account for up to two thirds of cases in patients older than 70 years. Common causes of diastolic dysfunction include the following:

- Left ventricular hypertrophy
- Hypertension
- Coronary artery disease (CAD)

CAD causes the great majority of cases of systolic HF, followed by hypertension and dilated cardiomyopathies.

4. **What are the stages of HF?**
   Four stages of HF have been identified by the American College of Cardiology/American Heart Association: Stage A defines patients at high risk for HF but without structural heart disease or symptomatology; stage B defines patients with structural heart disease with no symptomatology attributed; stage C denotes patients with prior or current symptoms of HD with evidence of structural heart disease; and stage D denotes patients with refractory HF.

5. **What is the common functional classification system used for patients with HF?**
   It is the New York Heart Association (NYHA) functional classification. Patients are divided according to the degree of effort needed to elicit symptomatology.
   Class I: no functional limitation during ordinary activity
   Class II: symptoms on ordinary exertion
   Class III: symptoms on minimal exertion
   Class IV: symptoms at rest

6. **What aspects of the patient's history should be emphasized during the initial encounter in patients with HF?**
   Physical examination does not help in differentiating HF from systolic dysfunction versus HF with preserved systolic function. A history of the following should be sought:

- Hypertension
- Diabetes mellitus
- Hyperlipidemia
- Valvular heart disease
- Coronary artery disease
- Myopathy
- Rheumatic fever
- Radiation to the mediastinum
- Symptoms of sleep-disordered breathing
- Exposure to cardiac toxins
- Alcohol abuse
- Collagen vascular disease
- Exposure to sexually transmitted diseases
- Thyroid disease
- Pheochromocytoma
- Obesity

7. **What laboratory or imaging tests are useful in patients suspected of having HF?**
   One of the most valuable initial diagnostic tests is the echocardiogram with Doppler flows. It estimates the EF, which, if less than 40%, indicates systolic dysfunction. The echocardiogram also determines systolic and diastolic abnormalities and endocardial or pericardial disease.
   Laboratory testing may reveal the presence of conditions that can lead to, or worsen, HF. Initial evaluation should include a complete blood count, urinalysis, serum electrolytes, calcium, magnesium, glycohemoglobin, blood lipids, renal function, hepatic function, chest radiography, and 12-lead electrocardiogram.

8. **What is BNP?**

   BNP, or B-type natriuretic peptide, is a peptide produced by the heart in the ventricles. The congestion seen in patients with HF stretches heart chambers, enhancing BNP secretion into the bloodstream. Serum levels of BNP can be measured as a diagnostic test.

9. **What is the accuracy on BNP?**

   More than 10 studies have looked into the diagnostic characteristics of serum BNP in patients evaluated in emergency departments for shortness of breath.

   The higher the value of BNP, the more suggestive it is of HF. They were not able to find a threshold that indicated the presence of HF without a doubt. It was determined that values below 250 pg/mL made HF much less likely.

   In a recent clinical trial of patients presenting to the emergency department with dyspnea, BNP was 90% sensitive and 76% specific for HF when the cutoff was 100 pg/mL. Thus, BNP can be used in the urgent-care setting to help exclude HF as the cause of dyspnea, but it cannot be used in isolation to confirm HF.

10. **What factors other than HF can affect BNP levels?**

    BNP levels have been noted to be elevated in patients with the following conditions:
    - Advanced age
    - Kidney failure
    - Acute coronary syndromes
    - Lung disease with cor pulmonale
    - Acute pulmonary embolism
    - High cardiac output states

11. **What other laboratory tests can be helpful to measure in HF?**

    Given the high prevalence of coronary artery disease in patients with HF and low EF, myocardial markers, such as troponin-I, are often measured.

    Radionuclide ventriculography, magnetic resonance imaging, computed tomography of the heart, and heart catheterization can also be used to assess right and left ventricular function and evaluate chamber size, cardiac function, and wall motion.

12. **What is the cardiorenal syndrome?**

    The cardiorenal syndrome (CRS) is concomitant dysfunction of the heart and kidneys. Recently, a classification of this syndrome has been proposed.
    - Type 1 CRS is acute kidney dysfunction resulting from acute cardiac dysfunction; an example would be acute cardiogenic shock, leading to acute kidney injury.
    - Type 2 CRS is chronic cardiac dysfunction leading to chronic kidney disease (CKD), as in the individual with HF and progressive CKD.
    - Type 3 CRS is acute kidney injury leading to HF.
    - Type 4 CRS is chronic kidney disease leading to chronic dysfunction.
    - Type 5 CRS is concomitant disease in both organ systems, such as occurs when amyloidosis affects both the heart and kidneys.

    Some patients with HF have kidney dysfunction that can be attributed to medications (i.e., nonsteroidal anti-inflammatory drugs [NSAIDs], angiotensin-converting enzyme [ACE] inhibitors, angiotensin receptor blockers [ARB], or contrast agents used for imaging testing). See Chapter 14 for more detailed discussion.

13. **What is the best identifier of in-hospital mortality of patients with HF?**

    According to the ADHERE registry, admission with blood urea nitrogen (BUN) greater than 43 mg/dL was the best identifier of in-hospital mortality in patients with HF.

    In HF, arginine vasopressin (AVP), the antidiuretic hormone, is typically secreted owing to underfilling of the arterial circulation (nonosmotic vasopressin release). This hormone can contribute to hyponatremia by increasing water reabsorption in the collecting duct as a result of its effects on V2 receptors. It also increases urea reabsorption in the collecting duct, increasing BUN in serum.

14. **What is the treatment for chronic HF?**

When systolic dysfunction is present, even asymptomatic patients benefit from treatment, which is typically pharmacologic. Multiple medications are useful to treat HF. The most frequently recommended medications are the following:

1. **Diuretics:** These improve sodium excretion, exercise tolerance, and overall symptomatology. Loop diuretics should be used as a first-line therapy, and thiazides should be added for refractory volume overload. Furosemide should be started at 20 to 40 mg daily and titrated to achieve resolution of edema and improved breathlessness, while avoiding symptomatic hypotension and worsening renal perfusion.

2. **ACE inhibitors:** At least six ACE inhibitors are approved by the U.S. Food and Drug Administration for the management of HF: captopril, enalapril, lisinopril, quinapril, trandolapril, and fosinopril. These medications should be prescribed to all patients with systolic dysfunction unless there is a contraindication or the patient is intolerant. ACE inhibitors do not, however, reduce the need for diuretics. They should also be avoided if patients have experienced angioedema, severe renal failure with anuria. They should be prescribed with caution if the patient has very low blood pressure (systolic blood pressure <80 mm Hg), bilateral renal artery stenosis, history of significant hyperkalemia with K levels higher than 5.5 meq/L, or marked increase on serum creatinine (i.e., >3 mg/dL). Treatment should be started at low doses, with gradual increments and frequent assessment of kidney function (Table 27-1). ACE inhibitors slow the progression of cardiovascular disease by their pleiotropic effects, which include improved endothelial cell damage; antiproliferative effect on smooth muscle cells, neutrophils, and monocytes; and antithrombotic effects.

3. **ARBs:** These are now considered a reasonable alternative to ACE inhibitors (Table 27-2). The risks of hypotension, hyperkalemia, and renal dysfunction are greater when they are used in combination with ACE inhibitors or aldosterone receptor blockers.

TABLE 27-1. ANGIOTENSIN-CONVERTING ENZYME INHIBITORS		
Drug	**Initial Daily Dose**	**Maximum Daily Dose**
Captopril	6.25 mg 3 times	50 mg 3 times
Enalapril	2.5 mg twice	10–20 mg twice
Lisinopril	2.5 mg to 5 mg once	20–40 mg once
Perindopril	2 mg once	8–16 mg once
Quinapril	5 mg twice	20 mg twice
Ramipril	1.25 mg to 2.5 mg once	10 mg once
Trandolapril	1 mg once	4 mg once

TABLE 27-2. ARBs		
Drug	**Initial Daily Dose**	**Maximum Daily Dose**
Candesartan	4–8 mg once	32 mg once
Losartan	25–50 mg once	50–100 mg once
Valsartan	20–40 mg once	160 mg twice

4. **β-adrenergic receptor blockers:** Selective β1-receptor inhibitors (metoprolol succinate and bisoprolol fumarate) and an α1-, β1-, and β2-receptor inhibitor (carvedilol) have improved symptoms and EF in patients with moderate to severe symptoms. All patients with stable NYHA class II or III HF from systolic dysfunction should receive beta blockers (Table 27-3). One of the three beta blockers proven to reduce mortality should be used (bisoprolol, carvedilol, or sustained-release metoprolol succinate).
5. **Aldosterone antagonist:** This is recommended in patients with moderately severe to severe HF symptoms and systolic dysfunction, as long as serum creatinine is below 2.0 mg/dL and serum potassium is below 5.0 meq/L. Kidney function and electrolytes should be monitored closely when aldosterone antagonists are used. Eplerenone is another aldosterone receptor antagonist available in clinical practice (besides spironolactone) (Table 27-4).
6. **Hydralazine:** Hydralazine can be combined with nitrates to treat HF from systolic dysfunction. This combination improves survival, although it is less effective than ACE inhibitors, for most patients. This combination is especially useful to treat African Americans. It is also commonly used when renal insufficiency prevents or complicates the use of ACE inhibitors (Table 27-5).
7. **Cardiac resynchronization therapy:** This therapy is indicated in selected patients who meet the following criteria: QRS duration >120 msec, left ventricular ejection fraction ≤35%, sinus rhythm, and NYHA class III.
8. **Digitalis:** Use digitalis in patients with current or prior symptoms of HF to reduce hospitalization. Digoxin does not reduce mortality or lead to substantial changes in quality of life, however.

TABLE 27-3.   β-ADRENERGIC RECEPTOR BLOCKERS

Drug	Initial Daily Dose	Maximum Daily Dose
Bisoprolol	1.25 mg daily	10 mg daily
Carvedilol	3.125 mg twice daily	25–50 mg daily
Metoprolol (LA)	12.5–25 mg daily	200 mg daily

TABLE 27-4.   ALDOSTERONE ANTAGONIST

Drug	Initial Dose	Maximum Daily Dose
Spironolactone	25 mg daily or every other day	25 mg twice daily

TABLE 27-5.   HYDRALAZINE

Drug	Initial Dose	Maximum Daily Dose
Isosorbide dinitrate	10 mg 3 times daily	80 mg 3 times daily
Hydralazine	25 mg 3 times daily	150 mg 4 times daily

The following treatments are not recommended for HF:

1. **Long-term infusion of a positive inotropic drug:** Palliation for end-stage disease may be an exception.
2. **Triple neurohormonal blockade with ACE inhibitors, angiotensin receptor blockade, and beta blockers:** These usually should be avoided. Two clinical trials have shown that adding valsartan to ACE inhibitors and beta blockers for patients with HF worsens outcomes.
3. **Routine anticoagulation:** There is no indication for routine anticoagulation in patients with HF.
4. **Drugs that can adversely affect the patient's clinical status:** These include NSAIDs; most antiarrhythmic drugs; and most calcium channel blockers, especially diltiazem and verapamil.

15. **What are the contraindications for the use of β-blockers?**
   - Severe chronic obstructive pulmonary disease
   - First-degree atrioventricular (AV) block and second-degree AV block (Mobitz II or advanced)
   - Heart rate fewer than 50 beats/min
   - Systolic blood pressure <90 mm Hg

16. **Are calcium channel blockers contraindicated in patients with HF?**
   No clinical trials have proved a mortality benefit in patients with HF. Some calcium channel blockers, including verapamil and diltiazem, can lead to worsening HF and have been associated with an increased risk of adverse cardiovascular events.

   Amlodipine and felodipine have been studied in this population; they do not increase mortality. According to the American College of Cardiology and the American Heart Association, routine administration of calcium channel blockers is not indicated.

17. **What are the indications for an implantable cardioverter defibrillator (ICD)?**
   An ICD is recommended for patients who survive sudden cardiac death. In addition, patients who have survived a myocardial infarction with an EF less than 30% and patients with cardiomyopathy and an EF less than 35% benefit from ICD placement.

18. **What are the advantages and disadvantages of the use of diuretics in HF?**
   Loop diuretics are the mainstay of pharmacologic treatment for symptomatic management of HF (Table 27-6). Electrolyte disturbances can be seen with the use of these medications, especially hypokalemia, hypomagnesemia, and in some cases hyponatremia. Hypotension also could be seen in some patients, especially if they have decreased cardiac preload in the setting of low cardiac output. As stated earlier, kidney dysfunction can occur as a result of hypotension and decreased renal perfusion.

TABLE 27-6. COMMON DOSES FOR DIURETICS				
	Furosemide	Bumetanide	Torsemide	Mechanism of Diminished Response to Diuretic
Kidney failure				Impaired delivery to site
GFR 20–50 mL/min	80 mg	2–3 mg	20–50 mg	of action and reduced
GFR <20 mL/min	200 mg	8–10 mg	50–100 mg	filtered Na
Nephrotic syndrome with normal GFR	120 mg	3 mg	50 mg	Diminished kidney response
HF with normal GFR	40–80 mg	2–3 mg	20–50 mg	Diminished kidney response, decreased renal blood flow

GFR = glomerular filtration rate; HF = heart failure.

19. **How do you define diuretic resistance?**

Diuretic resistance is the persistence of edema and signs of hypervolemia in the setting of an adequate dose of diuretics (i.e., furosemide >120 mg daily or bumetanide >4 mg daily). A daily dose of furosemide >160 mg is associated with a 2-year survival of only 55%.

Loop diuretics inhibit the reabsorption of sodium, chloride, and potassium in the thick ascending loop of Henle. They must reach the urinary space to inhibit sodium and chloride transport. They reach the tubular lumen by active secretion and not by glomerular filtration or passive diffusion. In renal failure, organic anions compete for the receptor sites of these transporters, so higher doses are required to obtain adequate diuresis.

Thiazide diuretics become less effective when renal function worsens and are typically ineffective when the glomerular filtration rate (GFR) is less than 30 cc/min; this does not apply, however, when thiazides are combined with loop diuretics.

Bumetanide and torsemide are more completely absorbed than furosemide, and their absorption is less variable. Bumetanide's half-life is shorter than furosemide's, but the torsemide has a longer half-life; this may be clinically significant. Another factor that plays a role in diuretic resistance is bowel edema, which may impair the gastrointestinal absorption of diuretics. An increase in the dose or intravenous administration may be required.

When serious resistance occurs in the hospital, a continuous intravenous infusion of diuretics may be used. The dose of continuous infusion of furosemide ranges between 2 and 80 mg/hour; most patients receive 10 to 20 mg/hour. The dose of bumetanide ranges between 0.5 and 2.0 mg/hour (Table 27-7).

In some patients, high doses of loop diuretics do not overcome resistance. In these cases, adding a thiazide diuretic may be beneficial. This combination is often very effective. Metolazone, 5 to 10 mg by mouth daily, with furosemide 80 to 160 mg intravenously (IV) every 6 to 8 hrs, or chlorothiazide 500 to 1000 mg once or twice with a loop diuretic, are commonly used combinations in clinical practice.

20. **What factors precipitate hospitalization for HF?**
   - Noncompliance with medical regimen including sodium and fluid restriction
   - Acute myocardial infarction
   - Uncontrolled hypertension
   - Atrial fibrillation and other arrhythmias
   - Addition of negative inotropic agents, such as verapamil, diltiazem, and beta blockers
   - Pulmonary embolism
   - NSAIDs
   - Excessive alcohol or illicit drug use

TABLE 27-7. DOSES FOR CONTINUOUS IV INFUSION OF LOOP DIURETICS				
Diuretic	IV Loading Dose	CrCl <25 cc/min	CrCl 25–75 cc/min	CrCl >75 cc/min
Furosemide	40 mg	20 mg then 40 mg/hour	10–20 mg/hour	10 mg/hour
Torsemide	20 mg	10 mg then 20 mg/hour	5–10 mg/hour	5 mg/hour
Bumetanide	1 mg	1–2 mg/hour	0.5–1 mg/hour	0.5 mg/hour

IV = intravenous; CrCl = creatinine clearance.

- Endocrine abnormalities (e.g., diabetes mellitus, thyroid disease)
- Infections (e.g., pneumonia, viral illnesses)
- Anemia
- Use of thiazolidinediones (TZD)

About 50% of patients with acute HF are readmitted to the hospital within 6 months.

21. **What are the indications for admission to the hospital in patients with acute decompensated HF?**
    - Markedly decompensated HF with evidence of hypotension, worsening kidney function, or mental status changes
    - Dyspnea at rest
    - Hemodynamically significant arrhythmia (i.e., atrial fibrillation with rapid ventricular rate)
    - Acute coronary syndrome
    - Worsened congestion reflected by an increase in weight gain (i.e., >5 kg)
    - Signs or symptoms of pulmonary congestion (i.e., dyspnea, pulmonary edema on chest x-ray)
    - Significant electrolyte disorders, such as hyponatremia or hyperkalemia
    - Presence of comorbid conditions such as stroke, transient ischemic attacks, pulmonary embolus, diabetic ketoacidosis, or pneumonia

    The mortality after a hospital admission has been reported to be up to 8%, with 1-year mortality up to 60%.

    Four parameters have been identified with worse outcome in patients with acute HF:
    - BUN >43 mg/dL
    - Systolic pressure <115 mm Hg
    - Serum creatinine >2.75 mg/dL
    - Elevated troponin I level

22. **What are the treatment goals for patients admitted with acute decompensated HF?**
    According to the Heart Failure Society of America (HFSA) guidelines, treatment should achieve the following:
    - Improve symptoms
    - Improve volume status
    - Identify cause of HF
    - Identify precipitating factors
    - Optimize chronic outpatient oral therapy
    - Minimize side effects
    - Identify patients who can benefit from revascularization
    - Educate patients regarding medication use, compliance, and self-assessment.

23. **What is the treatment of HF in the acute setting?**
    Intravenous diuretics are recommended as the first-line therapy because they lower ventricular filling pressure directly, thereby reducing pulmonary congestion. These effects may reduce shortness of breath and improve kidney function. Patients with acute HF from either systolic or diastolic dysfunction are often treated with the following (Table 27-8):
    - Those with HF and evidence of severe volume overload should be treated with IV diuretics, provided the patient is not severely hypotensive or in cardiogenic shock. Recommended dose is furosemide 40 mg IV, bumetanide 1 mg IV, or torsemide 10 to 20 mg IV.
    - Supplemental oxygenation and assisted ventilation should be provided as needed.
    - Hypotension, associated with hypoperfusion and evidence of elevated cardiac filling pressures (e.g., elevated jugular venous pressure, elevated pulmonary artery wedge pressure), should be treated with intravenous inotropic agents or vasopressors to maintain systemic perfusion and preserve end-organ performance.
    - In the absence of hemodynamic instability or hyperkalemia, ACE inhibitors or ARBs and the beta blockers should be continued. However, patients who develop progressive CRS may need these drugs withheld temporarily.

TABLE 27–8. PHARMACOLOGIC AGENTS IN THE MANAGEMENT OF DECOMPENSATED HEART FAILURE

Medication	Initial Dose	Dose Range	Comments
Vasodilators			
Nitroprusside	0.3–0.5 αg/kg/min	0.3–5 αg/kg/min	Caution in acute myocardial ischemia
Nitroglycerin	10–20 µg/min	20–400 αg/min	Watch for hypotension, severe headache
Nesiritide	No bolus	0.005–0.03 αg/kg/min	Maximum dose of 0.03 αg/kg/min. Follow kidney function closely
Inotropes			
Dopamine	2–5 αg/kg/min	2–20 αg/kg/min	Caution for arrhythmia May increase mortality
Dobutamine	1–2 αg/kg/min	1–20 αg/kg/min	Caution for arrhythmia May increase mortality
Milrinone	50 αg/kg IV loading dose over 10 min; then 0.25 α/kg/min to 1.0 αg/kg/min	0.10 αg/kg/min to 0.75 αg/kg/min	Caution for arrhythmia May increase mortality

- In patients with evidence of severely symptomatic fluid overload in the absence of hypotension, vasodilators such as intravenous nitroglycerin, nitroprusside, or nesiritide can be beneficial when added to diuretics or in those who do not respond to diuretics alone. Nesiritide, a recombinant form of human B-type natriuretic peptide, is a venous and arterial vasodilator that can decrease left atrial pressure and improve dyspnea. Its use, however, is limited, owing to concerns about deleterious effects on renal function and outcomes. The use of this medication has been limited to patients who are normotensive but clinically are hypervolemic despite adequate diuretic therapy.
- Ultrafiltration therapy is reasonable for patients with refractory congestion not responding to medical therapy.
- Mechanical assist devices may be required if patients do not respond to medical therapy. These include left ventricular assist devices; these are most commonly used as a bridge to heart transplantation.
- Inotropic therapy increases cardiac output, improving perfusion and relieving congestion. Milrinone dose must be adjusted in patients with renal disease as it is cleared by the kidneys. The use of these medications as a long therapy for HF increases mortality and increases the risk of arrhythmias and hypotension.

KEY POINTS: MANAGEMENT OF THE PATIENT WITH CONGESTIVE HEART FAILURE

1. Diuretic resistance is the persistence of edema and signs of hypervolemia in the setting of an adequate dose of diuretics (i.e., furosemide >120 mg daily or bumetanide >4 mg daily).

2. The most specific signs of decompensated heart failure (HF) are elevated jugular venous pressures and an S3 gallop (95% specificity).

3. B-type natriuretic peptide can be used in the urgent care setting to help exclude HF as the cause of dyspnea, but it cannot be used in isolation to confirm HF.

4. Thiazide diuretics become less effective when renal function worsens and are typically ineffective when the glomerular filtration rate is <30 cc/min; this does not apply, however, when thiazides are combined with loop diuretics.

5. Angiotensin-converting enzyme inhibitors slow the progression of cardiovascular disease by their pleiotropic effects, which include improved endothelial cell damage; antiproliferative effect on smooth muscle cells, neutrophils, and monocytes; and antithrombotic effects.

BIBLIOGRAPHY

1. Abraham WT, Elkayam U, Neibaur MT, et al. In-hospital mortality in patients with acute decompensated heart failure requiring intravenous vasoactive medications: An analysis from the acute decompensated heart failure registry (ADHERE). *J Am Coll Cardiol* 2005;46:57.
2. Brown JR, Uber PA, Mehra MR. The progressive cardiorenal syndrome in heart failure: Mechanisms and therapeutic insights. *Curr Treat Options Cardiovasc Med* 2008;10(4):342–348.
3. Cleland, JG, Coletta A, Witte K. Practical applications of intravenous diuretic therapy in decompensated heart failure. *Am J Med* 2006;119(12A):S26–236.
4. Cuffe MS, Califf RM, Adams KF Jr, et al. Short term intravenous milrinone for acute exacerbation of chronic heart failure: A randomized controlled trial. *JAMA* 2002;287:1541–1547.
5. Ellison DH: Intensive diuretic therapy: High doses, combinations, and constant infusions. In: Seldin D, Giebish G (eds.) *Diuretic Agents: Clinical Physiology and Pharmacology.* San Diego: Academic Press, 1997, pp. 281–300.
6. Fonarow GC, Adams KF Jr, Abraham WT, et al; ADHERE Scientific Advisory Committee, Study Group, and Investigators. Risk stratification for in-hospital mortality in acutely decompensated heart failure: classification and regression tree analysis. *JAMA* 2005;293(5):572–580.
7. Hunt SA, Abraham WT, Chin MH, et al. 2009 focused update incorporated into the ACC/AHA 2005. guidelines for the diagnosis and management of heart failure in adults: a report of the American College of Cardiology Foundation/ American Heart Association task force on practice guidelines: Developed in collaboration with the international society for heart and lung transplantation. *Circulation* 2009;119:e391.
8. Kapoor JR, Perazella, MA. Diagnostic and therapeutic approach to acute decompensated heart failure. *Am J Med* 2007;120(2):121–127.
9. Kirchner KA, Patel AR. Use of diuretics in chronic renal disease and nephritic syndrome. In: Seldin D, Giebish G (eds.) *Diuretic Agents: Clinical Physiology and Pharmacology.* San Diego: Academic Press, 1997, pp. 233–245.
10. Maisel AS, Krishnaswamy P, Nowak RM, et al.; Breathing Not Properly Multinational Study Investigators. Rapid measurement of B-type natriuretic peptide in the emergency diagnosis of heart failure. *N Engl J Med* 2002;347(3):161–167.
11. McKee PA, Castelli WP, McNamara PM, et al. *N Engl J Med* 1971;285(26):1441–1446, 1971.
12. Nohria A, Lewis E, Stevenson LW. Medical management of advanced heart failure. *JAMA* 2002;287:628–640.
13. Packer M, Poole-Wilson PA, Armstrong PW et al; ATLAS Study Group. Comparative effects of low and high doses of the angiotensin-converting enzyme inhibitor, lisinopril, on morbidity and mortality in chronic heart failure. *Circulation* 1999;100(23):2312–2318.
14. Ramani GV, Uber PA, Mehra MR. Chronic heart failure: Contemporary diagnosis and management. *Mayo Clin Proc* 2010;85(2):180–195.
15. Ronco C, Haapio M, House AA, et al. Cardiorenal syndrome. *J Am Coll Cardiol* 2008;52(19):1527–1539.
16. Rudy DW, Voelker JR, Greene PK, et al. Loop diuretics for chronic renal insufficiency: A continuous infusion is more efficacious than bolus therapy. *Ann Intern Med* 1991;115(5):360–366.
17. Sarraf M, Masoumi A, Schrier RW. Cardiorenal syndrome in acute decompensated heart failure. *Clin J Am Soc Nephrol* 2009;4:2013–2026.
18. Zile MR, Brutsaert DL. New concepts in diastolic dysfunction and diastolic heart failure: Part I: Diagnosis, prognosis, and measurements of diastolic function. *Circulation* 2002;105(11):1387–1393.

DRUG DOSING IN PATIENTS WITH CHRONIC KIDNEY DISEASE

Ryan S. Griffiths, MD, and Ali J. Olyaei, PharmD

1. **How can chronic kidney disease alter the pharmacokinetic behavior of most drugs?**
   Chronic kidney disease (CKD) directly and indirectly affects the pharmacokinetic properties of most drugs. Alterations of drug pharmacokinetics in patients with renal failure are based on changes in absorption, distribution, metabolism, and elimination.

2. **How can changes in absorption resulting from CKD alter the pharmacokinetic behavior of drugs?**
   Varying degrees of uremia may be present in CKD, particularly as patients progress toward end-stage renal disease (ESRD).
   - **Uremia:** This leads to a more alkaline saliva, which decreases absorption of drugs that need an acid milieu (e.g., iron supplements) and contributes to a higher gastric pH. Additionally, associated symptoms such as nausea and vomiting may lead to reduced mucosal contact time.
   - **Volume overload states:** Edema of the gastrointestinal tract will limit absorption.
   - **Drug interactions:** Many drugs used in the management of CKD limit drug absorption by forming nonabsorbable complexes (e.g., iron, phosphate-binding agents).
   - **Gastrointestinal neuropathy:** Uremia may decreases gastric emptying time, particularly in patients with diabetes. Today, diabetes is a leading cause of both CKD and ESRD.
   - **Hepatic first-pass metabolism:** This may be altered in stage 4 CKD and beyond. Decreased biotransformation of drugs to inactive metabolites will lead to increased levels in circulation.

3. **How can changes in distribution from CKD alter the pharmacokinetic behavior of drugs?**
   The volume of distribution (V_D) represents the ratio of administered dose to the resulting plasma concentration. The calculated V_D is a theoretic representation of the size of the anatomic space occupied by the drug if it were present throughout the body in the same concentration as that in the plasma. Drugs with a large V_D, such as digoxin, are distributed widely throughout the tissues and are present in relatively small amounts in the blood. Conversely, drugs that are less lipid-soluble and highly protein-bound will tend to have a lower V_D because they are more restricted to the vascular compartment.

   In patients with renal impairment, changes in drug distribution may arise from either fluid retention that may change the volume of distribution of water-soluble drugs (e.g., aminoglycosides) or reductions in the extent of protein binding in tissue and plasma. Malnutrition and proteinuria reduce the amount of protein available for protein binding, and uremia may alter the affinity of most drugs to albumin. Thus, the concentration of free drug will increase in these settings, which can result in increased free fraction and potential adverse drug reactions. Therapeutic drug monitoring (TDM) for free or unbound drug concentrations in patients with renal insufficiency or heavy proteinuria (e.g., free phenytoin levels) are an important consideration.

4. **How can changes in metabolism as a result of CKD alter the pharmacokinetic behavior of drugs?**
   Although renal elimination may be minimal for a drug as CKD progresses, dosing may still be difficult. CKD may increase, decrease, or have no effect on nonrenal clearance. Some drugs

are metabolized to active metabolites that are insignificant in those with normal renal function. However, in renal failure or CKD, accumulation of the active metabolites may cause serious adverse events. For example, morphine metabolizes to 3-morphine-gluconate with respiratory depression properties.

5. **How can changes in elimination as a result of CKD alter the pharmacokinetic behavior of drugs?**
Renal failure affects the clearance of predominantly renally excreted agents. Renal clearance could be estimated by the glomerular filtration rate (GFR). A reduction in GFR will generally lead to an increased half-life of a drug that is eliminated primarily by the kidney. GFR is usually expressed as a clearance, which is the amount of plasma from which the drug is cleared over unit time (e.g., milliliters per minute).

6. **What characteristics determine whether a drug is removed by dialysis?**
   - **Molecular size.** As a general rule, smaller molecular weight substances pass through the dialyzer membrane much more easily than larger size molecules. In general, free drug molecules with a molecular weight of less than 500 Daltons (D) are removed efficiently by hemodialysis.
   - **Protein binding.** Decreased protein binding may increase the amount of free drug available for removal during dialysis. In the setting of an overdose, the amount of ingested drug may exceed the normal protein-binding capacity. This would allow removal of the excess drug by hemodialysis, even though dialysis has a minimal effect when the drug is used at normal doses.
   - **Volume of distribution.** Drugs with large volumes of distribution are not removed effectively by dialysis. Lipid-soluble drugs usually have large volumes of distribution, making significant removal of the drug difficult because the plasma volume is rapidly replenished from other tissues (e.g., cyclosporine and digoxin).
   - **Water solubility.** Drugs with high water solubility will be dialyzed to a greater extent than those with high lipid solubility.
   - **Dialyzer membrane.** The pore size, surface area, and geometry are the primary factors in determining whether a dialysis membrane will clear a specific drug. Historically, standard dialysis membranes did not effectively remove vancomycin (molecular weight, 3300 D) given its size. Currently, high-flux membranes that remove larger molecular weight molecules have become standard of care in dialysis practice. Therefore, vancomycin and many other antibiotics are removed by these membranes. Dosing of these medications should be held until after dialysis on those days.
   - **Blood and dialysate flow rates.** Increased flow rates during hemodialysis will increase drug clearance. Patients who cannot tolerate standard blood flow rates will require less replacement dosing of a drug after hemodialysis.

7. **How is renal function assessed for drug dosing determination?**
The best way is to estimate the GFR. The gold standard is measurement of the clearance of inulin; however, this is cumbersome and impractical for clinical use. Measurement of the 24-hour creatinine clearance (CrCl) is no longer recommended for similar reasoning. This has lead to the development of equations to estimate GFR such as the Cockcroft-Gault and Modification of Diet in Renal Disease (MDRD) study. These equations use serum creatinine as one of the variables and both generally provide similar dosing recommendations. Adverse events such as drug accumulations are relatively uncommon when the GFR remains >50 mL/min.

It is still important to consider potential analytic interferences in these calculations based on the concurrent drug therapy. Some drugs may artifactually increase or decrease the measured serum creatinine concentration without directly influencing GFR. Drugs that inhibit the tubular secretion of creatinine will raise the serum level (e.g., trimethoprim, cimetidine, and probenecid).

8. **What commonly prescribed drugs are causes of hyperkalemia in patients with CKD and receiving dialysis?**

Many drugs used as therapy for CKD and associated conditions such as heart failure and hypertension can potentiate this serious complication. Often, it is combinations of these medications that lead to hyperkalemia. Potassium (K^+) supplements are used frequently in combination with diuretic therapy. Potassium-sparing diuretics (spironolactone, amiloride) inhibit renal elimination of K^+. Angiotensin-converting enzyme (ACE) inhibitors and angiotensin receptor blockers (ARBs) are common causes via alterations in the renin-angiotensin-aldosterone system (RAAS). Digoxin inhibits the basolateral Na-K ATPase in cardiac myocytes. Because of a narrow therapeutic window, overdose states are not uncommon and can result in elevated K^+. Acute and/ or chronic reductions in GFR in association with the previously mentioned medications can tip a patient into a hyperkalemic state by further reducing the ability to renally excrete K^+.

Several anti-infectious agents are frequently implicated. Trimethoprim can block electrolyte exchange in the collecting duct and lead to metabolic acidosis. These risks are increased as the GFR decreases further. It is generally avoided in the dialysis population because of this. Amphotericin B can cause K^+ shifts out of the cell. Penicillin infusion solutions contain a high amount of potassium for drug stability.

Finally, patients undergoing kidney transplant are becoming increasingly prevalent. All of them require immunosuppression, which usually involves a calcineurin inhibitor such as tacrolimus or cyclosporine. Both of these are associated with various electrolyte abnormalities, which include hyperkalemia.

9. **Which antimicrobials should be avoided prior to hemodialysis on scheduled dialysis days?**

Many antibacterial agents are water soluble, small molecules, and not highly protein bound, thus they are well dialyzed and will require supplementation postdialysis. Many of these agents are already administered in a reduced dose or frequency given the reduced renal clearance. Beta-lactam agents such as penicillins, cephalosporins, carbapenems, and monobactams are examples of such compounds. Aminoglycosides also exhibit similar properties. Carbapenem and imipenem can lower the seizure threshold and should be avoided in patients receiving dialysis altogether; meropenem in a reduced dose is a therapeutic alternative. Antifungals such as fluconazole may require supplemental dosing; however, the echinocandins (caspofungin, micafungin) and the amphotericin family do not. Antiviral agents should receive individual consideration given their varying properties. Entecavir and telbivudine appear to be removed by hemodialysis, whereas lamivudine does not.

10. **When is redosing or a supplemental dose required following hemodialysis?**

Dialysis clearance must increase total clearance by at least 30% to be considered clinically significant and to require a replacement dose after hemodialysis. The physicochemical characteristics as discussed previously determine the extent that a drug may be affected by dialysis.

11. **How should aminoglycosides be adjusted for hemodialysis?**

First, patient's dosing weight should be determined. Use ideal body weight (IBW) unless total body weight (TBW) is less. Nonobese is defined as follows:
- TBW <30% more than ideal body weight
- IBW (males) = 50 kg + (2.3 × height in inches >60 inches)
- IBW (females) = 45 kg + (2.3 × height in inches >60 inches)
- In patients who are obese, adjust IBW: ABW (kg) = IBW + 0.4 (TBW − IBW), where ABW is actual body weight.
  Second, select the appropriate loading and maintenance doses:
- Loading dose should be considered in life-threatening infection (for gentamicin and tobramycin, give 2.5 mg/kg; for amikacin give 7.5 mg/kg as a loading dose).
- Select appropriate maintenance dose according to indications (Table 28-1).

TABLE 28-1. AMINOGLYCOSIDE DOSING IN PATIENTS UNDERGOING DIALYSIS

	Dose and Frequency in Patients Undergoing Dialysis		
Drug	Hemodialysis (Dose Postdialysis)	Peritoneal Dialysis (Every 48 Hours)*	Continuous Renal Replacement Therapy (Every 24 Hours)
Gentamicin	1.5–2 mg/kg	1.5–2 mg/kg	1.5–2 mg/kg
Serious infection	1 mg/kg	1 mg/kg	1 mg/kg
Urinary tract infection	1 mg/kg	1 mg/kg	1 mg/kg
Synergy			
Tobramycin	1.5–2 mg/kg	1.5–2 mg/kg	1.5–2 mg/kg
Urinary tract infection	1 mg/kg	1 mg/kg	1 mg/kg
Amikacin	7.5 mg/kg	7.5 mg/kg	7.5 mg/kg

12. **What adjustments should be made for administering vancomycin to patients receiving hemodialysis?**
It is important to load patients receiving dialysis with 15 to 20 mg/kg based on actual body weight. Maintenance doses will depend on the dialysis membrane used during hemodialysis (Table 28-2).

13. **What adjustments should be made for patients with diabetes?**
The breakdown of insulin decreases as kidney function deteriorates. Patients with diabetes must be monitored for symptoms of hypoglycemia because their insulin requirement may decrease concurrently. Sulfonylureas that are excreted primarily by the kidneys can accumulate and result in a prolonged hypoglycemic effect. For example, glyburide is metabolized to active metabolites with hypoglycemic properties. A substitute to a drug with greater hepatic excretion such as glipizide should be considered when GFR is reduced to less than <50 mL/min. Metformin should be avoided in the presence of renal impairment because of the risk of lactic acidosis. All package inserts classify renal impairment as a serum creatinine ≥1.5 mg/dL in males or ≥1.4 mg/dL in females. Clinically, however, a GFR of 60 mL/min or less has become a recommended corollary (Table 28-3).

14. **How does narcotic pain management differ in patients with CKD?**
Meperidine should be avoided in patients with renal failure because of accumulation of its metabolite (normeperidine), which undergoes renal elimination. Normeperidine also has an excitatory effect on the central nervous system (CNS) and causes seizures if it accumulates.
　　Propoxyphene should also be avoided in patients with renal failure because of the accumulation of a metabolite (norpropoxyphene). Both can cause ventricular arrhythmias as a result of class IA antiarrhythmic properties. Another complication, propoxyphene-induced hypoglycemia, can be seen in patients with renal insufficiency.
　　Morphine should be used with caution in patients with renal failure. Morphine undergoes glucuronidation to morphine-6-glucuronide (M6G) and morphine-3-glucuronide. M6G accumulates in renal failure and is a more potent analgesic than the parent compound. In patients with ESRD, the half-life of M6G is estimated to be 38 to 103 hours.
　　Codeine is metabolized in the liver to codeine-6-glucuronide, norcodeine, and morphine. A dose reduction of 50% is generally recommended in renal failure.

TABLE 28-2. VANCOMYCIN ADMINISTRATION IN PATIENTS UNDERGOING DIALYSIS			
	Hemodialysis (HD) (High Flux)	Continuous Venovenous Hemofiltration (HD, Hemodiafiltration)	Peritoneal
Loading dose	15–20 mg/kg dose based on actual body weight (ABW) Note: Not to exceed 1500 mg May consider 20 mg/kg in severe infections (i.e., meningitis, severe sepsis, endocarditis, osteomyelitis, and hospital-acquired pneumonia [HAP])	15–20 mg/kg dose based on ABW Note: Not to exceed 1500 mg May consider 20 mg/kg in severe infections (i.e., meningitis, severe sepsis, endocarditis, osteomyelitis, HAP)	Not necessary
Maintenance dose (postdialysis)	<75 kg: 500 mg after HD for predialysis level <20 > 75 kg: 1000 mg after HD for predialysis level <20	10–15 mg/kg every 24 hours Note: May consider higher doses in patients who are obese not to exceed 1500 mg IV q24h	IP (intraperitoneal): 30 mg/kg loading dose 15 mg/kg every 3–5 days Note: Patients that are not anuric may need to adjust dosing frequency because there is residual renal function Intravenous (IV): 15–20 mg/kg per dose
Serum level monitoring	Draw serum level prior to the 2nd HD session, then get random levels with AM labs on HD days only (or q48 hrs) Note: Subsequent serum levels should be drawn prior to every or every other HD session	Draw serum level prior to the 2nd or 3rd dose (approx 24 hours after last dose) Note: May draw random daily levels with AM labs	IP: Draw serum trough level 72 hours after loading dose IV: Draw serum trough level 48–72 hours after initial dose
Dosing based on serum levels	If pre-HD level is: > 20: hold dose 10–20: give dose after HD (based on weight) < 10: administer another loading dose after HD	If serum level is: > 20: hold dose 10–20: continue with q24h dosing < 10: 15–20 mg/kg loading dose → consider more frequent dosing or increasing the dose	If level is: >20: hold dose <20: administer another dose

	Normal Renal Function	Chronic Kidney Disease Stages 3–5	Hemodialysis
TABLE 28-3.	**MEDICATION ADJUSTMENTS FOR PATIENTS WITH DIABETES**		
Metformin	500–2000 mg/day	Avoid	Avoid (lactic acidosis)
Rosiglitazone	4–8 mg/day	Caution	Caution (heart failure and fluid retention)
Pioglitazone	15–30 mg/day	Caution	Caution (heart failure and fluid retention)
Glyburide	2.5–10 mg bid	50%	Avoid
Glipizide	5–20 mg bid	100%	50%
Glimepiride	1–8 mg/day	50%	Avoid
Nateglinide	120–180 tid	100%	100%
Rapaglinide	0.5–4 mg tid	100%	100%
Sitagliptin	100 mg daily	50 mg/day	25 mg/day

Hydromorphone is considered to be relatively safe and effective in patients with renal failure. It is metabolized in the liver to hydromorphone-3-glucuronide followed by a reduction to 6-a-hydroxyhydromorphone and 6-b-hydroxyhydromorphone, both of which are less potent analgesics than the parent drug. Seizure activity and cognitive impairment have been reported in patients with renal failure receiving high-dose hydromorphone therapy.

Fentanyl is another good option for pain management in patients with renal failure, even though the kidneys eliminate both the parent drug and its metabolites.

15. **How is dosage of anticonvulsants adjusted in patients with CKD?**
Phenytoin is a highly protein-bound drug. In patients receiving dialysis or in patients with CKD and significant proteinuria the free fraction of phenytoin (free phenytoin) is elevated, although plasma phenytoin levels seem low. If not adjusted, total phenytoin levels are of little value. In patients receiving dialysis, the monitoring of free concentration is recommended for a target plasma concentration of 1 to 2 mcg/mL.

If unable to obtain a free phenytoin level, the following equations can be used to adjust the serum concentrations based on either reduced albumin levels or presence of renal failure (CrCl <10 mL/min).

- Hypoproteinemia: $C_{adjusted} = C_{measured}/[(0.2 \times albumin) + 0.1]$
- Acute kidney injury and dialysis: $C_{adjusted} = C_{measured}/[(0.1 \times albumin) + 0.1]$

16. **List the common drug interactions for cyclosporine and tacrolimus in kidney transplant recipients.**
Many drugs are known to interact with calcineurin inhibitors (cyclosporine and tacrolimus); some agents are more problematic than others. Antiepileptic medications such as phenytoin, carbamazepine, and phenobarbital; antituberculosis agents such as rifampin, rifabutin, and isoniazid (INH); and herbal supplements such as St. John's wort are well-known inducers of the cytochrome P-450 (CYP3A4) pathway and would decrease plasma concentrations of calcineurin inhibitors. Thus, these drug–drug interactions may increase the risk of acute

rejection following transplantation. The use of these agents in combination with calcineurin inhibitors requires dose escalation and careful therapeutic drug monitoring.

Coadministration of calcineurin inhibitors with agents that strongly inhibit the CYP3A4 enzymatic system may conversely result in nephrotoxicity. Nefazodone, nondihydropyridine calcium channel blockers (verapamil, diltiazem), antibiotics (erythromycin, clarithromycin, telithromycin, but not azithromycin), antifungal agents (ketoconazole, fluconazole, itraconazole, voriconazole), and grapefruit are strong CYP3A4 inhibitors. Grapefruit and grapefruit juice are known inhibitors of the cytochrome P-450 pathway and should be avoided in transplant patients and patients with CKD taking statins and calcium channel blockers.

17. **What are the common risk factors for aminoglycoside renal toxicity?**
Dose and duration of therapy, advanced age, use of other nephrotoxic agents (cyclosporine, tacrolimus, vancomycin), sepsis, hypotension, dehydration, and intravenous radiologic contrast medium have been reported as important risk factors in the development of aminoglycoside-induced nephrotoxicity. However, when confounding factors are adjusted using multivariate analysis, only dose, duration, advanced age, and baseline creatinine level have been associated with nephrotoxicity.

18. **What drugs have been associated with or precipitate nephrolithiasis?**
Several agents can crystallize in the urine, such as indinavir, acyclovir, sulfadiazine, and triamterene. Stones related to these drugs usually involve the crystalline structure. Nephrolithiasis has been reported with prolonged use of ceftriaxone in children. Large amounts of vitamin C intake in men have been associated with an increased risk of calcium-based stone formation, presumably related to its metabolism to oxalate. Initiation of uricosuric therapy with probenecid can precipitate uric acid stone formation. Loop diuretics (e.g., furosemide) can also play a role as a result of increased urinary calcium excretion and volume contraction related to diuresis. Conversely, thiazide-type diuretics reduce urinary calcium excretion.

KEY POINTS: DRUG DOSING IN PATIENTS WITH CHRONIC KIDNEY DISEASE

1. Renal disease alters pharmacokinetic and pharmacodynamic of most commonly used drugs.
2. Patient with chronic kidney disease (CKD) are at greater risk of adverse drug reactions and drug interactions.
3. Pharmacologic agents that could cause hyperkalemia in patients with CKD and undergoing dialysis should be used with caution.
4. Consider a loading dose of antibiotic in the treatment of serious infection and adjust dosage according to renal function to avoid toxicities.
5. Drug-induced kidney injury should be differentiated from other form of renal impairment.

19. **How can ACE inhibitors and ARBs cause renal dysfunction while being protective in diabetic nephropathy?**
ACE inhibitors and ARBs exert their effects by blocking the RAAS pathway. The pharmacodynamic effects of these agents are achieved by inhibiting the vasoconstrictive effect of angiotensin II at the efferent arteriole in the glomerulus. RAAS blockade at the glomerular structure of the nephron reduces glomerular capillary pressure, which has been shown to be associated with reductions in proteinuria, an important surrogate outcome for renal function. As a result of the reduced filtration fraction associated with this hemodynamic change, an

increase in the baseline serum creatinine concentration prior to drug initiation of 30% is generally determined acceptable. Increases in creatinine beyond this are suggestive of atherosclerotic renal artery stenosis and should be further evaluated.

Unfortunately, this same "protective" mechanism limits the kidney's ability to autoregulate its blood flow in times of stress such as severe infection or hypotension. Patients who incur these complications are at increased risk for acute kidney injury from renal hypoperfusion (ischemia). These drugs should be promptly discontinued if this clinical scenario becomes apparent. After a return to homeostasis, reinitiation of the drug can be considered.

20. **What is the association between proton pump inhibitors (PPIs) and acute interstitial nephritis (AIN)?**
The PPIs (i.e., omeprazole and lansoprazole) are fast becoming one of the most common causes of drug-induced AIN. The first documented case was in 1992. Since then, numerous case series with biopsy-proven disease have been published. The interaction appears to be a class effect because all PPIs have been documented to cause AIN. The onset of disease is idiosyncratic in that the development of symptoms has ranged from 1 week to 18 months after drug initiation. PPI-induced AIN generally does not manifest as the typical hypersensitivity reaction. The PPI should be withdrawn upon suspicion of this diagnosis. However, although most patients do recover kidney function, many are left with some level of chronic kidney disease.

21. **What are the dosing recommendations and indications for use of bisphosphonates in states of renal injury?**
In general, most of the data for the use of bisphosphonates in patients with varying degrees of acute kidney injury (AKI) have come from trials looking at treatment of hypercalcemia associated with multiple myeloma and other malignancies. Treatment of osteoporosis with bisphosphonates in CKD and dialysis populations remains controversial. Metabolic changes in bone morphology associated with CKD further complicate the definition of osteoporosis and thus the validity of the indication for these therapies in this population (Table 28-4).

TABLE 28-4.	DOSING RECOMMENDATIONS FOR BISPHOSPHONATES IN RENAL INJURY		
	Hypercalcemia in Acute Kidney Injury	Chronic Kidney Disease Stages 3–5	Hemodialysis
Pamidronate (Avedia)	OK	Avoid—associated with development of focal segmental glomerulosclerosis	OK—for 1 dose of 30 mg if failing other therapies
Alendronate (Fosamax)	—	Avoid in glomerular filtration rate <30–35	Avoid
Ibandronate (Boniva)	OK		Avoid
Risedronate (Actonel)	—		Avoid
Zoledronic acid (Zometa)	Use with caution	Avoid	Avoid

22. **What are the dosing recommendations for enoxaparin and other low molecular weight heparin in CKD?**

Enoxaparin dose should be adjusted for the treatment of the most common thrombotic disorders in patient with chronic kidney disease. For patients with stable estimated GFR less than 30 mL/min, the dose should be adjusted to 1 mg/kg per day and heparin assay (low molecular weight heparin) should be monitored twice a week initially, then weekly after 2 weeks of treatment. The heparin level should be drawn 4 hours after the dose and the dose should be adjusted to heparin level of 0.7 to 1.1. Unfractionated heparin should be considered the alternative of choice for patients with unstable renal function or undergoing dialysis.

23. **Discuss the dosing of antigout drugs in adults with CKD.**

Gout is a common inflammatory arthritis disorder in patients with CKD. Although NSAIDs are the drugs of choice for the treatment of acute attack in patients with normal renal function, NSAIDs should be avoided or used with caution in patients with CKD. Corticosteroids orally, intravenously, intra-articularly, or indirectly via adrenocorticotropic hormone (ACTH) can be given safely in this setting. Colchicine also can be used for the treatment of gout flare-up; however, the dose should be adjusted to 0.5 mg orally 2 to 3 times per day for patients with estimated GFR between 10 and 50 mL/min. Intravenous colchicines is contraindicated in CKD because of the associated risk for multiorgan failure. Recombinant urate oxidase (rasburicase) can be used in patients with hyperuricemia and have failed other standard oral antihyperuricemic drug therapy. No dosage adjustment is required in this setting (Table 28-5).

TABLE 28-5. DOSAGE RECOMMENDATIONS FOR ANTIGOUT DRUGS IN CHRONIC KIDNEY DISEASE (CKD)			
	Normal Renal Function	**CKD Stages 3–5**	**Hemodialysis**
Allopurinol	300–400 mg	25%–50%	25%
Colchicine	1 mg, then 0.5 mg q8h	25%	Avoid
Corticosteroids	40 mg	100%	100%
Febuxostat	40–80 mg/day	100%	NA
Rasburicase	0.15–0.2 mg/kg	100%	100%

BIBLIOGRAPHY

1. Aymanns C, Keller F, Maus S, et al. Review on pharmacokinetics and pharmacodynamics and the aging kidney. *Clin J Am Soc Nephrol* 2010;5(2):314–327.
2. Brater DC. Drug dosing in patients with impaired renal function. *Clin Pharmacol Ther* 2009;86(5):483–489.
3. Brewster UC, Perazella MA. Proton pump inhibitors and the kidney: Critical review. *Clin Nephrol* 2009;68:65–72.
4. Choi G, Gomersall CD, Tian Q, et al. Principles of antibacterial dosing in continuous renal replacement therapy. *Crit Care Med* 2009;37(7):2268–2282.
5. Li AM, Gomersall CD, Choi G, et al. A systematic review of antibiotic dosing regimens for septic patients receiving continuous renal replacement therapy: Do current studies supply sufficient data? *J Antimicrob Chemother* 2009;64(5):929–937.
6. Mushatt DM, Mihm LB, Dreisbach AW, et al. Antibiotic dosing in slow extended daily dialysis. *Clin Infect Dis* 2009;49(3):433–437.
7. Narva AS. Assessment of kidney function for drug dosing. *Clin Chem* 2009;55(9):1609–1611.
8. Olyaei AJ, Bennett WM. Drug dosing in the elderly patients with chronic kidney disease. *Clin Geriatr Med* 2009;25(3):459–527.
9. Spruill WJ, Wade WE, Cobb HH III. Continuing the use of the Cockcroft-Gault equation for drug dosing in patients with impaired renal function. *Clin Pharmacol Ther* 2009;86(5):468–470.
10. Stevens LA, Levey AS. Use of the MDRD study equation to estimate kidney function for drug dosing. *Clin Pharmacol Ther* 2009;86(5):465–467.
11. Verbeeck RK, Musuamba FT. Pharmacokinetics and dosage adjustment in patients with renal dysfunction. *Eur J Clin Pharmacol* 2009;65(8):757–773.

IV. PRIMARY GLOMERULAR DISORDERS

MINIMAL CHANGE DISEASE

Elaine S. Kamil, MD

CHAPTER 29

1. **What are the diagnostic criteria for nephrotic syndrome?**
   Nephrotic syndrome is a syndrome that results from severe proteinuria. Heavy glomerular protein losses (≥ 3.5 g in an adult or >40 mg/m^2/hour in a child) lead to the other three criteria for nephrotic syndrome: hypoalbuminemia, hyperlipidemia, and usually edema. From a practical standpoint, measuring a urine total protein/creatinine ratio is preferable to collecting a 24-hour urine for protein. A ratio of ≥ 3.5 correlates with nephrotic-range proteinuria.

2. **What is minimal change disease (minimal change nephrotic syndrome)?**
   Minimal change disease (MCD) is a disorder of glomeruli that leads to heavy proteinuria. Renal biopsy shows normal glomeruli by light microscopy but will show effacement of the podocyte foot processes by electron microscopy. Immunofluorescent microscopy typically is negative, although some patients may show staining for immunoglobulin M (IgM) in the mesangial regions of the glomeruli. Technically, a patient cannot be said to have MCD with certainty without having had a kidney biopsy. However, so many young children with nephrotic syndrome have MCD that kidney biopsies are only performed in those children with atypical findings or in those who are resistant to immunosuppressive therapy. Older adolescents and adults are diagnosed with MCD after a kidney biopsy is performed.

3. **How likely is MCD to be the cause of nephrotic syndrome in any individual?**
   MCD is the cause of nephrotic syndrome in about 90% of children younger than age 6, in about 65% of older children, and in about 20% to 30% of adolescents. In adults only about 10% to 25% of nephrotic syndrome results from MCD, but it represents the third most common cause of nephrotic syndrome in adults after membranous nephropathy and focal, segmental glomerulosclerosis.

4. **What causes MCD?**
   MCD is an immune-mediated disease, felt to be mediated by a circulating factor capable of inducing proteinuria. Presumably the circulating factor is secreted by lymphoid cells, and it functions as a vascular permeability factor that directly affects the function of the podocytes. Although the majority of cases of MCD are idiopathic, MCD, particularly in adults, may be associated with neoplastic disease such as lymphoma, toxic or allergic reactions to drugs, certain infections, allergies, or other autoimmune disorders.

5. **How common is MCD?**
   The prevalence of MCD in children is about 16 per 100,000 children, but it is much less prevalent in adults.

6. **What is the typical clinical presentation of MCD?**
   Patients with MCD typically present with mild to severe edema. Because the onset with periorbital edema commonly follows an upper respiratory infection in young children, nephrotic syndrome may sometimes be confused with an allergic reaction until a more thorough evaluation is performed. In the youngest children there is a 2:1 male to female

prevalence, but by adolescence and beyond males and females are equally affected. Other symptoms can include abdominal pain, diarrhea, poor appetite, and decreased urine output. Rarely, a patient may present with sepsis.

7. **How is MCD diagnosed?**
MCD presents with nephrotic syndrome. However, the child who presents with typical features (see question 1) of nephrotic syndrome is presumed to have MCD and does not undergo a kidney biopsy unless there are unusual factors such as resistance to prednisone therapy, hypertension, decreased kidney function, or hypocomplementemia.

8. **What is the standard initial therapy for MCD in children?**
The cornerstone of therapy of typical nephrotic syndrome in young children is high-dose glucocorticoids. Children treated with a longer initial course of prednisone are less likely to experience frequent relapses than those children treated with a more abbreviated course of steroid therapy. Children older than 4 years of age are treated with 60 mg/m^2 daily given early in the morning for 6 weeks followed by 40 mg/m^2 every other morning for an additional 6 weeks. Children younger than age 4 receive the same initial 6-week course of daily prednisone but then should receive a slower taper of 60 mg/m^2 every other morning for 4 weeks, tapering further by 10 mg/m^2 every 4 weeks for an additional 20 weeks. About 95% of young children will experience a complete remission of the nephrotic syndrome within 4 weeks; 75% will respond within 2 weeks.

9. **What is the standard initial therapy for MCD in adults?**
Prednisone is also the standard initial therapy for adults with MCD. Adults with MCD tend to require a longer course of prednisone before remission is attained. The optimal initial prednisone regimen varies somewhat among nephrologists, but typically a single morning dose of 1 mg/kg/day, maximum of 80 mg, is continued for a minimum of 8 weeks. For those patients not in remission at 8 weeks, daily prednisone may be continued for another 2 months until remission is attained. A gradual taper is then recommended on an every-other-day schedule until the patient is tapered off over many months. The slow taper is recommended to sustain the remission and to reduce the likelihood of problems with adrenal insufficiency.

10. **How do you define remission in nephrotic syndrome?**
Typically patients with nephrotic syndrome are taught to monitor their urine protein at home using dipsticks. A complete remission is defined in children as a urine dipstick of trace to negative OR a urine protein/creatinine ratio of <0.2. In adults a complete remission is defined as a reduction of proteinuria to ≤300 mg of urinary protein in a 24-hour period; however, a urine protein/creatinine ratio of <0.2 is also an appropriate benchmark for adults. A partial remission is defined as a ≥50% reduction in urinary protein in 24 hours or a 24 hour urine protein of <3.5 g with an associated normal serum albumin. Patients with MCD almost always experience a complete as opposed to a partial remission. Normalization of serum albumin quickly follows the reduction in proteinuria, but the hyperlipidemia may take several months to normalize.

11. **What other supportive therapies are useful for MCD?**
A no-added-salt diet is always recommended for patients with MCD—it will reduce edema formation and reduce the tendency to develop hypertension. In addition, angiotensin-converting enzyme (ACE) inhibitors and/or angiotensin receptor blockers (ARBs) are useful in ameliorating proteinuria and are the first choice for the treatment of hypertension if it appears in these patients. Oral diuretics may be used with caution in patients with moderate edema. For those patients with severe edema accompanied by ascites, scrotal or labial edema, and/or pleural effusions, intravenous infusions of 25% salt-poor albumin may be helpful. A dose of 1 g/kg, up to a maximum of 50 g, is infused over 2 to 4 hours once or twice a day, followed by intravenous furosemide at a dose of 1 mg/kg. Caution must be observed in the patient with oliguria because that patient could have had an acute kidney

injury, making him or her unresponsive to the diuretic and susceptible to mobilization of peripheral edema leading to the risk of pulmonary edema with respiratory compromise.

12. **What is the typical course for a patient with MCD?**
The majority of children (60% to 75%) with MCD experience relapses of the disease, and sometimes they are frequent—three or more relapses per year. Relapses tend to be precipitated by infections, particularly upper respiratory infections, or by allergies. About 50% to 75% of adults who respond to steroids will have a relapse, and 10% to 25% become frequent relapsers. A minority of patients develop steroid dependence of variable severity where the patient cannot be tapered off the prednisone. The steroid dependence can vary from being maintained in remission on low-dose, alternate-day steroids to requiring high-dose, daily steroids to maintain a remission.

13. **How are relapses of MCD treated?**
Relapses of MCD are treated with the same initial doses of corticosteroids as the initial episode of nephrotic syndrome but for a more abbreviated course, at least in children. Children are treated with daily steroids until the urine is negative for protein for 3 days. The prednisone dose is then lowered to 40 mg/m^2 every other morning for 4 weeks with either a rapid taper over 2 months or a slow taper over 6 to 12 months. The rapidity of the taper is usually based on the patient's prior response to tapering. Adults who relapse are also re-treated with a regimen similar to the initial corticosteroid protocol outlined previously.

14. **If the patient responds to steroids but develops steroid toxicity or steroid dependence, what other treatment options are there?**
Several treatment options are available for the child or adult with steroid toxicity or steroid dependence, each with its own unique risk-benefit profile. The goal of therapy for these patients is to avoid the complications of nephrotic syndrome (see question 16) by maintaining a remission while minimizing the toxicities of therapy. The first therapy used for these patients is alternate-day prednisone therapy, tapered slowly to the lowest dose that will maintain a remission. If that fails, other options include 12-week courses of oral cyclophosphamide (or chlorambucil), longer courses (1–2 years) of cyclosporine, mycophenolate mofetil, azathioprine, tacrolimus, or levamisole. These medications should only be prescribed by physicians who are familiar with their toxicities.

15. **If the patient is steroid resistant, what are the treatment options?**
The patient who is steroid resistant should have a kidney biopsy if one has not yet been performed. The biopsy may show focal, segmental glomerulosclerosis; MCD; or membranous nephropathy. Treatment options include a course of high-dose intravenous methylprednisolone, oral cyclosporine, or tacrolimus. Mycophenolate mofetil may also be tried. Some newer reports have shown some promise with rituximab, a CD20 monoclonal antibody, but those reports are still preliminary.

16. **What are the complications of MCD?**
The complications of MCD are those of nephrotic syndrome or are related to the toxicities of the treatments used. For the patient with frequent relapses, there is a delicate trade-off between the complications of the disease and the side effects of the medications. MCD may have life-threatening complications. These include the risks of overwhelming infection, thromboembolic phenomenon, and the cardiovascular complications related to hyperlipidemia. The cause of the increased risk of infection is multifactorial but is in part related to loss of opsonizing factors in the urine. Opsonizing factors are particularly important in defense against encapsulated bacteria such as *Pneumococcus* and *Hemophilus influenzae*. Another risk factor for infection in the patient with MCD is the frequent occurrence of hypogammaglobulinemia in these patients, especially during episodes of relapse. There is an increased risk of serious bacterial infections when the plasma IgG levels fall below 400 mg/dL and a very increased risk when levels fall below 200 mg/dL. In a patient with low IgG levels and sepsis, or in those patients with chronic hypogammaglobulinemia, intravenous gamma globulin may be used.

Thromboembolism may be seen in patients with MCD, more commonly in the adult with MCD than in the child with MCD. Children are more prone to sagittal sinus thrombosis, pulmonary artery thrombosis, or inferior vena caval thrombosis, whereas adults with MCD are more prone to deep vein or renal vein thrombosis. The hypercoagulable state in MCD results from several factors including increased clotting factor synthesis (fibrinogen, II, V, VII, IX, X, XIII), urinary losses of anticoagulants (antithrombin III), platelet abnormalities (thrombocytosis, increased aggregability), hyperviscosity, and hyperlipidemia.

Patients in a severe relapse have an increased risk of developing an acute kidney injury secondary to decreased renal perfusion and edema of the renal interstitium. Acute kidney injury is usually reversible in this setting, but intravenous albumin therapy should not be given during an episode of acute kidney injury because of the risk of its use leading to pulmonary edema.

Chronic hyperlipidemia in the patient with MCD can lead to the accelerated development of arteriosclerosis.

17. **What steps can be taken to reduce the complications of MCD?**
The complications of nephrotic syndrome can be avoided by keeping the patient in remission whenever possible. The risk of some of the infectious complications can be avoided by making sure that patients receive vaccines against all infectious agents that can cause life-threatening infections. All adults and all children older than 2 years of age should receive the 23-valent pneumococcal vaccine. All patients with MCD should receive a yearly influenza vaccine. Children should receive all of their childhood vaccines with deferral of live virus vaccines (measles-mumps-rubella, varicella) until they are in remission off of immunosuppressive medications. The administration of live virus vaccine may be associated with a relapse, but that risk is minimal when compared with the risk of vaccine-preventable disease. Adults and children with MCD should also have the status of their immunity against varicella determined by checking a varicella-zoster IgG titer. Varicella infections in individuals who are immune compromised, including those individuals taking prednisone, may be fatal. If the patient does not have a protective titer against varicella, vaccine should be given if possible. If the patient cannot receive vaccine because of continued immunosuppression, varicella-zoster immune globulin (VZIG) should be administered as soon as possible after exposure to an individual with chicken pox. If a patient who is immunosuppressed develops chicken pox or zoster, he or she should receive immediate treatment with intravenous acyclovir.

A reduction in thromboembolic complications can be attempted by being vigilant for situations where thromboembolism is more of a risk, particularly protecting the intravascular volume of a critically ill patient in relapse. Central venous catheters should be avoided whenever possible in this patient population. If a patient experiences a thromboembolic event, treatment should include heparin or low molecular weight heparin, followed by warfarin for 6 months. Prophylactic anticoagulation therapy should be administered for future relapses in these patients.

Chronic hyperlipidemia, if present, warrants therapy in adults; there are little data on its use in children at this point but should only be considered in children who are chronically hyperlipidemic. Hypertension is best treated initially with an ACE inhibitor and/or an ARB, which should help reduce the risk of cardiovascular complications later.

18. **What is the prognosis for a patient with MCD?**
The vast majority of children with MCD have a favorable prognosis. In children a prompt remission within 7 to 9 days of steroid therapy, the absence of microhematuria, and age greater than 4 years at presentation predict fewer relapses. By 10 years from diagnosis, only 16% of children with MCD are still experiencing relapses. Many children will "outgrow" their disease by or during adolescence, although some continue to experience relapses into adulthood. The long-term cardiovascular risk in children with MCD who have experienced long periods of steroid therapy and periods of hyperlipidemia and hypertension is largely unknown. In adults with MCD the most important prognostic factor is the patient's initial response to steroid therapy and whether he or she can experience extended periods of time off steroids, which carry a more serious toxicity profile in adults.

KEY POINTS: MINIMAL CHANGE DISEASE

1. Minimal change disease (MCD) is the cause of nephrotic syndrome in about 90% of children younger than age 6, in about 65% of older children, and in about 20% to 30% of adolescents. In adults, only about 10% to 25% of nephrotic syndrome results from MCD, but it represents the third most common cause of nephrotic syndrome in adults after membranous nephropathy and focal, segmental glomerulosclerosis.

2. MCD is an immune-mediated disease, felt to be mediated by a circulating factor capable of inducing proteinuria. Presumably the circulating factor is secreted by lymphoid cells, and it functions as a vascular permeability factor that directly affects the function of the podocytes.

3. Patients with MCD typically present with mild to severe edema. Because the onset with periorbital edema commonly follows an upper respiratory infection in young children, nephrotic syndrome may sometimes be confused with an allergic reaction until a more thorough evaluation is performed.

4. The cornerstone of therapy of typical nephrotic syndrome in young children is high-dose glucocorticoids. Children treated with a longer initial course of prednisone are less likely to experience frequent relapses than those children treated with a more abbreviated course of steroid therapy. Prednisone is also the standard initial therapy for adults with MCD. Adults with MCD tend to require a longer course of prednisone before remission is attained.

5. The vast majority of children with MCD have a very favorable prognosis. In children a prompt remission within 7 to 9 days of steroid therapy, the absence of microhematuria, and age greater than 4 years at presentation predict fewer relapses.

BIBLIOGRAPHY

1. Brenchly PEC. Vascular permeability factors in steroid-sensitive nephrotic syndrome and focal, segmental glomerulosclerosis. *Nephrol Dial Transplant* 2003;18:vi21.
2. Filler G. Treatment of nephrotic syndrome in children and adults, controlled trials. *Nephrol Dial Transplant* 2003;18:vi75.
3. Gipson DS, Massengil SF, Yao L, et al. Management of childhood onset nephrotic syndrome. *Pediatrics* 2009;124(2):747–757.
4. Glassock RJ. Secondary minimal change disease. *Nephrol Dial Transplant* 2003;18:vi52.
5. Hogg R, Portman RJ, Milliner D, et al. Evaluation and management of proteinuria and nephrotic syndrome in children: Recommendations from a pediatric nephrology panel established at the National Kidney Foundation Conference on Proteinuria, Albuminuria, Risk Assessment, Detection, and Elimination (PARADE). *Pediatrics* 2000;105:1242–1249.
6. Kamil ES. Minimal change disease. In: Lerma EV, Berns JS, Nissenson AR (eds.). *Current Diagnosis and Treatment Nephrology and Hypertension.* New York: McGraw-Hill Company, 2009, pp. 217–221.
7. Kyrieles HA, Lowik MM, Pronk I, et al. Long-term outcome of biopsy-proven, frequently relapsing minimal change nephrotic syndrome in children. *Clin J Am Soc Nephrol* 2009;4(10)1593–1600.
8. Mathieson PW. Immune dysregulation in minimal change nephropathy. *Nephrol Dial Transplant* 2003;18:vi26.
9. Nakayama M, Katafuchi R, Yanase T, et al. Steroid responsiveness and frequency of relapse in adult-onset minimal change nephrotic syndrome. *Am J Kidney Dis* 2002;39:503–512.
10. Tse KC, Lam MF, Yip PS, et al. Idiopathic minimal change nephrotic syndrome in older adults: Steroid responsiveness and pattern of relapses. *Nephrol Dial Transplant* 2003;18:1316.
11. Hodson E, Willis N, Craig J. Corticosteroid therapy for nephrotic syndrome in children. *Cochrane Database of Systematic Rev* (4):CD001533, 2007.
12. Palmer SC. Nand K. Strippoli GF. Interventions for minimal change disease in adults with nephrotic syndrome. *Cochrane Database of Systematic Rev* (1):CD001537, 2008.
13. Hodson EM. Willis NS. Craig JC. Interventions for idiopathic steroid-resistant nephrotic syndrome in children. [Review] [Update of *Cochrane Database Syst Rev* 2006;(2):CD003594.

CHAPTER 30

FOCAL SEGMENTAL GLOMERULOSCLEROSIS

Patrick E. Gipson, MD, and Debbie S. Gipson, MD

1. **What is focal segmental glomerulosclerosis?**
   Focal segmental glomerulosclerosis (FSGS) is a glomerular disease currently defined by its particular histopathologic presentation. As such, it represents a spectrum of idiopathic and secondary diseases affecting the kidney in a similar way. Idiopathic or primary FSGS is diagnosed, by definition, in patients without a known cause. Secondary FSGS may arise from various kidney insults that lead to a common endpoint of glomerular damage. These secondary insults include viral infection (HIV, parvovirus), drugs (heroin, pamidronate), postinflammatory conditions (autoimmune diseases), vascular issues (atheroembolic disease, hypertension, sickle cell), obesity, reflux nephropathy, and genetic mutations. The common factor in these conditions is the damage to the glomerular structure.

2. **How common is FSGS?**
   FSGS is the underlying cause of up to 2.3% of all patients with end-stage renal disease (ESRD) in the United States and up to 10.8% of those younger than age 24. In adults, it is the fourth most common cause of ESRD, following diabetes, hypertension, and glomerulonephritis not otherwise specified. Among children it is the second leading cause of ESRD, following congenital kidney anomalies. It has become the most common diagnosed primary glomerular disease reported in most published kidney biopsy series. The incidence of FSGS is estimated at 1.8/100,000 per year, with reported racial differences for lifetime risk estimated as 1:588 for whites and 1:139 for blacks.

3. **What is the clinical presentation of FSGS?**
   FSGS may present as a full-blown nephrotic syndrome with edema, hypoalbuminemia, and hypercholesterolemia, or it may present in a patient with hypertension or normotension with mild proteinuria and no systemic symptoms. Children are more likely to present with nephrotic syndrome, but the entire spectrum of FSGS occurs in both children and adults. Kidney function as assessed by glomerular filtration rate may be normal but is impaired in up to 60% at presentation. ESRD at presentation is rare. Microscopic hematuria is present in up to 50% of cases, but gross hematuria is rare.

   Clinical clues may help distinguish whether a patient has primary or secondary FSGS. Patients with primary FSGS more often have low serum albumin levels (<3 g/dL) and edema, whereas patients with secondary FSGS more often present with albumin levels >3.5 g/dL, without edema, and with some historical evidence of a predisposing primary condition or exposure.

4. **What is the cause of primary FSGS?**
   By definition, the cause of primary (idiopathic) FSGS is unknown. There are likely several different causes. Research has focused on possible immune defects, such as T-cell dysregulation and the presence of a "permeability factor," a soluble substance that induces proteinuria. Several genetic mutations associated with FSGS have been found in genes coding for structural and functional components of the glomerular podocyte, and further research in this area will likely reveal additional causes of FSGS.

5. **What are known genetic defects leading to sporadic and familial FSGS?**
    Over the past decade much of the biology of the glomerular filtration barrier has been elucidated, and defects in multiple structural and functional components of this barrier have been implicated in FSGS. These include mutations in genes NPHS2 (podocin), NPHS1 (nephrin), ACTN4 (alpha-actinin 4), TRPC6, CD2AP, PLCE1 WT1, INF2, and MYH9. Mutations in tRNAleu, COQ2, ITGB4, and LMXB1 have been noted in syndromic conditions that have FSGS as part of their presentation.

    ACTN4, TRPC6, and INF2 were first implicated in studies of affected adults from families with an autosomal-dominant transmission of FSGS. Familial FSGS of childhood onset has been associated with NPHS1, NPHS 2, and PLCE1 mutations transmitted in an autosomal recessive pattern.

    The prevalence of specific gene mutations in patients with FSGS seems to depend on the ethnic makeup of the cohort being studied. NPHS2 mutations have been seen in up to 26% of patients from families of European descent with familial FSGS, and perhaps 19% of sporadic cases in that population, but such mutations seem to be a rare cause of FSGS in Asian and African American populations. However, risk alleles in chromosome 22 have recently been identified in the nonmuscle myosin heavy chain IIA coding gene MYH9 and apolipoprotein L1 (APOL1) in cohorts of African descent with ESRD and FSGS and may be a primary cause of what has previously been considered a secondary form of FSGS caused by hypertension. The APOL1 polymorphisms appear to convey protection against Trypanosoma brucei which may account for the high frequency in populations of African descent. At present, the APOL1 polymorphisms appear to be most strongly linked to FSGS among patients of African descent, but the mechanisms of injury are not yet determined.

    Genotype/phenotype correlations for most of these genetic mutations are still being investigated and have not yet reached the point where they are routinely helpful for guiding clinical care. This may change if more robust correlations are able to inform prognosis, risk of relapse in allografts, or response to specific therapy.

    Genovese G, Tonna SJ, Knob AU, Appel GB, et al. A risk allele for focal segmental glomerulosclerosis in African Americans is located within a region containing APOL1 and MYH9. *Kidney Int* 2010;78:698–704.

6. **How is FSGS diagnosed?**
    The cause of proteinuria and nephrotic syndrome may be identified with the aid of specific history, physical, and laboratory and radiographic studies. However, only a kidney biopsy will confirm the diagnosis of FSGS.

    Prior to biopsy, children and adolescents with asymptomatic proteinuria should be evaluated for orthostatic proteinuria. This benign condition is diagnosed with a normal first morning urine protein/creatinine ratio.

    Patients presenting with sustained proteinuria, whether nephrotic (>3 g/day) or subnephrotic, will typically be evaluated for secondary forms of glomerular disease, including screens for systemic illnesses that may have a kidney component. Hepatitis B and C and HIV should be excluded by serology. Antinuclear antibody level should be obtained to screen for lupus. Complement C3 levels may be low in membranoproliferative glomerulonephritis (MPGN), lupus, and postinfectious glomerulonephritis. In appropriate-age adults, urine and protein electrophoresis and/or serum free light-chain measurements should be obtained to evaluate for paraproteinemias. Kidney ultrasound is useful to exclude obstructive disease and as a prescreen for potential biopsy.

    Because of the focal nature of FSGS, an initial biopsy may reveal only changes on electron microscopy consistent with minimal change disease (MCD), with the diagnosis of FSGS being confirmed only from a subsequent biopsy undertaken after persistent failure to respond to therapy.

7. **What are the pathologic findings in FSGS?**
    As noted by its descriptive name, FSGS at least initially involves sclerotic lesions in only a segmental part of some glomeruli. Electron microscopy may confirm these changes and show more global foot process effacement. Some small studies have suggested that the

extent of foot process effacement, other measurements such as foot process width, and overall glomerular size may assist in distinguishing primary from secondary forms of FSGS.

As the disease progresses, involvement of more glomeruli and sclerosis of entire glomeruli may occur. Tubular atrophy is a frequent finding that likely results from the primary glomerular lesion. Generally no significant immunoglobulin deposits are noted with primary FSGS, and their presence suggests an alternative etiology.

8. **Does histopathology predict prognosis?**
   There are five variants of primary FSGS based solely on histologic description: collapsing, tip, cellular, perihilar, and FSGS not otherwise specified. These variants may carry prognostic significance. Collapsing FSGS appears to represent a particularly virulent form of FSGS, tending to present with profound proteinuria and to progress more rapidly to ESRD. The tip variant may have a better response to steroid therapy and a better prognosis if it responds to therapy. Increased tubular atrophy and interstitial scarring also portend worse prognosis.

9. **What is the clinical course of FSGS?**
   Primary FSGS has a variable course whose prognosis can be somewhat predicted based on the degree of proteinuria at presentation, the amount of tubulointerstitial fibrosis noted on kidney biopsy, proteinuria reduction in response to therapy, and histologic variant. Spontaneous remission is rare. Therapy may result in complete remission (normal urinary protein excretion), partial remission (with at least 50% reduction in protein excretion relative to presentation), or resistance to therapy. Patients with complete remission have an expected 90% 10-year kidney survival. Those with a partial remission have up to an 80% 10-year kidney survival. For patients with proteinuria in the nephrotic range that is resistant to treatment, the probability of progressing to ESRD within 10 years is approximately 50%. As in many kidney diseases, patients who present with an elevated serum creatinine have a poorer prognosis for kidney survival.

10. **What therapies are indicated for primary FSGS?**
    Therapy targeted at a presumed immunologic basis of FSGS has been used clinically and in controlled and uncontrolled trials. Corticosteroids induce remission in 20% to 30% of patients. Treatment may begin with daily dosing and then progress to alternate-day therapy for primary FSGS. The duration of treatment may affect response to therapy with a typical course of 3 to 6 months.

    Cyclosporine, tacrolimus, and mycophenolate mofetil have been reported to be effective in case reports. Cyclosporine and tacrolimus been evaluated in a small number of randomized trials, with a combined complete and partial remission rate of 70%.

    Several case reports indicate the successful use of rituximab and plasmapheresis therapy in resistant FSGS, but as yet there are no randomized controlled studies and no reports of long-term outcomes of these therapies.

    Angiotensin-converting enzyme (ACE) inhibitor/angiotensin receptor blocker (ARB) therapy has been shown to be beneficial in reducing proteinuria and slowing the decline in kidney function in several proteinuric kidney diseases. There is only one randomized control trial of ACE therapy in adults with FSGS and one in children with steroid-resistant nephrotic syndrome. These studies document a reduction in urinary protein excretion by approximately 30%. Long-term data to assess a benefit in preventing a decline in kidney function are not available. Regardless, ACE inhibitor/ARB therapy is considered standard care for proteinuria control and hypertension management.

    Therapy for dyslipidemia is also a component of standard therapy in patients with nephrotic syndrome with a goal to improve nephrotic syndrome–associated dyslipidemia and to potentially mitigate the cardiovascular morbidity risk in those with progressive kidney dysfunction.

Diuretics are indicated for control of edema in patients with nephrotic syndrome. Intravenous albumin infusion with diuretic therapy may be beneficial to control severe edema in select patients with nephrotic syndrome, but it has not been shown to have significant additive benefit in controlled trials and carries with it the risk of pulmonary edema and hypertensive crisis.

11. **What are the therapeutic options for secondary forms of FSGS?**
Treatment of the secondary forms of FSGS is directed at the primary disease. In addition, therapies directed toward reducing proteinuria, controlling blood pressure, and minimizing further cardiovascular or kidney insults should be implemented.

12. **Should those with FSGS be on a special diet?**
The contribution of low-protein diets in slowing the progression of proteinuric kidney diseases has been suggested in adults, but care needs to be taken, especially in those with profound proteinuria, to balance concerns about protein malnutrition with concerns regarding disease progression. Protein-restricted diets are not recommended for children or adolescents. For patients with hypertension, and those profoundly nephrotic, low-salt diets should be emphasized.

13. **What is the role of the primary care physician in a patient with FSGS?**
Monitoring for adequacy of blood pressure therapy and lipid therapy, for signs of progressive edema and for side effects of specific immunosuppressive therapy, requires coordination between the primary care physician and nephrologist. Maintenance of appropriate immunizations is important, especially pneumococcal and influenza immunizations for patients with nephrotic syndrome of those who are immunosuppressed.

14. **What are indications for referral to a nephrologist?**
A patient with orthostatic proteinuria can be followed by the primary care physician. However, if abnormal proteinuria is demonstrated on overnight or first morning urine samples, creatinine is elevated, or edema or hypoalbuminemia is noted, referral is indicated.

15. **Are there special issues in patients with FSGS with respect to transplantation?**
Recurrence of primary FSGS in the kidney allograft occurs at a high rate. It may occur immediately after transplant, or it may take months or years to recur. Patients who initially present with profound proteinuria and/or rapid development of ESRD from FSGS are at higher risk for recurrence of FSGS when transplanted, with a recurrence rate of up to 70% in this group.

The presence of native kidneys with sufficient function to produce urine can complicate the evaluation of recurrence. A typical early marker for FSGS recurrence in the kidney allograft is proteinuria. Distinguishing proteinuria originating from the native kidneys from the allograft is difficult to impossible without a transplant allograft biopsy. This, and increased risk of graft thrombosis and infection in patients who are clinically nephrotic, may be an indication for some patients with FSGS to undergo medical or surgical nephrectomy prior to transplantation.

Patients with FSGS may receive an allograft from either deceased donors or living related donors. Early concern regarding the potential for an increased risk of recurrence when using living related donors seems to have been laid to rest.

Plasmapheresis has been used in the immediate pre- and post-transplant period in an attempt to remove the substances responsible for inducing proteinuria and recurrent FSGS. This approach has not been evaluated in randomized studies but may be of benefit in prevention or treatment of early FSGS recurrence.

KEY POINTS: FOCAL SEGMENTAL GLOMERULOSCLEROSIS

1. Focal segmental glomerulosclerosis (FSGS) represents a spectrum of idiopathic and secondary diseases affecting the glomerulus and the kidney in a similar way.

2. In adults, FSGS is the fourth most common cause of end-stage renal disease.

3. FSGS may present as either subnephrotic- or nephrotic-range proteinuria, with or without hypertension.

4. Mutations in multiple genes that direct the structure and function of the glomerular basement membrane have been implicated in familial and sporadic FSGS.

5. Angiotensin-converting enzyme inhibitor/angiotensin receptor blocker therapy and treatment of hyperlipidemia associated with FSGS are presumed to be beneficial therapies for most patients with FSGS based on studies of proteinuric kidney diseases, although there are little data from randomized trials specifically addressing these therapies in FSGS.

6. Primary FSGS has a high incidence of recurrence in allografts, and recurrence may lead to loss of the allograft.

BIBLIOGRAPHY

1. Cattran D, Appel G, Hebert L, Hunsicker L, et al. A randomized trial of cyclosporine in patients with steroid-resistant focal segmental glomerulosclerosis. *Kidney Int* 1999;56:2220–2226.
2. Choudhry S, Bagga A, Hari P, et al. Efficacy and safety of tacrolimus versus cyclosporine in children with steroid-resistant nephrotic syndrome: A randomized controlled trial. *Am J Kidney Dis* 2009;53(5):760–769.
3. Chun MJ, Korbet SM, Schwartz MM, et al. Focal segmental glomerulosclerosis in nephrotic adults: presentation, prognosis, and response to therapy of the histologic variants. *J Am Soc Nephrol* 2004;15:2169–2177.
4. D'Agati VD, Fogo AB, Bruijn JA, et al. Pathologic classification of focal segmental glomerulosclerosis: A working proposal. *Am J Kidney Dis* 2004;43(2):368–382.
5. Hickson LJ, Gera M, Amer H, et al. Kidney transplantation for primary focal segmental glomerulosclerosis: Outcomes and response to therapy for recurrence. *Transplantation* 2009;87:1232–1239.
6. Kitiyakara C, Eggers P, Kopp JB. Twenty-one–year trend in ESRD due to focal segmental glomerulosclerosis in the United States. *Am J Kidney Dis* 2004;44(5):815–825.
7. Nayagam LS, Ganguli A, Rathi M, et al. Mycophenolate mofetil or standard therapy for membranous nephropathy and focal segmental glomerulosclerosis: A pilot study. *Nephrol Dial Transplant* 2008;23:1926–1930.
8. Ponticelli C, Rizzon G, Edefonti A, et al. A randomized trial of cyclosporine in steroid-resistant idiopathic nephrotic syndrome. *Kidney Int* 1993;43:1377–1384.
9. Swaminathan S, Leung N, Lager DJ, et al. Changing incidence of glomerular disease in Olmsted County, Minnesota: A 30-year renal biopsy study. *Clin J Am Soc Nephrol* 2006;1:483–487.
10. Thomas DB, Franceschini N, Hogan SL, et al. Clinical and pathologic characteristics of focal segmental glomerulosclerosis pathologic variants. *Kidney Int* 2006;69:920–926.
11. Troyanov S, Wall CA, Miller JA, et al. Focal and segmental glomerulosclerosis: Definition and relevance of a partial remission. *J Am Soc Nephrol* 2005;16:1061–1068.
12. USRDS Annual Data Report, 2009.
13. Usta M, Ersoy A, Dilek K, et al. Efficacy of losartan in patients with primary focal segmental glomerulosclerosis resistant to immunosuppressive treatment. *J Intern Med* 2003;253:329–334.
14. Yi Z, Li Z, Wu X-C, et al. Effect of fosinopril in children with steroid-resistant idiopathic nephrotic syndrome. *Pediatr Nephrol* 2006;21:967–972.

CHAPTER 31

MEMBRANOUS NEPHROPATHY

Alfonso Eirin, MD; Maria Valentina Irazabal Mira, MD; and Fernando C. Fervenza, MD, PhD

1. **What is membranous nephropathy?**

   Membranous nephropathy (MN) is a common immune-mediated glomerular disease that remains the leading cause of nephrotic syndrome in white adults. It is a histologic diagnosis based on the presence of immunoglobulins (Ig), usually IgG and C3, deposition along the capillary walls on immunofluorescence microscopy and subepithelial deposits along the glomerular basement membrane on electron microscopy.

   Medawar W, Green A, Campbell E, et al. Clinical and histopathologic findings in adults with the nephrotic syndrome. *Ir J Med Sci* 1990;159(5):137–140.

2. **What antigens are involved in the immune complex deposits?**

   The nature of these antigens and their source are starting to be clarified. Debiec et al. reported a case of a pregnant woman who gave birth at gestational week 38 to a male infant in which a severe form of MN developed prenatally. Further evaluation revealed that antineutral endopeptidase (NEP) antibodies, produced by the mother who was NEP deficient, were transplacentally transferred to her fetus and were the cause of the MN. In addition, David Salant's group has shown that sera from approximately 70% of patients with MN specifically detect a 200-kDa human glomerular antigen identified as the M-type phospholipase A2 receptor (PLA2R). Antibodies against aldolase reductase and superoxide dismutase have also been described in MN. Although these findings do not explain the cause on all cases of MN, they suggest that antibodies against podocyte proteins are responsible for causing MN.

   Beck LH Jr, Bonegio RG, Lambeau G, Beck DM, Powell DW, Cummins TD, Klein JB, Salant DJ. M-type phospholipase A2 receptor as target antigen in idiopathic membranous nephropathy. *N Engl J Med* 2009 Jul 2;361(1):11–21.

   Debiec H, Guigonis V, Mougenot B, et al. Antenatal membranous glomerulonephritis due to anti-neutral endopeptidase antibodies. *N Engl J Med* 2002;346(26):2053–2060.

   Prunotto M, Carnevali ML, Candiano G, et al. Autoimmunity in membranous nephropathy targets aldose reductase and SOD2. *J Am Soc Nephrol* 2010;21(3):507–519.

3. **What are the clinical manifestations?**

   At presentation, 60% to 70% of patients will have the nephrotic syndrome, with the remaining 30% to 40% of patients presenting with proteinuria <3.5g/24 hours found at the time of a routine examination in an otherwise asymptomatic patient. Although more than 90% of patients have no evidence of impaired renal function at the time of presentation, hypertension at onset is found in 10% to 20% of patients. The presence of microscopic hematuria is common (30%–40%), but macroscopic hematuria and red cells casts are rare and suggest a different diagnosis. Findings at physical examination may vary from mild peripheral edema to full-blown nephrotic syndrome, including ascites and pericardial and pleural effusions.

   Cattran DC. Idiopathic membranous glomerulonephritis. *Kidney Int* 2001;59(5):1983–1994.

   Couser WG, Shankland SJ. Membranous nephropathy. In: Johnson RJ, Feehally J (eds.). *Comprehensive Clinical Nephrology*, 2nd ed. Philadelphia: Elsevier, 2003, pp. 295–307.

   Fervenza FC, Sethi S, Specks U. Idiopathic membranous nephropathy: diagnosis and treatment. *Clin J Am Soc Nephrol* 2008; 3(3)905–919.

4. **What are some of the differential diagnoses?**
   Membranous nephropathy occurs as an idiopathic (primary) or secondary disease. Secondary membranous nephropathy is caused by autoimmune diseases (e.g., systemic lupus erythematosus, autoimmune thyroiditis), infection (e.g., hepatitis B and C), drugs (e.g., penicillamine, gold, nonsteroidal anti-inflammatory drugs), and malignancies (e.g., colon cancer, lung cancer). In patients older than age 60, MN is associated with malignancy in 7% to 15% of patients.

5. **What are the renal biopsy findings?**
   The diagnosis of membranous nephropathy is based on the following findings: (1) thickened glomerular basement membrane (GBM), often showing pinholes and spikes on silver and periodic acid-Schiff stains, and occasionally subepithelial fuchsinophilic deposits on trichrome stains; (2) immunofluorescence microscopy showing granular immunoglobulin (Ig), usually IgG and C3, along the capillary walls; and (3) subepithelial deposits on electron microscopy (EM). In early stages of the disease, light microscopy may be completely normal.

6. **How is the disease classified?**
   Based on the location of the deposits on electron microscopy, membranous nephropathy has been divided into four stages: stage I, sparse small deposits without thickening of the GBM; stage II, more extensive subepithelial deposits with formation of basement membrane spikes between the deposits and thickening of the GBM; stage III, combination of stage II along with deposits completely surrounded by basement membrane (intramembranous deposits); and stage IV, incorporation of deposits in the GBM and irregular thickening of the GBM. These stages, however, have no correlation with clinical outcome.

7. **Is pathology helpful in identifying secondary causes of MN?**
   From the pathology standpoint, it is important to determine whether the MN may result from a secondary cause such as an autoimmune disease, neoplasia, infection, or drugs. Although it is often difficult to determine whether the MN is idiopathic or secondary, certain features are helpful in identifying a secondary cause. Features in favor of a secondary cause, in particular an autoimmune disease, include the following:
   - Proliferative features (mesangial or endocapillary)
   - Full-house pattern of Ig staining including staining for C1q on immunofluorescence microscopy
   - Glomerular deposits predominantly containing immunoglobulins other than IgG4
   - Electron-dense deposits in the subendothelial location of the capillary wall and mesangium or along the tubular basement membrane and vessel walls
   - Endothelial tubuloreticular inclusions on EM (EM showing only few superficial scattered subepithelial deposits may suggest a drug-associated secondary MN)

   Markowitz GS. Membranous glomerulopathy: Emphasis on secondary forms and disease variants. *Adv Anat Pathol* 2001;8:119–125.

8. **What is the clinical course of membranous nephropathy?**
   Membranous nephropathy is a chronic disease, with spontaneous remission and relapses clearly documented. The clinical course is characterized by great variability in the rate of disease progression, and the natural course is difficult to assess in part because of the selection criteria, geographic variability, and genetic characteristics of the subjects presented in the different studies. Although in most patients the disease progresses relatively slowly, approximately 40% of patients eventually develop end-stage renal disease (ESRD). Because of its frequency MN remains the second or third cause of a primary glomerulopathy leading to ESRD.

   Ruggenenti P, Chiurchiu C, Brusegan V, et al. Rituximab in idiopathic membranous nephropathy: A one-year prospective study. *J Am Soc Nephrol* 2003;14(7):1851–1857.

   Cattran DC. Membranous nephropathy: Quo vadis? *Kidney Int* 2002;61(1):349–350.

9. **Are there any factors associated with poor outcome?**
   A number of factors have been associated with worse outcome in patients with MN including advanced age, male sex, severity of initial proteinuria, and renal insufficiency. In addition,

histologic changes, such as tubular interstitial damage, and glomerulosclerosis have been implicated in poor prognosis. Unfortunately, these factors are all qualitative and not sufficient to predict outcome in all patients.

10. **What should be considered in a patient with MN and rapid loss of kidney function?**

In a few cases, when progressive loss of renal function occurs faster than usual, a superimposed condition, such as acute renal injury, acute interstitial nephritis, renal vein thrombosis, or urinary tract obstruction, may be the cause. In addition, rapidly progressive glomerulonephritis (RPGN) should be considered. The mechanisms involved in RPGN include immune complex-mediated systemic lupus erythematosus (SLE), postinfectious glomerulonephritis, IgA nephropathy, focal segmental glomerulosclerosis (FSGS), systemic vasculitis, pauci-immune crescentic glomerulonephritis, vasculitis mediated by antiglomerular basement membrane (anti-GBM) antibodies, and crescentic glomerulonephritis.

Austin HA, Illei GG. Membranous lupus nephritis. *Lupus* 2005;14:65–71.

Doi T, Kanatsu K, Nagai H, et al. An overlapping syndrome of IgA nephropathy and membranous nephropathy? *Nephron* 1983;35:24–30.

Hall AM, Symington EM, Sampson AS, et al. Crescentic transformation of membranous glomerulopathy: A reversible condition. *Nephrol Dial Transplant* 2006;21:1136–1137.

Hull RP, Goldsmith JA. Nephrotic syndrome in adults. *BMJ* 2008;336:1185–1189.

James SH, Lien YH, Ruffenach SJ, et al. Acute renal failure in membranous glomerulonephropathy: A result of superimposed crescentic glomerulonephritis. *J Am Soc Nephrol* 1995;6:1541–1546.

John R, Herzenberg AM. Renal toxicity of therapeutic drugs. *J Clin Pathol* 2009;62:505–515.

Kanjanabuch T, Kittikowit W, Eiam-Ong S. An update on postinfectious glomerulonephritis worldwide. *Nat Rev Nephrol* 2009;5:259–269.

Klassen J, Elwood C, Grossberg AL, et al. Evolution of membranous nephropathy into anti-glomerular-basement-membrane glomerulonephritis. *N Engl J Med* 1974;290:1340–1344.

Koomans HA. Pathophysiology of acute renal failure in idiopathic nephrotic syndrome. *Nephrol Dial Transplant* 2001;16:221–224.

Kutcher R, Cohen JR, Gordon DH. Glomerulonephritis and nephrotic syndrome complicated by renal vein thrombosis and pulmonary emboli: Report of two cases. *Am J Roentgenol* 1977;128:447–449.

Tse WY, Howie AJ, Adu D, et al. Association of vasculitic glomerulonephritis with membranous nephropathy: A report of 10 cases. *Nephrol Dial Transplant* 1997;12:1017–1027.

11. **Is it possible to accurately predict those patients who will progress to ESRD?**

Finding useful markers that predict this group has been difficult. Thus far, the best model for the identification of patients at risk was developed with data derived from the Toronto Glomerulonephritis Registry. This model takes into consideration the initial creatinine clearance (CrCl), the slope of the CrCl, and the lowest level of proteinuria during a 6-month observation period. Recent studies suggest that urinary excretion of $\alpha1$ microglobulin, β microglobulin, and IgG could predict outcome in MN. However, these parameters have yet to be validated, and these tests are not available to the nephrology community in general.

Branten AJ, du Buf-Vereijken PW, Klasen IS, et al. Urinary excretion of beta2-microglobulin and IgG predict prognosis in idiopathic membranous nephropathy: a validation study. *J Am Soc Nephrol* 2005;16(1):169–174.

Cattran DC, Pei Y, Greenwood CM, et al. Validation of a predictive model of idiopathic membranous nephropathy: Its clinical and research implications. *Kidney Int* 1997;51(3):901–907.

Pei Y, Cattran D, Greenwood C. Predicting chronic renal insufficiency in idiopathic membranous glomerulonephritis. *Kidney Int* 1992;42(4):960–966.

12. **How does the Toronto model work?**

Based on this model, patients who present with a normal CrCl, proteinuria ≤4 g/24 hours, and stable renal function over a 6-month observation period have an excellent long-term prognosis and are classified as at low risk for progression. Patients with normal renal function and whose CrCl remains unchanged during 6 months of observation but continue to have proteinuria >4 g but <8 g/24 hours have a 55% probability of developing chronic renal insufficiency and are classified as medium risk for progression. Patients with persistent proteinuria >8 g/24 hours, independent of the degree of renal dysfunction, have a 66% to 88% probability of progression to chronic renal failure within 10 years and are classified in the high risk for progression category.

13. **Why do so many patients still progress to ESRD?**
Growing evidence implicates proteinuria as major player in the development of progressive tubular injury, interstitial fibrosis, and glomerular filtration rate loss. It is well recognized that the higher the sustained levels of proteinuria, the faster the decline in renal function. That relation is not only true for patients with MN, but also for other proteinuric renal diseases including FSGS and diabetic nephropathy.

Chun MJ, Korbet SM, Schwartz MM, et al. Focal segmental glomerulosclerosis in nephrotic adults: Presentation, prognosis, and response to therapy of the histologic variants. *J Am Soc Nephrol* 2004;15(8):2169–2177.

Hovind P, Tarnow L, Rossing P, et al. Improved survival in patients obtaining remission of nephrotic range albuminuria in diabetic nephropathy. *Kidney Int* 2004;66(3):1180–1186.

Zandi-Nejad K, Eddy AA, Glassock RJ, et al. Why is proteinuria an ominous biomarker of progressive kidney disease? *Kidney Int Suppl* 2004;92:S76–89.

14. **What are the complications of MN?**
In addition to progression to ESRD, patients with membranous nephropathy who remain nephrotic are at an increased risk for thromboembolic events, with an incidence as high as 50% in patients with severe proteinuria. There is also an increased risk for cardiovascular events in these patients.

Ordoñez JD, Hiatt RA, Killebrew EJ, et al. The increased risk of coronary heart disease associated with nephrotic syndrome. *Kidney Int* 1993;44(3):638–642.

Wagoner RD, Stanson AW, Holley KE, et al. Renal vein thrombosis in idiopathic membranous glomerulopathy and nephrotic syndrome: incidence and significance. *Kidney Int* 1983;23(2):368–374.

Wheeler DC, Bernard DB. Lipid abnormalities in the nephrotic syndrome: causes, consequences, and treatment. *Am J Kidney Dis* 1994;23(3):331–346.

15. **What is the conservative therapy of membranous nephropathy?**
Conservative therapy consists of restricting dietary protein intake (0.8 g/kg ideal body weight per day of high-quality protein) and controlling blood pressure (target blood pressure is ≤125/75 mm Hg), hyperlipidemia, and edema.

16. **What are the preferred agents to control blood pressure in these patients?**
Angiotensin-converting enzyme (ACE) inhibitors and angiotensin receptor blockers (ARBs) are effective antihypertensive agents that can reduce proteinuria and slow renal progression of renal disease in patients with nephropathy with and without diabetes, and for these reasons they are the preferred agents to treat hypertension in membranous nephropathy. However, the antiproteinuric effect of ACE inhibitors or ARBs is modest (<30% decrease) and is more significant in patients with lower levels of proteinuria. More recently, the addition of aliskiren (renin inhibitor) to optimal antihypertensive therapy was shown to reduce the mean urinary albumin-to-creatinine ratio by 20% in the randomized, placebo-controlled aliskiren in the Evaluation of Proteinuria in Diabetes (AVOID) trial. However, until longer term studies are carried out, it will remain unknown whether aliskiren in combination with optimal antihypertensive therapy will result in a well-tolerated, durable therapy.

Ambalavanan S, Fauvel JP, Sibley RK, et al. Mechanism of the antiproteinuric effect of cyclosporine in membranous nephropathy. *J Am Soc Nephrol* 1996;7(2):290–298.

Gansevoort RT, Heeg JE, Vriesendorp R, et al. Antiproteinuric drugs in patients with idiopathic membranous glomerulopathy. *Nephrol Dial Transplant* 1992;7(Suppl 1):91–96.

Parving HH, Persson F, Lewis JB, et al. Aliskiren combined with losartan in type 2 diabetes and nephropathy. *N Engl J Med* 2008;358(23):2433–2346.

Ruggenenti P, Mosconi L, Vendramin G, et al. ACE inhibition improves glomerular size selectivity in patients with idiopathic membranous nephropathy and persistent nephrotic syndrome. *Am J Kidney Dis* 2000;35(3):381–391.

17. **How effective are lipid-lowering drugs in patients with MN?**

Lipid abnormalities associated with proteinuria are likely important players in the high cardiovascular risk in patients with proteinuria and thus provide an important target for treatment. A number of studies have demonstrated the efficacy of statins improving the lipid profile and in reducing cardiovascular morbidity and mortality in patients with hyperlipidemia and hypertension and in patients with chronic kidney disease. Statins have a synergistic antiproteinuric effect when combined with ACE inhibitors, but this effect is small and mainly observed in patients with proteinuria <3 g/24 hours.

Bianchi S, Bigazzi R, Caiazza A, et al. A controlled, prospective study of the effects of atorvastatin on proteinuria and progression of kidney disease. *Am J Kidney Dis* 2003;41(3):565–570.

Fried LF, Orchard TJ, Kasiske BL. Effect of lipid reduction on the progression of renal disease: A meta-analysis. *Kidney Int* 2001;59(1):260–269.

18. **Is anticoagulation recommended for patients with MN?**

Patients with severe nephrotic syndrome are at increased risk for thromboembolic complications, and prophylactic anticoagulation has been shown to be beneficial in reducing fatal thromboembolic episodes in patients who are nephrotic with MN without a concomitant increase in the risk of bleeding in retrospective reviews. Although no consensus has emerged regarding whether prophylactic anticoagulation should be used, the majority of physicians would consider to anticoagulate patients with MN who are severely nephrotic (proteinuria >10 g/day and serum albumin <2.5 g/day). Both heparin and low molecular weight heparin reduce proteinuria, but this effect has not been routinely used in the care of patients with MN.

Sarasin FP, Schifferli JA. Prophylactic oral anticoagulation in nephrotic patients with idiopathic membranous nephropathy. *Kidney Int* 1994;45:578–585.

19. **What is the role of immunosuppressive agents in the treatment of MN?**

The use of immunosuppression in the setting of idiopathic MN is controversial, especially because of the variable natural history of the disease and of drug toxicity. Immunosuppression is generally reserved for those patients with deteriorating renal function or heavy proteinuria that persists positive despite conservative therapy. Various agents have been used including corticosteroids; cytotoxic agents such as cyclophosphamide, chlorambucil, and azathioprine; or calcineurin inhibitors (e.g., cyclosporine, tacrolimus). In addition, mycophenolate mofetil alone does not work; however, a combination of mycophenolate mofetil with high-dose steroids is effective, but relapses are frequent.

Ballarin J, Poveda R, Ara J, et al. Treatment of idiopathic membranous nephropathy with the combination of steroids, tacrolimus and mycophenolate mofetil: results of a pilot study. *Nephrol Dial Transplant* 2007;22(11):3196–3201.

Praga M, Barrio V, Juárez GF, Luño J, et al. Tacrolimus monotherapy in membranous nephropathy: a randomized controlled trial. *Kidney Int* 2007;71(9):924–930.

Cattran DC, Appel GB, Hebert LA, Hunsicker LG, et al. Cyclosporine in patients with steroid-resistant membranous nephropathy: a randomized trial. *Kidney Int* 2001;59:1484–1490.

Ponticelli C, Zucchelli P, Passerini P, et al. A 10-year follow-up of a randomized study with methylprednisolone and chlorambucil in membranous nephropathy. *Kidney Int* 1995;481600–1604.

Ponticelli C, Altieri P, Scolari F, et al. A randomized study comparing methylprednisolone plus chlorambucil versus methylprednisolone plus cyclophosphamide in idiopathic membranous nephropathy. *JASN* 1998;9:444–450.

20. **Is there any role for mycophenolate mofetil (MMF) in the treatment of MN?**

The efficacy and safety of MMF for patients with MN have been evaluated by Branten et al., who reported no significant differences in remission of proteinuria at 12 months in patients with MN and renal insufficiency when compared with combined use of high-dose corticosteroids and MMF treatment (1 g twice daily) to high-dose corticosteroids and cyclophosphamide (1.5 mg/kg/day). However, relapses were much more common in the MMF-treated group. Most recently, Senthil Nayagam et al. demonstrated that a 6-month course of combined glucocorticoids with MMF is as effective as the conventional treatment for primary treatment of MN in the short term. However, Dussol et al. randomly assigned

36 patients with MN and nephrotic syndrome to receive conservative therapy in combination with MMF (2 g/day) ($n = 19$) or conservative therapy alone ($n = 17$) for 12 months and found that the probability of complete or partial remission did not differ between the two groups. In the opinion of the authors, MMF monotherapy is ineffective in MN.

Branten AJ, du Buf-Vereijken PW, Vervloet M, et al. Mycophenolate mofetil in idiopathic membranous nephropathy: A clinical trial with comparison to a historic control group treated with cyclophosphamide. *Am J Kidney Dis* 2007;50(2):248–256.

Dussol B, Morange S, Burtey S, et al. Mycophenolate mofetil monotherapy in membranous nephropathy: A 1-year randomized controlled trial. *Am J Kidney Dis* 2008;52(4):699–705.

Senthil Nayagam L, Ganguli A, Rathi M, et al. Mycophenolate mofetil or standard therapy for membranous nephropathy and focal segmental glomerulosclerosis: A pilot study. *Nephrol Dial Transplant* 2008;23(6):1926–1930.

Branten AJ, du Buf-Vereijken PW, Vervloet M, et al. Mycophenolate mofetil in idiopathic membranous nephropathy: A clinical trial with comparison to a historic control group treated with cyclophosphamide. *Am J Kidney Dis* 2007;50(2):248–256.

Choi MJ, Eustace JA, Gimenez LF, et al. Mycophenolate mofetil treatment for primary glomerular diseases. *Kidney Int* 2002;61(3):1098–1114.

21. **What are the follow-up strategies regarding cancer in patients with MN?**
Patients with MN have an increased incidence of malignancies, which persists on an annual basis for a period of 15 years after the kidney disease is diagnosed. Therefore, patients with MN should be regularly screened for the development of cancer for many years after the diagnosis of MN. Lefaucheur et al. suggested that age, smoking, and the presence of glomerular leukocytic infiltrates strongly increase the likelihood of malignancy in these patients. Also, they reported a strong relationship between reduction of proteinuria and clinical remission of cancer in patients with cancer-associated MN.

Bjørneklett R, Vikse BE, Svarstad E, et al. Long-term risk of cancer in membranous nephropathy patients. *Am J Kidney Dis* 2007;50(3):396–403.

Lefaucheur C, Stengel B, Nochy D, et al. Membranous nephropathy and cancer: Epidemiologic evidence and determinants of high-risk cancer association. *Kidney Int* 2006;70(8):1510–1517.

22. **What percentage of patients relapse after complete remission or partial remission?**
About 40% of MN cases will relapse subsequent to a complete remission. The great majority of those who relapse, however, will relapse only to subnephrotic-range proteinuria and will have stable function long term. These patients can be retreated with immunosuppressive therapy.

23. **Are any new therapies available?**
Rituximab is a monoclonal antibody that binds the CD20 antigen on B cells, thereby deleting them. Preliminary data suggest that treatment with rituximab is effective in remission of proteinuria in ~60% of these patients. However, recent reports regarding the development of unusual infections, such as progressive multifocal leukoencephalopathy following rituximab, raise the need for caution prior to its widespread use, especially because no randomized control trial have been performed in MN. Synthetic adrenocorticotropic hormone (ACTH) administered for 1 year also has been shown to decrease proteinuria in patients with membranous nephropathy. Adverse effects associated with the use of ACTH included dizziness, glucose intolerance, diarrhea, and the development of bronze-colored skin, which resolved after the end of the therapy. However, synthetic ACTH is not available in the United States.

Berg AL, Arnadottir M. ACTH-induced improvement in the nephrotic syndrome in patients with a variety of diagnoses. *Nephrol Dial Transplant* 2004;19(5):1305–1307.

Berg AL, Nilsson-Ehle P, Arnadottir M. Beneficial effects of ACTH on the serum lipoprotein profile and glomerular function in patients with membranous nephropathy. *Kidney Int* 1999;56(4):1534–1543.

Fervenza FC, Cosio FG, Erickson SB, et al. Rituximab treatment of idiopathic membranous nephropathy. *Kidney Int* 2008;73(1):117–125.

Fervenza FC, Abraham RS, Erickson SB, et al. Rituximab therapy in idiopathic membranous nephropathy: a 2-year study. *Clin J Am Soc Nephrol* 2010;5(12):2188–2198.

Ponticelli C, Passerini P, Salvadori M, et al. A randomized pilot trial comparing methylprednisolone plus a cytotoxic agent versus synthetic adrenocorticotropic hormone in idiopathic membranous nephropathy. *Am J Kidney Dis* 2006;47(2):233–240.

Ruggenenti P, Chiurchiu C, Brusegan V, et al. Rituximab in idiopathic membranous nephropathy: A one-year prospective study. *J Am Soc Nephrol* 2003;14(7):1851–1857.

24. **Does MN recur after kidney transplantation?**

MN can recur after kidney transplantation, causing proteinuria, allograft dysfunction, and graft failure. Recently, we assessed the incidence of MN recurrence utilizing surveillance graft biopsies in patients with MN. The initial clinical manifestations of recurrent MN were mild or absent, whereas light microscopic changes were subtle or absent at the time of diagnosis. All patients had granular GBM deposits of IgG but little or absent C3 by immunofluorescence. Subepithelial deposits were observed in all cases by electron microscopy. In conclusion, 42% of patients who had undergone kidney transplant show a recurrence in the allograft, and the recurrence most often occurs during the first year following transplantation. In addition, the initial clinical and histologic manifestations in those patients are subtle but the disease is progressive.

Dabade TS, Grande JP, Norby SM, et al. Recurrent idiopathic membranous nephropathy after kidney transplantation: A surveillance biopsy study. *Am J Transplant* 2008;8(6):1318–1322.

KEY POINTS: MEMBRANOUS NEPHROPATHY

1. Membranous nephropathy (MN) remains the leading cause of nephrotic syndrome in white adults. Patients who remain nephrotic are likely to progress to ESRD and are also at an increased risk for thromboembolic and cardiovascular events.

2. Recent findings about antibodies against podocyte proteins such as M-type phospholipase A2 receptor (PLA2R) suggest that these antibodies may be responsible for causing some cases of MN.

3. Membranous nephropathy occurs as an idiopathic (75% of cases) or secondary disease (autoimmune diseases, infection, and malignancies), where up to 70% of patients will have nephrotic syndrome at the time of presentation. It is a chronic disease, with spontaneous remission and relapses clearly documented.

4. The best model for the identification of patients at risk for progressing to end-stage renal disease was developed by the Toronto Glomerulonephritis Registry. This model considers the initial creatinine clearance (CrCl), the slope of the CrCl, and the lowest level of proteinuria during a 6-month observation period.

5. Conservative therapy consists of restricting dietary protein intake and controlling blood pressure, hyperlipidemia, and edema. Angiotensin-converting enzyme inhibitors and angiotensin receptor blockers are effective antihypertensive medication. However, their antiproteinuric effect is poor (average proteinuria reduction is ~30%), and they work best in patients with lower degrees of proteinuria.

6. The use of immunosuppression in the setting of idiopathic MN should be reserved for those patients with deteriorating renal function and/or heavy proteinuria that persist despite conservative therapy.

7. Current data suggest that new therapeutic agents such as rituximab and synthetic adrenocorticotropic hormone are effective in reducing proteinuria while having few adverse effects.

8. Membranous nephropathy can recur after kidney transplantation in approximately 42% of patients, causing proteinuria, allograft dysfunction, and graft failure. Recurrence most often occurs during the first year.

9. The relationship between anti-PLA$_2$R antibody levels in patients with MN and clinical response to different treatment modalities needs to be evaluated further.

CHAPTER 32

IgA NEPHROPATHY AND HENOCH-SCHÖNLEIN DISEASE

Daniel C. Cattran, MD, and Angela Alonso Esteve, MD

1. **What is immunoglobulin A nephropathy?**

   Immunoglobulin A nephropathy (IgAN) is the most common biopsy-proven primary glomerulonephritis in the world. IgAN shows geographic and ethnic variations, being much more common in Asians and Caucasians and rare in those of African ancestry. It shows a 2:1 male to female predominance and a peak incidence in clinical presentation in the second and third decades of life. Its diagnosis is confirmed by the deposition on immunofluorescence of the immunoglobulin IgA in the mesangial area of the kidney.

2. **What are the typical biopsy findings?**

   On light microscopy (LM), mesangial cellular proliferation and matrix expansion are the classic findings. In cases with rapid deterioration in renal function, more diffuse proliferation of both the endocapillary and mesangial cells can be seen. In addition, segmental necrosis and crescents may be associated with this clinical scenario. Pathology features, common to all patients with advanced glomerular diseases, can be seen in IgA nephropathy including glomerulosclerosis, tubular atrophy, and interstitial fibrosis.

   On immunofluorescence (IF), the defining hallmark of IgAN is the presence of prominent, globular mesangial dominant or codominant (most commonly with IgG) deposits of IgA.

   On electron microscopy (EM), electron-dense mesangial deposits are the typical finding. Paramesangial and subendothelial extension of the deposits may be present but are uncommon.

3. **What is the pathogenesis of IgA nephropathy?**

   A unifying theory of the pathogenesis has not been fully elucidated. The available data suggest that tissue injury can be initiated by the deposition in the mesangium of abnormally glycosylated IgA1 immune complexes. It remains a major question why in some patients—and not in others—this triggers a local immune response leading to the production of cytokines and growth factors and subsequent inflammatory cell recruitment, then mesangial cell proliferation and matrix formation.

4. **What is the etiology of IgA nephropathy?**

   The etiology of primary IgA nephropathy is unknown in the majority of cases. The molecular mechanisms involved in the development of the dysregulation of the mucosal-type IgA immune response that results in the production of the aberrant IgA are not completely understood. It is likely that there are contributions from both genetic and environmental factors. Both infectious agents and allergens are capable of driving the production of the abnormally glycosylated IgA product.

   Many families with multiple affected members have been described and a specific chromosomal abnormality has been identified, but none of the genomewide linkage studies reported to date have identified a causal gene. In most of the reported kindreds with IgAN, transmission is consistent with an autosomal-dominant pattern with incomplete penetrance. The variability in penetrance may indicate that additional environmental or genetic factors are necessary to produce the clinical phenotype.

   In the majority of cases of IgAN, specific familial or genetic patterns are not present, and IgA nephropathy is considered a sporadic disease.

5. **Is IgA nephropathy associated with any other conditions?**
Yes. Although IgAN is most commonly a primary (idiopathic) disorder, there are some well-established associations. The most common are liver cirrhosis (both alcohol and virus induced), celiac disease, HIV infection, inflammatory bowel disease, and some rheumatic conditions.

IgAN has also been described in association with minimal change disease, membranous nephropathy, and antineutrophil cytoplasmic antibody (ANCA)-positive vasculitis.

6. **How does IgA nephropathy present?**
About 30% to 50% of patients present with recurrent gross hematuria, typically within a few days of an upper respiratory infection. Classically known as "synpharyngetic hematuria," this presentation is more common in children and young adults than in the older affected population. Dull flank pain and low-grade fever may be present, and this pattern mimics either urinary tract infection or urolithiasis.

About 30% to 40% of patients with IgAN are asymptomatic and its presence is detected on routine examination of the urine (positive for microscopic hematuria with or without mild proteinuria [<300 mg/day]). Systemic hypertension may also be found. Nephrotic-range proteinuria or lesser degrees of proteinuria without hematuria are unusual but may occur.

In less than 5% of patients, IgAN can present with acute oliguric renal failure. It is felt that the renal failure is most commonly secondary to tubular obstruction and/or damage by red cell casts that form related to the gross hematuria. Crescentic glomerulopathy in IgA nephropathy can produce the same clinical phenotype and should be considered whenever an acute deterioration of renal function occurs. This is a relatively rare clinical presentation, and a kidney biopsy may be required to separate acute tubular damage from crescentic glomerulonephritis. This is particularly important given their outcome and that management is so distinctly different.

At least 20% of patients with IgAN present with chronic kidney disease as a result of longstanding but undiagnosed disease. The clinical phenotype usually includes hypertension, mild to moderate proteinuria, and hematuria of undetermined duration in combination with varying degrees of chronic kidney disease.
Rarely, IgAN can present with malignant hypertension.

7. **What is the differential diagnosis of synpharyngitic hematuria?**
The onset of hematuria shortly after a respiratory infection is common to both IgAN and postinfectious GN. However, the latent period from infection to gross hematuria averages 1 to 3 days in IgAN versus 10 to 14 days in poststreptococcal GN. Postinfectious GN can also be distinguished from IgAN by the presence of hypocomplementemia and the elevation of antistreptococcal antibodies.

8. **How is the IgAN diagnosis established?**
Even if IgAN is suspected on the basis of the clinical and laboratory findings, the diagnosis can only be confirmed by the findings on kidney biopsy. The presence of mesangial proliferation and matrix expansion on LM with dominant or codominant deposition of IgA on immunofluorescence microscopy confirms the diagnosis.

9. **What is the role of serum IgA in the diagnosis and monitoring of the disease?**
Although increased levels of serum IgA can be found in up to 50% of cases, this finding is not specific and has no diagnostic or prognostic value. The potential diagnostic usefulness of galactose-deficient IgA1 measurement needs further evaluation.

10. **Should a kidney biopsy always be performed?**
No. Asymptomatic patients with isolated hematuria or mild proteinuria (<500 mg/day) usually follow a benign course. General interventions known to slow progression used in other cases of chronic kidney disease should be implemented. Thus, the histologic findings at this stage of the disease are not likely to alter therapy, and a kidney biopsy is not necessary. The decision

to perform a biopsy in these cases even when IgAN is highly suspected is a matter of debate and varies widely among nephrologists and geographic region.

Regardless of whether a kidney biopsy is performed, ongoing follow-up of these patients is imperative because its evolution to a more concerning phenotype may occur at any time and is unpredictable. Kidney biopsy is generally recommended in patients with an unexplained serum creatinine above normal for age and sex and/or proteinuria (>500–1000 mg/day).

11. **What is the prognosis of IgAN?**

Most patients who present with isolated hematuria and no proteinuria have a low risk of progression provided these laboratory features do not change.

Among patients who develop significant persistent proteinuria (>500–1000 mg/day) approximately 25% to 30% will require renal replacement therapy within 20 to 25 years of presentation. A higher percentage will require renal replacement therapy if they have persistent higher-grade proteinuria (>2–3 g/day) with or without hypertension, especially if resistant to treatment.

Spontaneous improvement in laboratory findings in those with isolated hematuria (without significant proteinuria or impairment of glomerular filtration rate [GFR]) has been reported. It appears to be more common in children and has been estimated between 5% and 30% of such cases.

There is a geographic variability in IgAN prognosis that is in large part explained by lead-time bias related to differing clinical threshold for performing a renal biopsy. Calculating the influence of other factors such as genetics, diet, or treatment is relevant but currently impossible to quantitate.

12. **Do any renal biopsy findings predict outcome?**

Yes, several variables have been found to correlate with renal outcome. The most recent classification (the Oxford classification) suggests that there is predictive value, independent of the clinical parameters related to the degree of mesangial proliferation, presence of endocapillary proliferation, segmental glomerulosclerosis, and the degree of tubular atrophy/interstitial fibrosis. This classification has yet to be validated. Although uncommon, crescent formation also confers a poor renal prognosis. Extension of the IgA deposits into the subendothelial location of the capillary wall has also been associated with a worse prognosis.

13. **Are there clinical features predictive of outcome?**

Yes, in fact, they are known to have a stronger predictive value than the histologic ones. The level of sustained proteinuria over time has been shown to be the strongest predictor of progression. Regardless of the level of proteinuria at presentation, achieving a complete (proteinuria <300 mg/day) or partial remission (proteinuria <1 g/day) substantially reduces the rate of progression of the kidney disease. Mean arterial pressure over time has also been identified as an important predictor.

Whether isolated hematuria or recurrent macroscopic hematuria are prognostic indicators is still debated. It is possible that recurrent gross hematuria may leave subclinical renal damage that eventually will result in tubular interstitial scarring and a worse long-term outcome, but currently there is little evidence to support that contention.

14. **Is there a specific treatment for IgAN?**

There is no known treatment that specifically modifies the presumed pathogenesis of IgAN. Nonimmune-modulating treatment with renin-angiotensin system (RAS) blockade is still the best evidence-based intervention for slowing IgAN progression. The blood pressure target should be <125/75 to 130/80 mm Hg in adults (and similar targets adjusted appropriately for body size and age). The aim should be to reduce the proteinuria to 500 to 1000 mg/day. Maximal doses of angiotension-converting enzyme (ACE) inhibitors or angiotensin receptor blockers (ARB) may be necessary, and even a combination of these agents may be considered if these blood pressure and proteinuria targets have not been achieved. This combination may carry increased risk of adverse events and careful monitoring is required.

KEY POINTS: IgA NEPHROPATHY AND HENOCH-SCHÖNLEIN DISEASE

1. Immunoglobulin a nephropathy (IgAN) is the most common biopsy-proven primary glomerulonephritis in the world.

2. The classical presentation is painless gross hematuria 1 to 3 days after an upper respiratory infection.

3. When accompanied only by microscopic hematuria, the long-term prognosis of IgA nephropathy is excellent.

4. Persistent proteinuria >1 g per day and/or hypertension is associated with up to 50% likelihood of developing end-stage renal disease within 10 years.

5. Renin-angiotensin system blockade with angiotensin-converting enzyme inhibition and/or angiotensin receptor blockade has been proven in randomized controlled trials both in children and adults to improve prognosis.

15. **Should all patients with IgAN receive treatment?**
No. The approach to therapy in individual patients should take into account their relative risk of progression based on their clinical and pathology findings.
- Patients with isolated hematuria, no proteinuria, and normal GFR do not require treatment, but monitoring every 6 to 12 months for potential indicators of worsening disease (such as increasing proteinuria, blood pressure, and/or serum creatinine) is warranted.
- For patients with persistent proteinuria (>500–1000 mg/day), angiotensin inhibition is recommended with ACE inhibitors and/or ARB therapy, aiming for reduction in proteinuria to <500 to 1000 mg/day. Although there is no definitive evidence supporting the adjunctive use of fish oil supplements, many physicians advocate this therapy because of their lack of toxicity and because they may provide a nonspecific anti-inflammatory/vasoprotective effect.

16. **When should immunosuppressive therapy be considered?**
Corticosteroids in monotherapy:
- A 6-month trial of corticosteroids may be warranted in patients with sustained proteinuria >1 g/day despite optimal blood pressure control and maximal RAS blockade.
- In patients presenting with nephrotic syndrome and histologic findings consistent with minimal change disease (MCD), corticosteroids prescribed in a manner similar to MCD alone will commonly induce a complete remission in proteinuria.
Combined immunosuppressive therapy:
- There is very little and only low-quality evidence to support the use of cyclophosphamide, mycophenolate mofetil, or azathioprine in IgAN. This form of therapy should only be considered in those patients with both clinical and pathology features suggestive of ongoing active disease:
    - Patients with crescentic glomerulonephritis and a clinically rapidly progressive course with or without a positive test for ANCA may be considered for therapy with intravenous pulse glucocorticoids plus cyclophosphamide.
   In patients with a documented progressive decline in renal function despite RAS blockade and a course of glucocorticoids and after demonstrating adequate renal histologic reserve (not an end-stage kidney) combined therapy with glucocorticoids and cyclophosphamide may be considered.
   In these circumstances, conversion to maintenance therapy with either mycophenolate mofetil (MMF) or azathioprine (AZA) should be considered after 3 months provided the serum creatinine has stabilized and proteinuria has decreased.

If there is no improvement in these parameters after the initial course of cyclophosphamide, a repeat renal biopsy should be considered before considering additional immunosuppression.

17. Is tonsillectomy recommended?

No. Although tonsillectomy has been performed as a treatment for IgAN, particularly in the Asian population, it is not a risk-free procedure and the evidence of its usefulness is weak.

18. Does IgAN recur after transplantation?

Yes. Although histologic recurrence (the presence of IgA on immunofluorescence staining) is seen with increasing frequency over time post-transplant, its clinical manifestations are usually unimportant and overall graft survival is similar to that of patients with other causes of their kidney failure.

19. What is Henoch-Schönlein purpura?

Henoch-Schönlein purpura (HSP) is a systemic leukocytoclastic vasculitis affecting small vessels characterized by IgA immune deposits. It typically presents in winter or fall, often triggered by an infection or allergic reaction. Classic presentation is a tetrad of skin rash, abdominal pain, arthralgias, and hematuria/proteinuria. It has a peak incidence at ages 4 to 6 and shows a 2:1 male/female predilection. It is the most common cause of vasculitis in children. The four classical clinical features are as follows:

- **Skin:** Palpable purpura affecting mainly forearms, lower limbs, and buttocks. Skin manifestations usually predominate in children.
- **Gastrointestinal:** Bowel vasculitis causing colicky abdominal pain. Gastrointestinal bleeding may occur.
- **Joints:** Symmetric polyarthralgia typically limited to knees and ankles.
- **Kidney:** Renal involvement, which may be clinically and pathologically indistinguishable from IgAN, is more common and severe in older children and adults.

20. What is the prognosis of HSP nephritis?

Most patients have a self-limiting course and a good prognosis. A minority of patients have persistent hematuria or proteinuria that may eventually lead to end-stage renal disease. In these patients, evolution and prognosis of the nephritis is comparable to that of patients with IgAN; thus the follow-up and approach to treatment should be similar. There is no evidence-based treatment, but steroids with or without other immunosuppressive agents may be a reasonable option for severe or progressive renal disease.

Recurrent/relapsing episodes can occur but may not predict a worse long-term outcome. The disease behavior after transplantation is similar to that of IgAN but occasionally can be severe and include crescentic features.

BIBLIOGRAPHY

1. Ballardie FW, Roberts IS. Controlled prospective trial of prednisolone and cytotoxics in progressive IgA nephropathy. *J Am Soc Nephrol* 2002;13:142–148.
2. Barratt J, Feehally J. IgA nephropathy. *J Am Soc Nephrol* 2005;16(7):2088–2097.
3. Bartosik LP, Lajoie G, Sugar L, et al. Predicting progression in IgA nephropathy. *Am J Kidney Dis* 2001;38(4):728–735.
4. Cattran DC, Coppo R, Cook HT, et al., A Working Group of the International IgA Nephropathy Network and the Renal Pathology Society. The Oxford classification of IgA nephropathy: rationale, clinicopathological correlations, and classification. *Kidney Int* 2009;76:534–545.
5. Coppo R, Andrulli S, Amore A, et al. Predictors of outcome in Henoch-Schönlein nephritis in children and adults. *Am J Kidney Dis* 2006;47:993–1003.
6. D'Amico G. Natural history of idiopathic IgA nephropathy and factors predictive of disease outcome. *Semin Nephrol* 2004;24:179–196.
7. Donadio JV, Grande JP. IgA nephropathy. *N Eng J Med* 2002;347(10):738–747.
8. Feehally J. Predicting prognosis in IgA nephropathy. *Am J Kidney Dis* 2001;38:881–883.
9. Frisch G, Lin J, Rosenstock J, et al. Mycophenolate mofetil (MMF) vs. placebo in patients with moderately advanced IgA nephropathy: A double-blind randomized controlled trial. *Nephrol Dial Transplant* 2005;20:2139–2145.

10. Geddes CC, Rauta V, Gronhagen-Riska C, et al. A tricontinental view of IgA nephropathy. *Nephrol Dial Transplant* 2003;18(8):1541–1548.
11. Gharavi AG, Moldoveanu Z, Wyatt RJ, et al. Aberrant IgA1 glycosylation is inherited in familial and sporadic IgA nephropathy. *J Am Soc Nephrol* 2008;19:1008–1014.
12. Kiryluk K, Gharavi AG, Izzi C, et al. IgA nephropathy—The case for a genetic basis becomes stronger. *Nephrol Dial Transplant* 2010;25:336–338.
13. Niaudet P, Habib R. Methylprednisolone pulse therapy in the treatment of severe forms of Schönlein-Henoch purpura nephritis. *Pediatr Nephrol* 1998;12:238–243.
14. Pozzi C, Andrulli S, Del Vecchio L, et al. Corticosteroids effectiveness in IgA nephropathy: Long-term results of a randomized controlled trial. *J Am Soc Nephrol* 2004;15:157–163.
15. Praga M, Gutiérrez E, González E, et al. Treatment of IgA nephropathy with ACE inhibitors: A randomized and controlled trial. *J Am Soc Nephrol* 2003;14:1578–1583.
16. Reich HN, Troyanov S, Scholey JW, et al. Remission of proteinuria improves prognosis in IgA nephropathy. *J Am Soc Nephrol* 2007;18:3177–3183.
17. Roberts I, Cook HT, Troyanov S, et al., A Working Group of the International IgA Nephropathy Network and the Renal Pathology Society. The Oxford classification of IgA nephropathy: Pathology definitions, correlations, and reproducibility. *Kidney Int* 2009;76:546–556.
18. Rodríguez-Iturbe B, Batsford S. Pathogenesis of poststreptococcal glomerulonephritis a century after Clemens von Pirquet. *Kidney Int* 2007;71(11):1094–1104.
19. Tang S, Leung JC, Chan LY, et al. Mycophenolate mofetil alleviates persistent proteinuria in IgA nephropathy. *Kidney Int* 2005;68(2):802–812.
20. Tumlin JA, Lohavichan V, Hennigar R. Crescentic, proliferative IgA nephropathy: Clinical and histological response to methylprednisolone and intravenous cyclophosphamide. *Nephrol Dial Transplant* 2003;18(7):1321–1329.

CHAPTER 33

MEMBRANOPROLIFERATIVE GLOMERULONEPHRITIS

Howard Trachtman, MD

1. **What is membranoproliferative glomerulonephritis?**

   Membranoproliferative glomerulonephritis (MPGN) is a rare form of glomerular disease that occurs in children and adults. It is a disease characterized by a unique histopathologic feature—namely, splitting of the glomerular basement membrane (GBM), with interposition of mesangial cells and extracellular matrix material. It is associated with variable degrees of endothelial and mesangial hypercellularity. Together with postinfectious glomerulonephritis, systemic lupus erythematosus (SLE), and cholesterol embolic disease, it is one of the glomerulopathies that is marked by hypocomplementemia.

2. **How does one make the diagnosis and classify MPGN?**

   Although one may suspect the disease in a patient with hematuria and/or proteinuria and a reduced C3 level, a kidney biopsy is required to confirm the diagnosis. Examination of the renal histopathology demonstrates a lobular appearance of the glomerular tuft, mesangial expansion and hypercellularity, and the characteristic "tram track" finding with a double contour of the GBM. Immunofluorescence staining is usually positive for C3, immunoglobulin G (IgG), and IgM in a capillary wall distribution. Classical complement cascade components are seen in type I but not types II and III MPGN.

   Primary MPGN is divided into three subtypes based on the nature and location of electron-dense deposits in addition to the expected changes in the GBM: type I, subendothelial deposits; type II, large, ribbonlike, intramembranous deposits, so-called dense deposit disease (DDD); and type III, subendothelial and subepithelial deposits. The deposits can be numerous or sparse in number. The deposits are homogeneous in density and have no defining ultrastructural appearance.

3. **What is the cause of MPGN?**

   MPGN can be primary (idiopathic) in nature. Alternatively, it can be secondary to a wide variety of medical conditions including infections (hepatitis B, hepatitis C, and bacterial endocarditis), autoimmune diseases (e.g., systemic lupus erythematosus), chronic liver disease (e.g., α1-antitrypsin deficiency), malignancies, lymphoproliferative disorders, plasma cell dyscrasias leading to monoclonal gammopathy, and essential cryoglobulinemia. MPGN has been associated rarely with Lyme disease and autoimmune thyroiditis and type I diabetes mellitus. Finally, some newer medications have been linked to type I MPGN, such as granulocyte colony stimulating factor.

4. **What is the incidence and prevalence of MPGN?**

   Primary MPGN is one of the least common causes of idiopathic nephrotic syndrome, accounting for at most 5% to 10% of cases. Therefore, the incidence is probably in the range of 1 to 2 per million population per year and as such qualifies for the federal designation as a rare disease. The incidence of MPGN may have declined over the past two decades. The secondary causes of MPGN have a less clearcut incidence because of varying patterns of performing a kidney biopsy in patients with urinary abnormalities and subtle changes in glomerular filtration rate (GFR). This may underestimate the incidence of this complication. The prevalence of MPGN exceeds the incidence because of the slow rate of progression of kidney injury. Nonetheless, MPGN is a rare cause of end-stage renal disease (ESRD) in children and adults, accounting for less than 5% of patients on dialysis or receiving a kidney transplant.

5. What is the clinical presentation of patients with MPGN?

MPGN can be present with the full spectrum of glomerular disease. Hematuria can be the sole manifestation in rare cases. A larger number of patients, 10% to 30%, have glomerular hematuria (including gross hematuria) and proteinuria with normal kidney function. A third group can present with new-onset nephrotic syndrome (40% to 70%), and a fourth group (20% to 30%) may have a full-blown nephritic picture with hypertension, azotemia, hematuria, and proteinuria. Anemia may be present that is out of proportion to the degree of kidney dysfunction.

6. Are there extrarenal manifestations of MPGN?

Patients with primary MPGN generally have complaints solely related to the kidney. However, patients with type II disease, which is more common in children compared to adults, manifest partial lipodystrophy in nearly 25% of cases. This is characterized by the gradual loss of subcutaneous fat tissue in the face and upper-body regions. There may be other rare associated findings in patients with MPGN such as macular degeneration and mild visual field and color defects. Retinal angiography demonstrates the presence of choroidal neovascularization.

Patients with secondary MPGN may have extrarenal abnormalities related to the underlying disease. For example, patients with MPGN in association with cryoglobulinemia may have ulcerative skin lesions, Raynaud's phenomenon, peripheral neuropathy, hepatomegaly, and signs of cirrhosis.

7. What is the natural history of MPGN?

Although spontaneous remission has been described occasionally in children and adolescents with MPGN, nearly 50% progress to ESRD over 10 to 15 years. At onset, an elevated serum creatinine concentration, nephrotic-range proteinuria, severe hypertension, crescents in >50% of glomeruli, diffuse interstitial fibrosis and tubular atrophy, and a reduced calculated GFR after 1 year of treatment are indicators of a poor outcome. The prognosis is worse in patients with primary versus secondary forms of MPGN. In addition, type II MPGN may have a more ominous long-term outlook compared to types I and III disease. In general, the outcome of MPGN is comparable in adult compared to pediatric patients. Thus, 50% of patients progress to end-stage renal disease within 5 years of the diagnostic renal biopsy, and this percentage increases to 64% after 10 years of follow-up. The features associated with a poor prognosis are similar to those noted in pediatric patients.

8. Are there any patient groups at special risk of developing MPGN or developing adverse long-term outcomes?

MPGN appears to involve children and adults of both genders and all ethnic groups, and the prognosis is comparable in all patient groups.

9. What is the appropriate workup for patients with MPGN?

The critical test needed to confirm the diagnosis of MPGN is hypocomplementemia—namely, reduced C3 and CH50 levels, which is confirmed in 80% to 90% of cases. The C4 level is also low in approximately 40% of those with type I MPGN. This is less common in those with type II or III MPGN. Measurement of all components of the complement cascade to distinguish between the different types of MPGN is usually not performed in clinical chemistry laboratories and is only available in select research facilities. C3 nephritic factor activity should be assayed in all forms of primary and secondary MPGN. In adults with cryoglobulinemia, testing should be performed for hepatitis B and C infection. Hepatitis serology should be evaluated in pediatric patients with MPGN even in the absence of mixed cryoglobulinemia. Other laboratory abnormalities will be present depending on the underlying disease.

10. **Are there any unique laboratory tests that are relevant to patients with MPGN?**
C3 nephritic factor activity, an autoantibody to C3bBb the alternate pathway C3 convertase, is more common in type II disease—60% to 70% of patients, compared to 20% to 25% of patients with types I or III disease. C3 nephritic factor can be measured in a hemolytic- or a solid-phase assay. This autoantibody is also detectable in up to 50% of patients with secondary forms of MPGN. Patients with type III MPGN may have a nephritic factor of the terminal complement pathway that stabilizes properdin-dependent C5 convertase.

11. **What is the pathogenesis of MPGN?**
In primary forms of MPGN, the mechanism of disease centers around abnormal activation of the complement cascade. There are three distinct patterns of complement activation in the three types of MPGN. In type I disease, the process is initiated by immune complex deposition within the kidney and involvement of the classical pathway. The source of the immune complexes is unknown in the idiopathic form of the disease. Patients have low levels of C3, C4, C6, C7, and/or C9. In the type II variant, the continuous overactivity of the complement cascade involves an amplification loop in the alternative pathway, characterized mainly by markedly depressed C3 levels. An IgG or IgM autoantibody, termed C3 nephritic factor, is present in the majority of patients with dense deposit disease. Finally, type III MPGN appears to have features in common with type I disease and evidence of activation of the terminal complement pathway with low C3, C5, and properdin levels. In the secondary forms of MPGN, it is presumed that there is immune-complex–mediated activation of the complement cascade.

12. **Is there a genetic contribution to MPGN?**
Abnormal complement activation in MPGN can occur as a consequence of genetic mutations that yield reduced levels of endogenous inhibitors of the alternate pathway such as factor H or because of the presence of a circulating autoantibody that stabilizes C3 convertase. MPGN occurs in patients who carry homozygous mutations in factor H. Other genetic causes of MPGN include isolated C4 deficiency.

13. **What is the first-line treatment for MPGN?**
Children who are clinically well and free of any symptoms and who have only minor urinary abnormalities generally do not require aggressive therapy. These patients may be treated with antihypertensive agents, specifically angiotensin-converting enzyme inhibitors or angiotensin receptor blockers, to reduce proteinuria and prevent progressive renal damage. Those with more severe disease are treated with prolonged alternate daily therapy with oral steroids, prednisone 40 to 60 mg/m^2 or 2.0 to 2.5 mg/kg every other day for an average period of 6.5 years with an improved outcome compared to historical controls or patients treated at other centers. Repeat biopsies performed after 2 years of therapy indicated an increase in open capillary loops and a reduction in mesangial matrix expansion. An increase in glomerulosclerosis may be seen despite clinical improvement. The efficacy of therapy was greater in patients who began treatment within 1 year of disease onset and in those whose GFR is well preserved (i.e., >70 mL/min/1.73 m^2).

    In adults, there is widespread concern about the risks of prolonged steroid therapy. Therefore, the current evidence-based medicine recommendation is to prescribe steroids only for adults with nephrotic syndrome or impaired kidney function. Treatment is maintained for 6 months. Patients with asymptomatic urinary findings or who fail to respond to steroids should be treated conservatively. Angiotensin-converting enzyme inhibitors have been demonstrated to be effective in reducing proteinuria in patients with MPGN. Combined therapy with dipyridamole, cyclophosphamide, and warfarin does not appear to be beneficial, and this treatment is no longer recommended.

    In patients with hepatitis C infection and MPGN, interferon-α therapy for 6 to 12 months can achieve remission in 60% of patients. However, nearly all will relapse within 3 to 6 months. Addition of ribavirin to the regimen may improve the response.

14. **What are the second-line therapies for MPGN?**
There is a compelling argument in favor of optimal control of blood pressure, preferably with an angiotensin-converting enzyme inhibitor or angiotensin receptor blocker. Plasmapheresis has been reported to be a useful therapy in small numbers of patients with severe idiopathic MPGN and acute renal failure or rapidly deteriorating disease. Mycophenolate mofetil has been tried in patients with cryoglobulinemic MPGN related to hepatitis B infection. Although treatment resulted in reduced proteinuria, viral replication was induced by the drug. Therefore, caution is advisable when considering this immunosuppressive agent for the treatment of MPGN. Cyclosporine is another alternative form of immunosuppressive therapy that may be beneficial in patients with refractory MPGN; however, it has not been studied systematically in a large case series.

KEY POINTS: MEMBRANOPROLIFERATIVE GLOMERULONEPHRITIS

1. Membranoproliferative glomerulonephritis (MPGN) is diagnosed based on a kidney biopsy with renal histopathology demonstrating a lobular appearance of the glomerular tuft; mesangial expansion and hypercellularity; the characteristic "tram track" finding with a double contour of the glomerular basement membrane; and immunofluorescence staining that is usually positive for C3, immunoglobulin G (IgG), and IgM in a capillary wall distribution.

2. There are three subtypes: type I, subendothelial deposits; type II, large, ribbonlike, intramembranous deposits, so-called dense deposit disease (DDD); and type III, subendothelial and subepithelial deposits.

3. MPGN can be primary (idiopathic) in nature or secondary to a wide variety of medical conditions including infections, autoimmune diseases, chronic liver disease, malignancies, lymphoproliferative disorders, plasma cell dyscrasias, and essential cryoglobulinemia.

4. Primary MPGN is one of the least common causes of idiopathic nephrotic syndrome, accounting for at most 5% to 10% of cases and an incidence in the range of 1 to 2 per million population per year.

5. Spontaneous remission is rare and nearly 50% of patients with MPGN progress to end-stage renal disease over 10 to 15 years.

6. Children with severe disease are treated with prolonged alternate daily therapy with oral steroids, prednisone 40 to 60 mg/m^2 or 2.0 to 2.5 mg/kg every other day for an average period of 6.5 years with an improved outcome compared to historical controls or patients treated at other centers. The role of therapy is less clear in adults.

15. **What is the role of kidney transplantation in the treatment of patients with MPGN?**
Kidney transplantation is a viable treatment for patients with MPGN who progress to ESRD. However, there is a variable risk of recurrent disease in both primary and secondary categories of disease. In patients with primary MPGN, the recurrence rate is approximately 20% to 40% in those with type I and III disease and up to 80% to 90% in those with type II (dense deposit disease). In those with secondary disease, the recurrence is directly linked to control of the underlying illness. The risk of recurrent disease may be marginally higher in recipients of living-donor kidneys. Recurrent disease usually leads to allograft loss.

16. **Are there novel therapies for MPGN in development?**
Agents to block the abnormal activation of the alternate pathway of complement including eculizumab, a monoclonal antibody to C5a and recombinant factor H, are being considered as

potential treatments for primary MPGN, especially type II disease. In secondary disease, removal of cryoglobulins with cryofiltration is an experimental modality that may work by removing cryoglobulins from the circulation.

BIBLIOGRAPHY

1. Alchi B, Jayne D. Membranoproliferative glomerulonephritis. *Pediatr Nephrol* 2010;25(8):1409–1418.

2. Appel GB, Cook T, Hageman G, et al. Membranoproliferative glomerulonephritis type II (Dense deposit disease): An update. *J Am Soc Nephrol* 2005;16:1392–1404.

3. Cansick JC, Lennon R, Cummins CL, et al. Prognosis, treatment and outcome of childhood mesangiocapillary (membranoproliferative) glomerulonephritis. *Nephrol Dial Transplant* 2004;19:2769–2777.

4. Levin A. Management of membranoproliferative glomerulonephritis: Evidence-based recommendation. *Kidney Int* 1999;55(Suppl 70):S41–S46.

5. Lorenz EC, Sethi S, Leung N, et al. Recurrent membranoproliferative glomerulonephritis after kidney transplantation. *Kidney Int* (online publication February 3, 2010).

6. McEnery PT, McAdams AJ, West CD. The effect of prednisone in a high-dose, alternate-day regimen on the natural history of idiopathic membranoproliferative glomerulonephritis. *Medicine* 1986;64:401–424.

7. Nasr SH, Valeri AM, Appel GB, et al. Dense deposit disease: Clinicopathologic study of 32 pediatric and adult patients. *Clin J Am Soc Nephrol* 2009;4:22–32.

8. Tarshish P, Bernstein J, Tobin JN, et al. Treatment of mesangiocapillary glomerulonephritis with alternate-day prednisone: A report of the International Study of Kidney Diseases in Children. *Pediatr Nephrol* 1992;6:123–130.

9. Yanagihara T, Hayakawa M, Yoshida J, et al. Long-term follow-up of diffuse proliferative membranoproliferative glomerulonephritis type 1. *Pediatr Nephrol* 2005;20:585–590.

DIABETIC NEPHROPATHY

Yalemzewd Woredekal, MD, and Eli A. Friedman, MD

CHAPTER 34

1. **Concurrent with the global pandemic of diabetes, has the incidence rate of end-stage renal disease resulting from diabetic nephropathy increased?**
As shown in Figure 34-1, in the United States, although the number of persons whose end-stage renal disease (ESRD) was attributed to diabetes (prevalence) has continuously expanded, the incidence rate of new-onset ESRD per 100,000 persons with diabetes has sharply decreased since 1995. This observation was first reported in the *Morbidity and Mortality Weekly Report* (MMWR) published by the U.S. Centers for Disease Control and Prevention (CDC) in November 2005.

   Although a rationale for this "good news" was not proposed, the MMWR commented: "Although the number of new cases of ESRD in persons with diabetes increased overall, the incidence of ESRD-DM among persons with diabetes is not increasing among black, Hispanics, men, and persons aged 65–74 years, and is declining among persons aged <65 years, women, and whites." Using as denominator all persons known to have diabetes with new incidence of ESRD as numerator revealed a remarkable sharply downward slope from a peak of 305 per 100,000 in 1996 to 232 in 2002 ($p < 0.01$).

   Through 2009 the trend continued, indicating that as the total U.S. population continues to increase, the number of people with diabetes also grows; however, the proportion (rate) of individuals with diabetes who will develop ESRD should, by trend analysis, continue to

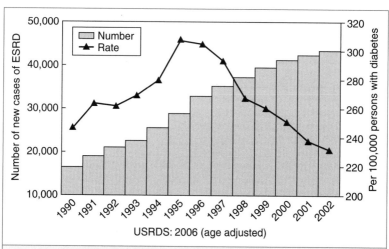

Figure 34-1. New-onset end-stage renal disease in persons with diabetes. (From Burrows NR, Wang J, Geiss LS, et al. Incidence of end-stage renal disease among persons with diabetes—United States, 1990–2002. *MMWR* 2005;54:1097–1100.)

decline. No evidence-based explanation for this welcome change is established, although crediting widely practiced renoprotection regimens is attractive.

Burrows NR, Wang J, Geiss LS, et al. Incidence of end-stage renal disease among persons with diabetes—United States, 1990–2002. *MMWR* 2005;54:1097–1100.

Miyata T, de Ypersele Strihou. Renoprotection of angiotensin receptor blockers: Beyond blood pressure lowering. *Nephrol Dial Tranplant* 2006;21(4):846–849.

2. **Has the pathogenesis of diabetic nephropathy been clarified?**

The pathogenesis of diabetic nephropathy is likely a result of genetic predisposition and the interplay between hemodynamic and metabolic pathways. A leading metabolic factor involved in the development of diabetic nephropathy is hyperglycemia. Glucose in high concentration is toxic to cells, altering cell growth and gene and protein expression, while increasing extracellular matrix and growth factor production. Hyperglycemia may also induce multiple adverse effects indirectly through activation and formation of metabolic end molecules such as oxidative and glycation products and by activation of protein kinase C (PKC), transforming growth factor beta (TGF-β), and the renin-angiotensin system. Illustrating the many mechanisms involving diverse pathways that have been studied to explore the pathogenesis of diabetic nephropathy are the following examples:

- **Advanced glycosylated end products:** Chronic hyperglycemia leads to formation of nonenzymatic glycated proteins referred to as advance glycosylated end products (AGEs). AGEs are formed from the nonenzymatic reactive binding (glycation) of sugar-derived carbonyl groups with a reactive amino group resulting in formation of an unstable Schiff base with subsequent Amadori rearrangement to form a more stable ketoamine. In cultured glomerular endothelial and mesangial cells, in vitro, glycated albumin, and AGE-rich proteins enhance expression of type IV collagen and TGF-β and increase PKC activity, contributing to glomerular sclerosis and tubulointerstitial damage by means of an abnormal extracellular matrix (ECM) production. Attempts to block either AGE formation or its action by inhibition of AGE interaction with its receptor have been conducted. Although highly promising in rodents with induced diabetes, clinical trials of aminoguanidine, an AGE blocker, were discontinued after noting that it caused deranged liver function tests. Other AGE blockers are currently in trials.

- **TGF-β:** In vitro, TGF-β modulates ECM production in glomerular, mesangial, and epithelial cells. In addition, TGF-β inhibits synthesis of collagenase and stimulates the production of metalloproteinase inhibitors, which could lead to reduced degradation of ECM. In renal biopsies from diabetic persons with nephropathy, increased TGF-β immunostaining has been described both in glomeruli and the tubulointerstitium. These findings have also been reported in other renal disease characterized by accumulation of ECM. Increased renal production of TGF-β and increased urinary TGF-β levels, findings noted in patients with type 2 diabetes, as correlates of urinary albumin excretion (UAE).

- Increased renal production of TGF-β as well as increased urinary TGF-β levels have been reported in patients with type 2 diabetes, their amount correlates with the quantity of urinary albumin excretion (UAE).

- **Protein kinase C (PKC):** Activation of PKC is strongly implicated in the pathogenesis of diabetic nephropathy. Hyperglycemia is the predominant stimulus that induces activation of distinct PKC isoforms within a cell, each mediating specific functions probably via different subcellular localization. PKC activation increases production of cytokines and extracellular matrix and vasoconstrictor endothelin-1. These changes contribute to basement membrane thickening, vascular occlusion, and increased cell membrane permeability.

Ruboxistaurin, a PKC β-specific inhibitor, is now in phase II clinical trials in diabetic retinopathy and cardiac ventricular hypertrophy. Inhibiting these perturbed metabolic pathways may afford a potential therapy for diabetic nephropathy; however, clinical trial results have thus far been less than gratifying. A pilot study of ruboxistaurin demonstrated stabilization of nephropathy in patients with type 2 diabetes. In this study, 123 patients with early diabetic nephropathy (albuminuria of 200–2000 mg/g and serum creatinine ≤ 1.7 mg/dL

[150 μmol/L] in women, and ≤2.0 mg/dL [177 μmol/L] in men) receiving stable doses of angiotensin-converting enzyme (ACE) inhibitors or angiotensin II receptor blockers (ARBs) were randomly assigned to receive ruboxistaurin, 32 mg/day or placebo. After 1 year, active treatment was associated with reduction in albuminuria and stabilization of glomerular filtration rate (GFR) without change in albuminuria or worsening of GFR in the placebo group. Mean blood pressure at baseline and end of study were similar in the two groups. Active trials of PKC inhibition underscore the potential treatment of diabetes with pharmaceutical agents that can protect against end-organ disease without the requirement for euglycemia.

Chen S, Chohen MP, Lautenslager GT. Glycated protein stimulates TGF-beta production and protein kinase activity in glomerular endothelial cells. *Kidney Int* 2001;59:1213–1221.

Katherene R, Tuttle MD, George L, et al. The effect of Ruboxistaurin on nephropathy in Type 2 diabetes. *Diabetes Care* 2005;28:2686–2690.

Marti HP, Lee L, Kashgarian M, et al. Transforming growth factor-beta during diabetic renal hypertrophy. *Kidney Int* 1994;46:431–442.

3. **Does genetic predisposition have a role in diabetic nephropathy?**
Nephropathy is a common complication of diabetes, but only a subset of patients with diabetes may prove to be susceptible to the development of diabetic nephropathy for reasons still to be clarified. After 10 to 15 years of diabetes, 30% to 50% of patients with type 1 diabetes and approximately 50% of all patients with type 2 diabetes show evidence of clinical nephropathy. Inexplicably, there remain patients who, despite prolonged hyperglycemia and poor blood pressure control, do not develop overt diabetic nephropathy. The strongest evidence for an inherited susceptibility to diabetic nephropathy comes from studies showing that some families of patients with type 1 or type 2 diabetes evince an increased risk of renal disease.

Segregation analysis has shown that diabetic offspring of parents with diabetes and proteinuria have three to four times the prevalence of nephropathy compared to siblings from parents with diabetes but without overt renal disease. The risk is even higher if both parents have nephropathy compared with the risk when only one parent has renal disease. This leads to the suggestion that the predisposition to diabetic nephropathy may be inherited as a dominant trait.

The prevalence of diabetic nephropathy varies significantly among different ethnic groups. For example, African American, Indo-Asians, and Native Americans have a substantially higher risk of the development of nephropathy than do matched white patients.

Earle KK, Porter KA, Osberg J. Variation in the progression of diabetic nephropathy according to racial origin. *Nephrol Dial Transplant* 2001;16:286–290.

Fogarty DG, Hanna LS, Wantman M, et al. Segregation analysis of urinary albumin excretion in families with type 2 diabetes. *Diabetes* 2000;49:765–775.

Quinn M, Angelico MC, Warram JH, et al. Familial factors determine the development of diabetic nephropathy in patients with IDDM. *Diabetologia* 1996;39:940–945.

4. **Will improved glycemic control modulate the rate of decline in GFR during the course of diabetic nephropathy?**
The effect of glycemic control on the rate of decline of renal function remains controversial. Observational data show that poor glycemic control, indicated by hemoglobin A1c (HbA1c) levels greater than 8%, is associated with a faster rate of decline in GFR, but only minimal interventional data demonstrate that improvement of glycemic control reduces the rate of renal function loss. A 5-year longitudinal observational study of 2613 patients with type 2 diabetes found no reduction in cardiovascular complications attained by "tight glycemic control" (HbA1c of less than 7.0%) in those who began the study with a high prevalence of comorbidities (total illness burden index). By contrast, those subjects who began the study with minimal or less severe comorbidities evidenced benefit in terms of fewer cardiovascular complications with tight glycemic control.

A number of small renal biopsy studies have provided information on the benefits of glycemic control on renal structure. In a 2- to 3-year study of patients with type 1 diabetes and microalbuminuria managed with intensive insulin treatment versus conventional treatment, indicated by an overall lower HbAic, the intensive insulin treatment group had a slower progression of microalbuminuria to proteinuria. Although basement membrane thickness increased in both groups, it increased most in those receiving conventional therapy. Similarly, mesangial matrix volume fraction increased only in those receiving conventional therapy.

Normalization of glycemic control in young adults with type 1 diabetes by solitary pancreas transplantation did cause regression of nephropathy in subjects with microalbuminuria or normal albuminuria. Although structural regression of glomerulopathy was not noted after 5 years of euglycemia, in kidney biopsies after 10 years there was reduction in glomerular and tubular basement membrane thickening and a decrease in mesangial fractional volume, mostly because of a reduction in mesangial matrices.

Bangstad HJ, Osterby R, Dahl-Jorgensen K, et al. Improvement of blood glucose control in IDDM patients retards the progression of morphologic changes in early diabetic nephropathy. *Diabetologia* 1994;37:483–490.

Fioretto P, Mauer SM, Sutherland DE, et al. Reversal of lesions of diabetic nephropathy after pancreas transplantation. *N Engl J Med* 1998;339:69–75.

5. **Is there additional benefit gained from using a combination of ACE inhibitors and ARBs in slowing progression of diabetic nephropathy?**
   The mainstay of antihypertensive therapy in patients with diabetes has evolved to be inhibition of the renin-angiotensin system involving the use of ACE inhibitors and/or ARBs. Large, well-designed prospective studies document the beneficial effect of ACE inhibitors or ARBs alone in patients with cardiovascular and renal diseases resulting from diabetes or other disorders affecting the kidneys. Several small studies support the inference that combining ACE inhibitors and ARBs provides additional benefit in diabetic nephropathy over either class of drug given alone. A meta-analysis looked at 10 trials comparing 156 patients who received ACE inhibitors and ARBs and 159 received ACE inhibitors only for 8 to 12 weeks, finding that the ACE inhibitors plus ARB combination reduced the amount of daily proteinuria to a greater extent than did ACE inhibitors alone. This benefit was associated with small improvements in GFR, serum creatinine, potassium, and blood pressure, although the changes were noted to be trends rather than statistically validated differences.

   Jennings DL, Kalus JS, Coleman CI, et al. Combination therapy with an ACE inhibitor and an angiotensin receptor blocker for diabetic nephropathy: A meta analysis. *Diabet Med* 2007;24:486–493.

   Mogensen CE, Neldam S, Tikkamen I, et al. Randomized controlled trial of dual blockade of rennin-angiotensin system in patients with hypertension, microalbuminuria, and non-insulin dependent diabetes. The Candesartan and Lisinopril microalbuminuria (CALM) study. *BMJ* 2000;321:1440–1444.

   Rossing K, Jacobsen P, Pectraszek L, et al. Renoprotective effects of adding angiotensin II receptor blocker to maximal recommended doses of ACE inhibitors in diabetic nephropathy: A randomized double-blind crossover trial. *Diabetes Care* 2003;26:2268–2274.

6. **Has the natural history of diabetic kidney changed?**
   Whether the result of effective measures of "renoprotection" or other factors yet to be identified, there have been numerous remarkable changes over the past decade in the course of diabetic nephropathy. As depicted in Figure 34-2, the rate of stroke, limb amputations, and ESRD, major complications previously viewed as inevitable in type 2 diabetes, has progressively declined over the past decade. For example, the sequence of microalbuminuria presaging macroalbuminuria followed by azotemia and ultimately renal failure is no longer an inevitable sequence of the detection of early renal malfunction. Illustrating this reality is a recent observational report of the course of a cohort of 79 of 109 patients with type 1 diabetes who developed new-onset microalbuminuria and were then followed for an average of 12 years. Surprisingly, according to former reports, only 12 of 23 patients who progressed to advanced chronic kidney disease (CKD stage 3–5) developed macroalbuminuria as a component of renal failure. Mogensen, one of the first to recognize that microalbuminuria represented an early and typically ominous sign of coming severe kidney disease in type 1 diabetes, warns of the necessity for repeated

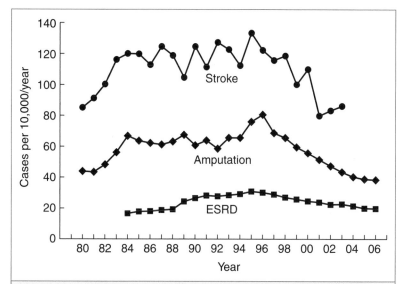

Figure 34-2. Incident rate/year of complications in U.S. persons with diabetes, 1980–2006. The data depict a decline of three major complications (stroke, limb amputation, and end-stage renal disease) in patients with type 2 diabetes since 1996. (Data from Centers for Disease Control and Prevention. National diabetes fact sheet: General information and national estimates on diabetes in the United States, 2007. Atlanta, GA: U.S. Department of Health and Human Services, Centers for Disease Control and Prevention, 2008.)

modification in standards of care for management of diabetes caused by shifting paradigms in diabetic renal disease.

Mogensen CE. Twelve shifting paradigms in diabetic renal disease and hypertension. *Diabetes Res Clin Pract* 2008;82S:S2–S9.

Perkins BA, Ficociello LH, Roshan B et al. In patients with type 1 diabetes and new-onset microalbuminuria the development of advanced chronic kidney disease may not require progression to proteinuria. *Kidney Int* 2010;77:57–64.

7. **Is diabetic nephropathy always preceded by diabetic retinopathy?**
   There may be different correlations between retinopathy and nephropathy during the course of type 1 versus type 2 diabetes. Large surveys of patients with type 1 diabetes indicate a high correlation between prevalent nephropathy and retinopathy. Both cross-sectional (Finnish Diabetic Nephropathy, $n = 3968$ adult patients with type 1 diabetes) and longitudinal (Diabetes Control and Complications Trial, $n = 1246$ adult patients with type 1 diabetes) studies found that short adult stature is associated with increased rates of both retinopathy and nephropathy and increased risks of prevalent diabetic nephropathy (odds ratio [OR] 1.71, 95% CI 1.44–2.02) and prevalent laser-treated retinopathy (1.66, 1.43–1.93) compared with other patients. No observational studies, however, recount the order of first detection of nephropathy and retinopathy in the same cohort of patients with type 1 diabetes. In type 2 diabetes, a study of 221 Japanese patients with advanced nephropathy found minimal discordance in the concurrence of nephropathy and retinopathy; five (4.1%) patients, all men aged 50 to 70, did not have retinopathy. Depending on the definitions used for retinopathy and nephropathy, the relative order of onset of the two microvascular complications continues to be undefined.

Kanauchi M, Kawano T, Uyama H, et al. Discordance between retinopathy and nephropathy in Type 2 diabetes. *Nephron* 1998;80:171–174.

Waden J, Forsblom C, Thorn LM, et al. Adult stature and diabetes complication in patients with type 1 diabetes: The FinnDiane Study and the diabetes control and complications trial. *Diabetes* 2009;58:1914–1920.

8. **Will proteomics have any role in management of diabetic nephropathy?**

Each cell produces thousands of proteins that in total are termed a proteome. Unlike the genome, which is constant irrespective of cell type, proteomes vary by cell type. Following the previously unimaginable impact of DNA testing on the professions of criminology and security and medicine, proteomics, the rapidly evolving ability to detect and correlate minute amounts of protein in serum, urine, feces, and expired air with the presence and progression of specific diseases, is transforming the practice of medicine. Using high-resolution capillary electrophoresis coupled with electrospray ionization mass spectrometry, both early detection and prediction of prognosis in diabetic nephropathy were possible by evaluating urinary biomarkers in 305 individuals with diabetic and nondiabetic proteinuric renal disease. Among subjects with diabetes, 102 biomarkers differed significantly between those with and without nephropathy, permitting 97% sensitivity and specificity in identifying their CKD as a result of diabetes. Foreshadowing what might be learned from proteomic analysis of individuals at risk for type 2 diabetes, the analysis of single-nucleotide polymorphisms (SNPs) in the peroxisome proliferator-activated receptor-delta gene (PPARD; i.e., rs1053049, rs6902123, and rs2267668) predicted improvement of mitochondrial function, aerobic physical fitness, and insulin sensitivity consequent to lifestyle intervention in addition to shifts in distribution of adiposity, hepatic fat storage, and relative muscle mass. How a proteomic urine study might affect our care of patients with diabetes is evident from a study of stored urine samples obtained from Pima Indians with type 2 diabetes 10 years after their entry into a registry when they had no evidence of diabetic nephropathy (serum creatinine levels <1.2 mg/dL and urine albumin excretion <30 mg/g). Using surface-enhanced laser desorption/ionization time-of-flight mass spectrometry to compare 14 individuals who progressed to nephropathy with 14 who did not, 714 unique urine protein peaks were detected and organized into a 12-peak "signature," permitting correct prediction of nephropathy (89%) with 93% sensitivity. In this context, the genesis of proteinuria in individuals with type 1 diabetes was studied by comparing the urine proteome in 12 healthy nondiabetic individuals with the urine proteome in 12 subjects with type 1 diabetes and normal urinary albumin excretion rates and 12 subjects with type 1 diabetes who had microalbuminuria. Megalin and cubilin, two multiligand receptors expressed in kidney proximal tubule cells that enable reuptake of filtered albumin and megalin/cubilin ligands, were significantly increased in those with type 1 diabetes and microalbuminuria compared with the other two groups. Whether this finding is causative of or a response to microalbuminuria has yet to be determined. Similarly, to distinguish the pathobiology of early nephropathologic changes in diabetes, urinary proteomes were identified using fluorescence-based difference gel electrophoresis and mass spectrometry techniques to identify novel biomarkers in urine from individuals with type 2 diabetes expressing normoalbuminuria, microalbuminuria, and macroalbuminuria compared with a control group without diabetes. E-cadherin, a specific biomarker, was also studied by Western blot in urine samples and immunohistochemistry in renal biopsies. Compared with nondiabetic control subjects, urinary E-cadherin was upregulated 1.3-fold, 5.2-fold, and 8.5-fold in those with diabetes and normoalbuminuria, microalbuminuria, and macroalbuminuria, respectively. The sensitivity and specificity of urinary E-cadherin for diagnosis of diabetes were 78.8% (95% CI, 74%–83%) supporting the quest for urine biomarkers capable of detecting the onset of diabetic nephropathy. Although proteomic methods to compare diseased and disease-free individuals have been applied to plasma and urine samples directly by either chemical labeling methods or label-free comparative analysis of proteins in the mass spectrometer, it is unlikely that a single protein initiates disease progression. Decoding which proteins signal and/or induce nephropathy in diabetes is the current quest of multiple investigators. This approach may transform patient care in diabetes to a "science" based on proteomics and urinomics.

Out HH, Can H, Spentzos D, et al. Prediction of diabetic nephropathy using urine proteomic profiling 10 years prior to development of nephropathy. *Diabetes Care* 2007;30:638–643.

Rossing K, Mischak H, Dakna M, et al.; on behalf of the PREDICTions Network. Urinary proteomics in diabetes and CKD. *J Am Soc Nephrol* 2008;19:1283–1290.

Thamer C, Machann J, Stefan N, et al. Variations in PPARD determine the change in body composition during lifestyle intervention: A whole-body magnetic resonance study. *J Clin Endocrinol Metab* 2008;93:1497–1500.

Thongboonkerd V. Searching for novel biomarkers and new therapeutic targets of diabetic nephropathy using proteomics approaches. *Contrib Nephrol* 2008;160:37–52.

Thrailkill KM, Nimmo T, Bunn RC, et al. Microalbuminuria in type 1 diabetes mellitus is associated with enhanced excretion of the endocytic multiligand receptors megalin and cubilin. *Diabetes Care* 2009;32:1266–1288.

9. **Does kidney biopsy help in managing diabetic nephropathy?**
Until recently, the value of and need for a kidney biopsy in planning therapy for diabetes complicated by proteinuria and/or azotemia was considered self-evident. Although currently kidney biopsy retains its preeminent role in distinguishing multiple proteinuric disorders from diabetic glomerulopathy, near-term challenge to the diagnostic primacy of renal biopsy is probable.

First, the similar histopathology between diabetic nodular intercapillary sclerosis defined by Kimmelstiel and Wilson and nodular glomerulosclerosis observed in dysproteinemias, lobular membranoproliferative glomerulonephritis, glomerular deposition disease, and chronic hypoxic states can confound recognition of the rare disorder idiopathic nodular glomerulosclerosis, which is diagnosed in the absence of these conditions. Second, the diagnosis of diabetic nephropathy is overused because many patients have diabetes and kidney disease from other causes. Last, as discussed in Question 8, the introduction of proteomics and urinomics permits highly specific identification of renal histopathologic disorders and has been demonstrated to proffer highly accurate predictive analysis of renal allograft biopsies that is forcing revision of "established criteria" for rejection and may yield the desired information without the surgical risks of biopsy.

Chang CS, Yang AH, Chang CH. Nodular glomerulosclerosis mimicking diabetic nephropathy without overt diabetes mellitus. *Clin Nephrol* 2005;64:300–304.

Kasmani R, Thiyagarajan T, Narwal-Chadha R, et al. The other end of spectrum in hypertension "Idiopathic nodular glomerulosclerosis." *Internal Urol Nephrol* 2010;42(3):857–859.

Kimmelstiel P, Wilson C. Benign and malignant hypertension and nephrosclerosis. A clinical and pathological study. *Am J Pathol* 1936;12:45–48.

Reeve J, Einnecke G, Mengel M, et al. Diagnosing rejection in renal transplants: A comparison of molecular and histopathology-based approaches. *Am J Transplant* 2009;9:1802–1810.

10. **Which renal replacement therapy is best for patients with diabetes and ESRD?**
Each patient with irreversible uremia must choose further management from a menu of four main choices: (1) no additional medical intervention (passive suicide), (2) peritoneal dialysis, (3) hemodialysis, or (4) renal transplantation. Although no prospective randomized trials have been conducted, mainly because of the ethical issues involved in removing patient choice, evaluations of equivalent patient cohorts strongly support the view that in terms of patient survival and/or degree of rehabilitation, the best option for patients with diabetes and ESRD is renal transplantation.

Until it was clearly established that long-term survival was possible in those patients whose kidney failure was caused by diabetes, a strong negative bias excluded those with kidney failure as a complication of diabetes from dialysis treatment. An early (1972), mainly negative, report in the *Journal of the American Medical Association* entitled "The Sad Truth about Hemodialysis in Diabetic Nephropathy" based on a 1-year mortality of 78% concluded the following: "Dialysis in diabetes may be considered as a palliative measure with little likelihood of long-term survival or improvement in quality of life."

In the 1970s and early 1980s many transplant programs excluded patients with diabetes and ESRD from consideration for renal transplantation. However, in centers that did perform transplants in patients with diabetes during this period, survival exceeded that of patients with diabetes continuing dialysis. Currently regimens of improved glycemic and hypertensive control have reduced macrovascular and microvascular diabetic and uremic complications facilitating longer patient survival in which kidney transplantation is established as the preferred treatment for patients with diabetes and ESRD.

Although survival of patients with diabetes and ESRD with a kidney transplant is continuously improving, according to the U.S. Renal Data System national registry, it continues to be 10% to 20% lower, after 5 years, than in other causes of renal disease. The most recent analysis of patient's survival in kidney transplant recipients with diabetes noted 90.6% 1-year survival and 79.5% 3-year survival for recipients of deceased donor grafts, and 96.4% 1-year and 88.3% 3-year survival for those receiving a living donor transplant. The annual death rate of transplant recipients is approximately one third in patients with diabetes who remain on dialysis. A strict outcome comparison, however, demands recognition of the reality that a strong selection bias extracts the fittest patients for kidney transplants, leaving a residual pool of those patients undergoing dialysis who have advanced comorbidities that preempted a transplant to continue on dialysis.

Kolff WJ. The sad truth about hemodialysis in diabetic nephropathy. *JAMA* 1972;222:1386–1389.

U.S. Renal Data System, *USRDS 2009 Annual Data Report: Atlas of End-Stage Renal Disease in the United States*, Volume 3. Bethesda, MD: National Institutes of Health, National Institute of Diabetes and Digestive and Kidney Diseases, 2009.

11. Is hemoglobin A1c applicable as an indicator of metabolic control in diabetes after onset of renal failure?

Following careful review of pertinent studies, Kovesdy, Park, and Kalantar-Zadeh conclude that it is "unclear" whether glycemic control in patients with advanced CKD, including those with ESRD sustained by maintenance dialysis treatment, is "beneficial." The term "burnt-out diabetes" was applied to that condition in which "complex changes in glucose homeostasis related to decreased kidney function and to dialytic therapies" may induce spontaneous resolution of hyperglycemia modulating hemoglobin A1c levels. In stages 4 and 5 of CKD and ESRD, current markers of glycemic control in patients with diabetes require prospective studies to affirm their value in predicting microvascular and macrovascular complications.

Percentages of HbA1c and glycated hemoglobin (GA%), both markers of glycemic control in diabetes, were compared in patients with diabetes undergoing maintenance hemodialysis ($n = 415$) and peritoneal dialysis ($n = 55$), with 49 control diabetic subjects without signs of nephropathy. As expected, serum glucose levels were higher in patients undergoing hemodialysis (169.7 mg/dL) and peritoneal dialysis (168.6 mg/dL) compared with those without nephropathy (146.1 mg/dL). GA% was also significantly higher ($p < 0.02$) in patients undergoing hemodialysis (20.6%) and peritoneal dialysis (19.0%) than in controls (8.0%). Paradoxically, HbA1c was lower in both cohorts of patients undergoing dialysis—hemodialysis (6.78%), peritoneal dialysis (6.87%)—than in controls (7.3%). The investigators concluded that HbA1c "significantly underestimates glycemic control in peritoneal and hemodialysis patients relative to GA%." Whether monitoring of metabolic control in patients undergoing dialysis with diabetes should be based on glycated hemoglobin or glycated albumin, a molecule that has also been advocated as superior to HbA1c, is a question worthy of future prospective controlled studies.

Freedman BI, Shenoy RN, Planer JA, et al. Comparison of glycated albumin and hemoglobin A1c concentrations in diabetic subjects on peritoneal and hemodialysis. *Perit Dial Int* 2010;30:72–79.

Kovesdy CP, Park JC, Kalantar-Zadeh K. Glycemic control and burnt-out diabetes in ESRD. *Semin Dial* 2010;23(2):148–156.

Park HI, Kim YS, Lee J, et al. Performance characteristics of glycated albumin and its clinical usefulness in diabetic patients on hemodialysis. *Korean J Lab Med* 2009;29:406–414.

KEY POINTS: DIABETIC NEPHROPATHY

1. The global pandemic of diabetes raised diabetes to first place among causes of renal failure throughout the world.

2. Both genetic predisposition and behavior (lifestyle) interplay in the pathogenesis of diabetic nephropathy.

3. Hyperglycemia stimulates potentially injurious oxidative products such as protein kinase C and transforming growth factor beta.

4. Diabetic retinopathy is present in more than 95% of individuals with diabetic nephropathy.

5. Growing treatment of hyperglycemia and hypertension reduced the incidence of renal failure in persons with diabetes.

6. Metabolic control in patients undergoing maintenance dialysis requires a more specific indicator than currently measured HbA1c.

12. **Might a new classification of diabetic nephropathy improve patient understanding and management?**

In both systemic lupus erythematosus and renal allograft rejection, classification of kidney pathology fostered design and testing of specific clinical regimens that facilitate direct comparisons of therapeutic interventions. Recently, the Research Committee of the Renal Pathology Society devised a consensus classification combining type 1 and type 2 diabetic nephropathies. Although assessment of the utility of this classification must await its use and analyses of generated reports, it may prove helpful to examine the pathologic findings that experts thought might distinguish progressive stages of diabetic nephropathy. Overriding the future of any classification system that is dependent on kidney biopsies is the issue raised in Questions 8 and 9 of whether proteomic analysis of urine and/or plasma samples might end the need for tissue sampling.

The proposed classification of diabetic nephropathy applies to both types 1 and 2 of diabetes, designating four hierarchical glomerular lesions that are evaluated separately from interstitial and vascular changes. Class I requires glomerular basement membrane thickening (electron microscopy) associated with mild, nonspecific changes by light microscopy. Class II is assigned to mild (IIa) or severe (IIb) mesangial expansion without nodular sclerosis or global glomerulosclerosis in more than 50% of glomeruli. When at least one glomerulus exhibits the nodular sclerosis described as a Kimmelstiel-Wilson nodule, the severity is assigned to Class III. Class IV, termed "advanced diabetic glomerulosclerosis in which more than 50% of glomeruli have global glomerulosclerosis," is a finding that, in the presence of other evidence both clinical and/or pathologic, indicates that the sclerosis results diabetic nephropathy.

Whether this new classification is either adopted or proves useful is as of this writing uncertain.

Tervaert TW, Mooyaart AL, Amann K, et al. Pathologic classification of diabetic nephropathy. *J Am Soc Nephrol* 2010;21:556–563.

CHAPTER 35

LUPUS NEPHRITIS

William L. Whittier, MD, and Edmund J. Lewis, MD

1. **How common is systemic lupus erythematosus (SLE), and how often is lupus nephritis present in patients with SLE?**
   The prevalence of SLE in the United States averages 40/100,000 (0.04%), has a peak age of onset of 20 to 40 years, and is more common in women and certain ethnic groups (especially African Americans). Renal involvement occurs in 20% to 60% of patients with SLE, and the kidney is the most common major organ affected.

2. **What is the single most important test to order to determine if a patient with SLE needs further evaluation for lupus nephritis?**
   A urinalysis should be performed at every visit in patients with SLE because lupus nephritis may be asymptomatic or intermittent. The presence of protein or blood on dipstick and/or the presence of red blood cells (RBCs) or RBC casts on microscopic examination requires further workup for lupus nephritis. Glycosuria and sterile pyuria can also represent renal involvement. Proteinuria, if present on dipstick, should be quantified, preferably with a 24-hour urine collection. The presence of any blood, protein, or casts in the urine warrants further nephrologic evaluation.

3. **How does a patient with lupus nephritis present clinically?**
   Although renal involvement may be the first sign of SLE in an individual patient, lupus nephritis typically becomes clinically apparent as a manifestation of the systemic disease. Some patients with lupus nephritis are asymptomatic, but classically, patients will have a variety of systemic manifestations including but not limited to cutaneous abnormalities, fever, malaise, weight loss, synovitis, Raynaud's phenomenon, serositis, pericarditis, retinopathy, thrombotic microangiopathy, and/or neuropsychiatric involvement. Hematologic abnormalities may be present such as leukopenia, anemia, and/or thrombocytopenia. Evidence of immunologic activity in the serum is usually present as antinuclear antibodies (ANA), antibodies to double-stranded DNA (anti-dsDNA) and Smith (anti-Sm), and hypocomplementemia (see Serologic Evaluation). The pattern of clinical activity varies between patients but characteristically is one of relapsing and remitting disease. Only 5% to 10% of patients with discoid lupus will develop SLE, and, if so, seldom develop nephritis. Certain medications, such as hydralazine or procainamide, may cause drug-induced systemic lupus but are only rarely associated with lupus nephritis.
   In patients with renal involvement, presentation can range from subtle disease such as asymptomatic microscopic hematuria and proteinuria on urinalysis with normal renal function to nephritic and/or nephrotic syndrome and rapidly progressive glomerulonephritis with renal failure and hypertension. The nephrotic syndrome is present in approximately 25% of patients during their disease course. Microscopic hematuria is commonly associated with proteinuria and rarely found in isolation. Renal failure, defined by an elevated serum creatinine, is present in approximately 25% to 50% of patients with lupus nephritis.

4. **If my patient with lupus has hematuria or proteinuria, what immunologic serology should I order to determine if lupus nephritis is present or active?**
   The only definitive way to determine if lupus nephritis is present or active is to perform a kidney biopsy. However, certain immunologic serology is useful to establish parameters of

activity that can be helpful to diagnosis SLE and/or monitor relapses or response to treatment. Serologic evaluation should include ANA, anti-Sm, anti-Ro/SSA, anti-La/SSB, anti-ribonucleoprotein (anti-RNP), anti-dsDNA, complement components, rheumatoid factor, and antiphospholipid antibodies. This serology may be positive in a variety of diseases other than SLE, but anti-Sm is quite specific for SLE. Anti-dsDNA antibodies, when present, are strongly associated with lupus nephritis. Hypocomplementemia and anti-dsDNA antibodies will typically correlate with disease activity.

5. **When does a kidney biopsy need to be performed in the setting of SLE?**
Any patient suspected of having lupus nephritis should be further evaluated with a kidney biopsy. This procedure is considered when abnormalities are present on urinalysis, such as protein, blood, or casts, often coupled with abnormal serology or reduced renal function. Severe involvement, such as nephrotic syndrome or nephritic syndrome with or without renal failure, will require a kidney biopsy for further evaluation. Even when subtle abnormalities are present (i.e., normal renal function with or without hematuria and less than 1 g of proteinuria/day), severe lupus nephritis may be present on kidney biopsy. Thus, a kidney biopsy should be performed to establish a diagnosis, determine prognosis, and guide therapy. Many patients may require more than one biopsy during their disease course. This procedure may be necessary to alter therapy because the characteristics of lupus nephritis may change over time or to determine if there is late progression of the disease, which may not be amenable to further immunosuppressive treatment.

6. **What are the pathologic features of lupus nephritis?**
Based on pathologic features in the glomeruli on kidney biopsy, two modern classifications for lupus nephritis exist (Tables 35-1 and 35-2). In addition, the presence of tubuloreticular inclusions in the glomerular capillary endothelial cell on electron microscopy are relatively specific for lupus nephritis.

7. **Do the lupus nephritis classifications provide information on treatment, pathogenesis, and/or prognosis?**
Both classifications provide valuable information on how to treat patients with lupus nephritis. Classes III (segmental proliferative) and IV (diffuse proliferative), and Class V (membranous), if it has concomitant features of III and IV, all are considered severe lupus nephritis, which generally requires aggressive immunomodulatory therapy, whereas pure mesangial (II) or

TABLE 35-1. THE WORLD HEALTH ORGANIZATION CLASSIFICATION OF LUPUS NEPHRITIS	
I	Normal glomeruli
II	Pure mesangial alterations
III	Focal segmental glomerulonephritis
IV	Diffuse glomerulonephritis
V	Diffuse membranous glomerulonephritis
Va	Pure membranous glomerulonephritis
Vb	Associated with lesions of category II
Vc	Associated with lesions of category III
Vd	Associated with lesions of category IV
VI	Advanced sclerosing glomerulonephritis

TABLE 35-2.   THE INTERNATIONAL SOCIETY OF NEPHROLOGY/RENAL PATHOLOGY SOCIETY (ISN/RPS) CLASSIFICATION OF LUPUS NEPHRITIS

I	Minimal mesangial lupus nephritis
II	Mesangial proliferative lupus nephritis
III	Focal lupus nephritis (<50% of glomeruli)
IV	Diffuse lupus nephritis (≥50% of glomeruli)
IV-S	Diffuse segmental lupus nephritis (<50% glomerular surface area)
IV-G	Diffuse global lupus nephritis (≥50% glomerular surface area)
V	Membranous lupus nephritis
VI	Advanced sclerosing lupus nephritis

pure membranous (V) requires less. The World Health Organization (WHO) classification categorizes information about the pathogenesis of the lesions (i.e., immune complex mediated or nonimmune complex mediated). The WHO classification also helps delineate prognosis because patients with severe lupus nephritis have a worse prognosis than those without severe lupus nephritis. In addition, those patients with diffuse proliferative lesions are generally more likely to achieve a remission and less likely to progress to end-stage kidney failure than those patients with severe segmental lesions (Table 35-3).

8. **What nephropathology occurs in patients with SLE that is not part of the classic lupus nephritis?**
Although glomerular inflammatory involvement is the prototypical example of lupus nephritis, the tubules, interstitium, and vasculature of the kidney can also be affected. Frequently patients are taking nonsteroidal anti-inflammatory agents, which can cause acute tubular necrosis and interstitial nephritis. Antiphospholipid antibodies may give rise to a thrombotic microangiopathy. The epithelial cells in the glomerular capillaries may also become effaced, termed podocytopathy, which typically gives rise to the dramatic onset of the nephrotic syndrome, similar to the clinical presentation of minimal change disease.

9. **How is lupus nephritis managed?**
Although the clinical presentation (signs, symptoms, serologic and urine tests) is an important part of determining the therapy of lupus nephritis, the information gained from a kidney biopsy is the most useful determinant to make a treatment decision for this disease. The biopsy will differentiate severe active lupus nephritis (diffuse or segmental proliferative glomerulonephritis with or without membranous) from milder (mesangial glomerulonephritis) or inactive forms.
    Treatment of severe active lupus nephritis (Table 35-4) is separated into an induction phase, of which the goal is to induce a remission, and a maintenance phase, of which the goal is to maintain remission and prevent relapse. Because lupus nephritis is a rare and heterogeneous disease, a standard treatment algorithm does not exist, and treatment is presently individualized. However, based on evidence from clinical trials, the therapeutic options for the induction phase are high-dose prednisone coupled with cyclophosphamide, mycophenolate mofetil, or (rarely) azathioprine. Cyclosporine is another option for induction, typically when membranous glomerulonephritis is present. Plasmapheresis has been proven to be ineffective when added to induction with cyclophosphamide and prednisone. The length of induction depends on the method of administration and the response or side effects to the therapy but is typically from

TABLE 35-3.   FACTORS FOR PROGRESSION TO KIDNEY FAILURE IN LUPUS NEPHRITIS

Clinical Factors at Baseline:
Elevated serum creatinine
Hypertension
Nephrotic-range proteinuria
Anemia
Race: African American or Hispanic
Anti-Ro/SSA antibodies

Clinical Factors on Followup:
Delay in treatment
Frequency and severity of relapse
Failure to achieve complete or partial remission
Increasing serum creatinine

Histopathologic:
Severe lupus nephritis
    Severe segmental has higher risk than diffuse proliferative
    Membranous lesions with either segmental or diffuse proliferative lesions have
        higher risk than isolated membranous lesions
Presence of crescents
Tubulointerstitial disease
High chronicity index
Thrombotic microangiopathy

2 to 12 months of therapy. Therapeutic choices for the maintenance phase, which occurs after successful induction and lasts several years (perhaps for life), include mycophenolate mofetil, azathioprine, rarely cyclosporine, or low-dose alternate-day prednisone.

If cyclophosphamide is chosen for induction, prevention of potential infectious complications such as *Pneumocystis* pneumonia can be achieved with trimethoprim-sulfamethoxazole. Prevention of gonadal toxicity can be attempted with leuprolide for woman and testosterone for men. Gonadal cryopreservation should be considered prior to therapy.

Extrarenal manifestations and symptoms should be identified and treated appropriately. Use of an angiotensin-converting enzyme (ACE) inhibitor or angiotensin II receptor blocker (ARB) and control of blood pressure are essential. Managing sequelae of the nephrotic syndrome, such as hyperlipidemia and edema, can be achieved with lipid-lowering agents and diuretics coupled with a low-sodium diet.

10. **What tests are useful to monitor response to treatment?**
Urine studies that should be routinely followed include a urinalysis (dipstick and microscopic evaluation) to monitor for hematuria and proteinuria. The urine protein should also be routinely quantified because lack of improvement may be a sign of unresponsiveness. Serum chemistries, renal function, albumin, and immune serology (ANA, dS-DNA, complement components) should be assessed at every visit.

11. **What is the typical response to treatment?**
There are many variables predictive of outcome, but with severe lupus nephritis and normal renal function, 60% to 85% of patients will achieve a complete or partial remission in 3 to 6 months with induction therapy. This response rate is less likely with abnormal renal function. Because

---

TABLE 35-4.   IMMUNOMODULATORY TREATMENT OPTIONS FOR SEVERE LUPUS NEPHRITIS

INDUCTION

High-dose steroids (e.g., intravenous [IV] methylprednisolone initially or oral prednisone 1 mg/kg not to exceed 80 mg daily, tapering at 4 weeks depending on response) plus one of the following:

Oral cyclophosphamide* 2 mg/kg daily (not to exceed 200 mg daily) for 6 to 12 weeks, dose adjusted based on white blood cell count nadir

High-dose IV cyclophosphamide* 0.5 to 1.5 g/m^2 body surface area (BSA) monthly for 6 months and two more quarterly doses. Dose not to exceed 1.5 g/m^2 BSA and adjusted based on white blood cell count

Low-dose IV cyclophosphamide* 500 mg/m^2 BSA every 2 weeks for six doses

Oral mycophenolate mofetil 2 to 3 g daily in two divided doses

MAINTENANCE

Choices of maintenance therapy are as follows:

Oral mycophenolate mofetil 0.5 to 3 g daily in two divided doses with prednisone taper

Oral azathioprine 1 to 3 mg/kg body weight daily with prednisone taper

Cyclosporine dosed 2 to 4 mg/kg/day to keep trough levels 75 to 200 ng/mL with low-dose prednisone

Oral prednisone 10 to 20 mg on alternate days

*Dose adjustment for kidney dysfunction is recommended.

---

renal function correlates directly with response to therapy, early diagnosis of lupus nephritis with a kidney biopsy is imperative. Overall, 5% to 22% of patients with lupus nephritis will progress to end-stage renal disease. Other clinical factors associated with progression are failure to achieve an initial remission, nephrotic-range proteinuria, hypertension, anemia, the presence of anti-Ro/SSA antibodies, and African American or Hispanic ethnicity. Pathologic features associated with a poor prognosis are the presence of crescents, severe segmental lesions with or without membranous nephritis, and extensive tubulointerstitial disease (see Table 35-3).

12. **What are common complications of immunomodulatory therapy?**
    Complications can be categorized as short or long term. Short-term complications directly related to the immunomodulating agents include bone marrow suppression and infectious complications. Gonadal failure and hemorrhagic cystitis can occur with cyclophosphamide. Gastrointestinal toxicity, such as early satiety, nausea, and diarrhea, is common with use of mycophenolate mofetil. High-dose prednisone is associated with cushingoid features, weight gain, cutaneous changes such as striae and acne, hypertension, osteopenia, and exacerbation of peptic ulcer disease. Long-term complications are generally correlated with a higher cumulative dose of cyclophosphamide and include malignancies, bone marrow suppression, gonadal failure, and infectious complications. Avascular necrosis and osteopenia are also related to long-term prednisone use.

13. **Is it advisable for my patient with lupus nephritis to get pregnant? How should pregnant patients be managed differently?**
    Both SLE and lupus nephritis commonly occur in women of childbearing age. Women with lupus nephritis have higher rates of maternal complications during pregnancy, including preeclampsia (difficult to distinguish between a lupus flare) and preterm delivery. Fetal complications are also more common, such as low birthweight or even fetal loss. Patients

with antiphospholipid antibodies are prone to develop spontaneous abortions and fetal loss. Anti-Ro/SSA and Anti-La/SSB antibodies can cross the placenta and cause cutaneous neonatal lupus and/or congenital heart block.

Prepregnancy counseling is recommended. The maternal–fetal risk of complication is lower in patients with normal renal function, normal blood pressure, a lack of antiphospholipid antibodies, and inactive disease.

If pregnancy is a consideration or if it occurs, a multidisciplinary approach with an obstetrician who specializes in high-risk pregnancies is recommended. Assessment for lupus serology, proteinuria, renal function, and systemic and pulmonary hypertension is necessary. Medications should be carefully reviewed, and, if possible, those that have high teratogenic potential should be discontinued in favor of those that have less. Medications used frequently that exhibit teratogenicity include cyclophosphamide, mycophenolate mofetil, ACE inhibitors and ARBs, and HMG-CoA reductase inhibitors. However, the outcome of the pregnancy is directly related to maternal health, and if severe lupus nephritis develops or flares during pregnancy, these medications may be considered to prevent the onset of renal failure.

KEY POINTS: LUPUS NEPHRITIS

1. A urinalysis should be performed on every patient with systemic lupus erythematosus (SLE) at each visit, and abnormalities in the urine should be confirmed and evaluated by a nephrologist. Immunologic serology for SLE and serum chemistries are also useful to differentiate if lupus nephritis is present.

2. Early diagnosis of lupus nephritis is imperative because renal function at the time of biopsy correlates with remission.

3. A kidney biopsy can be performed to determine diagnosis, treatment, and/or prognosis. A biopsy can help differentiate between severe and mild lupus glomerulonephritis, which requires different therapy.

4. Therapy of severe active lupus nephritis is with immunosuppressive medications. Prednisone, cyclophosphamide, mycophenolate mofetil, azathioprine, or cyclosporine are choices that may be used to induce or maintain remission.

5. Because SLE and lupus nephritis frequently occur in women of childbearing age, special considerations and counseling should be given prior to pregnancy if possible. A multidisciplinary approach is recommended.

14. **Can lupus nephritis recur following transplantation?**
Yes. In transplanted patients with ESRD from lupus nephritis undergoing transplant biopsy for renal failure, hematuria, or proteinuria, recurrent lupus nephritis is present in 11% to 52% of biopsies but rarely leads to graft loss unless there is concomitant chronic allograft nephropathy. In addition, based on the larger series, recurrent lupus nephritis does not have an impact on patient survival.

15. **How often will patients with ESRD from lupus nephritis experience extrarenal flares?**
Extrarenal flares were initially thought to be extremely infrequent once a patient starts dialysis, a process termed "burnout." This may be related to the relative immunodeficiency of uremia and/or dialysis, or it may just characterize the progressive course of lupus. However, in general, patients receiving peritoneal dialysis do not experience fewer extrarenal flares, and modern epidemiologic studies have revealed a persistence of lupus activity, both symptomatically and serologically, in patients undergoing hemodialysis. This may be related to improved dialysis techniques and biocompatibility of dialysis membranes.

BIBLIOGRAPHY

1. Appel GB, Contreras G, Dooley MA, et al. Mycophenolate mofetil versus cyclophosphamide for induction treatment of lupus nephritis. *J Am Soc Nephrol* 2009;20:1103–1112.
2. Austin HA III, Illei GG, Braun MJ, et al. Randomized, controlled trial of prednisone, cyclophosphamide, and cyclosporine in lupus membranous nephropathy. *J Am Soc Nephrol* 2009;20:901–911.
3. Behara VY, Whittier WL, Korbet SM, et al. Pathogenetic features of severe segmental lupus nephritis. *Nephrol Dial Transplant* 2009;25(1):153–159.
4. Birmingham DJ, Rovin BH, Shidham G, et al. Spot urine protein/creatinine ratios are unreliable estimates of 24 h proteinuria in most systemic lupus erythematosus nephritis flares. *Kidney Int* 2007;72:865–870.
5. Burgos PI, Perkins EL, Pons-Estel GJ, et al. Risk factors and impact of recurrent lupus nephritis in patients with systemic lupus erythematosus undergoing renal transplantation: Data from a single US institution. *Arthritis Rheum* 2009;60:2757–2766.
6. Cervera R, Khamashta MA, Font J, et al. Systemic lupus erythematosus: clinical and immunologic patterns of disease expression in a cohort of 1,000 patients. The European Working Party on Systemic Lupus Erythematosus. *Medicine* (Baltimore) 1993;72:113–124.
7. Chan TM, Li FK, Tang CS, et al. Efficacy of mycophenolate mofetil in patients with diffuse proliferative lupus nephritis. Hong Kong-Guangzhou Nephrology Study Group. *N Engl J Med* 2000;343:1156–1162.
8. Chen YE, Korbet SM, Katz RS, et al. Value of a complete or partial remission in severe lupus nephritis. *Clin J Am Soc Nephrol* 2008;3:46–53.
9. Christopher-Stine L, Siedner M, Lin J, et al. Renal biopsy in lupus patients with low levels of proteinuria. *J Rheumatol* 2007;34:332–335.
10. Churg J, Bernstein J, Glassock RJ. *Renal Disease: Classification and Atlas of Glomerular Diseases.* 2nd ed. New York: Igaku-Shoin, 1995.
11. Contreras G, Pardo V, Leclercq B, et al. Sequential therapies for proliferative lupus nephritis. *N Engl J Med* 2004;350:971–980.
12. Daugas E, Nochy D, Huong DL, et al. Antiphospholipid syndrome nephropathy in systemic lupus erythematosus. *J Am Soc Nephrol* 2002;13:42–52.
13. Ginzler EM, Dooley MA, Aranow C, et al. Mycophenolate mofetil or intravenous cyclophosphamide for lupus nephritis. *N Engl J Med* 2005;353:2219–2228.
14. Goral S, Ynares C, Shappell SB, et al. Recurrent lupus nephritis in renal transplant recipients revisited: it is not rare. *Transplantation* 2003;75:651–656.
15. Houssiau FA, Vasconcelos C, D'Cruz D, et al. The 10-year follow-up data of the Euro-Lupus Nephritis Trial comparing low-dose and high-dose intravenous cyclophosphamide. *Ann Rheum Dis* 2010;69:61–64.
16. Korbet SM, Lewis EJ, Schwartz MM, et al. Factors predictive of outcome in severe lupus nephritis. Lupus Nephritis Collaborative Study Group. *Am J Kidney Dis* 2000;35:904–914.
17. Korbet SM, Schwartz MM, Evans J, et al. Severe lupus nephritis: racial differences in presentation and outcome. *J Am Soc Nephrol* 2007;18:244–254.
18. Kraft SW, Schwartz MM, Korbet SM, et al. Glomerular podocytopathy in patients with systemic lupus erythematosus. *J Am Soc Nephrol* 2005;16:175–179.
19. Levey AS, Lan SP, Corwin HL, et al. Progression and remission of renal disease in the Lupus Nephritis Collaborative Study. Results of treatment with prednisone and short-term oral cyclophosphamide. *Ann Intern Med* 1992;116:114–123.
20. Lewis EJ, Hunsicker LG, Lan SP, et al. A controlled trial of plasmapheresis therapy in severe lupus nephritis. The Lupus Nephritis Collaborative Study Group. *N Engl J Med* 1992;326:1373–1379.
21. Lewis EJ, Schwartz MM, Korbet SM, et al. (eds.). *Lupus Nephritis: Second Edition.* Oxford, England: Oxford Clinical Nephrology Series, 2010.
22. Moroni G, Doria A, Mosca M, et al. A randomized pilot trial comparing cyclosporine and azathioprine for maintenance therapy in diffuse lupus nephritis over four years. *Clin J Am Soc Nephrol* 2006;1:925–932.
23. Moroni G, Quaglini S, Banfi G, et al. Pregnancy in lupus nephritis. *Am J Kidney Dis* 2002;40:713–720.
24. Moroni G, Tantardini F, Gallelli B, et al. The long-term prognosis of renal transplantation in patients with lupus nephritis. *Am J Kidney Dis* 2005;45:903–911.
25. Najafi CC, Korbet SM, Lewis EJ, et al. Significance of histologic patterns of glomerular injury upon long-term prognosis in severe lupus glomerulonephritis. *Kidney Int* 2001;59:2156–2163.
26. Ribeiro FM, Leite MA, Velarde GC, et al. Activity of systemic lupus erythematosus in end-stage renal disease patients: Study in a Brazilian cohort. *Am J Nephrol* 2005;25:596–603.
27. Rodby RA, Korbet SM, Lewis EJ. Persistence of clinical and serologic activity in patients with systemic lupus erythematosus undergoing peritoneal dialysis. *Am J Med* 1987;83:613–618.
28. Weening JJ, D'Agati VD, Schwartz MM, et al. The classification of glomerulonephritis in systemic lupus erythematosus revisited. *J Am Soc Nephrol* 2004;15:241–250.

DYSPROTEINEMIAS OR LIGHT CHAIN DISEASES

Ashley B. Irish, MBBS, and Rajalingam Sinniah, MD, PhD

CHAPTER 36

1. **What is myeloma?**

   Myeloma is a hematologic malignancy comprising about 1% of malignancies. It consists of an excess of bone marrow–derived plasma cells with two cardinal features: dysregulated overproduction of a monoclonal immunoglobulin (the paraprotein or M-protein) and associated light chains (kappa [κ] and lambda [λ]) with bone destruction usually manifest as osteolytic lesions. The International Myeloma Working Group (2003) and Mayo Clinic Diagnostic Criteria for symptomatic myeloma require all of the following: a serum or urine monoclonal protein, increased bone marrow (clonal) plasma cells ($\geq$10%) or biopsy-proven plasmacytoma, and end-organ damage not explained by other pathology (hypercalcemia, renal failure, anemia, lytic bone disease). The most common class of whole immunoglobulin (Ig) is IgG followed by IgA and IgD. In some patients only an associated light chain (LC) component is detected. It is a disease of the elderly, with the median age of diagnosis being older than 65 years of age. At diagnosis, nearly half of patients have biochemical evidence of renal damage and up to 10% present with severe renal failure requiring urgent dialysis. Renal failure is most common in patients with IgD and LC myeloma.

2. **In what ways does myeloma cause acute kidney injury?**

   Myeloma can cause acute kidney injury (AKI) in several ways and it is the renal tubule that is most affected. The most common histologic finding is myeloma cast nephropathy (MCN) characterized by eosinophilic acellular casts, with brittle cracks commonly in the distal tubules and collecting ducts, and to a lesser extent, in the proximal tubules with epithelial cell necrosis and thinning and dilatation of the lumina. The casts are surrounded by inflammatory cells including macrophages, multinucleated giant cells, and polymorphonuclear neutrophils. There is interstitial edema and inflammation and in the later stages interstitial fibrosis (Fig. 36-1). The casts usually stain for a monoclonal light chain. In some cases casts are absent but the interstitial inflammation and fibrosis are present. Less commonly, injury relates to acute tubular necrosis precipitated by sepsis or hypotension, hyperuricemia related to high cell turnover, Fanconi syndrome from proximal tubular dysfunction, and other specific disorders that have glomerular involvement known as amyloidosis and monoclonal immunoglobulin deposition diseases (MIDD). The use of renal biopsy to distinguish between these potential etiologies and to guide therapy is frequently required.

3. **What can precipitate AKI in myeloma?**

   Patients with myeloma are particularly vulnerable to factors that cause volume depletion or sudden reductions in glomerular filtration. This is because these changes reduce tubular flow and increase the exposure of the tubule to high single-nephron light chain concentrations. Classically, hypercalcemia related to plasma cell–mediated bone destruction and release of calcium causes volume depletion and vasoconstriction and is present in around 15% of patients at diagnosis. Nonsteroidal agents prescribed for bone pain and intravenous contrast agents used for diagnostic investigations also abruptly reduce glomerular filtration and are associated with acute renal failure, which is sometimes irreversible. Sepsis resulting from chemotherapy and reduced immunoglobulin levels is also associated with AKI.

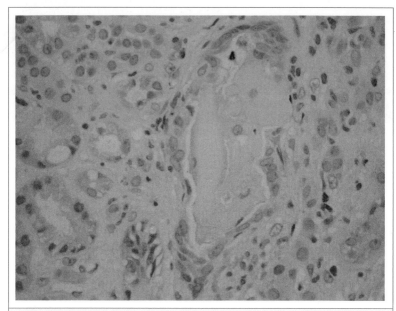

Figure 36-1. Myeloma/light chain cast nephropathy. The tubular cast shows attached giant and inflammatory cells and distension of the lumen. There is interstitial inflammatory cellular infiltration (hematoxylin and eosin ×40).

4. **What clinical and laboratory clues suggest myeloma as the cause of acute kidney injury?**

   Patients with myeloma most frequently present with the signs and symptoms of renal failure, anemia, or malignant bone pain, typically low back pain unrelieved by rest or simple analgesics. Myeloma should be suspected when the patient has any severe cytopenia (anemia, thrombocytopenia, or pancytopenia resulting from marrow invasion by plasma cells), relatively preserved albumin-corrected calcium (from bone release of calcium), immunoparesis (when all immunoglobulin classes are reduced), or an increased globulin fraction as a result of the excessively high monoclonal whole immunoglobulin. Urinalysis, although important, may be misleading because the increased urinary excretion of light chains associated with myeloma is not detected by testing for albumin (e.g., Albustix) but only for total protein (e.g., sulfosalicylic acid test) or by specific urine electrophoresis and immunofixation. The diagnosis of myeloma in renal disease is now rapidly and preferentially made by the measurement of the serum free light chain (sFLC) ratio (see Question 12).

5. **What specific laboratory diagnostic tests are used for myeloma?**

   Serum protein electrophoresis (SPE) by separation of protein upon an agarose gel can detect the whole immunoglobulin in the range of 1 to 5g/dL but only detects increased LC in patients who have very high levels of LC-only myeloma and is semi-quantitative. Serum immunofixation electrophoresis (IFE) is around 10 times more sensitive for immunoglobulins and LC but is not quantitative. Urine IFE requires concentrated urine samples for the detection of free light chains and can detect low levels of LC yet remains less sensitive than sFLC measurement because sFLC are elevated before urine overflow may occur.

6. **What is the value of a bone marrow biopsy in patients with myeloma and AKI?**

   Bone marrow biopsy is usually performed to confirm marrow involvement by plasma cells and for quantification and determination of clonality. The bone marrow shows displacement of the normal marrow by plasma cells, which ranges from complete replacement by sheets of tumor cells or as nodular aggregates. The mature plasma cells have eccentric nuclei with "clock-face" chromatin and plentiful cytoplasm, and the immature forms are pleomorphic with abnormal nuclear forms. Immunoperoxidase stains show the tumor cells to stain positive with CD138 and a monoclonal light chain restriction (Fig. 36-2).

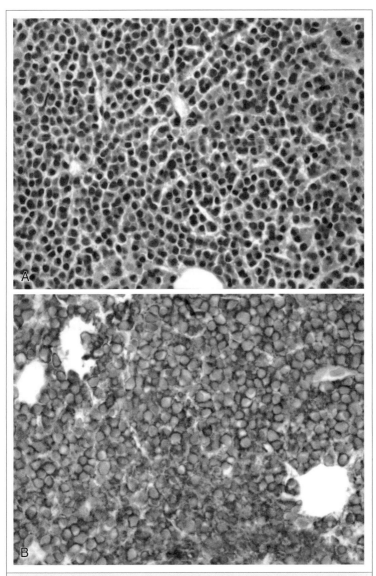

Figure 36-2. *A,* Multiple myeloma. The bone marrow is replaced by plasma cells showing nuclear chromatin clumping and eccentric nuclei (hematoxylin and eosin ×40). *B,* Multiple myeloma. Immunoperoxidase staining for CD138 and monoclonal antibodies will show membrane and cytoplasm staining (immunoperoxidase stain with monoclonal antibody ×20).

7. **When should I perform a renal biopsy in patients with myeloma and AKI?**
In patients with biochemically proven myeloma and AKI who do not show a prompt response to hydration and correction of precipitants, a diagnostic renal biopsy to determine the cause of renal failure is usually, but not always, recommended because of variability in renal etiology and the importance of ensuring a correct histologic diagnosis. The type and stage of disease (especially the degree of tubular fibrosis) may influence the choice of chemotherapy and adjunctive treatments such as high cut-off (HCO) dialysis and plasmapheresis. Often, the diagnosis of myeloma is made or suggested by the renal biopsy as the first investigation and subsequently confirmed with protein chemistry. In this situation the necessity of a bone marrow biopsy is determined by diagnostic and therapeutic need and may be required for prognosis to guide chemotherapy and determine eligibility for specific drug trials.

8. **How do I treat myeloma cast nephropathy?**
Myeloma cast nephropathy is a medical emergency and requires immediate diagnosis and early institution of therapy to prevent irreversible renal failure. Once the diagnosis is made (or suspected) there are two key strategies. The first is to remove any precipitants (e.g., sepsis, nonsteroidal anti-inflammatory drugs, hypercalcemia) and increase urine flow to reverse or prevent oliguria. The toxicity of LC in the tubules in part relates to their concentration, and increasing tubular flow reduces this. Volume expansion with normal saline (or sodium bicarbonate in the presence of acidosis) and maintenance of a high urine flow (ideally 3 L a day) with adequate oral fluids are required. Reversal of hypercalcemia with volume expansion and bisphosphonates with reduced dosing and infusion rates (as a result of tubular toxicity in renal failure) is also indicated. The use of furosemide may worsen cast formation and induce volume depletion and should be used with caution. The second key strategy is the early use of chemotherapy (see Question 9) to reduce the LC load. Dexamethasone, 20 mg bid, which induces apoptosis of plasma cells, can be immediately commenced to rapidly lower the serum LC load while additional chemotherapy agents are considered.

KEY POINTS: MYELOMA

1. Patients with myeloma are particularly vulnerable to factors that cause volume depletion or sudden reductions in glomerular filtration. This is because these changes reduce tubular flow and increase the exposure of the tubule to high single-nephron light chain concentrations.

2. Patients with myeloma most frequently present with the signs and symptoms of renal failure, anemia, or malignant bone pain, typically low back pain unrelieved by rest or simple analgesics.

3. Urinalysis, although important, may yield misleading results because the increased urinary excretion of light chains associated with myeloma is not detected by testing for albumin (e.g., Albustix) but only for total protein (e.g., sulfosalicylic acid test) or by specific urine electrophoresis and immunofixation.

4. In patients with biochemically proven myeloma and acute kidney injury who do not show a prompt response to hydration and correction of precipitants, a diagnostic renal biopsy to determine the cause of renal failure is usually, but not always, recommended because of variability in renal etiology and the importance of ensuring a correct histologic diagnosis.

5. Myeloma cast nephropathy is a medical emergency and requires immediate diagnosis and early institution of therapy in order to prevent irreversible renal failure.

6. Dexamethasone 20 mg bid, which induces apoptosis of plasma cells, can be immediately commenced to rapidly lower the serum LC load while additional chemotherapy agents are considered.

9. **What chemotherapy is used in patients with myeloma and AKI?**
Although incurable, recent advances in chemotherapy and the use of autologous stem cell transplantation (ASCT) have improved patient survival significantly. ASCT is now the procedure of choice for eligible patients and the avoidance of alkylating agents such as melphalan that impair stem cell harvest is preferred. Chemotherapy targeting rapid plasma cell killing and LC lowering include the reversible proteasome inhibitor bortezomib (which does not need dose adjustment in renal failure) given cyclically alone or in conjunction with agents such as Adriamycin (doxorubicin). Lenalidomide, a newer derivative of thalidomide, has also shown great benefit for rapid lowering of LC but requires dose adjustment in renal failure because of myelosuppression. Determining the optimal chemotherapy requires close collaboration between nephrologists and hemato-oncologists to individualize management decisions according to age and comorbidity, suitability for ASCT, eligibility for trials, and application of plasma exchange or HCO dialysis.

10. **Why are light chains toxic to the kidney?**
Kidney injury is principally related to the light chain component of myeloma because, unlike immunoglobulins, LC are freely filtered at the glomerulus and reabsorbed in the proximal tubule. Under normal conditions only small amounts of LC are filtered and reabsorbed, but in myeloma the amount of LC may rise to extreme levels that overwhelm the capacity and function of the proximal tubular cell (and induce proximal tubular injury) and pass to the distal tubule where, in certain conditions and with certain LC, they can complex with uromodulin (Tamm-Horsfall protein) to form insoluble casts that obstruct the tubule, rupture the basement membrane, and induce an inflammatory response. Not all LC are toxic, however, and some patients can excrete large quantities without AKI. Specific molecular variants of the LC molecule seem associated with the tendency to form specific forms of kidney injury such as myeloma cast nephropathy or amyloidosis.

11. **What are Bence-Jones proteins?**
Excessive production and filtration of LC can overwhelm proximal tubular reabsorption and result in an increase in urinary excretion. Detection of urine LC by primitive techniques of boiling and precipitation were one of the earliest descriptions of myeloma disease "mollities ossium" and its manifestations published in 1847 by Dr. Henry Bence Jones. Subsequently Korngold and Lapiri (designated Kappa and Lambda) raised antisera against the two LC domains. Bence-Jones proteins are urinary free light chains detected by urinary protein electrophoresis and immunofixation.

12. **Why measure serum free light chains?**
Historically the biochemical methods to diagnose myeloma and especially light chains via protein chemistry have been problematic, have been slow to perform, and lacked both sensitivity and specificity. The measurement of serum FLC by nephelometry is rapid (hours); more sensitive (1–3 mg/L); and, along with an SPE (to determine the presence or a whole immunoglobulin component), will diagnose the majority of patients with myeloma, amyloidosis, and other MIDD. An abnormal sFLC ratio (normal κ/λ 0.26–1.65) occurs as a result of overproduction of a single κ or λ clone (with suppression of the other) and this excess is detectable in the serum before urinary tubular catabolism is exceeded and before the SPE or IFE is abnormal. In patients with chronic kidney disease, significant accumulation of sFLC occurs (approximately five-fold) as a result of reduced excretion, and the normal range is adjusted to reflect this (κ/λ 0.37–3.17) so as not to incorrectly classify patients with a monoclonal gammopathy. In patients with myeloma and severe AKI from MCN, however, the absolute level of the abnormal sFLC always exceeds 1000 mg/L and the ratio is abnormal in 100% of cases. The measurement of urine FLC does not improve diagnostic yield, and the measurement of sFLC instead of urine IFE is now incorporated into many hematologic guidelines. Serial measurements of FLC also provide real-time and quantitative monitoring of response to chemotherapy and dialysis because of the short half-life (hours) of the sFLC compared with whole immunoglobulins (3 weeks) when measured by SPE.

KEY POINTS: LIGHT CHAINS

1. Kidney injury is principally related to the light chain component of myeloma because, unlike immunoglobulins, light chains are freely filtered at the glomerulus and reabsorbed in the proximal tubule.

2. The measurement of serum free light chain by nephelometry is rapid (hours); more sensitive (1–3 mg/L); and, along with a serum protein electrophoresis (to determine the presence or a whole immunoglobulin component), will diagnose the majority of patients with myeloma, amyloidosis, and other monoclonal immunoglobulin deposition diseases.

13. **Does plasmapheresis remove free light chains in myeloma?**
Patients with AKI as a result of cast nephropathy in myeloma have very high circulating and tissue FLC because of uncontrolled production and impaired excretion. Reduction of this burden by enhanced nonrenal clearance while awaiting clinical benefit from chemotherapy may allow renal recovery. Conventional dialysis has very low FLC clearance and plasmapheresis has therefore been used to improve plasma clearance. Modeling of clearance suggests that plasmapheresis can reduce the FLC load, but because there is a high extravascular refilling and exchanges are limited to around 3.5 L volumes, it requires daily treatment. Variability in therapeutic application and treatment times probably accounts for the failure of most trials to demonstrate a convincing benefit of plasmapheresis. Comparison with daily dialysis using HCO membranes (see Question 14) suggests plasmapheresis is inferior and should be utilized as adjunctive therapy only when HCO dialysis is unavailable. Plasma exchange is still beneficial in patients with symptoms and signs of hyperviscosity (e.g., in IgA myeloma and Waldenström macroglobulinemia [WM]) when rapid lowering of whole immunoglobulins is required to alleviate symptoms.

14. **What form of dialysis is best for patients with myeloma?**
The use of dialysis is required in up to 10% of new patients with myeloma and AKI. Most often this is hemodialysis via central venous catheters. Until recently, only 15% of patients recovered renal function and there was a high mortality. However, long-term use of both peritoneal dialysis and hemodialysis has been used, and survival on dialysis, although reduced, depends on adequate control by chemotherapy of the myeloma. Sepsis remains a considerable risk, and aggressive measures to reduce this should be considered such as early placement of an arteriovenous fistula and antibiotic locking of lines. Recently, the use of HCO membranes for hemodialysis has offered a novel method to provide hemodialysis with removal of very large amounts of sFLC over extended dialysis of 8 hours duration and in conjunction with chemotherapy, especially bortezomib, improve renal recovery rates to more than 70%. The HCO membrane allows extended clearance of molecules up to 50 kD (FLC are around 25–50 kD) and provides effective clearance, although it requires albumin replacement and careful patient monitoring.

15. **What is MGUS?**
Monoclonal gammopathy of unknown significance (MGUS) is defined as a paraprotein <3 g/dL, with <10% plasma cells in the bone marrow and no evidence of end-organ damage (no anemia, lytic bone lesions, hypercalcemia, or renal disease attributable to the paraprotein). Nearly 3% of individuals older than age 70 have an MGUS, and about 1% of patients with MGUS progress to symptomatic myeloma each year and annual follow-up is required. Patients with a higher level of paraprotein (>1.5 g/dL), non-IgG paraproteins, and an abnormal sFLC ratio at diagnosis are more likely to progress. Patients with MGUS usually have no or low levels of Bence-Jones proteins.

16. **If I screen a patient with newly found renal impairment and find a monoclonal protein, how do I know if he or she has myeloma-induced renal disease?**
    This older age group also has high disease prevalence for diabetes and hypertension, and screening for alternative causes for renal dysfunction in this group will find patients with an MGUS. The duration of the clinical history of renal impairment and extent of diabetic complications are helpful in differentiating cause. In general, patients with MGUS have low levels of monoclonal protein (<3 g/dL), a normal FLC ratio, absence or low level of urine light chains, and no clinical evidence of myeloma (no osteolytic lesions, anemia, or hypercalcemia). In some cases, bone marrow or diagnostic renal biopsy after a period of observation may be required if doubt persists.

17. **What is Waldenström macroglobulinemia, and does it cause AKI?**
    Waldenström macroglobulinemia is a clonal IgM monoclonal protein secreting lymphoid and plasma cell disorder. It usually manifests with anemia and fatigue but also may cause constitutional symptoms of fever, weight loss, and sweats; organ involvement with hepatosplenomegaly and lymphadenopathy; peripheral neuropathy; and features of hyperviscosity and cryoglobulinemia (rash). The diagnosis requires a monoclonal IgM protein and a bone marrow with >10% lymphoplasmacytic cell infiltration. Usually the FLC component is kappa only, and urinary kappa light chains can be found in around 70% of cases. Renal involvement with WM is uncommon and classic myeloma cast nephropathy does not occur. Renal involvement is glomerular and presents with hematuria/proteinuria, impaired renal function, and rarely nephrotic syndrome. Histologically it takes the form of an immune-mediated glomerulonephritis with IgM deposition and/or features of cryoglobulinemia with intraglomerular thrombi. Treatment is required when significant end-organ damage or symptoms require and should be targeted according to the severity of illness and age of the patient. Plasma exchange, rituximab, alkylating agents (chlorambucil), and the purine nucleoside analogues (fludarabine, cladribine) alone or in combination can be used.

KEY POINTS: MGUS AND WM

1. In general patients with monoclonal gammopathy of unknown significance have low levels of monoclonal protein (<3 g/dL), a normal free light chain ratio, absence or low level of urine light chains, and no clinical evidence of myeloma (no osteolytic lesions, anemia, or hypercalcemia). In some cases bone marrow or diagnostic renal biopsy after a period of observation may be required if doubt persists.

2. Renal involvement with Waldenström macroglobulinemia is uncommon, and classic myeloma cast nephropathy does not occur.

18. **Do plasmacytomas involve the kidneys?**
    Plasmacytomas are solitary lesions of clonal plasma cells in bone or soft tissues (especially the upper respiratory tract) without plasma cell involvement of the bone marrow or any other features of myeloma. Approximately 50% have a small monoclonal serum protein. They do not involve the kidneys, although they can subsequently progress to myeloma. Elevated sFLC ratio at diagnosis is associated with a higher risk of progression.

19. **What is POEMS syndrome?**
    The acronym POEMS refers to *P*olyneuropathy, *O*rganomegaly, *E*ndocrinopathy, *M*onoclonal protein and *S*kin involvement. This is a very rare disease and requires a monoclonal plasma cell disorder with a progressive sensorimotor peripheral neuropathy and at least one other

key criterion, particularly the presence of Castleman's disease (angiofollicular lymph node hyperplasia) or osteosclerotic myeloma. In general, renal involvement is not a usual feature and when present is unrelated to light chain deposition. Definitive therapy is uncertain but may involve radiotherapy and chemotherapy regimens directed toward the myeloma component.

20. **What is amyloidosis?**
Amyloidosis describes diseases characterized by the abnormal deposition of fibrils in extracellular tissues derived from an abnormal protein bound to serum amyloid P protein. When this abnormal protein is a light chain (usually λ) it is known as primary or AL amyloidosis. Other causes include the hereditary/genetic (AH; e.g., transthyretin) or secondary amyloidosis when chronic inflammation (e.g., familial Mediterranean fever, or FMF) is associated with increased serum amyloid A protein (AA amyloid). These fibrils form tissue deposits within the body, especially the kidney, heart, liver, nerves, and gut. Although associated with myeloma in around 10% of patients, the majority present with organ dysfunction as a result of tissue infiltration rather than bone destruction.

21. **What are the histologic features of amyloidosis?**
Macroscopically the kidneys are enlarged, firm, and pale and may be waxy. On light microscopy AA and AL amyloid have the same morphologic features and involve mainly the glomerulus and blood vessels, with less involvement from the tubulointerstitium. The glomerular deposits are seen predominantly in the mesangium as amorphous acidophilic deposits, weakly PAS positive and negative or weakly positive with Silver stain (Fig. 36-3A). There is usually extension of the deposits along the peripheral capillary wall and the deposits form delicate spikes on the outer surfaces. The classical diagnostic test is the Congo red stain, which shows an orange-red color and apple-green birefringence when examined by polarized microscopy. Potassium permanganate bleaches AA amyloid. Specific immunohistochemistry tests identify immunoglobulin light chains or amyloid A protein, with the majority of AL amyloidosis caused by lambda light chain deposits. Electron microscopy shows the distinctive amyloid fibrils, which are nonbranching, are randomly arranged, measure 9 to 12 nm, and have electrolucent cores but cannot distinguish between AA, AL, and AH amyloidosis (Fig. 36-3B).

22. **How does amyloidosis present?**
Patients with amyloidosis usually present with edema and nephrotic syndrome. However, restrictive cardiomyopathy, hepatomegaly (from infiltration), and peripheral neuropathy (carpal tunnel syndrome) are also common presentations. Severe edema, often with anasarca and pleural effusions, is common, and other clinical signs include easy bruising and macroglossia. Involvement of the adrenal glands can cause primary hypoadrenalism. In some cases, amyloid is confined to a single organ including bowel, bladder and upper airways; these localized disorders are not usually associated with renal disease. AA amyloid is usually associated with a chronic illness such as rheumatoid arthritis, bronchiectasis, or FMF.

23. **What is the diagnostic test for amyloidosis?**
Although the diagnosis is suggested by the finding of heavy albuminuria and bland urine sediment, a tissue biopsy is required to diagnose amyloidosis and distinguish between the various types (AL, AA, and AH). Amyloid deposits can also be found in virtually all other organs including the rectum, abdominal fat pad, and the bone marrow, and these are sometimes biopsied in preference to the kidney. The combination of SPE and serum FLC will be abnormal in 98% of patients with primary amyloidosis as a result of an LC disorder because of the increase in the abnormal (usually λ) sFLC.

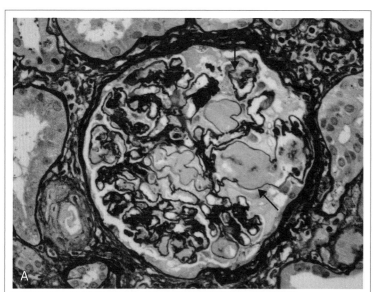

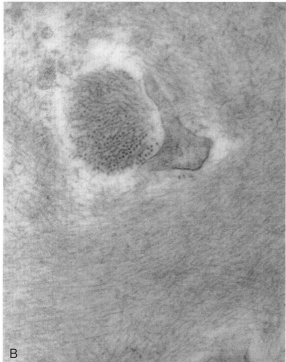

Figure 36-3. *A,* Amyloidosis. The glomerulus shows marked mesangial expansion with amorphous deposits with loss of mesangial argyrophilia (*arrows*). Similar deposits are present in the arteriole (methenamine silver with PAS counter stain ×40). *B,* Amyloidosis. Electron microscopy shows randomly arranged parallel bundles of straight fibrils (magnification ×12,500).

KEY POINTS: AMYLOIDOSIS

1. These fibrils form tissue deposits within the body, especially the kidney, heart, liver, nerves, and gut. Although associated with myeloma in around 10% of patients, the majority present with organ dysfunction resulting from tissue infiltration rather than bone destruction.

2. Patients with amyloidosis usually present with edema and nephrotic syndrome.

3. The combination of serum protein electrophoresis and serum free light chain (sFLC) will be abnormal in 98% of patients with primary amyloidosis resulting from a light chain disorder because of the increase in the abnormal (usually λ) sFLC.

24. **How can we treat amyloidosis?**
Primary amyloidosis frequently occurs in elderly patients, and therapy requires chemotherapy and/or ASCT to effect survival by reducing or eliminating the plasma cell clone responsible. Survival is based on age and extent of tissue involvement, with cardiac involvement suggesting a particularly poor prognosis. Prednisolone and melphalan have modest benefits on survival, and newer LC-focused strategies including ASCT derived from studies in myeloma are now being tried. The management of AA amyloid requires treatment of the underlying secondary disorder; for AH treatment depends on the specific genetic mutation, and liver transplantation may be curative in some cases.

25. **What is dialysis (beta-2 microglobulin) amyloidosis?**
β_2-microglobulin (β_2M) is a 12 kD LC component of the major histocompatibility complex (MHC) class 1 molecule and is synthesized by all cells that express MHC-1. Similar to LC, it is freely filtered and reabsorbed in the PTC. It accumulates in renal failure, and its clearance in patients with end-stage renal disease (ESRD) receiving dialysis is dependent on dialyzer type (clearance), duration, and ultrafiltration volume. Elevated β_2M in patients with ESRD managed by either hemodialysis or peritoneal dialysis is amyloidogenic and can deposit in soft tissues, especially in or around joints and cartilage, after binding to collagen types 1 and 2. This tissue deposition occurs early in dialysis (based on staining of tissues) and exceeds 90% of patients after 10 years, but the clinical syndrome rarely presents before 5 years of dialysis and most commonly presents after 10 years of dialysis. The clinical syndromes include carpal tunnel disorder, destructive arthropathy (especially hands, shoulders, and spine), bone cysts, and fractures. Radiologically bone cysts (e.g., carpal bones) and periarticular lucencies are noted. Although other organs are often involved (gut, heart, lung), on postmortem examination this is much less commonly clinically apparent. Gastrointestinal hemorrhage and bowel infarction have been most frequently described. The diagnosis is made clinically and radiologically, but examination of tissue samples at joint replacement or carpal tunnel surgery stain positively with Congo red and specific anti β_2M antibody. Treatment (and prevention) is aimed at improving clearance of β_2M by attention to increased dialysis clearance using high-flux membranes and increased hours. Renal transplantation is associated with rapid symptomatic benefit but only gradual clearance of deposits and bone healing.

26. **What are the monoclonal immunoglobulin deposition diseases?**
The MIDD describe another histologic and clinical variant of abnormal tissue deposition resulting from a monoclonal-free LC (or rarely the heavy chain [HC] component of immunoglobulin alone or in combination with LC), which has some characteristics similar to amyloid in that abnormal extracellular protein deposition occurs, yet the microstructure differs because these proteins do not form fibrils and the deposits do not stain with Congo red. Typically, LCDD (also known as Randall's disease) is associated with specific variants of the κ-LC variable region domain (types I and IV), which bind strongly and accumulate along the tubular and glomerular basement membrane but also deposit in the mesangium where they

induce production of extracellular matrix and typical nodular glomerular lesions. The clinical presentation of both LCDD and HCDD is similar and is usually with a glomerulonephritis or nephritic picture—hypertension, hematuria, and proteinuria with renal impairment. Cardiac and hepatic involvement may also occur. Therapy is directed toward treatment of the LC with steroids and myeloma chemotherapy including ASCT; clinical response is variable. Renal transplantation has a high risk of recurrent disease.

27. **What are the features of light chain deposition disease on renal biopsy?**
Light chain deposition disease (LCDD), heavy chain deposition disease (HCDD), and light and heavy chain deposition disease (LHCD) show the same morphologic features. The glomerular changes are heterogeneous and range from mild mesangiopathic changes to a mesangiocapillary (membranoproliferative) pattern with features similar to diabetic nodular glomerulosclerosis (Kimmelstiel-Wilson type) but do not stain strongly positive with Silver stains. They are Congo red negative, and immunofluorescence microscopy shows monoclonal light chain deposits in the glomerular basement membrane, Bowman capsule, and the cortical and medullary tubular basement membranes (Fig. 36-4). Electron microscopy shows a band of dense granules usually in the inner position of the lamina densa of the glomerular basement membrane and the outer aspect of the tubular basement membrane.

28. **What are fibrillary and immunotactoid glomerulonephritis?**
Fibrillary and immunotactoid glomerulonephritis are very uncommon nonamyloid (Congo red negative) forms of immunoglobulin-associated renal disease with abnormal tissue deposits from fibrils. Similar to LCDD, they usually present with a glomerulonephritis picture (hematuria and proteinuria, hypertension, and renal impairment). They can only be distinguished from LCDD by renal biopsy and especially electron microscopy, where the size and characteristics of the deposits differ (Table 36-1). Fibrillary glomerulonephritis does not usually associate with a paraprotein and has polyclonal IgG deposits, whereas immunotactoid disease may be

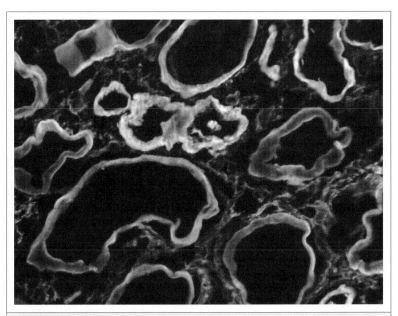

Figure 36-4. Light chain deposition disease. There is a heavy concentration of single light chain deposits along the outer aspect of the tubular basement membrane (immunofluorescence microscopy with antibody to single light chain ×25).

TABLE 36–1. THE CLINICAL AND HISTOLOGIC CHARACTERISTICS OF THE DYSPROTEINEMIAS

	Myeloma	Amyloidosis (AL/AA/AH)	LCDD	Fibrillary Glomerulonephritis	Immunotactoid Glomerulonephritis	Waldenström Macroglobulinemia
Clinical presentation	Acute kidney injury	Nephrotic syndrome	Nephritic syndrome	Nephritic syndrome	Nephritic syndrome	Nephritic or nephrotic hyperviscosity
Urinalysis	Bland or proteinuria (no or minimal albumin)	Bland predominant albuminuria	Hematuria Proteinuria casts	Hematuria Proteinuria casts	Hematuria Proteinuria casts	Hematuria Proteinuria casts
Serum paraprotein class	IgD/IgA/IgG	None	None	Uncommon	IgG	IgM
Serum free light chains	κ and λ	λ > κ (primary) None (secondary/ hereditary)	κ > λ (LCDD)	Unknown	Unknown	κ
Histology						
Light microscopy	Interstitial fibrosis, edema, inflammation, and giant cells with distal casts	All show similar features with acidophilic deposits in the mesangium, peripheral capillaries, and blood vessels	Heterogeneous most severe pattern is membranoproliferative (mesangio-capillary) with nodularity	Heterogeneous Mesangial to membrano-proliferative pattern	Heterogeneous Proliferative to membrano-proliferative pattern	Subendothelial deposits and thrombi

Congo red stain	Negative	All positive	Negative	Negative	Negative	Negative
Immunofluorescence	κ or λ only	λ > κ	κ > λ	Polyclonal IgG κ and λ	Monoclonal IgGκ or IgGλ ± IgM	IgM ± IgG
Complement C3	Negative	All negative	Negative	Positive	Positive	Positive
Electron microscopy	Tubular crystals	All show similar random fibrils 8–12 nm	Amorphous dense deposits	Random fibrils 15–30 nm	Parallel microtubules 10–90 nm	Dense deposits ± cryoglobulin microtubules

Nephrotic syndrome = edema, hypoalbuminemia, and heavy albuminuria.
Nephritic syndrome = hematuria and proteinuria, hypertension, renal impairment.

associated with hematologic disorders (lymphoma, leukemia) and have monoclonal IgGλ or IgGκ deposits and in some cases a circulating paraprotein. Treatment of fibrillary disease is often attempted with steroids and cytotoxics, but response is poor. Immunotactoid disease may respond to treatment of the underlying hematologic disorder. Progression to end-stage renal disease is frequent and can occur within a few years.

29. **Can patients with chronic renal failure and dysproteinemias receive a kidney transplant?**
Despite significant advances in diagnosis and chemotherapy, most patients with myeloma, amyloidosis, or LCDD are older and have significant comorbidity, and the disease remains incurable with a high chance of recurrence. Hence, kidney transplant is rarely considered appropriate. A smaller group of younger patients with myeloma, after successful induction therapy and ASCT, may be considered suitable if prolonged disease remission (approximately 3 years) by standard criteria and normalization of the sFLC ratio are achieved. In the absence of active LC myeloma, the risk of recurrent cast nephropathy is low. Surveillance after renal transplant for disease recurrence is indefinite and would involve regular estimation of sFLC ratio because this is the most sensitive and specific marker of disease recurrence and provides an estimate of the risk of allograft injury. The results for LCDD suggest a very high risk of early and aggressive disease recurrence after renal transplant in the absence of prolonged disease remission and ASCT. Rare cases of renal transplantation in primary amyloid after chemotherapy and ASCT are also reported.

BIBLIOGRAPHY

1. Criteria for the classification of monoclonal gammopathies, multiple myeloma and related disorders: A report of the International Myeloma Working Group. *Br J Haematol* 2003;121:749–757.
2. Hutchison CA, Cockwell P, Reid S, et al. Efficient removal of immunoglobulin free light chains by hemodialysis for multiple myeloma: In vitro and in vivo studies. *J Am Soc Nephrol* 2007;18:886–895.
3. Hutchison CA, Basnayake K, Cockwell P. Serum free light chain assessment in monoclonal gammopathy and kidney disease. *Nat Rev Nephrol* 2009;5:621–627.
4. Kumar SK, Rajkumar SV, Dispenzieri A, et al. Improved survival in multiple myeloma and the impact of novel therapies. *Blood* 2008;111:2516–2520.
5. Rajkumar SV, Dispenzieri A, Kyle RA. Monoclonal gammopathy of undetermined significance, Waldenström's macroglobulinaemia, AL amyloidosis and related plasma cell disorders: Diagnosis and treatment. *Mayo Clin Proc* 2006; 81(5):693–703.
6. Bradwell AR. *Serum Free Light Chain Analysis*, 5th ed. Birmingham UK: The Binding Site Ltd, 2008.
7. Sanders PW, Booker BB. Pathobiology of cast nephropathy from human Bence-Jones proteins. *J Clin Invest* 1992;89:630–639.
8. Ludwig H, Drach J, Graf H, et al. Reversal of acute renal failure by bortezomib-based chemotherapy in patients with multiple myeloma. *Haematologica* 2007;92(10):1411–1414.
9. Heher EC, Spitzer TR, Goes NB. Light chains: Heavy burden in kidney transplantation. *Transplantation* 2009;87(7):947–952.
10. Lin J, Markowitz GS, Valeri AM, et al. Renal monoclonal immunoglobulin deposition disease: The disease spectrum. *J Am Soc Nephrol* 2001;12:1482–1492.
11. Churg J, Bernstein J, Glassock R, et al. (eds.). *Renal Disease: Classification and Atlas of Glomerular Diseases.* New York: Igaku-Shoin, 1995.
12. Jennette JC, Olson JL, Schwartz MM, et al. (eds.). *Heptinstall's Pathology of the Kidney.* Philadelphia: Lippincott Williams & Wilkins, 2007.

CHAPTER 37

ANTI-GLOMERULAR BASEMENT MEMBRANE DISEASE AND GOODPASTURE'S SYNDROME

Eleri Williams, MRCP, and Neil Turner, PhD

1. **Who was Ernest Goodpasture?**

   Dr. Ernest Goodpasture was an American physician and pathologist born in Tennessee in 1886. His scientific research was principally in the field of infectious diseases. He developed a pioneering method for cultivating viruses in chicken eggs, which eventually allowed the development of vaccines for many viruses including smallpox and influenza. Despite his hugely influential contributions to research in infectious diseases, he is best remembered in the wider medical community for giving his name to the eponymous Goodpasture's syndrome. During the 1919 influenza pandemic, Goodpasture was stationed at the Chelsea Naval Hospital near Boston and was responsible for performing autopsies on victims of the influenza pandemic. He described the case of an 18-year-old man with lung hemorrhage and crescentic nephritis at autopsy. Nearly four decades later, in 1958, two pathologists described a group of nine patients with similar findings and applied Goodpasture's name to the entity. According to one biographer, Goodpasture did not approve of the association of his name with this syndrome.

2. **What is Goodpasture's syndrome and how does it differ from Goodpasture's disease?**

   Goodpasture's syndrome describes the clinical presentation of a rapidly progressive glomerulonephritis and alveolar hemorrhage. There are several causes, outlined in Table 37-1.

   Anti-glomerular basement membrane (anti-GBM) disease, also known as Goodpasture's disease, is an autoimmune disorder characterized by the presence of autoantibodies directed against a target restricted to the glomerular and a few other specialized basement membranes.

TABLE 37-1. CAUSES OF RPGN-LUNG HEMORRHAGE (GOODPASTURE'S SYNDROME)
Goodpasture's disease (anti-GBM disease)
ANCA-associated small-vessel vasculitis
Microscopic polyangiitis
Wegener's disease
Drug associated: hydralazine, penicillamine
Uncommonly in other vasculitis
Systemic lupus erythematosus
Henoch-Schönlein purpura
Behçet's disease
Mixed essential cryoglobulinaemia
Rheumatoid vasculitis
RPGN, rapidly progressive glomerulonephritis; GBM, glomerular basement membrane; ANCA, antineutrophilic cytoplasmic antibodies.

It manifests as a highly aggressive crescentic glomerulonephritis often associated with lung hemorrhage. It is a cause of Goodpasture's syndrome. Other causes are more common than anti-GBM disease itself, with systemic vasculitis accounting for about two thirds of cases.

The terminology can be confusing, and the Goodpasture eponym is best reserved for anti-GBM disease.

3. **What other conditions present with acute renal and respiratory failure?**
The pulmonary-renal syndrome refers to conditions manifesting as acute renal and respiratory failure. It is important to distinguish these from the syndrome of lung hemorrhage and rapidly progressive glomerulonephritis. The first two causes in Table 37-2 are common.

4. **How common is Goodpasture's disease?**
Goodpasture's disease is a rare condition, with an estimated incidence of one case per million, per annum in the United Kingdom. The disease is more common in white races and rare in South Asian and African races, although it is recognized in China. The disease may occur from childhood to old age; the youngest reported case is in an 11-month-old infant, and cases in patients in their eighties have been reported. The disease is more common in young men, and this age and gender distribution is dissimilar to those of other organ-specific autoimmune disorders. The peak incidence is bimodal with peaks in the third and sixth decades.

5. **How does Goodpasture's disease present clinically?**
Goodpasture's disease is characteristically the most rapidly progressive of all the causes of crescentic nephritis and can cause complete loss of renal function over days. It often presents at a time of disease acceleration.

Early symptoms are often nonspecific, with malaise, arthralgia, and weight loss typical, but often mild. This paucity of systemic symptoms results in the illness initially being perceived as minor until rapidly progressive pulmonary or renal disease develops.

The prevalence of pulmonary hemorrhage in anti-GBM disease is around 50%. This typically presents as hemoptysis, but significant pulmonary hemorrhage may occur in its absence. Hemoptysis can be minor or severe and can precede the diagnosis by several years. Those presenting early with pulmonary disease may have only mild renal involvement.

Renal presentations are more common in nonsmokers and older patients. They may notice macroscopic hematuria and complain of loin pain associated with renal swelling. Symptoms of uremia and fluid overload may predominate in advanced renal impairment. The classical presentation of lung hemorrhage and advanced renal impairment needs to be differentiated from other causes of the pulmonary-renal syndrome.

TABLE 37-2. OTHER CAUSES OF THE PULMONARY-RENAL SYNDROME
Pulmonary edema secondary to hypervolemia in acute kidney injury of any cause
Severe cardiac failure with pulmonary edema
Infections with pulmonary syndrome and acute interstitial nephritis
Hantavirus
Leptospirosis
Legionella
Paraquat poisoning
Thrombosis of renal vein/inferior vena cava with pulmonary emboli
Anti-phospholipid syndrome with pulmonary emboli
Thrombotic microangiopathy (HUS) with acute lung syndrome
Fibrillary glomerulonephritis

6. **What preliminary investigations should be performed in suspected Goodpasture's disease?**
    Renal failure may be advanced at the time of presentation, and laboratory tests will demonstrate elevated creatinine and urea levels. Anemia is a common feature, typically microcytic, and often represents subclinical pulmonary hemorrhage. Acute inflammatory markers may be moderately elevated. A sudden unexplained drop in hemoglobin can herald the presence of a significant hemorrhage.

    The urine sediment is active, with evidence of red cell casts on microscopy. Heavy proteinuria is not a typical feature.

    Ultrasonographic imaging of the kidneys typically shows structurally normal or enlarged kidneys.

    Changes in the chest radiograph are seen in most cases of pulmonary hemorrhage. There is usually shadowing involving the central lung fields, with peripheral and upper lobe sparing. The abnormalities are commonly symmetric. There is a spectrum of changes that range from small, ill-defined nodules to confluent consolidation. Shadowing is rarely limited or entirely confined by a fissure and is rarely only apical. Such radiographs would suggest infection, lone or superimposed. These changes will generally begin to resolve within 48 hours and are often cleared by 2 weeks.

    The most specific test for fresh pulmonary hemorrhage is an acute increase in the gas transfer factor as measured on pulmonary function testing. The additional free hemoglobin within the alveoli is able to bind to inspired CO and so increase values of KCO. This is in contrast to the typical situation in renal failure in which the KCO is about 30% lower that predicted. KCO is also reduced in pulmonary edema.

7. **How is a diagnosis of Goodpasture's disease established?**
    Anti-GBM antibodies, either circulating or fixed to the GBM, are the hallmark of anti-GBM disease. Solid-phase immunoassays are used to detect circulating antibodies. However, a renal biopsy is essential to the diagnosis of Goodpasture's disease and has prognostic and diagnostic implications. Direct immunofluorescence on the renal biopsy is the most sensitive technique for identifying pathogenic antibodies, and this is the main method of diagnosis in most centers.

8. **What are the biopsy findings of Goodpasture's disease?**
    Even in the absence of clinical evidence of renal disease, the glomeruli are often abnormal. Segmental mesangial matrix expansion and hypercellularity are the earliest changes. This progresses to a focal and segmental proliferative glomerulonephritis with increased numbers of neutrophils in the glomeruli. In advanced disease, there is a diffuse nephritis with segmental or total necrosis and extensive crescent formation. Linear binding of antibody to the GBM is found in all patients.

9. **How is Goodpasture's disease treated?**
    The rationale behind the treatment of Goodpasture's disease is the removal of circulating antibodies and simultaneous inhibition of their synthesis. Most centers now use protocols based on those developed in the mid-1970s, involving a combination of cyclophosphamide, oral corticosteroids, and plasma exchange (Table 37-3). Prior to the development of such treatment, the condition was commonly fatal. Similar regimes are used to treat other rapidly progressive glomerulonephritides.

    Plasma exchange acts to lower antibody titers rapidly. Immunoadsorption onto protein A columns is an alternative method utilized in some centers. The use of plasma exchange alone has only a transient effect on antibody titers, and there is no place for its use in isolation in current regimens. Cyclophosphamide is a cytotoxic drug, which can be given orally or as pulsed IV doses. Oral corticosteroids may be used in preference to pulsed IV corticosteroids, which increase the risk of infection, the most common cause of early complications and death after the first week.

TABLE 37–3. PROTOCOL FOR TREATING GOODPASTURE'S DISEASE

- Prednisolone 1 mg/kg/24 hours orally
- Cyclophosphamide 2.5 mg/kg/24 hours orally rounded down to nearest 50 mg (usual maximum 150 mg)
- Daily exchange of 4 L of plasma for 5% human albumin for 14 days or until circulating antibody is suppressed; fresh frozen plasma is administered concurrently in the presence of pulmonary hemorrhage

---

Such an aggressive treatment regimen carries considerable risks, and patients with likely irrecoverable renal disease in whom lung hemorrhage is not a feature may be best managed conservatively with renal replacement therapy. Additional supportive measures are important, including avoiding vascular catheter-associated infections, adequate dialysis with avoidance of overhydration, monitoring of white cell count after cyclophosphamide, pneumocystis prophylaxis, measures to prevent gastric bleeding, and protection against osteoporosis.

Without treatment, Goodpasture's disease carries a poor prognosis. Early renal disease may be reversed, but patients with isolated renal disease may present late, which is associated with a poorer renal outcome. For those patients who survive the early insult of lung hemorrhage, the lung lesions of Goodpasture's disease almost completely resolve. Long-term radiologic changes or pulmonary function deficits are unusual.

10. **What is the target of anti-GBM antibodies in Goodpasture's disease?**
Anti-GBM antibodies are targeted toward the Goodpasture antigen, a molecule specific to the basement membrane of certain organs. This has been identified as the carboxy-terminal globular (NC1) domain of a tissue-specific type IV collagen isoform, the $\alpha 3$ chain. Basement membranes are specialized extracellular structures found at the junction between cells and connective tissue stroma. Most of the molecules are common to all basement membranes, but others have a restricted distribution. This basement membrane collagen isoform is expressed in the GBM, the alveolar basement membrane, and in other specialized basement membranes that appear not to be usually accessible to the autoimmune response.

11. **Are patients with Goodpasture's disease and renal failure suitable for renal transplantation?**
Many patients with previous Goodpasture's disease have gone on to receive successful renal transplants. Disease recurrence and graft loss are well described, however, particularly where circulating antibodies are present at the time of transplantation. Pulmonary hemorrhage is rare in these circumstances. Renal transplantation should be postponed until at least 6 months after the disappearance of circulating antibodies by immunoassay. In patients with persisting antibodies in whom early transplantation is desirable, similar treatment to that used at presentation can be given in preparation. With current immunosuppressive regimens, disease recurrence should be rare. Linear fixation of IgG to the GBM can, however, occur without overt disease. Renal function and urinary sediment should be closely monitored in these patients, along with monitoring of anti-GBM titers.

12. **What is "double positivity"?**
Numerous reports have documented the association of Goodpasture's disease and antineutrophil cytoplasmic antibodies (ANCA)-associated small-vessel vasculitis. In most of these cases, the ANCA has had specificity for myeloperoxidase. Many patients have had clinical features of vasculitis. These patients are labeled "double positive." The incidence of double positivity for both autoantibodies has varied in different studies. In most published

series, the anti-GBM antibody titers in patients who are double positive are relatively lower. Some reports suggest a better prognosis for patients who are double positive who present with oliguria or severe renal impairment; others have contradicted this finding. It is thought that the anti-GBM response could occur in patients who are genetically predisposed following damage to the alveolar or glomerular basement membrane by a small-vessel vasculitis. Rare reports describe cases where the clinical history suggests that the anti-GBM disease antedated the development of vasculitis.

13. **What other diseases are associated with Goodpasture's disease?**
A number of diseases have been shown to be recurrently associated with Goodpasture's disease (Table 37-4).

14. **Is there an association between cigarette smoking and pulmonary hemorrhage in Goodpasture's disease?**
Yes, there is a clear association between cigarette smoking and pulmonary hemorrhage in Goodpasture's disease. Recurrence of pulmonary hemorrhage has been observed following resumption of smoking in patients in whom the disease was in clear remission. There are descriptions of cases of pulmonary hemorrhage with a history of exposure to other inhaled toxins, including gasoline or other hydrocarbons. There is no such association between smoking and pulmonary hemorrhage in patients with small-vessel vasculitis. The mechanism for this association is not fully understood but may reflect the fact that the endothelium lining the alveolar capillaries constitutes a significant barrier to the circulating antibody, and a second insult is required to permit their passage.

15. **Are there other environmental triggers to the development of Goodpasture's disease?**
There is evidence to support the role of environmental factors in the development of Goodpasture's disease, including clustering of cases in mini-outbreaks, anecdotal reports of associations with inhaled toxins, and discordance in identical twins. However, no specific triggers have been identified, partly because of the difficulty in distinguishing true etiologic agents from those that merely aggravate pre-existing disease. In experimental models, nonspecific irritants such as gasoline act to precipitate pulmonary hemorrhage in the presence of circulating anti-GBM antibodies.

Several case reports and case-control studies have linked exposure to organic solvents and hydrocarbons with glomerulonephritis, some specifically to Goodpasture's disease, but the evidence for causation is weak.

TABLE 37-4. DISEASES RECURRENTLY ASSOCIATED WITH GOODPASTURE'S DISEASE	
Disease	**Number of Patients***
ANCA-associated vasculitis	Hundreds
Membranous nephropathy	<20
Diabetes mellitus	10
Malignancy	10
Lithotripsy	3

ANCA = antineutrophilic cytoplasmic antibodies.
*Total number of reports in the world literature.

16. **Is there a genetic predisposition to Goodpasture's disease?**
Goodpasture's disease is associated with specific HLA class II antigens. This is a feature shared with other organ-specific autoimmune diseases. The majority of patients carry human leukocyte antigen (HLA)-DR15; those who do not typically carry DR4. DR7 confers a strong protective effect.

17. **What is the link between Goodpasture's disease and Alport's syndrome?**
The Goodpasture antigen is absent or diminished in most patients with the hereditary nephritis Alport's syndrome. Transplant of a normal kidney can therefore allow the development of anti-GBM antibodies to foreign antigens in the donor kidney. Immunoglobulin G fixation to the GBM without renal damage may be common, but a small number of patients develop crescentic nephritis. This is typically not associated with lung hemorrhage. The histologic features are typical of spontaneous Goodpasture's disease, although the target of autoantibodies is usually the $\alpha 5$, rather than the closely related $\alpha 3$, chain of type IV collagen that is the target in Goodpasture's disease. In the majority of cases the transplanted kidney is irreversibly damaged.

KEY POINTS: ANTI-GLOMERULAR BASEMENT MEMBRANE DISEASE AND GOODPASTURE'S SYNDROME

1. Goodpasture's disease is the most aggressive and rapidly progressive glomerulonephritis encountered in clinical practice. Crescentic nephritis may be accompanied by life-threatening pulmonary hemorrhage.

2. It is caused by autoimmunity to a component of glomerular basement membrane (GBM) (the Goodpasture antigen) that is also found in the alveolar basement membrane.

3. Treatment with cyclophosphamide, steroids, and plasma exchange can arrest the disease, but renal damage may be irrecoverable.

4. The Goodpasture antigen and related collagen chains are missing in many patients with Alport's syndrome, who can then occasionally develop an anti-GBM response to the normal antigens in a transplanted kidney.

BIBLIOGRAPHY

1. Phelps RJ, Turner AN. Goodpasture's syndrome and anti-GBM disease. In Feehally J, Johnson R (eds.). *Comprehensive Clinical Nephrology*, 3rd ed. London: Mosby International, 2007.

2. Turner AN, Edinburg Royal Infirmary Renal Unit. Goodpasture's Disease. Available at: www.edren.org/pages/edreninfo/goodpastures-anti-gbm-disease/goodpastures-disease-more-info.php.

VASCULITIDES

Vimal K. Derebail, MD, and Patrick H. Nachman, MD

CHAPTER 38

1. **Which of the vasculitides are often associated with glomerular disease?**
   The small-vessel vasculitides are most often associated with glomerular disease (Fig. 38-1). Henoch-Schönlein purpura and cryoglobulinemia are associated with immune complex deposition. Pauci-immune glomerulonephritis demonstrates little to no immune deposits and is seen in the antineutrophil cytoplasmic autoantibody (ANCA) syndromes, including Wegener's granulomatosis, microscopic polyangiitis, Churg-Strauss syndrome, and renal-limited pauci-immune necrotizing and crescentic glomerulonephritis.

   Polyarteritis nodosa, a medium-vessel vasculitis typically affecting medium-sized or small arteries and sparing arterioles, capillaries, and venules, does not cause glomerulonephritis but may cause ischemic renal injury via inflammation of the larger renal vessels.

2. **What features distinguish the small-vessel vasculitides?**
   Although the small-vessel vasculitides have significant overlap in their manifestations, features that distinguish them have been used in proposed classification schemes:
   - *Wegener's granulomatosis* is associated with granulomatous inflammation that may affect lower and upper respiratory tracts, often causing sinus symptoms and glomerulonephritis.
   - *Microscopic polyangiitis* also leads to necrotizing vasculitis of small vessels and often leads to glomerulonephritis, pulmonary capillaritis, and pulmonary hemorrhage. Notably, granulomatous inflammation is absent.
   - *Churg-Strauss* also demonstrates granulomatous inflammation of small and medium-sized vessels and involves the respiratory tract. The distinguishing histologic feature is that of eosinophil-rich inflammation with peripheral eosinophilia. Patients also have severe asthma.
   - *Henoch-Schönlein purpura* demonstrates immunoglobulin A (IgA) immune deposits with vasculitis affecting small vessels. In addition to glomeruli, skin and gastrointestinal involvement are common. Patients often have arthralgias or arthritis.
   - *Cryoglobulinemia* leads to skin and glomerular lesions with cryoglobulin immune deposits in affected small vessels.

3. **What findings in the urinalysis suggest renal involvement from vasculitis?**
   Microscopic hematuria, typically with dysmorphic red blood cells and red blood cell casts, suggests renal vasculitis. Proteinuria is often present but is usually subnephrotic. Inflammation in the form of white blood cells in the urine may also be an accompanying feature.

4. **What serologic markers may be helpful in distinguishing the renal vasculitides?**
   Complement levels may be depressed in patients with cryoglobulinemia and other vasculitides including systemic lupus erythematosus (SLE) and postinfectious glomerulonephritis. These are typically normal in the other small-vessel vasculitides. Although somewhat technically difficult, cryoglobulins may be directly measured in serum. Antinuclear antibodies (ANA) suggest connective-tissue related disorders, such as SLE, and may be further distinguished

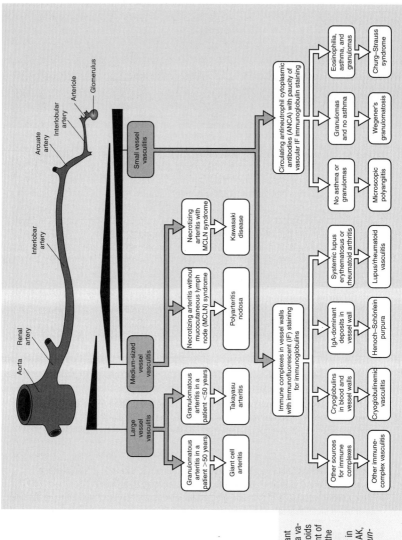

Figure 38-1. Renal vasculitis: The predominant distribution of renal vascular involvement by a variety of vasculitides. The heights of the trapezoids represent the relative frequency of involvement of different portions of the renal vasculature by the three major categories of vasculitis. (Adapted from Jennette JC, Falk RJ. Renal involvement in systemic vasculitis. In: Greenberg A, Cheung AK, Coffman TM, et al. (eds.). *National Kidney Foundation Nephrology Primer*, 2nd ed. San Diego: Academic Press, 1998, pp. 200–207.)

by testing for antibodies to extractable nuclear antigens (ENA). Patients with small-vessel vasculitis (pauci-immune necrotizing glomerulonephritis, Wegener's granulomatosis, microscopic polyangiitis, and Churg-Strauss syndrome) often have positive ANCAs. Anti-glomerular basement membrane (GBM) antibodies are detected in patients with renal-limited anti-GBM disease and patients with Goodpasture's syndrome (associated with pulmonary hemorrhage). There is broad overlap in the clinical presentation of the various small-vessel vasculitides. In addition, overlap syndromes can occur. For instance, one third of patients with anti-GBM disease will also have circulating ANCA, typically directed against myeloperoxidase (MPO). In addition to the clinical presentation and serologic studies, a renal biopsy is usually indicated to provide a definitive diagnosis and provide valuable information on the extent of glomerular injury and of glomerular and interstitial scarring.

5. **What is the relevance of ANCAs?**
ANCAs are present in 90% of patients with pauci-immune glomerulonephritis, seen in Wegener's disease, microscopic polyangiitis, and renal-limited disease. ANCAs are also present in about 40% of patients with the Churg-Strauss syndrome. They are typically *absent* in patients with polyarteritis nodosa (PAN). Immunofluorescence is most sensitive to the detection of ANCA and demonstrates distinct patterns, either a *cytoplasmic* pattern (C-ANCA) or *perinuclear* pattern (P-ANCA).

The antigen specificity of C-ANCA is usually directed to a neutrophil and monocyte protease-proteinase-3 (PR-3), whereas P-ANCAs are usually directed to myeloperoxidase. Although both MPO and PR-3 may be seen in any of the described manifestations, MPO (P-ANCA) is more common in patients with microscopic polyangiitis, and PR-3 (C-ANCA) is more common in Wegener's granulomatosis. Approximately 50% of patients with Churg-Strauss disease will manifest ANCA that may be directed to either MPO or PR-3. Again, 10% of patients with pauci-immune glomerulonephritis do not demonstrate ANCA despite renal biopsy findings consistent with this diagnosis.

In vitro and in vivo studies support a pathogenic role of ANCAs. These antibodies have been demonstrated to activate neutrophils and monocytes, leading to degranulation at the vessel wall and resulting in endothelial cell damage. In vivo, the transfer of mouse anti-MPO IgG to MPO-competent mice results in pauci-immune necrotizing and crescentic glomerulonephritis and pulmonary vasculitis that is similar to the human disease, thus demonstrating the ability of these antibodies to confer disease. This same animal model has recently been used to demonstrate an important role of complement activation via the alternative pathway in the pathogenesis of MPO-ANCA glomerulonephritis.

A potential new subtype of ANCAs was recently described. Antibodies directed to lysosomal membrane protein-2 (LAMP-2) were detected in more than 90% of patients with pauci-immune glomerulonephritis in one series. These antibodies may provide further insight into the pathogenesis of ANCA vasculitis; however, their frequency and role in vasculitis have not been confirmed and their utility in clinical practice has not been established.

6. **Which of the renal vasculitides are associated with pulmonary-renal syndrome?**
Pulmonary-renal syndrome describes the presentation of acute glomerulonephritis with pulmonary or alveolar hemorrhage, as demonstrated by radiographic demonstration of pulmonary infiltrates and varying degrees of hypoxia, hemoptysis, and anemia. It is a life-threatening complication of small-vessel vasculitis.

The ANCA small-vessel vasculitides are the most common cause of pulmonary-renal syndrome. Goodpasture's disease, or anti-GBM disease, may also present with pulmonary hemorrhage and concomitant rapidly progressive glomerulonephritis. This syndrome may also be seen in patients with SLE and similar connective tissue diseases, Henoch-Schönlein purpura, and cryoglobulinemia.

Patients with this presentation should also be evaluated for other conditions accompanying renal failure that may have similar presentations including pneumonia and pulmonary embolus.

7. **What primary rapidly progressive glomerulonephritis may occur in conjunction with ANCA glomerulonephritis?**
Goodpasture's disease or anti-GBM disease may occur concurrently with ANCA small-vessel vasculitis. Approximately 20% to 30% of patients with anti-GBM disease also have positive ANCA testing, more commonly for P-ANCA (or MPO), although C-ANCA has also been reported. In patients with a history of anti-GBM disease who develop recurrent signs of disease, ANCA testing should be obtained, even if originally negative, because relapsing anti-GBM disease is rare. The outcome of patients with both antibodies appears to be worse than those with ANCA disease alone.

8. **What are the histologic findings of a renal biopsy in patients with ANCA vasculitis?**
Renal biopsy usually demonstrates the presence of focal segmental to global fibrinoid necrosis and crescent formation affecting variable proportions of glomeruli. By both immunofluorescence and electron microscopy, glomeruli demonstrate few or no immune depositions, lending to the term pauci-immune glomerulonephritis and distinguishing ANCA vasculitis from other diseases that may produce similar features by light microscopy, such as anti-GBM disease or immune complex-mediated glomerulonephritis (e.g., lupus nephritis). The glomerular lesions are usually associated with little or no endocapillary proliferation.

9. **What drugs have been implicated in inducing ANCA vasculitis?**
The development of vasculitis with ANCAs has been associated with many agents. The most commonly implicated drug is the antithyroid medication propothiouracil (PTU), with other thyroid agents including methimazole and carbimazole also implicated. Other agents reported to be associated with ANCA vasculitis include hydralazine, minocycline, allopurinol, phenytoin, and penicillamine, among others. Withdrawal of the offending agent is at times sufficient to prompt resolution of the vasculitis, whereas in some instances, immunosuppressive therapy is necessary.

10. **What are the medical therapies for the treatment of ANCA vasculitis?**
Treatment of the ANCA vasculitides centers on the use of immunosuppressive therapies. Initial therapy, or induction, involves use of corticosteroids and cytotoxic agents, primarily cyclophosphamide. Pulsed intravenous cyclophosphamide is preferred to daily oral therapy because of the lower incidence of neutropenic sepsis and a markedly reduced total cumulative dose. Limiting the cumulative dose of cyclophosphamide is aimed at reducing rates of myelosuppression, infection, infertility, and malignancy.
    Methotrexate has been advocated for induction in patients with less severe presentations and preserved renal function, although relapse rates may be higher in these patients. Rituximab, a B-cell depleting agent, has been evaluated as a potential induction agent in lieu of cyclophosphamide or as an adjunct agent, but its utility in these roles remains to be determined.
    Following induction of remission after 3 to 6 months of cyclophosphamide therapy, azathioprine or mycophenolate mofetil are used as maintenance therapy. At present, the optimal duration of maintenance therapy remains uncertain.
    Relapses of disease are often treated with repeat pulse dosing of corticosteroids and cyclophosphamide. Disease that is refractory to corticosteroids and cyclophosphamide has been treated with several medical regimens including intravenous immunoglobulin (IVIg), B-cell depletion with rituximab, plasmapheresis, and tumor necrosis factor-α (TNF-α) blockade with infliximab. However, data for use of these agents in this fashion have been primarily in the form of case reports or case series.

11. **What are the indications for the use of plasma exchange therapy in the treatment of ANCA vasculitis?**
Plasma exchange is thought to rapidly clear ANCA, coagulation factors, and inflammatory cytokines that may be pathogenic in vasculitis. At present, plasma exchange is recommended

in addition to corticosteroids and cyclophosphamide for patients presenting with advanced renal failure and/or pulmonary hemorrhage. The role of plasmapheresis as adjunctive therapy is not established for patients with less severe disease.

12. **What is the prognosis of patients with ANCA vasculitis?**
Most patients with pauci-immune glomerulonephritis have a good response to present induction therapy with nearly 85% achieving remission. With treatment with corticosteroids and cyclophosphamide, overall survival rates at 1 and 5 years are 85% and 75%, respectively. Mortality is significantly greater in older patients reaching approximately 23% at 1 year for those older than age 60 and nearly 44% for those older than age 70. The presence of diffuse alveolar hemorrhage is associated with an eight-fold increased risk of death, whereas the serum creatinine level at presentation is the major predictor of renal outcome. Although pulmonary hemorrhage is a major cause of death in the early weeks after presentation, the major causes of "late" death are infections and cardiovascular disease.

Relapsing disease, unfortunately, occurs in almost 50% of patients at 5 years; most respond to therapy but do receive recurrent exposure to immunosuppression and cytotoxic agents.

Approximately 20% of patients who survive initial disease presentation will eventually develop end-stage renal disease.

13. **Which features predict relapse of the ANCA vasculitis?**
Patients with PR-3 ANCA are more than one and a half times as likely to relapse when compared to those with MPO ANCA. Additionally, pulmonary involvement has been associated with higher rates of relapse. Upper airway involvement has also been implicated as a risk factor for relapse, which was linked to nasal carriage of *Staphylococcus aureus,* also suggested as a risk factor for relapsing disease. The persistence of detectable anti-PR3 antibodies at the end of induction therapy is also associated with a two- to three-fold increase in the risk of subsequent relapse.

14. **What is the recurrence rate of ANCA disease following renal transplantation?**
Recurrent vasculitis occurs in about 17% of patients with ANCA vasculitis following renal transplantation. The mean time to recurrence is roughly 31 months, although recurrence has been reported within days and up to 13 years after transplantation. Of those who develop a recurrence, 60% will have glomerulonephritis (either alone or with extrarenal disease), whereas 40% will have only extrarenal disease.

Once remission is achieved, there is no evidence to delay transplantation for any particular waiting period or until ANCA testing is negative.

15. **Is venous thromboembolism (deep venous thrombosis or pulmonary embolus) a concern in patients with ANCA disease?**
Venous thromboembolism is an increasingly recognized complication of ANCA vasculitis. A high rate of events has been reported in both PR-3 and MPO ANCA disease, with about 10% of patients developing symptomatic venous thromboembolism (VTE) and an incidence of approximately seven events/100 person years. VTE events occur more frequently at time of active disease.

The pathogenesis of VTE in this population remains unclear, but there is speculation that ANCA disease may induce endothelial damage and hypercoagulability. A recent report has demonstrated the concurrent presence of antibodies complementary to PR-3 and reactive to plasminogen. These antibodies delay fibrinolysis in vitro and may provide insight into the pathogenesis of VTE in ANCA disease.

16. **What is the associated risk of malignancy for patients with ANCA treated with cyclophosphamide?**
The increased risk for cancer among patients with ANCA treated with cyclophosphamide has been relatively well-established. The most recent data have demonstrated an increased risk for nonmelanoma skin cancer, bladder cancer, and acute myelogenous leukemia (AML).

Both bladder cancer and AML appear to occur primarily among those treated with a cumulative cyclophosphamide dose >36 g and have a latency period of ≥7 years.

Additionally, bladder and skin cancers also seemed to present more commonly among those treated with azathioprine or mycophenolate maintenance therapies.

KEY POINTS: VASCULITIDES

1. Small-vessel vasculitis affecting the kidney frequently presents with microscopic hematuria, typically with dysmorphic red blood cells and red blood cell casts, a variable degree of proteinuria, and a rapid decline in glomerular filtration rate.

2. Antineutrophil cytoplasmic autoantibodies (ANCA) are present in 90% of patients with pauci-immune necrotizing glomerulonephritis, seen in Wegener's granulomatosis, microscopic polyangiitis, Churg-Strauss syndrome, and renal-limited disease.

3. Goodpasture's disease or anti-glomerular basement membrane disease may occur concurrently with ANCA small vessel vasculitis.

4. In small-vessel vasculitis, the mainstay of therapy consists of corticosteroids and cyclophosphamide.

5. In ANCA small-vessel vasculitis, plasma exchange is presently recommended in addition to corticosteroids and cyclophosphamide for patients presenting with advanced renal failure and/or pulmonary hemorrhage.

6. A high rate of venous thromboembolism has been reported in ANCA vasculitis with about 10% of patients developing symptomatic events.

7. Patients with ANCA treated with cyclophosphamide demonstrate an increased risk for nonmelanoma skin cancer, bladder cancer, and acute myelogenous leukemia.

BIBLIOGRAPHY

1. Allenbach Y, Seror R, Pagnoux C, et al. High frequency of venous thromboembolic events in Churg-Strauss syndrome, Wegener's granulomatosis and microscopic polyangiitis but not polyarteritis nodosa: a systematic retrospective study on 1130 patients. *Ann Rheum Dis* 2009;68:564–567.
2. Bautz DJ, Preston GA, Lionaki S, et al. Antibodies with dual reactivity to plasminogen and complementary PR3 in PR3-ANCA vasculitis. *J Am Soc Nephrol* 2008;19:2421–2429.
3. Faurschou M, Sorensen IJ, Mellemkjaer L, et al. Malignancies in Wegener's granulomatosis: Incidence and relation to cyclophosphamide therapy in a cohort of 293 patients. *J Rheumatol* 2008;35:100–105.
4. Geetha D, Seo P. Renal transplantation in the ANCA-associated vasculitides. *Am J Transplant* 2007;7:2657–2662.
5. Huugen D, van Esch A, Xiao H, et al. Inhibition of complement factor C5 protects against anti-myeloperoxidase antibody-mediated glomerulonephritis in mice. *Kidney Int* 2007;71:646–654.
6. Jayne D. The diagnosis of vasculitis. *Best Pract Res Clin Rheumatol* 2009;23:445–453.
7. Jayne D. Treatment of ANCA-associated systemic small-vessel vasculitis. *APMIS* 2009;Suppl:3–9.
8. Jennette JC, Falk RJ. Small-vessel vasculitis. *N Engl J Med* 1997;337:1512–1523.
9. Jennette JC, Falk RJ. New insight into the pathogenesis of vasculitis associated with antineutrophil cytoplasmic autoantibodies. *Curr Opin Rheumatol* 2008;20:55–60.
10. Jennette JC, Falk RJ, Andrassy K, et al. Nomenclature of systemic vasculitides. Proposal of an international consensus conference. *Arthritis Rheum* 1994;37:187–192.
11. Kain R, Exner M, Brandes R, et al. Molecular mimicry in pauci-immune focal necrotizing glomerulonephritis. *Nat Med* 2008;14:1088–1096.
12. Kalluri R, Meyers K, Mogyorosi A, et al. Goodpasture syndrome involving overlap with Wegener's granulomatosis and anti-glomerular basement membrane disease. *J Am Soc Nephrol* 1997;8:1795–1800.
13. Merkel PA, Lo GH, Holbrook JT, et al. Brief communication: High incidence of venous thrombotic events among patients with Wegener granulomatosis: The Wegener's Clinical Occurrence of Thrombosis (WeCLOT) Study. *Ann Intern Med* 2005;142:620–626.
14. Niles JL, Bottinger EP, Saurina GR, et al. The syndrome of lung hemorrhage and nephritis is usually an ANCA-associated condition. *Arch Intern Med* 1996;156:440–445.

15. Pagnoux C, Hogan SL, Chin H, et al. Predictors of treatment resistance and relapse in antineutrophil cytoplasmic antibody-associated small-vessel vasculitis: Comparison of two independent cohorts. *Arthritis Rheum* 2008;58: 2908–2918.
16. Stassen PM, Derks RP, Kallenberg CG, et al. Venous thromboembolism in ANCA-associated vasculitis—Incidence and risk factors. *Rheumatology* (Oxford) 2008;47:530–534.
17. ten Holder SM, Joy MS, Falk RJ. Cutaneous and systemic manifestations of drug-induced vasculitis. *Ann Pharmacother* 2002;36:130–147.
18. Watts R, Lane S, Hanslik T, et al. Development and validation of a consensus methodology for the classification of the ANCA-associated vasculitides and polyarteritis nodosa for epidemiological studies. *Ann Rheum Dis* 2007;66:222–227.
19. Weidner S, Hafezi-Rachti S, Rupprecht HD. Thromboembolic events as a complication of antineutrophil cytoplasmic antibody-associated vasculitis. *Arthritis Rheum* 2006;55:146–149.
20. Xiao H, Schreiber A, Heeringa P, et al. Alternative complement pathway in the pathogenesis of disease mediated by anti-neutrophil cytoplasmic autoantibodies. *Am J Pathol* 2007;170:52–64.

CHAPTER 39

THROMBOTIC MICROANGIOPATHIES

Marina Noris, PhD, and Giuseppe Remuzzi, MD

1. **Define thrombotic microangiopathy.**
   The term thrombotic microangiopathy defines a lesion of the microvasculature characterized by detachment and swelling of the endothelium, deposition of amorphous material in the subendothelial space, and luminal platelet aggregation leading to microthrombosis with partial or complete obstruction of the vessel lumina.

2. **What are the clinical features of patients with thrombotic microangiopathies?**
   Thrombotic microangiopathies present with thrombocytopenia, anemia, fever, and neurologic and renal dysfunction. Anemia is severe and microangiopathic in nature (Coombs negative), with fragmented red blood cells (schistocytes) in the peripheral smear, high serum lactate dehydrogenase (LDH), circulating free hemoglobin, and reticulocytes.

3. **What are the most common clinical syndromes associated with thrombotic microangiopathy?**
   - Typical Shiga toxin-associated hemolytic uremic syndrome (Stx-HUS)
   - Atypical hemolytic uremic syndrome (aHUS)
   - Thrombotic thrombocytopenic purpura (TTP)

4. **Can we make a differential diagnosis of Stx-HUS, aHUS, and TTP?**
   Yes and no. In HUS (either Stx-HUS or aHUS) there is primarily glomerular endothelial cell injury, resulting in acute renal impairment, whereas in TTP there is predominantly brain microvascular endothelial cell injury, resulting in neurologic disturbance. However, HUS can involve brain manifestation and patients with TTP often have renal dysfunction, which makes it difficult to distinguish the syndromes on clinical ground only. The underlying pathophysiologic mechanisms are different in Stx-HUS, aHUS, and TTP:
   - **Stx-HUS:** This occurs secondary to infection by certain strains of *Escherichia coli* or *Shigella dysenteriae,* which produce powerful toxins, the Shiga-like toxins (Stxs) that damage glomerular endothelial cells.
   - **aHUS:** Most cases are associated with genetic abnormalities leading to hyperactivation of the alternative pathway of complement.
   - **TTP:** Most patients have severe deficient activity of ADAMTS13, a plasma metalloprotease that cleaves von Willebrand factor (vWF) multimers soon after their secretion by endothelial cells and generates the range of vWF multimers sizes that normally circulate in blood.

5. **What is the incidence of Stx-HUS, aHUS, and TTP in the general population?**
   - Stx-HUS: Two cases for 100,000 persons/year
   - aHUS: One to two cases for 1,000,000 persons/year
   - TTP: Two to four cases for 1,000,000 persons/year

6. **Does Stx-HUS manifest disproportionately in children and adults?**
   Yes. Stx-HUS occurs most frequently in children younger than age 5 years (80% to 90% of overall cases of Stx-HUS).

7. **Describe the clinical course of Stx-HUS.**
   Stx-HUS is characterized by prodromal diarrhea (often bloody) followed within 4 or 6 days by acute renal failure. Vomiting occurs in 30% to 60% of cases, and fever occurs in 30%. Most patients require red blood cell transfusions, half need dialysis, and 25% have neurologic involvement. Renal function commonly recovers in a few days, and 75% of patients retain normal renal function long term. However, 3% to 5% of patients still die during the acute phase.

8. **Does the presence of bloody diarrhea prodrome distinguish between Stx-HUS and aHUS?**
   Yes and no. Most but not all cases of Stx-HUS (about 80%) have prodromal diarrhea. However, diarrhea at onset is recorded in up to 40% of cases with aHUS.

9. **How should patients with Stx-HUS be treated?**
   Treatment is based on supportive management of anemia, renal failure, hypertension, and electrolyte and water balance. There is no indication for plasma therapy (plasma infusion or exchange) except in those cases (mainly in adults) with prolonged severe renal insufficiency and central nervous system involvement.

10. **Is there any indication for antibiotic therapy in Stx-HUS?**
    No. Antibiotics should not be administered to children with gastroenteritis by Stx-producing *E. coli* infection because they may increase the risk of HUS. Indeed, antibiotic-induced injury to the bacterial membrane might favor the acute release of large amounts of preformed Stxs. The only indication for antibiotics is for cases of hemorrhagic colitis caused by *Shigella* in developing countries, when early antibiotic treatment can shorten the duration of diarrhea, decrease the incidence of complications, and reduce the risk of transmission by shortening the duration of bacterial shedding.

11. **What are the genetic causes of aHUS and their prevalence?**
    Several genetic abnormalities have been described in association with aHUS, all of them leading to uncontrolled activation of the alternative pathway of complement. The prevalence of the specific abnormalities is as follows:
    - Mutations in *CFH* (encoding complement factor H): 20% to 30%
    - Deletion of *CFHR1* and *CFHR3* (associated with anti-CFH autoantibodies): 6% to 8%
    - Mutations in *MCP* (encoding membrane cofactor protein): 10% to 15%
    - Mutations in *CFI* (encoding complement factor I): 4% to 10%
    - Mutations in *C3* (encoding complement C3): 5% to 10%
    - Mutation in *THBD* (encoding thrombomodulin): 5%
    - Mutations in *CFB* (encoding complement factor B): 1% to 2%

12. **What is the penetrance of aHUS in carriers of mutations in complement genes?**
    Mutations in complement genes confer predisposition rather than cause aHUS and penetrance among carriers of mutations ranges 50% to 60%. Hence, carriers of the mutations do not necessarily develop aHUS, but instead can be told that overall they have an approximately 50% chance of developing the disease.

13. **Are there any conditions that trigger aHUS in mutation carriers?**
    A number of conditions that cause complement activation directly (bacterial or viral infections) or indirectly by causing endothelial insult (drugs, such as cyclosporine, mitomycin, quinidine, tacrolimus, and bleomycin, and pregnancy) trigger the acute episode in about 60% of cases.

14. **Does the underlying genetic defect have an impact on clinical outcome in aHUS?**
    Yes. The course and outcome are influenced by the genes involved. About 60% to 70% of patients with *CFH, CFI, C3, THBD,* and *CFB* mutations lose renal function or die during the

presenting episode or develop end-stage renal disease (ESRD) following relapses. However, *MCP* mutation carriers have a good prognosis and 80% of patients remain dialysis-free long term. Patients with anti-CFH autoantibodies have an intermediate phenotype (rate of ESRD long term: 30% to 40%).

15. **What are effective treatments in aHUS?**
Treatment is based on plasma infusion or exchange. Guidelines suggest that plasma therapy (plasma-exchange, 1–2 plasma volumes/day, plasma infusion, 20–30 mL/kg/day) should be started within 24 hours of diagnosis. Plasma exchange allows supplying larger amounts of plasma than would be possible with infusion while avoiding fluid overload. Plasma therapy should be performed daily for 5 days, then five times a week for 2 weeks, and then three sessions per week for 2 additional weeks. The duration of plasma therapies should be determined on the basis of individual response to therapy, and treatment should be continued until complete normalization of hematologic parameters.

In patients with anti-*CFH* antibodies, plasma therapy should be combined with oral prednisone or intravenous prednisolone in patients with evidence of hepatic dysfunction (both at the dose of 200 mg/day rapidly tapered to 60 mg/day and then more slowly by 5 mg/week).

16. **Is kidney transplant outcome different among patients with Stx-HUS and aHUS who progress to ESRD, and what is the impact of the genetic defect on transplant outcome in aHUS?**
Yes, it is very different. Renal transplantation is an effective and safe treatment for patients who have Stx-HUS and have progressed to ESRD. In children with Stx-HUS, the incidence of disease recurrence in the graft ranges from 0% to 10%, and graft survival at 10 years is even better than in children who receive a transplant for other causes of ESRD.

In contrast, the disease recurs in around 50% of patients with aHUS who undergo transplantation, and graft failure occurs in 80% to 90% of those with recurrent disease. The type of mutation may predict the outcome after transplantation. The recurrence rate is 50% to 90% in patients with genetic abnormalities in the circulating complement regulators and proteins (*CFH, CFI, CFB, C3*) but is less than 20% in patients with *MCP* mutations.

17. **Is a combined kidney and liver transplant an option for patients with aHUS at high risk for recurrence?**
Simultaneous kidney and liver transplantation has been performed in 10 patients with aHUS associated with *CFH* mutations and succeeded in seven, with good liver and kidney graft function on long term and no disease recurrence. However, the other three patients died as a result of early failure of the transplanted kidney. The substantial risks of combined kidney and liver transplantation require a careful assessment of potential benefits for candidate patients.

18. **Are there any new specific treatments for aHUS under investigation?**
Yes. A humanized anti-C5 monoclonal antibody, eculizumab, has been reported as a promising treatment in case reports of aHUS. Trials of eculizumab have commenced in patients who are plasma therapy-sensitive or plasma therapy-resistant and interim results provided further data on the efficacy of this drug in aHUS.

19. **What is known about the causes of ADAMTS13 deficiency in TTP?**
Two mechanisms for deficiency of ADAMTS13 activity have been identified in patients with TTP. Of patients, 60% to 80% have an acquired deficiency as a result of the formation of anti-ADAMTS13 autoantibodies (acquired TTP). About 5% to 10% of patients have a genetic ADAMTS13 deficiency as a result of homozygous or compound heterozygous mutations in *ADAMTS13* gene (congenital TTP).

20. **Is severe ADAMTS13 deficiency a specific marker of TTP?**
Yes and no. About 20% of patients with clinical features of TTP do not have severely deficient ADAMTS13 activity. In addition, patients with other disorders, such as sepsis and liver

cirrhosis, may have severe ADAMTS13 defects. Also, patients with clinical diagnosis of aHUS may completely lack ADAMTS13 activity, albeit less frequently. However, severe ADAMTS13 deficiency is the most important risk factor for TTP and documentation of ADAMTS13 deficiency can be important to confirm diagnosis.

21. **Is plasma therapy effective in TTP?**
Yes. Plasma therapy is a cornerstone in the treatment of all forms of TTP. Patients with congenital ADAMTS13 deficiency benefit from plasma infusion, whereas in patients with anti-ADAMTS13 antibodies plasma exchange may have the additional benefit of removing the antibodies from the patient's blood.

22. **Are corticosteroids and immunosuppressive therapy effective in TTP?**
Yes and no. Corticosteroids, combined with plasma exchange, might be of benefit in acquired TTP by inhibiting the synthesis of anti-ADAMTS13 antibodies. The rationale of combined treatment is that plasma exchange will have only a temporary effect on the autoimmune basis of the disease and addition of immunosuppressive treatment may cause a more durable response. However, there is no indication for administering corticosteroids to patients with congenital TTP.

23. **Is there good evidence supporting the use of rituximab in treating TTP associated with anti-ADAMTS13 antibodies?**
Yes. Prospective studies have successfully and safely used the anti-CD20 monoclonal antibody rituximab in patients whose disease had failed to respond to daily plasma exchange and corticosteroids and in patients with relapsed acute TTP who had demonstrated antibodies to ADAMTS13. Treatment was associated with clinical remission and disappearance of anti-ADAMTS13 antibodies. Rituximab has also been used electively to prevent relapses in patients with autoantibodies and recurrent disease.

KEY POINTS: THROMBOTIC MICROANGIOPATHIES

1. Hemolytic uremic syndrome (HUS) and thrombotic thrombocytopenic purpura (TTP) are thrombotic microangiopathies (TMAs) manifesting with thrombocytopenia and microangio-pathic hemolytic anemia.

2. The most common form of TMA is Shiga toxin-associated HUS, which is caused by strains of bacteria that produce exotoxins, the Shiga-like toxins causing endothelial damage. This form generally has a good outcome with supportive therapy alone.

3. Atypical forms of HUS are associated with hyperactivation of the alternative pathway of complement caused either by complement gene abnormalities or by autoantibodies against factor H. These forms have a poor outcome.

4. TTP is caused by deficiency in ADAMTS13, a plasma metalloprotease that cleaves von Willebrand factor multimers. The defect is caused either by ADAMTS13 gene mutations or by anti-ADAMTS13 autoantibodies.

5. In both atypical HUS and in TTP, the clinical outcome; response to therapy; and, in atypical HUS the outcome of kidney transplantation are greatly influenced by the specific underlying defect.

6. Immune-mediated HUS and TTP are caused by the formation of autoantibodies against complement or ADAMTS13, respectively.

7. Identification of the specific genetic defect underlying atypical hemolytic uremic syndrome is critical to predict outcome, response to therapy, and outcome of kidney transplantation.

BIBLIOGRAPHY

1. Besbas N, Karpman D, Landau D, et al. A classification of hemolytic uremic syndrome and thrombotic thrombocytopenic purpura and related disorder. *Kidney Int* 2006;70:423–431.
2. Bresin E, Daina E, Noris M, et al. Outcome of renal transplantation in patients with non-Shiga toxin-associated haemolytic uremic syndrome: Prognostic significance of genetic background. *Clin J Am Soc Nephrol* 2006;1:88–99.
3. Bresin E, Gastoldi S, Daina E, et al. Rituximab as pre-emptive treatment in patients with thrombotic thrombocytopenic purpura and evidence of anti-ADAMTS13 autoantibodies. *Thromb Haemost* 2009;101:233–238.
4. Caprioli J, Noris M, Brioschi S, et al. Genetics of HUS: The impact of MCP, CFH, and IF mutations on clinical presentation, response to treatment, and outcome. *Blood* 2006;108:1267–1279.
5. Delvaeye M, Noris M, De Vriese A, et al. Thrombomodulin mutations in atypical hemolytic-uremic syndrome. *N Engl J Med* 2009;361:345–357.
6. Galbusera M, Noris M, Remuzzi G. Thrombotic thrombocytopenic purpura—Then and now. *Semin Thromb Hemost* 2006;32:81–89.
7. George JN. Clinical practice. Thrombotic thrombocytopenic purpura. *N Engl J Med* 2006;354:1927–1935.
8. Jozsi M, Licht C, Strobel S, et al. Factor H autoantibodies in atypical hemolytic uremic syndrome correlate with CFHR1/CFHR3 deficiency. *Blood* 2008;111:1512–1514.
9. Levy GG, Nichols WC, Lian EC, et al. Mutations in a member of the ADAMTS gene family cause thrombotic thrombocytopenic purpura. *Nature* 2001;413:488–494.
10. Noris M, Remuzzi G. Atypical hemolytic uremic syndrome. *N Engl J Med* 2009;361:1676–1687.
11. Scheiring J, Andreoli SP, Zimmerhackl LB. Treatment and outcome of Shiga-toxin-associated hemolytic uremic syndrome (HUS). *Pediatr Nephrol* 2008;23:1749–1760.
12. Tsai HM, Lian EC. Antibodies to von Willebrand factor-cleaving protease in acute thrombotic thrombocytopenic purpura. *N Engl J Med* 1998;339:1585–1594.
13. Walport MJ. Complement. First of two parts. *N Engl J Med* 2001;344:1058–1066.

VI. INFECTION-ASSOCIATED GLOMERULONEPHRITIDES

POSTINFECTIOUS GLOMERULONEPHRITIS

Warren Kupin, MD

CHAPTER 40

1. **What is the definition of postinfectious glomerulonephritis?**
   Postinfectious glomerulonephritis (PIGN) describes a form of acute glomerulonephritis as a consequence of an extrarenal infection. In past years, this renal disease has been referred to as poststreptococcal glomerulonephritis (PSGN), and these terms are often used interchangeably. However, this is not an accurate designation because PSGN is a form of PIGN and has its own unique clinical presentation and natural history. The term PIGN refers to the glomerular disease that results from not just streptococcal infection, but also from a wide variety of gram-positive and gram-negative organisms, fungi, parasites, and viruses.

2. **Does the site of infection affect whether a patient will develop PIGN?**
   No. Infections at any site in the body have the potential to cause PIGN. Because the original description of this disease occurred after an episode of streptococcal pharyngitis, however, most physicians primarily associate this source of infection and the development of glomerulonephritis and are not aware that skin infections, pneumonia, any visceral abscesses, urinary tract infections, periodontitis, and endocarditis can lead to the same lesion. The important point to keep in mind is that it is not the type or source of the infection; rather, it is simply the presence of foreign antigens that arise from the infection coupled with the response of the immune system that lead to immune complex formation and glomerulonephritis.

3. **What is the typical time for presentation of PIGN after an infection?**
   The course of PIGN has been well documented for both the pharyngitis and skin infection sites of streptococcal infection. Typically, renal disease begins 10 to 14 days after the onset of streptococcal pharyngitis, whereas it takes about 21 days for the development of glomerulonephritis after a skin infection such as impetigo. The onset of glomerulonephritis after infection in other sites of the body also follows a course of between 2 to 4 weeks postinfection. These time patterns are critical because usually the infection has healed and only later on does the patient present with renal disease. As an example, sometimes the patient may have forgotten about having an upper or lower respiratory illness in the preceding 3 to 4 weeks, and it would appear that the glomerulonephritis has no link to any infectious event. A careful history and laboratory workup (described later) may help identify a cause of the renal disease.

4. **How does PIGN present clinically?**
   All types of acute glomerulonephritis, whether primary or secondary, present with combinations of the nephritic and nephrotic syndrome. The nephritic syndrome consists of the presence of an active urinary sediment containing red blood cell casts, white blood cells, red blood cells (dysmorphic), and proteinuria (less than 3.5 g/24 hours) coupled with acute renal injury, hypertension (HTN), and edema. Depending on the degree of basement membrane damage by the immune complexes, the magnitude of proteinuria can increase substantially even to the nephrotic range (>3.5 g/24 hours). Renal function is often significantly impaired with concomitant HTN and peripheral/pulmonary edema. Severe, uncontrolled HTN is a common feature in patients with acute glomerulonephritis and requires immediate control and management. The absence of HTN would be extremely unusual and

may warrant a reconsideration of the diagnosis. Another important pertinent negative in the presentation of these patients is that there is no evidence of a rash as one would see in allergic interstitial nephritis.

Many patients with PIGN present with "dark or tea-colored" urine as a result of the presence of significant microscopic hematuria. The color is only indicative of the effect of the pH on the free hemoglobin molecule, with an alkaline urine looking more bright red and an acidic urine showing a darker brownish hue for the same number of hemolyzed red blood cells. This onset of this "dark" urine with PSGN occurs 2 to 4 weeks after the infection.

5. **What laboratory findings are characteristic of PIGN?**
The development of glomerulonephritis results from immune complex deposition in the basement membrane of the glomerulus leading to loss of the filtration area and a breach of the integrity of the membrane for protein. These immune complexes consist of an antigen from the infection and usually an immunoglobulin G (IgG) antibody. The damage to the basement membrane from these complexes is often a result of local complement activation exclusively through the alternative pathway. This pathway leads to C3 cleavage and then the production of the membrane attack complex C5-9. Bypassed in this pathway is the activation of C4, which is only used in the classical complement pathway activation. Therefore, when PIGN is suspected, the measurement of serum complement both C3 and C4 is crucial. In PIGN, the C3 level will be low but the C4 level will be normal. If both C3 and C4 are low, then the diagnosis of PIGN is not supported and another source of immune complexes may be present that activate the classical complement pathway, such as cryoglobulinemia or systemic lupus erythematosus.

Microbiologic and radiologic tests for infection are frequently negative but should still be done. These studies would include a chest x-ray, blood, sputum, and pharyngeal and urine cultures in addition to a careful examination of the skin, anogenital region, and oral cavity for any signs of inflammation. If a streptococcal infection is suspected, then specific serologic assays are available such as the ASO titer. However, this test may be falsely negative and lacks the sensitivity to be used as a stand-alone test for streptococcal infection. A more sensitive screen for a recent streptococcal infection is the streptozyme test, which includes five different antibodies that will develop to this infection. These include ASO titer, anti-hyaluronidase (AHase), anti-streptokinase (ASKase), anti-nicotinamide adenine dinucleotidase (anti-NAD), and anti-DNAse B antibodies. The reason this test is important is because the source of the streptococcal infection will determine what pattern of antibodies will develop; for skin infections only the anti-DNAse and AHase are positive, whereas for a pharyngeal infection all five of these antibodies are usually present in various concentrations.

6. **What does the renal biopsy show in PIGN?**
The most common histology seen with all forms of PIGN is diffuse proliferative glomerulonephritis with significant endocapillary proliferation. By light microscopy, this lesion is characterized by involvement of almost all glomeruli with an influx of neutrophils into the glomerular capillaries and a proliferation of the capillary endothelial cells. The capillary lumens are virtually obliterated, reducing the area for ultrafiltration, which leads to a loss of glomerular filtration rate (GFR). By electron microscopy the etiology for the inflammation is seen by the presence of immune complexes in the subepithelial, subendothelial, and mesangial regions. The subepithelial deposits are often called "humps" because they protrude outward on top of the basement membrane. The presence of immune complexes results in a "granular" appearance by immunofluorescence using IgG and C3. Less frequent glomerular findings include a mesangial proliferative glomerulonephritis or a focal proliferative glomerulonephritis. It should be noted that a renal biopsy is usually not done in straightforward cases of PIGN because the treatment will not differ (as noted later). A renal biopsy is only recommended for those atypical cases when the clinical and laboratory features are not compatible with PIGN.

7. **Is there any treatment for PIGN?**

    The treatment for PIGN is primarily supportive because the infection is often not apparent any longer and the immune complex deposition in the kidney spontaneously resolves over time. For supportive therapy the major focus is on blood pressure and volume control. Remember, the tubules are relatively unaffected by the glomerular disease and there is a sodium avid state that accompanies the glomerular inflammation. The absorption of sodium and water leads to significant volume overload and salt-sensitive HTN. Therefore, in addition to the use of regular anti-HTN medication along with salt and water restriction, the early inclusion of loop diuretics is particularly efficacious in PIGN.

    The use of steroids or more aggressive forms of immunosuppression for PIGN has not been shown to alter the natural history of the disease and exposes the patient to the potential short- and long-term risks of immunosuppression. The only exception to this rule is the presence of severe crescentic glomerulonephritis. This subset of PIGN includes the standard features of diffuse proliferative glomerulonephritis coupled with the presence of crescents that arise from the parietal epithelium. Often these patients receive bolus steroids and anecdotal reports have used cytotoxic therapy, but there are no well-designed studies supporting these therapies.

8. **Do patients eventually go into remission, or is there evidence for permanent renal injury after PIGN?**

    The recovery of the kidney from PIGN follows a different time sequence when looking at the GFR, hematuria, and proteinuria. Of note, the acute renal injury begins to improve within 1 to 2 weeks of onset and the serum creatinine returns to its baseline level after 3 to 4 weeks. This improvement in GFR usually parallels the clearance of infiltrating neutrophils in the glomerulus and the decrease in the proliferation of endothelial cells.

    Proteinuria in PIGN is a result of the subepithelial immune complexes and will only improve as they are removed. As a result of their location, these immune complexes are cleared very slowly and proteinuria may persist for years after the initial episode. The hematuria seen in PIGN is a result of the subendothelial immune complexes, and these are more rapidly removed from the basement membrane. Consequently, hematuria will resolve within 3 to 6 months. It is recommended that failure to resolve the hematuria or proteinuria should warrant a biopsy to determine if another type of renal disease is present other than PIGN.

    It is essential to know that evidence of renal injury can persist for years after an episode of PIGN. The risk of developing chronic kidney disease and eventually end-stage renal disease from PIGN is almost unheard of in children, but in adults this can be seen in a minimum of 10% to 15% of cases.

9. **Are there any subgroups of patients that are more susceptible to develop PIGN after an infection?**

    It appears that socioeconomic conditions play a major role in the development of PIGN, especially after a streptococcal infection. At present the majority of cases of PIGN arise in Third World countries, in areas in which the population has been exposed to poor nutritional support and inadequate general sanitation. These conditions likely result in an immunocompromised state and a dysregulated response to infections. If an impaired immune system is a prerequisite in most cases for the development of PIGN, then additional high-risk populations can be identified, such as patients with a chronic illness like diabetes mellitus, HIV, or alcoholism and those receiving chemotherapy for malignancy.

    Specifically looking at PSGN, the overall incidence in children has decreased substantially over the past three decades, likely related to better pediatric care, early use of antibiotics, and improved nutrition worldwide. However, particularly in South America and Asia, PSGN remains a significant cause of acute renal failure in children.

    An interesting feature in patients with diabetes is that in many circumstances there was clear evidence of diabetic nephropathy in the background of PIGN. Consequently, just because a patient has one type of renal disease, that does not exclude the fact that they can develop a superimposed new form of kidney disease.

In the case of streptococcal infection, it is well established that only certain strains are nephritogenic for the pharyngeal or cutaneous sites. In addition, there must be a genetic susceptibility because even when there is an epidemic of a nephritogenic strain, the penetrance of the kidney disease is between 10% and 25%. Routine testing for nephritogenic strains of *Streptococcus* is not recommended, and the diagnosis and workup of PSGN are based on clinical and laboratory findings.

KEY POINTS: POSTINFECTIOUS GLOMERULONEPHRITIS

1. Infections at any site in the body have the potential to cause postinfectious glomerulonephritis (PIGN); however, because the original description of this disease occurred after an episode of streptococcal pharyngitis, most physicians primarily associate this source of infection and the development of glomerulonephritis.

2. The course of poststreptococcal glomerulonephritis has been well documented for both the pharyngitis and skin infection sites of streptococcal infection; renal disease begins 10 to 14 days after the onset of streptococcal pharyngitis, whereas it takes about 21 days for the development of glomerulonephritis after a skin infection. These time patterns are critical because usually the infection has healed and only later on does the patient present with renal disease.

3. The use of steroids or more aggressive forms of immunosuppression for PIGN has not been shown to alter the natural history of the disease and exposes the patient to the potential short- and long-term risks of immunosuppression. The only exception to this rule is the presence of severe crescentic glomerulonephritis.

4. It is essential to know that evidence of renal injury can persist for years after an episode of PIGN. The risk of developing chronic kidney and eventually end-stage renal disease from PIGN is almost unheard of in children, but in adults this can be seen in a minimum of 10% of cases.

10. **When PIGN follows an upper respiratory illness (URI), are any other differential diagnoses important to consider?**
One of the most difficult diagnostic situations occurs when patients develop renal disease after a URI. In addition to PIGN, there are two important differential diagnoses to consider: IgA nephropathy and membranoproliferative glomerulonephritis (MPGN). As previously discussed, PIGN occurs approximately 10 to 14 days or more after the infection has started and there may not be any evidence of the URI at the time renal disease develops. Alternatively, IgA nephropathy is called "synpharyngitic" because it is exacerbated at the time of the URI, usually within the first few days of onset. It is at this time that the patient will present with gross hematuria, HTN, and signs of acute renal injury such as edema. IgA is the antibody that exists on the mucous membranes, and any type of infection (viral, bacterial) will lead to overproduction of IgA and, in susceptible individuals, the development of immune complexes and glomerulonephritis. This concept is interesting because in PIGN, especially in PSGN, it is the actual strain of bacteria that is nephritogenic, whereas in IgA nephropathy it is more of a disease of the host having a dysregulated immune response to a nonspecific pathogen.
Clinically, IgA nephropathy relapses during the episode of URI and then afterward settles back into a background level of low-grade microhematuria and non-nephrotic proteinuria. Many patients have had unsuspected IgA nephropathy prior to the onset of the URI and it was the gross hematuria from the exacerbation of IgA nephropathy that brought the patient to the physician. The complement levels are normal in IgA nephropathy because the immune complexes are different than in PIGN. These IgA immune complexes only locally activate

complement through the alternate pathway (low C3) at the level of the mesangium and basement membrane and not by the classical pathway (low C3 and C4), as in PIGN.

MPGN can be an idiopathic disease in young adults, which is the very population that may present with a URI to the emergency room or physician's office. This disease is characterized by microhematuria and proteinuria, even in the nephrotic range. It is associated with activation of the alternate pathway leading to low systemic levels of C3. In contrast to IgA nephropathy, which also activates the alternate pathway but has normal systemic levels of C3, MPGN shows persistently low levels of C3, especially after the URI has resolved. The URI may transiently worsen the renal manifestations of MPGN; however, as compared to PIGN, even after the URI is resolved and months have passed, there remains significant hematuria and proteinuria with a low C3.

Key points in differentiating PIGN from IgA nephropathy and idiopathic MPGN are noted in Table 40-1.

TABLE 40-1. DIFFERENTIATING PIGN FROM IgA NEPHROPATHY AND IDIOPATHIC MPGN			
	PIGN	IgA Nephropathy	MPGN
Timing in relationship to a URI	10–14 days or more after the onset	"Synchronous" with the URI	"Synchronous" with the URI
Gross hematuria	30%–50%	>80%	10%–20%
Nephrotic syndrome	10%–20%	5%–10%	40%–60%
Hypertension	>80%	30%–50%	>80%
Serum complement	Classical pathway Low C3 and C4	Alternate pathway Locally in the kidney Normal C3 and C4	Alternate pathway Low C3 normal C4

PIGN = postinfectious glomerulonephritis; IgA = immunoglobulin A; MPGN = membranoproliferative glomerulonephritis; URI = upper respiratory illness.

BIBLIOGRAPHY

1. Kanjanabuch T, Kittikowit W, Eiam-Ong S. An update on acute postinfectious glomerulonephritis worldwide. *Nat Rev Nephrol* 2009;5:259–269.

2. Naicker S, Fabian J, Naidoo S, et al. Infection and glomerulonephritis. *Semin Immunopathol* 2007;29:397–414.

3. Nasr S, Markowitz G, Stokes M, et al. Acute postinfectious glomerulonephritis in the modern era. *Medicine* 2008;87:21–32.

4. Rodriguez-Iturbe B, Musser JM. The current state of poststreptococcal glomerulonephritis. *J Am Soc Nephrol* 2008;10:1855–1864.

5. Wen YK. Clinicopathological study of acute glomerulonephritis in adults. *Int Urol Nephrol* 2010;42(2):477–485.

6. Wen YK. The spectrum of adult postinfectious glomerulonephritis in the new millennium. *Ren Fail* 2009;31:676–682.

CHAPTER 41

VIRAL HEPATITIS–ASSOCIATED GLOMERULONEPHRITIS

Warren Kupin, MD

1. **What types of viral hepatitis are associated with glomerulonephritis?**

   Chronic hepatitis B or hepatitis C puts patients at risk of developing specific types of glomerular diseases. By definition, a carrier state for these viruses would be characterized by a positive polymerase chain reaction (PCR) assay showing active viral replication. Usually the PCR is not the first screening test for these viruses in clinical practice.

   For hepatitis B, the common markers used for routine screening include the hepatitis B surface antibody, hepatitis B core antibody, and the hepatitis B surface antigen. Patients positive for hepatitis B surface antigen and with negative hepatitis surface and core antibodies are very likely to have a chronic carrier state. The next confirmatory tests would be an assay for hepatitis B e antigen and the PCR assay. The presence or absence of hepatitis B e antigen will be very important in regard to the type of glomerular disease that may develop. Patients positive for both hepatitis B e antigen and hepatitis B surface antigen are highly infectious and have a greater risk of kidney disease.

   For hepatitis C, the most common initial screening test is the enzyme-linked immunosorbent assay (ELISA) for hepatitis C antibodies. In stark contrast to the importance of hepatitis B surface antibodies as an indicator of disease remission and the absence of a carrier state for hepatitis B, the presence of hepatitis C antibodies usually means the absence of viral control and a chronic carrier state for hepatitis C. Once detected, the next step would be a PCR assay to determine the viral load. There is a small subgroup of patients (5% to 7%) who do not mount an antibody response to hepatitis C and are chronic carriers by PCR. This is especially true for patients with end-stage renal disease (ESRD); therefore, if a renal lesion is suspicious for hepatitis C glomerulopathy (as discussed later), then a PCR should be done even if the ELISA is negative.

2. **Are the usual measurements of glomerular filtration rate (GFR) and proteinuria applicable to patients with chronic hepatitis?**

   We know that the serum creatinine concentration results from the metabolism of creatine, which is a nitrogenous organic acid stored in muscles and functions as an energy-providing catalyst. Creatine has two sources in the body: liver production and oral ingestion. About half the creatine comes from each source, which is extremely important when it comes to evaluating renal function in patients with chronic hepatitis. Most patients who are chronic carriers of either hepatitis B or C have significant inflammatory injury to the liver and may even have various stages of cirrhosis. Creatine production in the liver will then be significantly reduced, and this will lead to a lower muscle mass and a lower serum creatinine that would be expected for a person of any given gender or age. In the presence of cirrhosis, the synthesis of creatine can be reduced by more than 50% and the oral intake of creatine will also be reduced as a result of the overall state of malnutrition of these patients. The typical serum creatinine is usually 0.5 to 0.6 mg/dL in patients with cirrhosis, which is well below the normal expected maximum range for the general population (1.2 mg/dL for women and 1.5 mg/dL for men). Patients with liver disease can have a significant loss of GFR with a serum creatinine level within "the normal range" for the general population.

For this reason, all physicians managing patients with chronic hepatitis should monitor renal function by the use of either a 24-hour creatinine clearance or a calculated GFR from either the Modification of diet in Renal Disease Study (MDRD) or Cockcroft-Gault formulas. Although these methods have significant bias and may overestimate GFR, they are still the preferred means compared to the serum creatinine to monitor renal function in patients with liver disease.

In addition, all patients who are hepatitis carriers should be screened for proteinuria. A random urine protein/creatinine ratio or a 24-hour urine protein collection are equally valid ways to quantify proteinuria. In patients with severe jaundice, the colorimetric dipstick may give false readings for protein because of the bilirubin pigment in the urine, so every positive urine dipstick test for protein should be confirmed with a quantitative measurement.

3. **What type of glomerular lesions are seen with a chronic hepatitis B carrier state?**
The most common glomerular pathology seen with active hepatitis B antigenemia, is membranous nephropathy (MN). These patients can also develop polyarteritis nodosa, membranoproliferative glomerulonephritis (MPGN), IgA nephropathy, and focal segmental glomerulosclerosis (FSGS).

4. **How does hepatitis B cause each of these types of renal disease?**
The most common lesion seen is MN. Typically, this pathologic finding is considered to be idiopathic and is the most common cause of nephrotic syndrome in white people in the United States. However, worldwide, a chronic hepatitis B carrier state is an important secondary cause of MN. This lesion is a result of the deposition of immune complexes in the basement membrane of the glomerulus, specifically in the subepithelial space. This location is important because it tells us a great deal about the size of the immune complex— it has to be very small to pass through the basement membrane and end up on the outside of the capillary underneath the podocyte foot processes (subepithelial space). The only immune complex from hepatitis B that can do this is the hepatitis B e Ag-antibody complex. Therefore, the vast majority of patients with chronic hepatitis B antigenemia who develop MN are also positive for the hepatitis B e antigen.

For those patients who are carriers of hepatitis B but are only hepatitis B surface antigen positive and negative for hepatitis B e antigen, the renal lesion is not usually MN but MPGN. This is because the hepatitis B surface antigen-antibody immune complex is too large to filter through the basement membrane, so it lodges in the inner surface of the capillary wall (subendothelial space). The subsequent inflammation leads to proliferation and histologically appears as MPGN. In summary, the information in Table 41-1 is important to know.

TABLE 41-1. GLOMERULAR LESIONS CAUSED BY HEPATITIS B		
	Hepatitis B e Antigen Positive + **Hepatitis B Surface Antigen Positive**	**Hepatitis B e Antigen Negative** + **Hepatitis B Surface Antigen Positive**
Glomerular lesion	Membranous nephropathy	Membranoproliferative glomerulonephritis
Location of immune complexes	Subepithelial space	Subendothelial space

The liver is responsible for the metabolism of immunoglobulin A (IgA), so in the presence of significant liver injury, the circulating levels of IgA increase and may deposit in the kidney. These complexes first embed in the mesangium but may also be in the peripheral capillary loops. Clinically significant renal disease from this "secondary" deposition of IgA in the glomeruli in any patient with liver disease regardless of etiology is extremely rare.

Polyarteritis nodosa is a necrotizing vasculitis of medium-sized vessels that is not a direct form of glomerulonephritis. Rather, it affects the inflow circulation of the kidney and, as a result of fibrinoid necrosis and thrombosis of the larger muscular arteries of the kidney, there is glomerular ischemia and progressive kidney failure. The etiology for the vasculitis is the presence of hepatitis B surface antigen-antibody complexes in the blood vessel walls, causing complement activation and necrosis. The presence or absence of hepatitis B e antigen is not important in the genesis of this lesion.

Finally, recent reports have shown a higher than expected incidence of focal segmental glomerulosclerosis in patients with chronic hepatitis B antigenemia. Because there are no immune complexes in the kidney with FSGS, it is not clear why this pathologic entity develops. The hepatitis B virus may actually enter or deposit in renal tissue and lead to FSGS. However rare, it remains in the differential of any patient with hepatitis B and nephrotic syndrome.

5. **Can you determine what the renal disease is without a kidney biopsy in a patients with chronic hepatitis B?**

Ultimately, a kidney biopsy is needed to be absolutely confident of the diagnosis and treatment plan. A few clues may be present as the etiology. Patients with MN and FSGS are typically nephrotic with a bland urine sediment, whereas those patients with MPGN, IgA nephropathy, and polyarteritis nodosa are more likely going to have a nephritic sediment with a variety of casts (epithelial and red cell), dysmorphic red cells, white blood cells, and renal tubular cells.

6. **Is hepatitis B-related glomerular disease treatable?**

Because the generation of immune complexes requires active hepatitis B viral replication, it is clear that the primary goal of therapy is to directly treat the source of the antigens—the hepatitis B virus. Initially, lamivudine was the treatment of choice for suppressing the viral load and this agent had to be continued indefinitely to maintain a sustained viral response. Patients experiencing a complete suppression of viral replication have a remission of MN with normalization of their proteinuria, improved renal function, and a prolonged renal survival. Over time, as many as 50% of patients have developed mutational resistance to lamivudine and show a relapse of viremia. The current guidelines have replaced lamivudine with entecavir as the primary agent for treatment of active hepatitis B antigenemia. For MN, this is all the therapy that is needed along with the typical antiproteinuria therapy such as angiotensin-converting enzyme inhibitors and angiotensin receptor blockers. No steroids or other forms of immunosuppression are needed, and these agents may actually worsen the prognosis by increasing viremia.

For patients with MPGN, the data are not as clear, but theoretically control of viremia would be essential. Again, the use of steroids or other immunosuppressant agents is not efficacious in this lesion. IgA nephropathy as mentioned is rarely clinically important and would require specific therapy. Because the IgA deposits are a result of advanced liver disease, unless liver function improves, there will be a continuous presence of IgA in the kidney.

Polyarteritis nodosa is a different disease because it is a systemic vasculitis that can cause life-threatening widespread organ dysfunction. In hepatitis B it results from immune complexes, so once again, control of viremia is essential. However, if there is significant systemic vasculitis, then a temporary use of steroids and even immunosuppressive therapy may be needed. The risk of this option would be further increasing the hepatitis B viral load temporarily at the expense of reducing end-organ damage. This decision must be weighed carefully based on the severity of the vasculitis.

7. **What types of glomerular disease are caused by hepatitis C?**
The most common histologic change in the glomerulus of patients with chronic hepatitis C infection is type I membranoproliferative glomerulonephritis as a consequence of type II cryoglobulinemia. These patients may also develop membranous nephropathy, fibrillary glomerulonephritis, IgA nephropathy, and diabetic nephropathy.

8. **What is type I MPGN as a consequence of type II cryoglobulinemia?**
MPGN is a specific type of glomerular injury, in which there is damage to the basement membrane and an increase in the proliferation of endothelial cells and mesangial cells. Therefore, compared to MN, in which there is only thickening of the basement membrane as a result of immune complexes without proliferation, MPGN is clearly a more aggressive type of renal injury. MN would typically cause only the nephrotic syndrome, whereas MPGN would be accompanied by the nephritic syndrome with an "active" urinary sediment showing red cells casts, granular casts, dysmorphic red cells, and renal tubular epithelial cells.

MPGN, like MN, results from immune complexes, but they deposit in a distinct distribution. Hepatitis C results in the unique production of cryoglobulins that deposit in the kidney leading to MPGN. This is completely distinct from idiopathic MPGN, which may occur in children and young adults where the immune complexes are not a result of cryoglobulins and deposit in a different pattern. The cryoglobulins in hepatitis C are so large that they can not filter through the basement membrane, thereby becoming trapped in the subendothelial space. Their size forces them to protrude into the lumen of the capillary, and it almost looks like there are thrombi in the glomeruli capillaries. The entire capillary lumen may become filled with the cryoglobulin complex. In idiopathic MPGN, the immune complexes are also subendothelial but never so large as to cause compromise of the vascular lumen.

Cryoglobulins are immune complexes comprising certain types of antibody and antigens that precipitate on cooling and are classified based on the composition of the antibody involved and its target. When the antibody is composed of a single subtype (monoclonal) such as only an IgG or IgM and precipitates in the cold, it is called type I cryoglobulinemia. This often results from a hematopoietic malignancy. If there is an antibody that is monoclonal (IgM or IgG) and it targets another antibody that is polyclonal (IgG), this is called type II cryoglobulinemia. If there are two different polyclonal antibodies present that interact and form an immune complex, this is called type III cryoglobulinemia. Hepatitis C is characteristically associated with type II cryoglobulinemia.

Once a patient is infected with hepatitis C, the immune system tries to neutralize the virus by producing IgG antibodies against the surface antigens of the viral capsid. Unfortunately, although these antibodies are produced, they fail to neutralize the virus yet they circulate in the blood of patients chronically infected with hepatitic C. This is what is measured with the ELISA—non-neutralizing IgG antibodies against the hepatitis C capsid. What is unusual in hepatitis C is that the patient will make a rare type of monoclonal IgM antibody (IgM*k*) that directly targets the IgG the person has made against the virus. When one antibody attacks another antibody, the product is called an anti-idiotypic antibody. The IgM that is made in patients with hepatitis C is anti-idiotypic because it is directed against the IgG molecule. The cryoglobulin in hepatitis C is composed of a monoclonal IgM*k*, a polyclonal IgG, and viral capsid antigens. This is why it is so large and obstructs the lumen of the capillary. It is not known why only the IgM heavy chain and only the kappa light chains are made by the stimulated B cells from hepatitis C.

9. **Why do cryoglobulins form only with hepatitis C and not hepatitis B?**
Hepatitis B is a hepatotropic virus, meaning it selectively enters hepatic tissue but no other organ tissue. In contrast to HIV, it does not directly infect renal tissue to cause its damage to the kidney. Rather, it causes immune complexes that deposit in the kidney leading to MN. Hepatitis C is not only hepatotropic, but it is lymphotropic, having an affinity to bind to select receptors on B cells. The viral capsid antigens appear to be able to target B-cell receptors that are responsible for cell proliferation and disrupt the normal cell cycle. Infected B cells in

hepatitis C become clonal and produce a specific type of IgM antibody that has anti-idiotypic capacity. Hepatitis B and no other form of viral hepatitis has this ability to bind to and stimulate B cells, which is why cryoglobulins are unique to hepatitis C.

Over time, patients with hepatitis C who have cryoglobulinemia are at higher risk for the development of B-cell lymphoma. Type II cryoglobulinemia is a result of a clonal expansion of B cells and should be regarded as a premalignant disease. If these patients live long enough, approximately 6% will manifest evidence of a lymphoma.

10. **Do the cryoglobulins cause damage in any other organ system?**
Absolutely. The circulation of these type II cryoglobulins leads to inflammatory damage in the vascular system throughout the body, characterized by vasculitis. Specifically, these patients develop lower extremity skin lesions (palpable purpura); cerebral/cardiac/pulmonary/peripheral nerve infarction; and a constant inflammatory state of failure to thrive, malaise, and myalgias. Hepatitis C–related renal disease may appear as the only systemic manifestation of type II cryoglobulinemia but more often appears in the context of systemic disease. Once diagnosed with MPGN, a patient with hepatitis C should undergo a careful screening for systemic complications of this disorder.

11. **Other than a kidney biopsy, is there any other way to make the diagnosis of MPGN and cryoglobulinemia from Hepatitis C?**
Because the renal disease cannot occur in the absence of active hepatitis C viral replication, the first question to ask is as follows: "What is the status of the patient's hepatitis C?" Many of these patients are receiving interferon and ribavirin therapy and could be in partial or complete remission with very low viral loads. If these patients are nephrotic or have impaired renal function, then there will have to be an alternative explanation because it is not likely a result of MPGN from hepatitis C.

If the patient has active viral replication, then certain serologic testing may help confirm the diagnosis of MPGN/cryoglobulinemia. When immune complexes such as cryoglobulins deposit and initiate an inflammatory response, the mechanism by which they result in tissue damage is through the complement cascade. Cryoglobulins activate the classical complement pathway and lead to a significant reduction in the serum concentrations of C3 and C4. It is highly improbable that a patient could have renal disease because of type II cryoglobulins and not show complement activation. Ordering a C3 and C4 is essential in the workup of these patients.

A serum cryoglobulin level can be checked, but the turnaround time for this assay is not often rapid enough to help immediately with the diagnosis. More commonly, an indirect marker for the presence of cryoglobulins, called the rheumatoid factor, is measured. An antibody directed against another antibody is said to be anti-idiotypic and to possess "rheumatoid factor" activity. In patients with rheumatoid arthritis, these immune complexes likely result in the pathogenesis of the disease. In other diseases that manifest antibodies that are anti-idiotypic, the test for "rheumatoid factor" will be positive. A positive rheumatoid factor assay coupled with a low C3 and C4 is typical of active cryoglobulinemia.

12. **What is the treatment for MPGN in hepatitis C?**
The development of cryoglobulinemia is contingent on viral interaction with B cells and subsequent B-cell IgM production to form cryoglobulins. Therefore, reducing the viral load is the most critical step in controlling this disease process. Currently the only effective therapy for hepatitis C is the use of interferon with or without adjunctive ribavirin. This treatment must be attempted in patients with MPGN; otherwise, renal function will continue to decline leading to ESRD.

In certain circumstances, additional, more aggressive immunosuppressive therapy may be warranted in hepatitis C-related MPGN. These exceptions include the following: (1) a rapid decline of renal function with biopsy evidence of crescentic changes or (2) systemic vasculitis with life-threatening organ dysfunction. In these cases, simply controlling the virus will not pre-empt the damage occurring from the cryoglobulins that are already formed and circulating. The strategy will need to target removing the cryoglobulins that are circulating systemically so ongoing tissue injury can be attenuated and then inhibiting the new production of the IgM type II cryoglobulins.

Plasmapheresis has become the treatment of choice for severe cases of cryoglobulinemia and will effectively remove these immune complexes from the circulation. Concomitantly treatment should target the B cells that are producing the abnormal IGM antibodies. In past years, chemotherapy such as the use of cyclophosphamide was used to inhibit B-cell proliferation. This therapy was not specific to B cells and resulted in potentially serious collateral effects on other cell lines. The recent development of a monoclonal antibody that selectively removes B cells from the circulation has revolutionized the therapy of B-cell lymphomas and cryoglobulinemia. Rituximab is a monoclonal antibody that binds to a surface antigen only found on B cells (CD20) and leads to their destruction. This will markedly assist in stopping further cryoglobulin production as plasmapheresis works to remove the preformed antibodies.

13. **Why is diabetic nephropathy listed as a cause of nephrotic syndrome for patients with hepatitis C?**
In addition to the lymphotropic effect of hepatitis C, this virus also appears to bind to β islet cells. The interaction of the virus surface antigens with β islet cells in the pancreas initiates a sequence of events that leads to islet dysfunction and secondary diabetes. In addition, viral structural proteins interfere with the postreceptor response to insulin, leading to a combination of type I and type II diabetes in these patients.

Over years, the end-organ complications of diabetes can accrue, especially the development of diabetic nephropathy. Therefore, in a patient with hepatitis C and diabetes who presents with nephrotic syndrome and renal dysfunction, the differential diagnosis needs to include diabetic nephropathy. Clinically, the presence of low complement levels (C3 and C4) and an active urinary sediment possibly associated with systemic manifestations of vasculitis would all be supportive of hepatitis C–related cryoglobulinemia as opposed to diabetes.

The treatment of diabetic nephropathy in patients with hepatitis C is similar to that of diabetic nephropathy in the general population and includes inhibition of the renin-angiotensin-aldosterone system (RAAS), anti-hypertension control, and strict glucose control.

14. **Can patients with hepatitis B or hepatitis C glomerulopathies eventually undergo renal transplantation?**
As discussed earlier, both types of glomerulopathies that occur with hepatitis B or C are directly related to active viral replication. In the case of hepatitis B, it results from immune complexes, whereas in the case of hepatitis C it is associated with the development of cryoglobulinemia. If transplantation is considered in these cases, one of the first questions to ask is as follows: "What is the status of the liver involvement from these viruses?"

The answer to this question is crucial in order to define whether the patient needs a combined liver–kidney transplant or a kidney transplant only. The presence of cirrhosis on biopsy would automatically mandate that a combined transplant be performed. Without a liver biopsy it is not always possible to estimate whether or not cirrhosis is present. Evaluation of liver function studies, clotting parameters, and the presence or absence of portal hypertension are all useful in the clinical assessment for the presence of cirrhosis.

If the patient has stable liver function and no evidence of cirrhosis, then a kidney transplant alone can be considered. The second question to answer is as follows: "How active is the viral disease?" It would be counterproductive to transplant a patient and provide intensive immunosuppression if there is uncontrolled viral proliferation. The risks of exacerbating viral activity can lead to either post-transplant immune complex renal disease or post-transplant liver disease. One of the most common causes of death in patients with hepatitis C after transplantation is liver disease. There is an increased risk of hepatoma in patients with active hepatitis B or C, and routine monitoring of alpha fetoprotein levels is required during long-term followup.

The risk of recurrent disease (MPGN) in the allograft is particularly common in patients with hepatitis C. Because a sustained viral remission is difficult to achieve with hepatitis C in patients with ESRD even with prolonged interferon therapy, the most important goal is to modify the production of cryoglobulins and evidence of systemic disease. Transplantation can be successfully performed in the absence of cryoglobulins, but careful monitoring of liver function studies afterward is essential. Patients with hepatitis B are usually more easily managed with long-term viral suppressive doses of lamivudine or entecavir.

One of the most serious issues in offering renal transplantation to patients with hepatitis B or C is that interferon therapy is relatively contraindicated post-transplant because of the increased risk of rejection, particularly vascular rejection. Therefore, every effort to control viral activity pretransplant should be made.

15. **What are the really important secrets I need to know about hepatitis B– and C–related glomerulopathies?**
Table 41-2 summarizes the key aspects of these two lesions.

TABLE 41-2. KEY ASPECTS OF HEPATITIS B– AND C–RELATED GLOMERULOPATHIES		
	Hepatitis C	**Hepatitis B**
Primary glomerular disease	Type I membranoproliferative glomerulonephritis	Membranous nephropathy
Pathophysiology	Type II cryoglobulinemia	Hepatitis B e Ag-antibody immune complexes
Clinical findings	Nephritic syndrome	Nephrotic syndrome
Systemic manifestations	Vasculitis	None
Laboratory features	Low C3, C4 Positive rheumatoid factor	Normal complement levels
Treatment	Interferon	Entecavir
Malignancy potential	Hepatoma B-cell lymphoma	Hepatoma

KEY POINTS: VIRAL HEPATITIS-ASSOCIATED GLOMERULONEPHRITIS

1. The presence or absence of hepatitis B e antigen will be very important in regard to the type of glomerular disease that may develop. Patients positive for both hepatitis B e antigen and hepatitis B surface antigen are highly infectious and have a greater risk of kidney disease.

2. The typical serum creatinine is usually 0.5 to 0.6 mg/dL in patients with cirrhosis, which is well below the normal expected maximum range for the general population—1.2 mg/dL for women and 1.5 mg/dL for men. Patients with liver disease can have a significant loss of glomerular filtration rate with a serum creatinine level within "the normal range" for the general population.

3. For those patients who are carriers of hepatitis B but are only hepatitis B surface antigen positive and negative for hepatitis B e antigen, the renal lesion is not usually membranous nephropathy but membranoproliferative glomerulonephritis. This is because the hepatitis B surface antigen-antibody immune complex is too large to filter through the basement membrane, so it lodges in the inner surface of the capillary wall (subendothelial space).

16. **Is there anything else I need to know about hepatitis-induced renal disease?**
     Yes. Not every patient with hepatitis B or C who develops renal disease has a viral-induced glomerulopathy. Because both of these viruses cause renal disease as a result of active replication, it is not surprising that advanced liver disease is usually present when they lead to glomerulonephritis. Consequently, these patients will all have portal hypertension and cirrhosis, which adds another differential diagnosis into the picture: hepatorenal syndrome (HRS).

     Acute renal injury in patients with cirrhosis is often related to prerenal azotemia as a result of the diuretics used for mobilization of ascites and lower extremity edema and at the extreme can result from HRS. It is absolutely essential that physicians evaluating a patient with cirrhosis and known hepatitis B or C who has developed acute renal injury take into consideration the possibility of HRS. Differentiating hepatitis B or C glomerulonephritis from HRS can be done using routine laboratory and urinalysis tests. The following questions should be asked:

- **Is there proteinuria?** Patients with HRS by definition have to have <500 mg of protein excretion in 24 hours, as compared to patients with either hepatitis B– or C–related glomerulonephritis where the nephrotic syndrome is common.
- **What does the urine sediment show?** In patients with HRS, the urine sediment is bland with no cells or casts. In hepatitis C MPGN, the urine will be nephritic with red cell casts, dysmorphic red blood cells, white blood cells, and renal tubular epithelial cells, whereas for hepatitis B MN the urine will be nephrotic with fatty casts and oval fat bodies.
- **Is the FENa (Fractional Excretion of Sodium) helpful?** Unfortunately, the FENa in patients with HRS or any form of glomerulonephritis will be <1%, indicating a sodium avid state. The FENa is not useful in differentiating between these diagnoses.
- **What about serum complement levels?** In hepatitis C MPGN the levels of C3 and C4 will be very low, indicating active consumption by the cryoglobulins, and the rheumatoid factor will be elevated. For hepatitis B MN and HRS, the serum complement levels and rheumatoid factor will all be within normal limits.

BIBLIOGRAPHY

 1. Alpers CE, Smith KD. Cryoglobulinemia and renal disease. *Curr Opin Nephrol Hypertens* 2008;17(3):243–249.
 2. Ayodele OE, Salako BL, Kadiri S, et al. Hepatitis B virus infection: implications in chronic kidney disease, dialysis and transplantation. *Afr J Med Med Sci* 2006;35(2):111–119.
 3. Fabrizi F, Lunghi G, Messa P, et al. Therapy of hepatitis C virus-associated glomerulonephritis: Current approaches. *J Nephrol* 2008;21(6):813–825.
 4. Izzedine H, Sene D, Cacoub P, et al. Kidney diseases in HIV/HCV-co-infected patients. *AIDS* 2009;23(10): 1219–1226.
 5. Kamar N, Izopet J, Alric L, et al. Hepatitis C virus-related kidney disease: An overview. *Clin Nephrol* 2008;69(3): 149–160.
 6. Lai AS, Lai KN. Viral nephropathy. *Nat Clin Pract Nephrol* 2006;2(5):254–262.
 7. Martin P, Fabrizi F. Hepatitis C virus and kidney disease. *J Hepatol* 2008;49(4):613–624.
 8. Saadoun D, Delluc A, Piette JC, Cacoub P. Treatment of hepatitis C-associated mixed cryoglobulinemia vasculitis. *Curr Opin Rheumatol* 2008;20(1):23–28.
 9. Sansonno L, Tucci FA, Sansonno S, et al. B cells and HCV: An infection model of autoimmunity. *Autoimmun Rev* 2009;9(2):93–94.
10. Tang S, Lai FM, Lui YH, et al. Lamivudine in hepatitis B-associated membranous nephropathy. *Kidney Int* 2005;68(4):1750–1758.

CHAPTER 42

HIV-ASSOCIATED RENAL DISORDERS

Warren Kupin, MD

1. **What types of renal syndromes does HIV cause?**
    Renal disease in patients with HIV can manifest itself in many different clinical presentations including acid–base and electrolyte abnormalities and acute and chronic kidney disease. There is no difference in the basic approach in the evaluation of a patient with HIV compared to that of a patient who does not have HIV in the setting of renal disease in regard to differentiation of acute from chronic renal disease and in the categorization of acute kidney injury into prerenal, renal, and postrenal causes. However, there are a number of unique findings in patients with HIV that the clinician must be aware of that will aid in the diagnosis. These findings will be detailed in the following sections.

2. **How is renal disease first detected in patients with HIV?**
    For most physicians the presence of renal disease is first suggested by either an elevation of the serum creatinine or the presence of proteinuria.

3. **How accurate are these markers for detecting renal disease in patients with HIV?**
    It is now clear that the serum creatinine has significant limitations in many patients as a result of the dependence of this on gender, age, and underlying medical condition. Patients with HIV who are not receiving highly active retroviral therapy (HAART) may have marked reductions in muscle mass as a result of malnutrition and will have lower baseline serum creatinine levels than in the general population. It would not be unusual for a patient with advanced HIV to have a serum creatinine level of 0.9 mg/dL and yet have a significant reduction in glomerular filtration rate (GFR). Therefore, the use of a calculated GFR instead of relying on the serum creatinine level is now recommended as a screening tool in all patients with HIV by the Infectious Disease Society of America (IDSA) and the National Kidney Foundation (NKF). The two equations commonly used are the Cockcroft-Gault formula and the Modification of Diet in Renal Disease (MDRD) formulas, with the latter being routinely reported by most laboratories. A GFR of <60 cc/min by these methods should raise serious concern about the presence of either acute or chronic renal disease in a patient with HIV and requires additional investigation.

    A newer marker has been used to improve the sensitivity in detecting renal disease in patients with HIV and involves the serum level of a molecule called cystatin C. This enzyme, which is produced by all nucleated cells, has been suggested as being more accurate than the serum creatinine for determining early levels of renal injury. However, it appears that the inflammatory state of chronic HIV infection leads to increased production of cystatin C and this may limit its utility as a marker for kidney disease in this population. Many laboratories are now reporting both the serum creatinine level and the cystatin C level, and an elevation of either should be considered as evidence for important alterations in renal function in a patient with HIV.

    In addition to an impaired GFR as a sign of renal disease in patients with HIV, often a patient with HIV will first present with only proteinuria. One of the pathognomonic hallmarks of HIV-induced glomerular injury is proteinuria. The recommendations by the IDSA also state that all patients with HIV should have a dipstick urinalysis performed for detection of proteinuria. The finding of proteinuria is a significant predictor of increased morbidity and mortality in patients with HIV and it is essential to routinely check the urinalysis in this patient population at regular intervals. If the dipstick test result is positive, then a spot urine test for protein/creatinine ratio should be done to estimate the degree of proteinuria.

Recent studies have shown that microalbuminuria may be an important indicator of the presence of renal disease in patients with HIV, similar to the use of microalbuminuria in patients with diabetes. However, at the present time there are no guidelines that require the measurement of microalbuminuria for early detection of renal disease in this population.

In summary, all patients with HIV require a serum creatinine, an estimated GFR calculation, and a urinalysis dipstick for proteinuria at the initial visit and at regular intervals afterward to monitor for the development of renal disease.

4. **What are the common causes of acute kidney failure in patients with HIV?**
Approximately 6% of hospitalized patients with HIV have acute kidney failure, with a mortality risk that is five times higher than the general patient without HIV and with kidney injury. The most important approach in the assessment of acute kidney failure in a patient with HIV requires answers to the following questions: Is the patient receiving HAART? What is the viral control of HIV? The approach to acute kidney injury will be different based on the answers to these questions. If a patient is not receiving HAART and has uncontrolled HIV viremia, the most common causes of renal injury are related to systemic infection and volume depletion leading to prerenal azotemia. Uncontrolled infectious diarrhea with fever and large insensible fluid losses is a common presenting scenario in a patient with HIV who is HAART naïve. Patients with HIV frequently develop sepsis from pneumonia and other opportunistic infections complicated with hypotension leading to acute tubular necrosis (ATN).

In patients with infection who are HAART-naïve, multiple antibiotics are often used to cover bacterial, viral, fungal, and atypical infectious agents. Many of these antibiotics can result in acute renal injury, as noted in Table 42-1.

If the patient is receiving HAART therapy with a controlled viral load, then the development of acute renal injury may be secondary to the HAART drugs. It is essential that all physicians treating patients with HIV be familiar with the complications of HAART, including nephrotoxicity.

TABLE 42-1. ANTIBIOTICS CAN RESULT IN ACUTE RENAL INJURY	
Antibiotic	Renal Syndrome(s)
Amphotericin	ATN, type I renal tubular acidosis
Trimethoprim-sulfamethoxazole	Crystal-induced ATN, allergic interstitial nephritis
Penicillin/cephalosporin agents	Allergic interstitial nephritis
Aminoglycosides	ATN
Foscarnet	ATN
Pentamidine	ATN
Vancomycin	ATN
Ciprofloxacin	Crystal-induced ATN, allergic interstitial nephritis
Acyclovir	Crystal-induced ATN, allergic interstitial nephritis

ATN = acute tubular necrosis.

5. **How does HAART cause renal disease?**

The combination therapy used for management of HIV infection involves multiple classes of agents, including protease inhibitors, reverse transcriptase inhibitors, and entry blockers. Distinct syndromes are associated with certain classes of HAART that must be kept in mind (Table 42-2). The protease inhibitors can crystallize in the urinary tract and form either macroscopic stones resulting in urinary obstruction (hydronephrosis), or they may crystallize inside the tubules, causing microtubular obstruction and ATN (no hydronephrosis). Tenofovir is considered to be the prototypic agent causing tubular damage and ATN. Because the tubular injury is localized to the proximal tubule, a Fanconi syndrome may develop. Of note, long-term use of tenofovir may also lead to chronic kidney disease (CKD) with the development of irreversible interstitial fibrosis. It is estimated that 4% of stable patients receiving HAART on a tenofovir-based regimen may develop CKD. The GFR needs to be monitored routinely in all patients receiving HAART to detect early changes in renal function before irreversible damage occurs.

6. **What glomerular diseases are seen in patients with HIV?**

Proteinuria in patients with HIV is often a sign of glomerular disease, even if it is not within the nephrotic range. Although these lesions are classically associated with a 24-hour urine protein excretion of >3.5 g, it depends on when in their natural history they are found. It is now well proven that these glomerular diseases go through an initial phase of microalbuminuria (30-300 mg/24 hours) followed by macroalbuminuria (300 mg/24 hours), culminating in the nephrotic syndrome. Any level of proteinuria in a patient with HIV would be considered highly suspicious for one of the glomerular lesions (see later).

The two main glomerular syndromes directly related to HIV infection and their associated pathologic findings on biopsy are as follows:

- HIV-associated nephropathy (HIVAN): collapsing variant of focal segmental sclerosis (FSGS)
- HIV immune complex disease of the kidney (HIVICK): immunoglobulin A (IgA) nephropathy or a systemic lupus erythematosus (SLE)-like proliferative glomerulonephritis

Approximately 30% of patients with HIV are coinfected with hepatitis C and may develop glomerular disease not from HIV but from hepatitis C–related immune complex disease. In certain parts of the world, patients with HIV may also be coinfected with hepatitis B and subsequently develop a glomerular lesion related to that virus infection. These hepatitis-related glomerular lesions are as follows:

- Hepatitis C: membranoproliferative glomerulonephritis (MPGN) associated with cryoglobulinemia
- Hepatitis B: membranous nephropathy (MN)

TABLE 42-2. RENAL SYNDROMES ASSOCIATED WITH HAART		
HAART Class	**Representative Drugs**	**Renal Syndrome(s)**
Protease inhibitors	Indinavir, atazanavir, nelfinavir, saquinavir, ritonavir, amprenavir	Urolithiasis: obstructive uropathy
Nucleoside reverse transcriptase Inhibitors	Stavudine, zidovudine, didanosine, lamivudine	Mitochondrial cytopathy: hepatic steatosis, lactic acidosis, rhabdomyolysis, acute tubular necrosis
Nucleotide reverse transcriptase inhibitors	Tenofovir, adefovir	Fanconi syndrome, acute tubular necrosis, chronic kidney disease

When patients with HIV are treated with HAART, there is a high risk of developing diabetes mellitus. Recent studies show that patients with HIV successfully treated with HAART therapy now are developing renal biopsy evidence of diabetic nephropathy, especially if they are not under strict diabetic control. These patients will present with nephrotic-range proteinuria as a result of diabetic glomerulopathy.

When developing a differential diagnosis of proteinuria in a patient with HIV, the following questions are important to ask:

- Does the patient have active HIV viremia? If yes, consider HIVAN or HIVICK.
- Is the patient coinfected with hepatitis B or hepatitis C? If yes, consider MPGN or MN.
- Is the patient receiving HAART with secondary diabetes? If yes, consider diabetic nephropathy.

7. **What exactly is HIVAN?**

HIVAN is a unique glomerular disease that is specifically a result of the effects of active HIV viral replication in the kidney. It is characterized by four pathologic changes in the kidney:

1. Collapsing variant of focal sclerosis: hypertrophy and hyperplasia of the podocytes to the point that they literally cave in the capillary tuft and reduce the filtration area of the glomerulus
2. Microcystic dilation of the tubules: markedly enlarged dilated tubules that are not seen in any other form of renal disease
3. Interstitial nephritis: infiltration of the interstitial space of the kidney with CD8+ T cells
4. Tubuloreticular inclusion bodies: the presence of arrays of microparticles in tubular cells that result from high levels of cytokines

8. **How does HIVAN present clinically?**

HIVAN is almost exclusively found in African American patients (90%) with active HIV viral replication. It is rarely an early presentation in the course of HIV disease but results from untreated viremia. Most patients with HIVAN have a CD4 count <200 and a viral load of >400 copies/mL. How HIV is acquired is not important. There is a misconception that HIV related to intravenous drug use is more of a risk factor for HIVAN as compared to HIV acquired from blood transfusions or sexual exposure. The single most important risk factor is the presence of active infection (high viral load, low CD4 count) in a susceptible host (African American race).

9. **Are there any special clinical features of HIVAN that may help in establishing this diagnosis?**

Other than the race, there are two clinical findings that are often reported to favor a diagnosis of HIVAN as opposed to the other types of glomerular disease. The first is the absence of hypertension (HTN) in the setting of renal disease and proteinuria. Typically, FSGS and the glomerulopathies related to the viral hepatitides (hepatitis C or B) or diabetes are associated with moderate to marked HTN but not HIVAN. Patients with HIVAN have unexpectedly normal blood pressures because of the presence of vasodilatory cytokines that are produced in response to the HIV infection and a salt-losing state in the kidney also related to active HIV infection. More than 80% of patients with HIVAN have normal blood pressures in the setting of significant renal injury. Based on these data, the presence of HTN in a patient with HIV with renal disease should prompt a reconsideration of the diagnosis of HIVAN to an alternative etiology.

The second suggestive feature that may point to HIVAN is the presence of large echogenic kidneys on ultrasound. Most patients with nephrotic syndrome and progressive renal failure will have loss of renal size and mild echogenicity as a result of interstitial fibrosis. In HIVAN the presence of microcystic dilation may result in larger than expected kidney size at any level of kidney function and the degree of echogenicity is significantly more than that seen in other renal lesions. Therefore, the initial evaluation by ultrasound of a patient with HIV with proteinuria may already lead to a tentative diagnosis of HIVAN if these characteristic findings are reported. The ultrasound radiologist may be the first one to suggest a differential diagnosis of HIVAN based on these characteristic findings.

10. **How common is HIVAN?**

The natural history of untreated HIV in the United States and in Africa has shown that approximately 3% to 12% of African American patients will develop HIVAN. In the dialysis population, HIVAN is the third leading cause of end-stage renal disease (ESRD) in African American adults, after diabetes and HTN.

11. **What is the etiology of HIVAN?**

As discussed earlier, HIVAN is a direct result of active HIV infection. Current research shows that the HIV virus gains direct entry into renal tissue including the podocytes, mesangial cells, and tubular cells. Once inside the cells, the viral genome is translated and the gene products lead to alterations of cellular function and development. Some of the candidate genes whose products are responsible for HIVAN include negative factor for viral replication (NEF), transactivating factor (TAT), and virus protein R (VPR). Research studies are still investigating what types of receptors the virus uses to enter renal tissue. The viral gene proteins lead to an interruption of normal cell maturation and the infected cells de-differentiate into an immature cell phenotype. The delicate balance between cell growth and apoptosis is offset and, being unable to control their own proliferation, the podocytes increase in number and cause collapsing FSGS and the tubules dilate, forming the microcysts.

12. **What is HIVICK?**

HIVICK (HIV immune complex disease of the kidney) is another histologic variant of active HIV infection in the kidney. Two major types of immune complex diseases in the kidney are related to HIV infection: IgA nephropathy and diffuse proliferative glomerulonephritis. Idiopathic IgA nephropathy is the most common glomerular disease in the world and is characterized by IgA immune complexes in the mesangium and occasionally in the capillary loops. The antigen that is bound by the IgA immune complexes in idiopathic IgA nephropathy is not known. In patients with HIV, the HIV antigen p24 appears to be one of many different HIV related antigens that are targeted by IgA and deposit in the kidney.

Another immune complex disease of the kidney is an SLE-like glomerular disease: diffuse proliferative glomerulonephritis. This is called SLE-like because on histopathology staining there are immune complexes of IgG, IGM, C3, C4, and C1Q indicative of the classical complement pathway activation. This pattern is typical of SLE, yet these patients with HIV have no serologic signs of SLE—negative ANA, DSDNA, and normal complement levels.

In both types of HIVICK, the immune complexes are related to HIV-induced circulating immune complexes, and it would be a prerequisite to have active viremia. Why some patients develop HVAN and others develop HIVICK is not clear, and both syndromes are a result of a dysregulated immune response to HIV infection.

13. **Is HIVAN the most common lesion found in patients with HIV with proteinuria?**

Before the development and widespread use of HAART therapy, HIVAN was by far the most common cause of nephrotic syndrome in patients with HIV. However, this pattern has changed dramatically in the HAART era. HIVAN now accounts for only 40% to 50% of all cases of nephrotic syndrome with HIVICK, with classic FSGS and viral hepatitis-induced glomerulopathies accounting for the remaining 50% to 60%. A renal biopsy is usually recommended for patients with HIV with proteinuria because more often than not a renal lesion other than HIVAN is found.

14. **Is there a treatment for HIVAN?**

Successful therapy of any renal disease is dependent on the degree of reversible or irreversible lesions that are present. The most important predictor of response to therapy is the degree of interstitial fibrosis, which can only be ascertained from a renal biopsy. HIVAN is considered a treatable and potentially reversible disease if diagnosed at an early stage. Because HIVAN is a result of the direct infection of renal tissue and the gene products of the HIV genome, then eradication of active viremia should improve renal function.

HAART has resulted in regression of the glomerular and tubular lesions with remission of proteinuria and improvement of renal function. This benefit lasts only as long as viremia is controlled and relapses with discontinuation of HAART and a resurgence of viremia.

Although HIVICK lesions also result from active HIV infection, they do not appear responsive to HAART therapy. HIVAN results from direct infection of renal tissue with HIV, and this may make it more amenable to control with HAART. HIVICK results from peripheral generation of immune complexes and the renal damage is different than with HIVAN, so HAART is not as effective in this scenario.

In addition to HAART, short-term steroid therapy has been of benefit, especially in patients who have a significant interstitial infiltrate on biopsy. Steroids do not affect the collapsing glomerular lesion of FSGS, but they do reduce the inflammatory cytokine production in the interstitium and can improve renal function while HAART is initiated. Steroids have not been shown to be effective in HIVICK, most likely because of the lack of a significant component of interstitial nephritis in these patients.

Adjunctive therapy for nephrotic syndrome with inhibitors of the renin-angiotensin system—angiotensin-converting enzyme inhibitors and angiotensin receptor blockers—are effective in reducing proteinuria and delaying the progression of renal disease in HIVAN. These agents can be used at the time of diagnosis but are not considered to be first-line therapy. The most important initial treatment for HIVAN is HAART.

KEY POINTS: HIV AND THE KIDNEY

1. HIV-associated nephropathy (HIVAN) is a form of collapsing variant of focal segmental sclerosis (FSGS) and is only present in fewer than 50% of patients with HIV.

2. Patients with HIV are frequently coinfected with hepatitis C and/or B and may develop renal disease from these infections.

3. HIVAN occurs almost exclusively in African American patients with active viremia regardless of how they acquired HIV.

4. Patients with HIVAN are unexpectedly normotensive, often demonstrating large echogenic kidneys on ultrasound.

5. Highly active retroviral therapy (HAART)-related nephrotoxicity is a growing cause of acute renal injury and chronic kidney disease.

6. HAART is the primary treatment only for HIVAN and is not as successful in HIV immune complex disease of the kidney (HIVICK).

7. HIVICK is a distinct category of HIV glomerular disease as a result of immune complex deposition in the kidney.

8. Dialysis and transplantation are viable options for patients with HIV.

9. Acute kidney injury is extremely common in patients with HIV because of either prerenal azotemia or acute tubular necrosis.

10. Guidelines require all patients with HIV need to be regularly screened for renal disease with a glomerular filtration rate and urinalysis for proteinuria.

15. **If treatment fails, can a patient with HIV undergo long-term dialysis?**
As a result of the early poor long-term prognosis in patients with HIV before HAART was developed, it was thought that maintenance dialysis therapy would not be a viable option. This thinking has changed dramatically over the past 15 years since HAART has been routinely used in HIV. Currently approximately 1.6% of the ESRD population has HIV and their survival is

very similar to those patients without HIV if they are receiving HAART. Both types of dialysis modalities, hemodialysis or peritoneal dialysis, are equally effective options for patients with HIV.

16. **Can a patient with HIV be considered for kidney transplantation?**
The National Institutes of Health have sponsored a multicenter trial to evaluate the efficacy of transplantation in patients with HIV. The prerequisite for transplantation includes the use of HAART therapy with a CD4 count >400 and an undetectable viral load. There is experience with the use of both liver and kidney transplants in patients with HIV. The preliminary data show acceptable graft and patient survival with a higher risk of rejection, making transplantation an option in select patients with HIV. The pharmacologic management of HAART and immunosuppressive therapy is challenging because of the effect of HAART on the hepatic P450 enzyme system. These enzymes metabolize the primary immunosuppressive class used as maintenance therapy, the calcineurin inhibitors (tacrolimus, cyclosporine). As a result, these drugs may only need to be administered once a week and frequent drug level monitoring is essential. Patients with HIV have also been candidates for liver transplantation with similar equivalent results compared to patients who do not have HIV. At present, transplantation is a potential option in a subgroup of patients with HIV with ESRD.

BIBLIOGRAPHY

1. Atta MG. Diagnosis and natural history of HIV-associated nephropathy. *Adv Chronic Kidney Dis* 2010;17(1):52–58.
2. Bruggeman LA, Bark C, Kalayjian RC. HIV and the kidney. *Curr Infect Dis Rep* 2009;11(6):479–485.
3. Buskin SE, Torno MS, Talkington DF, et al. Trends in nephropathy among HIV-infected patients. *J Natl Med Assoc* 2009;101(12):1205–1213.
4. Dinavahi RV, Mehrotra A, Murphy BT, et al. Human immunodeficiency virus and renal transplantation. *Kidney Int* 2009;76(8):907–910.
5. Izzedine H, Sene D, Cacoub P, et al. Kidney diseases in HIV/HCV-co-infected patients. *AIDS* 2009;23(10): 1219–1226.
6. Jao J, Wyatt CM. Antiretroviral medications: adverse effects on the kidney. *Adv Chronic Kidney Dis* 2010;17(1): 72–82.
7. Kalim S, Szczech LA, Wyatt CM. Acute kidney injury in HIV-infected patients. *Semin Nephrol* 2008;28(6):556–562.
8. Post FA, Holt SG. Recent developments in HIV and the kidney. *Curr Opin Infect Dis* 2009;22(1):43–48.
9. Quaggin SE. Genetic susceptibility to HIV-associated nephropathy. *J Clin Invest* 2009;119(5):1085–1089.
10. Rachakonda AK, Kimmel PL. CKD in HIV-infected patients other than HIV-associated nephropathy. *Adv Chronic Kidney Dis* 2010;17(1):83–93.
11. Sawinski D, Murphy B. End-stage renal disease and kidney transplant in HIV-infected patients. *Semin Nephrol* 2008;28(6):581–584.
12. Symeonidou C, Hameeduddin A, Malhotra A. Imaging features of renal pathology in the human immunodeficiency virus-infected patient. *Semin Ultrasound CT MR* 2009;30(4):289–297.
13. Szczech LA. Renal disease: The effects of HIV and antiretroviral therapy and the implications for early antiretroviral therapy initiation. *Curr Opin HIV AIDS* 2009;4(3):167–170.
14. Winston JA. Estimating glomerular filtration rate in patients with HIV infection. *Semin Nephrol* 2008;28(6):576–580.
15. Wyatt CM, Klotman PE, D'Agati VD. HIV-associated nephropathy: Clinical presentation, pathology, and epidemiology in the era of antiretroviral therapy. *Semin Nephrol* 2008;28(6):513–522.
16. Yahaya I, Uthman AO, Uthman MM. Interventions for HIV-associated nephropathy. *Cochrane Database Syst Rev* 2009;4:CD007183.

VII. OTHER RENAL PARENCHYMAL DISEASES

FABRY DISEASE

Brian Kirmse, MD, and Robert J. Desnick, PhD, MD

CHAPTER 43

1. **What is Fabry disease?**

   Fabry disease is a multisystemic, X-linked, lysosomal storage disorder that results from the deficient activity of the enzyme α-galactosidase A (α-Gal A) and the lysosomal accumulation of its primary glycolipid substrate, globotriaosylceramide (GL-3). The progressive GL-3 accumulation, particularly in vascular endothelial lysosomes, leads to ischemia and occlusion of small vessels throughout the body. Clinical onset in affected males with the classic phenotype occurs in childhood or adolescence, characterized by painful acroparesthesias, gastrointestinal dysfunction, corneal dystrophy, absent or decreased sweat (anhidrosis or hypohidrosis), and cutaneous lesions (the angiokeratomas). With advancing age, the progressive vascular glycolipid accumulation leads to renal failure, cardiac disease, strokes, and early demise. Patients develop end-stage renal disease (ESRD) in the third to fourth decades of life. Female heterozygotes from classically affected families can be as severely affected as classically affected males or may be asymptomatic throughout life, primarily as a result of random X-chromosomal inactivation. Patients with the later-onset phenotype lack the manifestations of the classic early-onset phenotype and often are unrecognized. Previously undiagnosed males with Fabry disease have been identified in hemodialysis, cardiac, and stroke clinics by screening patients for markedly deficient plasma α-Gal A activity.

   Desnick RJ, Ioannou Y, Eng C. Fabry disease: α-Galactosidase A deficiency. In Scriver CR, Beaudet AL, Valle D and Sly WS (eds.). *Metabolic and Molecular Bases of Inherited Disease*, 8th ed. New York: McGraw-Hill, 2001, pp. 3733–3774.

   Linthorst GE, Bouwman MG, Wijburg FA, et al. Screening for Fabry disease in high risk populations: A systematic review. *J Med Genet* 2010;47:217–222.

   Nakao S, Kodama C, Takenaka T, et al. Fabry disease: Detection of undiagnosed hemodialysis patients and identification of a "renal variant" phenotype. *Kidney Int* 2003;64:801–807.

2. **What are the subtypes of Fabry disease?**

   The two major subtypes of Fabry disease are the classic and later-onset phenotypes. Affected males with the classic phenotype have little, if any, α-Gal A enzyme activity (<1% of mean normal), whereas males with the later-onset phenotype have residual enzymatic activity, typically >1% of mean normal activity. Heterozygous females from classic Fabry families have a wide range of clinical manifestations from asymptomatic to severely affected, whereas heterozygous females from later-onset families may have symptoms later in life, including cardiac and renal manifestations.

   Desnick RJ, Ioannou Y, Eng C. Fabry disease: α-Galactosidase A deficiency. In: Scriver CR, Beaudet AL, Valle D and Sly WS (eds.). *Metabolic and Molecular Bases of Inherited Disease*, 8th ed. New York, McGraw-Hill, 2001, pp. 3733–3774.

3. **What is the genetic basis of Fabry disease?**

   All cases of Fabry disease are caused by mutations in the gene encoding the lysosomal hydrolase α-Gal A. The α-Gal A gene is located on the long arm of the X chromosome (Xq22) and the disease is inherited as an X-linked trait. To date, more than 600 α-Gal A gene mutations have been described. Classically affected males have mutations that result in essentially no enzymatic activity, whereas patients with the later-onset phenotype have mutations that retain low levels of residual enzyme activity. There are no common α-Gal A mutations and most α-Gal A gene mutations occur in one or a few families. For both phenotypes, the sons of affected males will not have the disease, whereas all daughters will be heterozygotes. For heterozygous females, on average 50% of their sons will be affected and 50% will not inherit the disease. For daughters of heterozygotes, on average 50% will be heterozygotes and 50% will not inherit the disease gene.

4. **What is the metabolic abnormality in Fabry disease?**
The deficient or absent α-Gal A activity results in the accumulation of glycolipids with terminal α-linked galactose molecules. As noted earlier, the major accumulated glycolipid is globotriaosylceramide (GL-3). In addition, galabiosylceramide (GL-2), the blood group B glycolipid, and lyso-GL-3 accumulate in the lysosomes of various cell types. However, the major pathology leading to renal failure results from the accumulation in the microvascular endothelial cells. In addition, there is accumulation in podocytes, interstitial, mesangial, and tubular cells.

5. **What are the clinical findings in males with Fabry disease?**
Clinical manifestations in classically affected males begin in childhood or adolescence. Most often, the first symptoms are the painful acroparesthesias (especially during febrile illnesses); hypohidrosis; and gastrointestinal symptoms, including postprandial abdominal cramping, bloating, and diarrhea. Small petechiae-like angiokeratomas, the classic cutaneous vascular lesions, typically are present in the umbilical and swimsuit regions in childhood. Classically affected males also have a distinctive corneal dystrophy observed by slit-lamp microscopy, which does not affect vision. Microvascular involvement of the kidney begins in childhood; progresses to isothenuria, proteinuria, and tubular dysfunction; then, with advancing age, results in progressive renal disease and ESRD typically by age 35 to 45 years. Dialysis or renal transplantation are effective in correcting the renal disease, and renal transplants are not affected by the disease. All potential family donors should be evaluated to ensure that they are not affected or heterozygotes.

Other manifestations include lower extremity edema in the absence of significant renal disease, hypoproteinemia, or varices; the lymphedema results from the accumulation of GL-3 in the lymphatic vessels and nodes. Cardiac manifestations include arrhythmias (initially sinus bradycardia), valvular abnormalities, and left ventricular hypertrophy, which may lead to hypertrophic cardiomyopathy. Cerebrovascular disease manifests as transient ischemic attacks and stroke, which can lead to multi-infarct dementia. Progressive high-frequency hearing loss occurs in classically affected males in the third to fifth decades of life.

6. **What are the clinical findings in females with Fabry disease?**
The clinical manifestations in heterozygous females from classically affected families range from as severely affected as males to asymptomatic throughout life. The variation in manifestations is primarily a result of random X-chromosome inactivation. Renal manifestations in heterozygotes can include isosthenuria; proteinuria; and the presence of leukocytes, erythrocytes, and hyaline and granular casts in the urinary sediment. Approximately 10% of heterozygotes will progress to ESRD, according to U.S. and European registry data. Cardiac involvement, transient ischemic attacks, and strokes occur in older symptomatic heterozygotes. To date, most heterozygotes from later-onset families are asymptomatic for decades but can develop renal, cardiac, or cerebrovascular disease later in life.

7. **What is "renal variant" of Fabry disease?**
Screening of patients undergoing hemodialysis by determining their plasma α-Gal A activity revealed that about 0.2% to 1.0% of males had unrecognized Fabry disease. Most of these males lacked the acroparesthesias, angiokeratomas, hypohidrosis, and corneal opacities that typically brought classically affected males to medical attention. Most of these patients had the later-onset phenotype with α-Gal A missense mutations and residual α-Gal A activity. These males presented with kidney manifestations as early as the third or fourth decades of

life. "Renal variants" also may have cardiac involvement, typically left ventricular hypertrophy. These patients are now more correctly designated as having the later-onset phenotype. Recent newborn screening studies have revealed that the later-onset patients are more frequent than patients with the classic phenotype.

Hwu WL, Chien YH, Lee NC, Chiang SC, Dobrovolny R, et al. Newborn screening for Fabry disease in Taiwan reveals a high incidence of the later-onset GLA mutation c.936+919G>A (IVS4+919G>A). *Hum Mutat* 2009;30:1397–1405.

Linthorst GE, Bouwman MG, Wijburg FA, et al. Screening for Fabry disease in high risk populations: A systematic review. *J Med Genet* 2010;47:217–222.

Nakao S, Kodama C, Takenaka T, et al. Fabry disease: Detection of undiagnosed hemodialysis patients and identification of a "renal variant" phenotype. *Kidney Int* 2003;64:801–807.

Spada M, Pagliardini S, Yasuda M, et al. High incidence of later-onset Fabry disease revealed by newborn screening. *Am J Hum Genet* 2006;79:31–40.

8. **What other abnormalities may be associated with Fabry disease?**
Pulmonary involvement can manifest as dyspnea and wheezing, and pulmonary function tests may reveal an obstructive pattern. Most classically affected males and older heterozygotes may have tinnitus, bilateral hearing loss, and/or vertigo. Depression, anxiety, and fatigue are also seen in affected individuals and will negatively affect quality of life.

9. **What are the characteristic renal biopsy findings in Fabry disease?**
Renal insufficiency leading to failure results from GL-3 accumulation primarily in the microvascular endothelium. However, the most significant glomerular GL-3 involvement is in the podocytes, which is responsible for the proteinuria that occurs in affected males and symptomatic heterozygotes. In classically affected patients, glomerular interstitial and mesangial cells also progressively accumulate the glycolipid. To a lesser extent and in later stages of disease, the proximal tubules, histiocytes, and interstitial cells show glycolipid accumulation. Lipid-laden distal tubular epithelial cells will desquamate and can be detected by analysis of the urinary sediment. Nonspecific pathologic changes such as arteriolar sclerosis, glomerular atrophy and fibrosis, tubular atrophy, and diffuse fibrosis can be seen in the later stages of disease. Biopsies early in the disease course will show histologically the foamy inclusions in most cell types. The histology of the end-stage kidney is not diagnostic, and electron microscopy is needed to visualize the characteristic lamellar cytoplasmic inclusions in the renal lysosomes. Of interest, the renal involvement in the later-onset phenotype occurs primarily in the podocytes with little involvement of the glomerular vascular endothelial, interstitial, or mesangial cells.

10. **What treatment is available for Fabry disease?**
Enzyme replacement therapy (ERT) has been shown to stabilize and slow the progression of the renal disease. Two preparations are available: agalsidase-alpha (Replagal; Shire Pharmaceuticals) and agalsidase-beta (Fabrazyme; Genzyme Corp.). Only agalsidase-beta is U.S. Food and Drug Administration approved and commercially available in the United States. Agalsidase-beta delivered intravenously at 1 mg/kg every 2 weeks has been shown in randomized, double-blind, placebo-controlled clinical trials to clear the accumulated GL-3 from interstitial capillary endothelial cells of the kidney and to stabilize the estimated glomerular filtration rate. ERT with agalsidase-beta also cleared the GL-3 from the vascular endothelial cells in the heart and skin. A phase IV randomized, double-blind, placebo-controlled study in advanced patients with Fabry disease with mild to moderate renal insufficiency demonstrated that agalsidase-beta slowed the progression of renal dysfunction. Subsequent studies have shown that the addition of angiotensin-converting enzyme inhibitors or angiotensin II receptor blockade may augment the renal protective effects of enzyme replacement.

Banikazemi M, Bultas J, Waldek S, et al. Agalsidase-beta therapy for advanced Fabry disease: A randomized trial. *Ann Intern Med* 2007;146:77–86.

Eng C, Guffon N, Wilcox W, et al. Safety and efficacy of recombinant human alpha-Galactosidase A replacement therapy in Fabry's disease. *N Engl J Med* 2001;345:9–16.

Germain DP, Waldek S, Banikazemi M, et al. Sustained, long-term renal stabilization after 54 months of agalsidasebeta therapy in patients with Fabry disease. *J Am Soc Nephrol* 2007;18:1547–1557.

11. **When should enzyme replacement therapy be started, and what are the risks?**
    Published guidelines suggest that ERT be initiated at the time of diagnosis in males older than 16 and at the onset of significant symptoms in males younger than 16 and should be considered in asymptomatic males between the ages of 10 and 13 years. ERT is considered safe for use in children based on a pediatric trial. ERT should be started in heterozygous females with significant clinical symptoms or when there is evidence of organ involvement (i.e., proteinuria, cardiac dysfunction). ERT has been associated with reactions during the infusions for which medication with an antipyretic and antihistamine is recommended. Classically affected males typically develop immunoglobulin G antibodies to ERT, and the titers tend to decrease with continued treatment. These antibodies may be neutralizing but have not affected efficacy based on renal biopsies after 5 years of treatment.

Eng C, Germain D, Banikazemi M, et al. Fabry disease: Guidelines for the evaluation and management of multi-organ system involvement. *Genet Med* 2006;8:539–548.

Germain DP, Waldek S, Banikazemi M, et al. Sustained, long-term renal stabilization after 54 months of agalsidase beta therapy in patients with Fabry disease. *J Am Soc Nephrol* 2007;18:1547–1557.

Wraith JE, Tylki-Szymanska A, Guffon N, et al. Safety and efficacy of enzyme replacement therapy with agalsidase beta: An international open-label study in pediatric patients with Fabry disease. *J Pediatr* 2008;152:563–570.

KEY POINTS: FABRY DISEASE

1. Patients undergoing hemodialysis may have unrecognized Fabry disease, a treatable X-linked renal disease. The plasma α-galactosidase A assay reliably diagnoses affected males but not heterozygous females, who require mutation analysis for accurate diagnosis.

2. Enzyme replacement therapy in Fabry disease can clear the renal glycolipid accumulation and stabilize renal function; early treatment and adequate dose (1 mg/kg every other week) are important.

3. Females in families with X-linked Fabry disease can develop proteinuria and renal failure.

4. The differential diagnosis of postpartum proteinuria should include Fabry disease.

CHAPTER 44

CYSTIC DISEASES OF THE KIDNEYS

Marie C. Hogan, MD, PhD, and Vicente Torres, MD, PhD

1. **What are the major types of renal cystic diseases?**
   In addition to the inherited diseases listed in Table 44-1, other disorders need to be considered. In acquired renal cystic disease (ACKD) associated with longstanding renal insufficiency, the kidneys are initially small. With time they can enlarge and resemble those of autosomal-dominant polycystic kidney disease (ADPKD). Localized renal cystic disease, characterized by nonprogressive cystic transformation of a portion of a kidney, should be differentiated from asymmetric presentations of ADPKD, segmental multicystic dysplasia, and cystic neoplasms. In the absence of a family history of ADPKD, bilateral renal enlargement and cysts or the presence of multiple bilateral cysts with hepatic cysts together with the absence of other manifestations suggesting a different renal cystic disease provide presumptive evidence for the diagnosis.

2. **Which renal cystic diseases are the most common?**
   Simple renal cysts are the most common renal cystic abnormality and can be single or multiple. They are rare in children and individuals <30 years old, but the frequency increases with age. They may be solitary or multiple and contain fluid similar to plasma ultrafiltrate. In autopsy studies and as incidental computed tomography (CT) findings, they are found in up to 50% of patients aged 40 and older. Ultrasound is less sensitive than CT or magnetic resonance imaging (MRI) and turns up lower percentages. Simple renal cysts are acquired, although the contribution of genetic factors has not been studied. Tubular obstruction and ischemia might play a role in their pathogenesis. They rarely produce symptoms such as flank pain, abdominal discomfort, palpable mass, or hematuria; they also rarely result from complications or consequent to an enlarging cyst. There may be an association with hypertension. The Bosniak classification (Table 44-2) categorizes cystic lesions on the basis of their radiologic characteristics.

   ADPKD is the most common inherited cystic kidney disease, occurring in 1 in 400 to 1 in 1000 individuals. In the United States, approximately 500,000 people are affected, and ADPKD accounts for ~5% of end-stage renal disease (ESRD) in developed countries. It is characterized by progressive enlargement of kidney cysts and typically leads to renal failure by middle age. A family history of ADPKD may be present (but is not necessary). Most individuals with *PKD1* mutations have renal failure by the age of 70 years, whereas more than 50% of individuals with *PKD2* mutations have adequate renal function at the same age. Mean age of onset of ESRD is 54.3 years with a *PKD1* mutation and 74 years with *PKD2*.

   Harris PC, Torres VE. Polycystic kidney disease. *Ann Rev Med* 2009;60(1):321–337.

   Hateboer N, van Dijk MA, Bogdanova N, et al. Comparison of phenotypes of polycystic kidney disease types 1 and 2. *Lancet* 1999;353:103.

3. **What is the genetic basis of ADPKD?**
   This disease is genetically heterogenous, with two different genes identified for this disease. *PKD1* is located on the short arm of chromosome 16 and is responsible for ~85% of the disease. *PKD2* is located on chromosome 4 and accounts for ~15% cases. A third gene, which has not been cloned, may also cause a small number of cases. The greater severity of

---

TABLE 44-1.   CLASSIFICATION OF CYSTIC KIDNEY DISORDERS

Autosomal-dominant polycystic kidney disease (ADPKD)

Autosomal-recessive polycystic kidney disease (ARPKD)

Autosomal-dominant or X-linked diseases in the differential diagnosis of ADPKD
- Tuberous sclerosis complex (TSC)
- von Hippel-Lindau syndrome (VHL)
- Hepatocyte nuclear factor-1 associated nephropathy
- Familial renal hamartomas associated with hyperparathyroidism-jaw tumor syndrome
- Orofaciodigital syndrome (OFD)

Autosomal-dominant medullary cystic kidney disease (MCKD)

Hereditary recessive ciliopathies with interstitial nephritis and/or cysts
- Nephronophthisis (NPH)
- Joubert syndrome (JBTS)
- Meckel-Gruber syndrome (MKS)
- Bardet-Biedl syndrome (BBS)
- Alström syndrome
- Nephronophthisis variants associated with skeletal defects

Renal cystic dysplasias
- Multicystic kidney dysplasia

Other cystic kidney disorders
- Simple cysts
- Localized or unilateral renal cystic disease
- Medullary sponge kidney
- Acquired cystic kidney disease

Renal cystic neoplasms
- Cystic renal cell carcinoma
- Multilocular cystic nephroma
- Cystic partially differentiated nephroblastoma
- Mixed epithelial and stromal tumor

Cysts not of tubular origin
- Cystic disease of the renal sinus
- Perirenal lymphangiomas
- Subcapsular and perirenal urinomas

Pyelocalyceal cysts

Adapted from Grantham JJ, Torres VE. Cystic renal diseases. In Brenner BM (ed). *The Kidney,* 9th ed. Philadelphia: W.B. Saunders, 2010.
For a continuously updated list of laboratories providing clinical or research genetic testing, refer to www.genetests.org.

PKD1 results from the development of more cysts at an early age and not to faster cyst growth. Mutations in the PKD1 and PKD2 mutations are highly variable. It is thought that kidney cysts may develop from loss of functional polycystin with somatic inactivation of the normal allele consistent with a "two hit" mechanism, but other genetic mechanisms may play a role. The products of these genes, the polycystins, are localized in specialized structures that

---

TABLE 44-2.   THE BOSNIAK CLASSIFICATION

Category I: Benign simple cyst
- Cyst has a hairline-thin wall that does not contain septa, calcifications, or solid components.
- It parallels water density and does not enhance.

Category II: Benign cyst
- Cyst may contain a few hairline-thin septa in which "perceived" enhancement may be present.
- Fine calcification or a short segment of slightly thickened calcification may be present in the wall or septa. Uniformly high-attenuation lesions smaller than 3 cm (so-called high-density cysts) that are well marginated and do not enhance are included in this group. Cysts in this category do not require further evaluation.

Category IIF: (F stands for "follow-up")
- Cysts may contain multiple hairline-thin septa or minimal smooth thickening of the wall or septa.
- Perceived enhancement of the septa or wall may be present.
- The wall or septa may contain calcification that may be thick and nodular, but no measurable contrast enhancement is present.
- These lesions are generally well marginated.
- Totally intrarenal, nonenhancing, high-attenuation renal lesions larger than 3 cm are also included in this category. Such lesions require follow-up studies to prove benignity.

Category III: "Indeterminate" cystic masses
- Masses are thickened irregular or smooth walls or septa in which measurable enhancement is present.
- These lesions require surgery, although some will prove to be benign (e.g., hemorrhagic cysts, chronic infected cysts, and multiloculated cystic nephroma); some will be malignant, such as cystic renal cell carcinoma and multiloculated cystic renal cell carcinoma.

Category IV: Cystic renal cell carcinoma

Adapted from Israel GM, Bosniak MA. How I do it: Evaluating renal masses. *Radiology* 2005;236(2): 441–450.

---

sense the extracellular environment, such as primary cilia, focal adhesions, and adherens complexes, and recently in urinary exosomes (small particles shed in urine), and also appear to function by regulation of intracellular calcium homeostasis, which leads to alterations in intracellular calcium and cyclic adenosine monophosphate (cAMP) signaling.

4. **Does ADPKD have extrarenal manifestations?**
   - **Polycystic liver disease (PLD):** This is the most common extrarenal manifestation. It is associated with both *PKD1* and non-*PKD1* genotypes. The disease also occurs as a genetically distinct disease in the absence of renal cysts. Like ADPKD, autosomal-dominant polycystic liver disease is genetically heterogeneous, with two genes identified (*PRKCSH* and *SEC63*), which account for around one third of isolated cases. These individuals may have few renal cysts.
   - **Hepatic cysts:** The overall prevalence of hepatic cysts in patients with ADPKD was 83% using MRI. Hepatic cysts are also more prevalent and cyst volume is larger in women than in men. Women who have multiple pregnancies or who have used oral contraceptive drugs or estrogen replacement therapy have more severe disease, suggesting that hepatic-cyst

growth is estrogen dependent. In a minority of patients, it can result in severe PLD requiring surgical intervention.

- **Cysts in other organs:** Cysts of the seminal vesicles, pancreas, and arachnoid membrane occur in 40% (of men), 5%, and 8% of patients, respectively. Seminal vesicle cysts rarely result in infertility. Defective sperm motility is another cause of male infertility in ADPKD. Pancreatic cysts are almost always asymptomatic, with very rare instances of recurrent pancreatitis. Anecdotal case reports of intraductal papillary mucinous tumors or pancreatic carcinoma have been associated with ADPKD. Arachnoid membrane cysts are asymptomatic but can increase the risk of subdural hematomas. Meningeal diverticula can occur with increased frequency and rarely present with intracranial hypotension as a result of cerebrospinal fluid leak. Ovarian cysts are not associated with ADPKD.

- **Vascular manifestations:** Intracranial aneurysms are approximately five times more common than in the general population and can have significant morbidity/mortality associated with aneurysmal rupture. Other vascular manifestations include dolichoectasias, thoracic aortic and cervicocephalic artery dissections, and coronary artery aneurysms. They are caused by alterations in the vasculature directly linked to mutations in *PKD1* or *PKD2*. Polycystin-1 and polycystin-2 are expressed in vascular smooth muscle cells. Intracranial aneurysms occur in around 6% of patients with a negative family history of aneurysms and 16% of those with a positive history. They are most often asymptomatic. Focal findings such as cranial nerve palsy or seizure may result from compression of local structures. Rupture carries a 35% to 55% risk of combined severe morbidity and mortality. Mean age at rupture is lower than in the general population (39 years versus 51 years). Most patients have normal renal function, and ~30% have normal blood pressure at the time of rupture.

- **Cardiac manifestations:** Mitral valve prolapse is the most common valvular abnormality found in up to 25% of patients on echocardiography. Aortic insufficiency can occur in association with dilatation of the aortic root. Although these lesions can progress with time, they rarely need valve replacement. Screening echocardiography is not indicated unless a murmur is detected on clinical examination.

- **Diverticular disease:** Colonic diverticulosis and diverticulitis are more common in patients with ESRD with ADPKD than in individuals with other kidney diseases. Whether this heightened risk extends to patients before ESRD occurs is uncertain. The disease might become clinically significant in a few patients. Subtle alterations in polycystin function can enhance the smooth-muscle dysfunction from aging thought to underlie the development of diverticula.

- **Abdominal hernia:** Hernias (inguinal, incisional, and paraumbilical) are more frequent. These may lead to problems in people who are undergoing peritoneal dialysis.

Abderrahim E, Hedri H, Lâabidi J, et al. Chronic subdural haematoma and autosomal polycystic kidney disease: report of two new cases. *Nephrology* (Carlton) 2004;9(5):331–333.

Bae KT, Zhu F, Chapman AB, et al. Magnetic resonance imaging evaluation of hepatic cysts in early autosomal-dominant polycystic kidney disease: The Consortium for Radiologic Imaging Studies of Polycystic Kidney Disease cohort. *Clin J Am Soc Nephrol* 2006;1(1):64–69.

Davila S, Furu L, Gharavi AG, et al. Mutations in SEC63 cause autosomal dominant polycystic liver disease. *Nat Genet* 2004;36:575.

Drenth JPH, te Morsche RH, Smink R, et al. Germline mutations in PRKCSH are associated with autosomal dominant polycystic liver disease. *Nat Genet* 2003;33(3):345–347.

Everson GT, Taylor MR. Management of polycystic liver disease. *Curr Gastroenterol Rep* 2005;7(1):19–25.

Gabow PA, Johnson AM, Kaehny WD, et al. Risk factors for the development of hepatic cysts in autosomal dominant polycystic kidney disease. *Hepatology* 1990;11(6):1033–1037.

Griffin MD, Torres VE, Grande JP, et al. Vascular expression of polycystin. *J Am Soc Nephrol* 1997;8(4):616–626.

Heinonen PK, Vuento M, Maunola M, et al. Ovarian manifestations in women with autosomal dominant polycystic kidney disease. *Am J Kidney Dis* 2002;40(3):504–507.

Hossack KF, Leddy CL, Johnson AM, et al. Echocardiographic findings in autosomal dominant polycystic kidney disease. *N Engl J Med* 1988;319(14):907–912.

Inagawa T. Trends in incidence and case fatality rates of aneurysmal subarachnoid hemorrhage in Izumo City, Japan, between 1980–1989 and 1990–1998. *Stroke* 2001;32(7):1499–1507.

Lederman ED, McCoy G, Conti DJ, et al. Diverticulitis and polycystic kidney disease. *Am Surg* 2000;66(2):200–203.

Leier CV, Baker PB, Kilman JW, et al. Cardiovascular abnormalities associated with adult polycystic kidney disease. *Ann Intern Med* 1984;100(5):683–688.

Li A, Davila S, Furu L, et al. Mutations in PRKCSH cause isolated autosomal dominant polycystic liver disease. *Am J Hum Genet* 2003;72(3):691–703.

Lumiaho A, Ikäheimo R, Miettinen R, et al. Mitral valve prolapse and mitral regurgitation are common in patients with polycystic kidney disease type 1. *Am J Kidney Dis* 2001;38(6):1208–1216.

McCune TR, Nylander WA, Van Buren DH, et al. Colonic screening prior to renal transplantation and its impact on post-transplant colonic complications. *Clin Transplant* 1992;6(2):91–96.

Pirson Y, Chauveau D, Torres V. Management of cerebral aneurysms in autosomal dominant polycystic kidney disease. *J Am Soc Nephrol* 2002;13(1):269–276.

Qian Q, Li A, King BF, et al. Clinical profile of autosomal dominant polycystic liver disease. *Hepatology* 2003;37(1):164–171.

Qian Q, Li M, Zhou WJ, et al. Analysis of the polycystins in aortic vascular smooth muscle cells. *J Am Soc Nephrol* 2003;14(9):2280–2287.

Reynolds DM, Falk CT, Li A, et al. Identification of a locus for autosomal dominant polycystic liver disease, on chromosome 19p13.2-13.1. *Am J Hum Genet* 2000;67(6):1598–1604.

Scheff RT, Zuckerman G, Harter H, et al. Diverticular disease in patients with chronic renal failure due to polycystic kidney disease. *Ann Intern Med* 1980;92(2 Pt 1):202–204.

Schievink WI, Torres VE. Spinal meningeal diverticula in autosomal dominant polycystic kidney disease. *Lancet* 1997;349(9060):1223–1224.

Sharp CK, Zeligman BE, Johnson AM, et al. Evaluation of colonic diverticular disease in autosomal dominant polycystic kidney disease without end-stage renal disease. *Am J Kidney Dis* 1999;34(5):863–868.

Sherstha R, McKinley C, Russ P, et al. Postmenopausal estrogen therapy selectively stimulates hepatic enlargement in women with autosomal dominant polycystic kidney disease. *Hepatology* 1997;26(5):1282–1286.

Stamm ER, Townsend RR, Johnson AM et al. Frequency of ovarian cysts in patients with autosomal dominant polycystic kidney disease. *Am J Kidney Dis* 1999;34(1):120–124.

Tahvanainen P, Tahvanainen E, Reijonen H, et al. Polycystic liver disease is genetically heterogeneous: clinical and linkage studies in eight Finnish families. *J Hepatol* 2003;38(1):39–43.

Torres VE, Cai Y, Chen X, et al. Vascular expression of polycystin-2. *J Am Soc Nephrol* 2001;12(1):1–9.

Wijdicks EF, Torres VE, Schievink WI. Chronic subdural hematoma in autosomal dominant polycystic kidney disease. *Am J Kidney Dis* 2000;35(1):40–43.

5. **What are the clinical features of autosomal-recessive polycystic renal disease?**

Autosomal-recessive polycystic renal disease (ARPKD) is an autosomal-recessive disorder characterized by various combinations of bilateral renal cystic disease and congenital hepatic fibrosis. Although siblings may have the disease, it should not occur in the parents. The incidence is ~1 in 20,000 live births. Typically, ARPKD presents in infancy and childhood, where it causes significant renal and liver morbidity. All individuals with ARPKD will have liver involvement. Fusiform dilatation of the collecting tubules (to 1 to 2 mm in the cortex and medulla) characterizes the renal cystic disease. The liver disease consists of enlargement and fibrosis of portal areas, bile-duct proliferation, and hypoplasia of portal vein branches leading to portal hypertension; some patients have nonobstructive intrahepatic bile-duct dilatation (Caroli disease). Congenital hepatic fibrosis (CHF) and Caroli disease can also occur without other manifestations of ARPKD or other associated diseases—for example, the Meckel and Joubert syndromes and nephronophthisis (see Table 44-1).

ARPKD is generally considered to be the infantile form of polycystic kidney disease, with the majority of individuals presenting by the neonatal period with enlarged (up to 20 times normal), echogenic kidneys. On prenatal ultrasound, large, hyperechogenic kidneys and oligohydramnios are typical findings and most of these infants die in the perinatal period from respiratory insufficiency and complications of renal failure. More than half of the patients are detected late during pregnancy, and those who are undetected on prenatal evaluation usually survive the perinatal period. About half of all individuals with ARPKD have associated liver abnormalities such as hepatomegaly, increased echogenicity, or dilated intrahepatic bile ducts at initial presentation. A minority of affected individuals can present for the first time as older children or adolescents, usually with manifestations of portal hypertension as a result of CHF (gastrointestinal bleeding from varices, hepatosplenomegaly, or hypersplenism) or episodes of cholangitis resulting from Caroli disease. ARPKD is rarely diagnosed in adults. Genetic testing for ARPKD is available with a mutation detection rate of ~95%. All reported associated gene mutations are archived in the ARPKD mutation public database.

Adeva M, El-Youssef M, Rossetti S, et al. Clinical and molecular characterization defines a broadened spectrum of autosomal recessive polycystic kidney disease (ADPKD). *Medicine* 2006;85:1.

Blyth H, Ockenden BG. Polycystic disease of kidney and liver presenting in childhood. *J Med Genet* 1971;8(3):257–284.

Caroli J. Diseases of intrahepatic bile ducts. *Isr J Med Sci* 1968;4(1):21–35.

Desmet VJ. Congenital diseases of intrahepatic bile ducts: Variations on the theme ductal plate malformation. *Hepatology* 1992;16(4):1069–1083.

Fonck C, Chauveau D, Gagnadoux MF, et al. Autosomal recessive polycystic kidney disease in adulthood. *Nephrol Dial Transplant* 2001;16(8):1648–1652.

MacRae Dell K, Avner E. Autosomal Recessive Polycystic Kidney Disease. Gene Clinics, 2001. Available at http://www.geneclinics.org/.

Nadina Ortiz Brüchle D, Zerres K. Mutation Database Autosomal Recessive Polycystic Kidney Disease (ARPKD/PKHD1). 2010.

Osathanondh V, Potter E. Pathogenesis of polycystic kidneys. Type 1 due to hyperplasia of interstitial portions of the collecting tubules. *Arch Pathol* 1964;77:466–473.

Zerres K, Rudnik-Schöneborn S, Deget F, et al. Autosomal recessive polycystic kidney disease in 115 children: clinical presentation, course and influence of gender. *Acta Paediatr* 1996;85:437–445.

6. **Which imaging studies are used to diagnose cystic diseases of kidneys?**
    Ultrasound is commonly used because it is noninvasive and cost efficient and no radiation is administered. CT with contrast is another highly sensitive imaging modality and will provide additional useful information about the liver, pancreas, spleen, and other organs. Counseling should be done before performing imaging. CT scans are capable of detecting cysts as small as 3 mm. Contrast with CT should be avoided if there is significant renal impairment.
    A presumptive diagnosis of ADPKD may be considered in patients without a positive family history and the presence of bilateral and multiple cysts (10 or more per kidney). CT (with and without contrast) is also helpful in determination of prognosis and complications (e.g., nephrolithiasis, complex cysts, cyst wall calcification, or parenchymal calcifications) and will show the severity of renal cyst involvement and degree of relative parenchymal preservation in individuals with preserved renal function at the time of the initial evaluation. MRI can also be used in imaging in ADPKD and can be used as an alternative to CT, particularly in individuals who have renal insufficiency that precludes the use of iodinated contrast. Gadolinium is not required to differentiate cystic disease from noncystic renal parenchyma and should be avoided if there is significant renal impairment. MR does not detect stones. Using MRI data in an observational study in ADPKD, it was observed that kidneys increase on average 5.27% per year, but with a wide range of variability, and is more sensitive to detect disease progression occurring before a measurable decline in renal function. Consider a KUB (Kidneys, Ureter, and Bladder scan) and tomograms to differentiate between uric acid stones (radiolucent) and calcium stones (radiopaque). Dual-energy computed tomography (DECT) is another useful method to discriminate uric acid stones from other renal stones. Indium 111 scan is a helpful imaging modality to identify infected kidney or liver cysts. Positron emission tomography (PET) scans are also useful in identifying infected liver cysts. Recently, new diagnostic criteria for diagnosis of ADPKD by ultrasound in individuals at risk (individuals from families with ADPKD) has been developed (Table 44-3). Close attention to the family history of renal disease severity in ADPKD may also provide a simple means of predicting the mutated gene, which has prognostic implications. The presence of at least one affected family member who developed ESRD at age ≥55 is highly predictive of a *PKD1* mutation (positive predictive value

TABLE 44-3.   ULTRASOUND CRITERIA FOR THE DIAGNOSIS OF ADPKD

	Criteria	PKD1	PKD2	Unknown ADPKD Gene Type
REVISED UNIFIED DIAGNOSTIC CRITERIA FOR ADPKD				
15–29	≥3 cysts, unilateral or bilateral	PPV = 100% SEN 94.3%	PPV = 100% SEN 69.5%	PPV =100% SEN = 81.7%
30–39	≥3 cysts, unilateral or bilateral	PPV = 100% SEN = 96.6%	PPV = 100% SEN = −94.9%	PPV = 100% SEN = 95.5%
40–59	≥2 cysts in each kidney	PPV = 100% SEN = 92.6%	PPV = 100% SEN = 88.8%	PPV = 100% SEN = 90%
REVISED ULTRASOUND CRITERIA FOR EXCLUSION OF ADPKD				
15–29	≥1 cyst	NPV = 99.1% SPEC = 97.6%	NPV = 83.5% SPEC = 96.6%	NPV = 90.8% SPEC = 97.1%
30–39	≥1 cyst	NPV = 100% SPEC = 96%	NPV = 96.8% SPEC = 93.8%	NPV = 98.3% SPEC = 94.8%
40–59	≥1 cyst	NPV = 100% SPEC = 93.9%	NPV = 100% SPEC = 93.7%	NPV = 100% SPEC = 93.9%

ADPKD = autosomal-dominant polycystic kidney disease; PKD = polycystic kidney disease; PPV = positive predictive value; SEN = sensitivity; NPV = negative predictive value; SPEC = specificity.

Note: These criteria if applied to magnetic resonance imaging or computed tomography will result in false-positive diagnoses.

For at-risk subjects at or older than 60, four or more cysts per kidney have a sensitivity and specificity of 100%, whether in PKD1 or PKD2 (and therefore of unknown gene type as well).

100%; sensitivity 72%), whereas the presence of at least one affected family member who continues to have sufficient renal function or develops ESRD at age >70 is highly predictive of a *PKD2* mutation (positive predictive value 100%; sensitivity 74%).

Bleeker-Rovers CP, de Sévaux RG, van Hamersvelt HW, et al. Diagnosis of renal and hepatic cyst infections by 18-F-fluorodeoxyglucose positron emission tomography in autosomal dominant polycystic kidney disease. *Am J Kidney Dis* 2003;41(6):E18–21.

Grantham JJ, Torres VE, Chapman AB, et al. Volume progression in polycystic kidney disease. *N Engl J Med* 2006;354:2122.

Gupta S, Seith A, Sud K, et al. CT in the evaluation of complicated autosomal dominant polycystic kidney disease. *Acta Radiol* 2000;41(3):280–284.

Pei Y, Obaji J, Dupuis A, et al. Unified criteria for ultrasonographic diagnosis of ADPKD. *J Am Soc Nephrol* 2009;20(1):205–212.

Primak AN, Fletcher JG, Vrtiska TJ, et al. Noninvasive differentiation of uric acid versus non-uric acid kidney stones using dual-energy CT. *Acad Radiol* 2007;14(12):1441–1447.

Sallée M, Rafat C, Zahar JR, et al. Cyst infections in patients with autosomal dominant polycystic kidney disease. *Clin J Am Soc Nephrol* 2009;4(7):1183–1189.

7. **What is a complex renal cyst?**

   Complex renal cysts can be distinguished from simple cysts by using the Bosniak classification (Table 44-2). Clearly malignant cystic masses can have all the criteria of category III but also contain enhancing soft-tissue components adjacent to, but independent of, the wall or septum. These lesions include cystic carcinomas and require surgical removal.

8. **What are the most reliable diagnostic criteria to differentiate ADPKD from ARPKD?**

   ADPKD is typically an adult-onset disease characterized by progressive bilateral cystic development and enlargement of the kidneys. Kidney function as estimated by glomerular filtration rate (GFR) usually appears normal over many decades followed by a decline in GFR that occurs rapidly (4.4–5.9 mL/min/m² per year). The mean age of onset of ESRD is 59 years (quartiles 49 and 70 years) with ~15% retaining adequate renal function by 80 years. Occasionally ADPKD presents as very-early-onset disease, with features of renal enlargement in children younger than 18 months of age, in whom it may be confused with ARPKD.

   Individuals with ARPKD usually present in the neonatal period with enlarged echogenic kidneys with loss of cortico-medullary differentiation on ultrasound. Macroscopic cysts are not present at first visit. Fusiform dilatation of the collecting tubules characterizes the renal cystic disease of ARPKD as patients get older. With increasing age, kidneys become smaller and develop macroscopic cysts, nephrocalcinosis, and/or medullary calcifications (common). Hepatomegaly can be seen and liver biopsy may reveal congenital hepatic fibrosis (periportal fibrosis, bile-duct proliferation, and hypoplasia of portal vein branches leading to portal hypertension). Some patients have nonobstructive intrahepatic bile-duct dilatation (Caroli disease). A diagnosis of ARPKD or CHF can also be made in mutation-defined families in siblings who had inherited the mutant alleles using clinically available genetic testing.

9. **Is it possible to have a normal renal ultrasound and still have ADPKD?**

   In most cases, the diagnosis of ADPKD will be confirmed or ruled out on imaging testing. However, in individuals <30 years with a family history of the disease (especially people with *PKD2* mutations), the utility of ultrasound for disease exclusion may be limited where there is a negative or indeterminate scan. In these individuals, consider MRI, CT, or genetic testing. Genetic testing is available as a clinical test, and mutations can be identified in ~90% of confirmed cases. The ADPKD Mutation Database (http://pkdb.mayo.edu) lists known mutations of the *PKD1* and *PKD2* genes. Counseling should be done before imaging and/or genetic testing in those at risk.

10. **What are the most common clinical complications of ADPKD?**
    - **Hypertension:** Blood pressure >140/90 mm Hg is present in ~50% of patients aged 20 to 34 years with ADPKD and normal renal function and increases to nearly 100% of patients with ESRD. Left ventricular hypertrophy is common. Early detection and treatment of hypertension is important because cardiovascular disease is the main cause of death. Uncontrolled blood pressure increases the morbidity and mortality from valvular heart disease and aneurysms, increases the risk of proteinuria and hematuria, and increases speed of decline of renal function. Activation of the intrarenal renin-angiotensin system likely plays an important role.
    - **Pain:** Pain is the most common symptom (around 60%) reported by adult patients, and flank pain can frequently be an early symptom of ADPKD. Most often it is attributed to compression of surrounding structures by expanding cysts, but it can also be caused by hemorrhage into a cyst, cyst rupture, or infection; stones or tumor should be excluded. Acute pain may be associated with renal hemorrhage, passage of stones, and urinary tract infections. Most cyst hemorrhages resolve within 2 to 7 days. If symptoms last longer than 1 week or if the initial episode occurs after the age of 50 years, investigation to exclude neoplasm should be undertaken. Some patients develop chronic flank pain without identifiable etiology other than the cysts.
    - **Hematuria**: Both microscopic and macroscopic hematuria are common. A history of gross hematuria is associated with worse renal function at a given age.
    - **Nephrolithiasis:** About 20% of patients with ADPKD have kidney stones. The composition of these is typically uric acid or calcium oxalate. Low urine citrate and urine pH and decreased ammonia excretion are the main metabolic factors predisposing to stone formation. Urinary stasis secondary to the distorted renal anatomy may also contribute to

conditions for stone formation. A CT of the abdomen before and following contrast enhancement is the best imaging technique to detect small uric acid stones that may be very faint on plain films with tomograms and to differentiate stones from cyst wall and parenchymal calcifications. Stones may be missed if only a contrast-enhanced CT is obtained. Dual-energy CT can be used to distinguish between calcium and uric acid stones.

- **Urinary tract infection:** As in the general population, women are more frequently affected than men. Most are caused by *Enterobacteriaceae*. CT and MRI are useful to detect complicated cysts and provide anatomic definition, but the findings are not specific for infection. Nuclear imaging (^{67}Ga or ^{111}In-labeled leukocyte scans) may be helpful, but false-negative and false-positive results are possible. An 18-F-fluorodeoxyglucose (FDG) PET scan has become a promising agent for detection of infected cysts, but its use to diagnose kidney infections may be difficult because FDG is filtered by the kidneys, is not reabsorbed by the tubules, and appears in the collecting system. Cyst aspiration should be considered when the clinical setting and imaging are suggestive and blood and urine cultures are negative.
- **ESRD:** ESRD is the major late outcome of patients with ADPKD; 45% of patients with ADPKD develop renal insufficiency by 60 years of age and progress to dialysis or renal transplantation. A strong relationship exists between renal enlargement and renal function decline.
- **Recurrent UTI:** Of all patients 50% to 75% will experience at least one clinical urinary tract infection in their life, with the majority occurring in women.

Bleeker-Rovers CP, Vos FJ, Corstens FH, et al. Imaging of infectious diseases using [18F] fluorodeoxyglucose PET. *Q J Nucl Med Mol Imaging* 2008;52(1):17–29.

Elzinga LW, Bennett WM. Miscellaneous renal and systemic complications of autosomal dominant polycystic kidney disease including infection. In: Watson ML, Torres VE. *Polycystic Kidney Disease,* Vol. 1. Oxford, England: Oxford Medical Publications. 1996, pp. 483–499.

Grosjean R, Sauer B, Guerra RM, et al. Characterization of human renal stones with MDCT: Advantage of dual energy and limitations due to respiratory motion. *AJR Am J Roentgenol* 2008;190(3):720–728.

Kelleher CL, McFann KK, Johnson AM, et al. Characteristics of hypertension in young adults with autosomal dominant polycystic kidney disease compared with the general U.S. population. *Am J Hypertens* 2004;17 (11 Pt 1):1029–1034.

Matlaga BR, Kawamoto S, Fishman E. Dual source computed tomography: A novel technique to determine stone composition. *Urology* 2008;72(5):1164–1168.

Soussan M, Sberro R, Wartski M, et al. Diagnosis and localization of renal cyst infection by 18F-fluorodeoxyglucose PET/CT in polycystic kidney disease. *Ann Nucl Med* 2008;22(6):529–531.

11. **What are the indications for nephrectomy in ADPKD?**
    Nephrectomy may be indicated where there is severe renal hemorrhage that cannot be controlled, where there is a renal carcinoma, or in the situation where an individual with life-threatening infection is not responding to medical management. Pretransplant nephrectomy is not usually performed in order to avoid the anephric state. Consider pretransplant nephrectomy only if massively enlarged polycystic kidneys are present that create difficulty in determining a site for the new kidney transplant or if there are recurrent infections of native kidneys. Bilateral hand-assisted nephrectomy is associated with a lower complication rate than transabdominal bilateral nephrectomy.

12. **Are there any treatments for ADPKD?**
    Early detection and treatment of complications of ADPKD are likely to improve quality of life and life expectancy in affected individuals. Particular attention should be paid to cardiovascular complications, which are the most common cause of morbidity and mortality in ADPKD. Patients should be informed about the significance of systolic and diastolic blood pressure readings and how to take their own blood pressure and the targets of blood pressure–lowering therapies. Dietary guidelines should include restricting protein intake to 0.8 g/kg of ideal body weight per day and avoiding or limiting foods or medications containing caffeine, which increases cAMP. For patients with hypertension or hypercholesterolemia, advise sodium

restriction of 90 mEq per day and low cholesterol (<200 mg/day) diet. Control of hypertension to JNCVII (the Seventh Report of the Joint National Committee on Prevention, Detection, Evaluation, and Treatment of High Blood Pressure) targets (aim for target blood pressure of 130/80 or lower) is recommended using angiotensin-converting enzyme (ACE) inhibitors or angiotensin II receptor blockers. Consider β blockers in individuals with dilated aortic root or in those with supraventricular tachycardias associated with mitral valve prolapse. Refer to a nephrologist if impaired renal function to closely monitor the rate of renal function decline, adjust diet and antihypertensive medications, prepare for renal-replacement therapy, and manage metabolic abnormalities associated with chronic kidney disease progression. Refer individuals with ADPKD for kidney transplant evaluation before initiation of dialysis (i.e., estimated GFR of 15–25 mL/min, depending on the rate of decline of renal function).

Multiple potential therapies are also being evaluated in clinical trials. These include vasopressin 2 receptor antagonists and somatostatin analogues and mTOR (mammalian target of rapamycin) inhibitors. Most individuals with PLD require no treatment, but they should be advised to avoid estrogens and compounds that promote cAMP accumulation (e.g., caffeine). Histamine H_2 blockers and proton pump inhibitors may inhibit secretin production and fluid secretion into liver cysts. Occasionally, symptomatic PLD requires interventions to reduce cyst volume and hepatic size. Surgical procedures such as percutaneous cyst aspiration without or with sclerosis, laparoscopic cyst fenestration, combined liver resection and cyst fenestration, or liver transplantation may be indicated in a minority of cases.

13. **Which antibiotics should be used for treatment of urinary tract infection in patients with ADPKD?**
Urinary tract infections have increased morbidity in patients with ADPKD; therefore, they should all be treated promptly according to cultures and current treatment guidelines. Most are caused by *Enterobacteriaceae.* If the infection relapses after completing antibiotics, complications such as obstruction, cyst infection, or infected stone need to be excluded. If none is found, several months of continued antibiotic treatment may be needed to eradicate the infection. Quinolone antibiotics (e.g., ciprofloxacin or levofloxacin) are usually the antibiotics of choice because they are effective in treating gram-negative organisms and accumulate in cysts. Trimethoprim-sulfamethoxazole is an alternative.

Elzinga LW, Golper TA, Rashad AL, et al. Trimethoprim-sulfamethoxazole in cyst fluid from autosomal dominant polycystic kidneys. *Kidney Int* 1987;32(6):884–888.

Elzinga LW, Golper TA, Rashad AL, et al. Ciprofloxacin activity in cyst fluid from polycystic kidneys. *Antimicrob Agents Chemother* 1988;32(6):844–847.

14. **Which patients with ADPKD should be screened for intracranial aneurysms?**
Intracranial aneurysms occur in 6% of patients without a family history of aneurysms and in 16% of those with a family history. Widespread screening is not recommended because it yields small aneurysms with a low risk of rupture. Presymptomatic screening for intracranial aneurysm is appropriate in patients with a strong family history of ruptured intracranial aneurysm, high-risk occupations (e.g., pilots), and anticipated major surgical procedures with a risk of hemodynamic instability and for individuals who need reassurance. Magnetic resonance angiography is the imaging of choice. For any patient with known ADPKD who has new-onset or severe headache or other troubling central nervous system symptoms, a thin-cut noncontrast CT is more sensitive than MRI in the detection of acute intracranial bleed (subarachnoid hemorrhage). If the CT scan is negative and index of suspicion of intracranial bleed remains high, obtain a lumbar puncture, CT, or MR angiogram and consider other treatable causes of headache (e.g., cervicocephalic artery dissection, subdural hematoma, leaking spinal meningeal diverticulum, or uncontrolled hypertension).

15. **What are the clinical characteristics of tuberous sclerosis?**
Tuberous sclerosis complex (TSC) is an autosomal-dominant disorder with an incidence in newborns of 1:6000 that results from mutations in the *TSC1* or *TSC2* genes (encoding the

tumor suppressor proteins tuberin and hamartin, respectively) and is associated with hamartoma formation in multiple organ systems including the brain, heart, skin, eyes, kidney, lungs, and liver. These are frequently seen as facial angiofibromas, forehead patches, shagreen patches, subungual fibromas, hypomelanotic macules, cortical tubers, subependymal nodules, giant-cell astrocytomas, cardiac rhabdomyomas, and pulmonary lymphangioleiomyomatosis. The most frequent renal findings (developing in 50% to 80% affected individuals) are angiomyolipomas (AMLs) (usually multiple), renal cysts, and (rarely) renal cell carcinomas (RCC). AMLs are benign tumors composed of abnormal vessels, immature smooth-muscle cells, and fat cells. Renal lesions (usually AMLs) can cause clinical problems secondary to hemorrhage or by compression and replacement of healthy renal tissue, leading to renal failure. Although renal cancers affect only 2% to 3% of patients with TSC, because benign AMLs are so common, the challenge is to recognize a cancer in the setting of multiple benign AMLs in these patients. *TSC1* and *TSC2* gene mutation analyses are available as clinical tests.

The *TSC2* and *PKD1* genes lie adjacent to each other in a tail-to-tail orientation on chromosome 16 at 16p13.3. Deletions inactivating both genes are associated with polycystic kidneys diagnosed during the first year of life or early childhood (*TSC2/PKD1* contiguous gene syndrome). Therefore, TSC should be considered in children with renal cysts and no family history of PKD. Patients with the contiguous gene syndrome usually reach ESRD at an earlier age than that of patients with ADPKD alone.

Brook-Carter PT, Peral B, Ward CJ, et al. Deletion of the TSC2 and PKD1 genes associated with severe infantile polycystic kidney disease—A contiguous gene syndrome. *Nat Genet* 1994;8(4):328–332.

Sampson JR, Maheshwar MM, Aspinwall R, et al. Renal cystic disease in tuberous sclerosis: Role of the polycystic kidney disease 1 gene. *Am J Hum Genet* 1997;61:843.

16. **What are the major characteristics of von Hippel-Lindau disease?**
The incidence of von Hippel-Lindau disease (VHL) is 1:30 to 50,000. Clinical features include retinal and/or central nervous system hemangioblastomas, pheochromocytomas, pancreatic cysts, and epididymal cystadenoma. Renal involvement in VHL consists of multiple, bilateral, clear cell-lined cysts in 70% to 80% and multifocal and bilateral renal clear cell carcinoma in 40% to 60% of patients. VHL gene mutation analysis is available as a clinical test, and the VHL gene encodes a tumor suppressor protein.

17. **What are distinguishing radiographic characteristics of simple cysts?**
Differentiation of simple cysts from a RCC is a common problem. Ultrasonography, CT, or MRI is commonly required to characterize these lesions.
- **Ultrasound criteria for simple cyst:** The mass is round and sharply demarcated with smooth walls with no echoes (anechoic) within the mass and presence of a strong posterior wall echo indicating good transmission through the cyst and enhanced transmission beyond the cyst. If the ultrasound study is equivocal, then CT or MRI should be performed.
- **CT criteria:** The cyst is sharply demarcated from the surrounding parenchyma and has a smooth, thin wall. Fluid within the cyst is homogeneous, with a density of less than 20 Hounsfield units (similar to water); however, higher values may be seen with a benign proteinaceous or hemorrhagic cyst. There is no enhancement of the mass following the administration of intravenous contrast media, indicating the presence of an avascular lesion. Enhancement implies vascularity and strongly suggests a malignant lesion even in the absence of irregular margins.

18. **What is the nephronophthisis-medullary cystic kidney disease complex?**
The nephronophthisis (NPH) complex is a heterogenous group of autosomal-recessive diseases with an estimated prevalence of 1 in 50,000 live births. It accounts for approximately 5% of ESRD in North American children. The gene products in these diseases are located on primary cilia or centrosomes (Table 44-1). More than ten genes have been identified. Homozygous deletions in *NPHP1* account for approximately 21% of all NPH cases, whereas

the other genes contribute less than 3% each. No mutations in any of the known genes are found in approximately 70% of patients, indicating that many other genes remain to be discovered. Mutations in *NPHP2/INV* and less frequently *NPHP3* lead to renal failure between birth and age 3 years (infantile NPH), whereas mutations in the other genes, also including *NPHP3*, cause renal failure in the first three decades of life (juvenile NPH). Polyuria and polydipsia are the presenting symptoms. Hypertension is common in the infantile form but absent or, if present, not a prominent feature in the juvenile form. Sodium wasting is common. The urine sediment is characteristically benign. Proteinuria is absent or low grade. There is no microhematuria. Progression to end-stage renal failure occurs within the first 3 years in the infantile form and within the first two to three decades of life in the juvenile form. The radiologic appearance of early-stage nephronophthisis is nonspecific, with normal-shaped kidneys. Loss of corticomedullary differentiation on ultrasound is an early finding. Although nephronophthisis is considered a cystic kidney disease, cysts are seldom found on imaging at the initial stages of disease (although they are seen on kidney biopsy).

Medullary cystic kidney disease is an autosomal-dominant disorder characterized by cystic dilation of the medullary part of the collecting ducts and is associated with gout and hyperuricemia in some cases, and usually ESRD occurs between the ages of 20 and 50 years. So far, two loci on chromosomes 1 and 16 have been located. For the latter, mutations in the UMOD gene have been described. Ultrasound examination is nonspecific, similar to nephronophthisis. MRI is helpful, as is genetic testing.

The pathology of both diseases is similar, characterized by interstitial inflammation, tubular basement membrane disruption, interstitial fibrosis, cysts lined by a single epithelial layer, and nonspecific glomerular hyalinosis. The clinical manifestations of the disease reflect dysfunction of affected nephron segments, predominantly reduced concentrating ability, polyuria, polydipsia, hypovolemia, and hyponatremia early in the course of the disease. Subsequently, glomerular filtration declines as the glomerular hyalinosis develops and progresses. Both variants are characterized by multiple renal cysts arising from distal and collecting tubules located primarily at the corticomedullary junction and in the medulla. The cysts are characteristically small (approximately 2 cm), detectable on MRI, and contain fluid. However, almost 25% of patients will have no grossly identifiable cysts because of the small size of these cysts.

Dahan K, Devuyst O, Smaers M, et al. A cluster of mutations in the UMOD gene causes familial juvenile hyperuricemic nephropathy with abnormal expression of uromodulin. *J Am Soc Nephrol* 2003;14(11):2883–2893.

Hildebrandt F, Attanasio M, Otto E. Nephronophthisis: Disease mechanisms of a ciliopathy. *J Am Soc Nephrol* 2009;20(1):23–35.

Wolf MT, Mucha BE, Attanasio M, et al. Mutations of the uromodulin gene in MCKD type 2 patients cluster in exon 4, which encodes three EGF-like domains. *Kidney Int* 2003;64(5):1580–1587.

19. **How does medullary sponge kidney differ from other cystic diseases?**
The diagnosis of medullary sponge kidney (MSK) is based on the finding of dilated collecting ducts (precalyceal ducts) that may or may not contain calculi and/or nephrocalcinosis, and classic radiologic appearance is described as a "papillary blush" or "paint brush" on early and delayed films during intravenous urography (IVU). Occasionally cysts can be seen that reach 8 to 10 cm arising in the medullary-collecting ducts, and cysts in at least 50% of patients contain calcium deposits or stones. Hematuria, urinary tract infection, or obstruction may be seen. Multidetector CT urography is now the preferred imaging study for evaluating patients with renal stone disease, although resolution of the collecting system detail is superior with IVU. It provides both cross-sectional displays and images of the contrast-filled renal collecting systems, ureters, and urinary bladder. The classic appearance is a result of the direct result of pooling of contrast material within the anomalous dilated collecting ducts located within the tips of the renal papilla. The disease may affect one, both, or only portions of the kidneys. Most patients with MSK are asymptomatic and therefore remain undiagnosed. Alternatively, the condition is diagnosed when intravenous pyelography (IVP) is performed for flank pain or diagnosed incidentally when IVP is performed for indications other than renal colic. Although

the prevalence in the general population is unknown, 12% to 20% of calcium stone formers carry this diagnosis, and the diagnosis is made in 1 in every 200 IVPs. It is seen more commonly in women than men in this group. Low urinary excretion of citrate and magnesium is the typical metabolic abnormality seen in patients with MSK and helps distinguish these individuals from idiopathic calcium stone formers.

Yagisawa T, Kobayashi C, Hayashi T, et al. Contributory metabolic factors in the development of nephrolithiasis in patients with medullary sponge kidney. *Am J Kidney Dis* 2001;37(6):1140-1143.

KEY POINTS: CYSTIC DISEASES OF THE KIDNEYS

1. The presence of multiple bilateral renal cysts should raise suspicion of inherited renal cystic disease.

2. Physicians should be aware of other disease-associated systemic complications in autosomal-dominant polycystic kidney disease.

3. Improved diagnostic criteria have been developed for autosomal dominant polycystic kidney disease.

4. Genetic testing can be helpful in diagnosis of inherited forms of renal cystic disease.

5. Several promising therapies are in clinical trials for polycystic kidney disease.

20. **What is acquired cystic kidney disease?**
Acquired cystic kidney disease (ACKD) is characterized by small cysts distributed throughout the renal cortex and medulla of patients with ESRD unrelated to inherited renal cystic diseases. Thus family and clinical history are often the most helpful discriminators. It is commoner in men and women. ACKD develops in 7% to 22% of patients with renal failure and serum creatinine values exceeding 3 mg/dL before dialysis, and it develops in 35% with less than 2 years of dialysis, 58% with 2 to 4 years, 75% with 4 to 8 years, and 92% with dialysis for longer than 8 years. Kidneys are typically smaller than expected, but they may also increase in size and resemble those of ADPKD. Most patients are asymptomatic. Hemorrhage is often seen. The cysts can regress after successful renal transplant surgery, but conversely can develop in chronically rejected kidneys. Because RCC is an important complication of ACKD, CT screening has been recommended after 3 years of dialysis, followed by screening for neoplasm at 1- or 2-year intervals thereafter. Cyclosporine therapy in transplant recipients of a nonrenal organ is associated with a predisposition for kidney cyst development.

21. **Are renal tumors more common in patients with ESRD than in patients with ACKD?**
Yes. Screening for ACKD and RCC is recommended for patients at high risk or who have been on long-term dialysis and are kidney transplant recipients. The overall prevalence of RCC in patients receiving hemodialysis evaluated radiologically or at autopsy is approximately 1%. Carcinomas in individuals receiving dialysis are three times more common in the presence than in the absence of acquired renal cysts, and it is six times more common in large cystic kidneys than in small cystic kidneys. Overall, the incidence of renal malignancy in patients receiving hemodialysis has been estimated to be 50 to 100 times greater than in the general population. However, these cancers have a lower risk for metastasis and a better prognosis compared with RCCs not associated with ACKD. Renal cancer can occur without ACKD in ESRD, but this is less common. The predominant type appears to be papillary, with most of the other cases being clear cell type and less frequently other types or oncocytomas. The longer the duration of the individual on dialysis, the greater the risk of RCC and the higher the positive predictive value of screening ultrasound.

22. **How are tumors in patients with ACKD managed?**
Renal masses larger than 3 cm detected in ACKD are treated by excision. For tumors smaller than 3 cm, some physicians advise nephrectomy for the acceptable surgical candidate, whereas others recommend annual CT follow-up with resection if the lesions enlarge. Tumors occurring in patients with ACKD tend to be more indolent, as shown by better 5-year survival; they also are often smaller, multifocal, bilateral, and lower stage than sporadic RCCs and have a papillary histology, but they may still metastasize. Although most tumors grew at a rate of 0.5 to 1 cm per year, 25% of cases show rapid growth of 6 cm or more per year. Thus, all neoplasms in ESRD/ACKD behave similarly. The association with renal carcinomas in ACKD requires frequent and life-long monitoring of these kidneys by periodic CT or MRI.

Noronha IL, Ritz E, Waldherr R, et al. Renal cell carcinoma in dialysis patients with acquired renal cysts. *Nephrol Dial Transplant* 1989;4(9):763–769.

Schwarz A, Vatandaslar S, Merkel S, et al. Renal cell carcinoma in transplant recipients with acquired cystic kidney disease. *Clin J Am Soc Nephrol* 2007;2(4):750–756.

OTHER HEREDITARY RENAL DISEASES

Beth A. Vogt, MD

CHAPTER 45

1. **What is familial hematuria?**

   Familial hematuria is defined as a group of genetic kidney disorders that are characterized clinically by the onset of persistent microscopic hematuria during childhood. The unifying feature of these conditions is an abnormality in the network of type IV collagen in the glomerular basement membrane (GBM). The major forms of familial hematuria are Alport syndrome and thin basement membrane nephropathy (TBMN).

2. **How many children with asymptomatic microscopic hematuria will have familial hematuria?**

   Familial hematuria is found in an estimated 30% to 50% of children referred to a nephrology clinic for evaluation of persistent microscopic hematuria.

3. **What are the major clinical features in males with Alport syndrome?**

   Males with Alport syndrome have persistent microscopic hematuria beginning in infancy. Episodes of macroscopic hematuria may also be seen, but they become less frequent after adolescence. Proteinuria and progressive chronic kidney disease develop as early as the second decade of life but may not be present until well into adulthood. End-stage renal disease (ESRD) ultimately develops in virtually all affected males, but the rate of progression of kidney disease is variable between families. Overall, about 60% of males reach ESRD by age 30 years and 80% reach ESRD by age 40 years.

4. **What are the major clinical findings in females with Alport syndrome?**

   Females with Alport syndrome have a much milder course than males. Microscopic hematuria is present in 95% of females with Alport syndrome. Significant proteinuria and progressive kidney dysfunction occur in only 15% of females.

5. **What other abnormalities may be associated with Alport syndrome?**

   Measurable bilateral, high-frequency, sensorineural hearing loss typically occurs in late childhood in all males and a minority of females with Alport syndrome. Deafness ultimately develops in 80% of affected males. About 40% of males with Alport syndrome exhibit characteristic ocular abnormalities. Twenty percent of patients have white or yellow perimacular flecks, which increase in number with age. Twenty percent of patients have anterior lenticonus, a protrusion of the central area of the lens into the anterior chamber, which can result in recurrent corneal erosion. Leiomyomatosis and platelet abnormalities are occasionally seen.

6. **What are the characteristic kidney biopsy findings in Alport syndrome?**

   The pathognomonic renal biopsy finding in Alport syndrome is diffuse thickening of the GBM with splitting of the lamina densa, giving a basket-weave appearance on electron microscopy. In young patients, both thickening and thinning of the GBM may be present, causing difficulty in distinguishing early stages of Alport syndrome from TBMN. Light microscopy shows segmental or global glomerulosclerosis, interstitial fibrosis, and tubular atrophy.

7. **How is Alport syndrome inherited?**
   The most common form of Alport syndrome is X-linked Alport syndrome (XLAS), which comprises 80% of cases. Autosomal-recessive Alport syndrome (ARAS) comprises 15% of cases, and autosomal-dominant Alport syndrome (ADAS) comprises 5% of cases. Of children with XLAS, 10% to 15% have no family history of hematuria or kidney disease and are felt to represent de novo mutations.

8. **What are the genetic abnormalities in Alport syndrome?**
   XLAS results from one of a variety of mutations in the gene for the alpha-5 chain of type IV collagen *(COL4A5)* on the X chromosome. The result is the alteration of the structure of the alpha-5 collagen chain, preventing normal incorporation of alpha-A3 and alpha-A4 collagen chains into basement membranes. Mutations in the *COL4A3* and *COL4A4* genes on chromosome 2 have been reported in ARAS. Heterozygous mutations in *COL4A3* and *COL4A4* have been identified in ADAS.

9. **What treatment is available for Alport syndrome?**
   Currently, there is no definitive therapy for Alport syndrome. Treatment remains supportive in nature and should focus on control of hypertension and reduction of proteinuria to slow the progressive loss of kidney function over time. Angiotensin-converting enzyme inhibitors and/or angiotensin receptor blockers are useful agents. In addition, the metabolic consequences of chronic kidney disease should be carefully managed and all affected family members should be identified. In general, patients with Alport syndrome have good transplant outcomes.

10. **Are there any special complications in patients with Alport syndrome following kidney transplantation?**
    Post-transplant anti-GBM nephritis is a rare condition that occurs in 3% to 5% of transplanted males with Alport syndrome. The cause of this condition is an immunologic response by the recipient to the alpha-5 chain of type IV collagen, a previously unrecognized antigen in the transplant recipient. Post-transplant anti-GBM nephritis usually results in rapid allograft destruction despite aggressive therapy. The subset of patients at highest risk for this complication is males with significant deafness who develop ESRD before 30 years of age.

11. **What is TBMN?**
    TBMN is a form of familial hematuria characterized by persistent microscopic hematuria and occasionally episodic macroscopic hematuria. Proteinuria, hypertension, progressive loss of kidney function, and extrarenal abnormalities are not part of the clinical picture. The family history reveals individuals with persistent hematuria but none with associated end-stage kidney disease or hearing loss.

12. **What is the inheritance pattern of TBMN?**
    TBMN follows an autosomal-dominant pattern of inheritance. Recent studies have identified mutations in the type IV collagen gene (*COL4A3* and *COL4A4*) in some families, suggesting that TBMN and Alport syndrome may be related disorders.

13. **What are the renal biopsy findings in TBMN?**
    The pathognomonic renal biopsy finding in TBMN is uniform thinning of the GBM on electron microscopy, with attenuation of the lamina densa. Light and immunofluorescence microscopic analyses are usually normal.

14. **What is the natural history of TBMN?**
    In the majority of patients, TBMN is a benign condition in which progressive kidney failure does not occur. Rare patients, however, have been reported to develop significant proteinuria with loss of kidney function. For this reason, it is recommended that patients diagnosed with TBMN have yearly follow-up with urinalysis and blood pressure measurement.

15. **What is nephronophthisis?**
    Nephronophthisis (NPH) is an inherited cystic kidney disease characterized by chronic tubulointerstitial nephritis with eventual progression to end-stage kidney disease. NPH is believed to account for 5% of pediatric ESRD in the United States and 10% to 25% of pediatric ESRD in Europe and is therefore the most frequent genetic cause of ESRD in the first three decades of life. The three forms of NPH include infantile, juvenile, and adolescent, with variable age of onset. Juvenile NPH accounts for the majority of affected individuals.

16. **What are the clinical features of NPH?**
    Children with NPH display progressive polyuria and polydipsia, with characteristic night-time fluid intake beginning at about 6 years of age. Secondary enuresis may occur, as may impaired growth, fatigue, and pallor. Anemia is a prominent finding even before significant reduction in kidney function occurs. Progression to ESRD occurs on average at 13 years of age in children with juvenile NPH, age 1 year in infantile NPH, and age 19 years in adolescent NPH. Hematuria, proteinuria, urinary tract infection, and hypertension are uncommon.

17. **What is the genetic basis of NPH?**
    NPH is inherited in an autosomal-recessive fashion. To date, eight genes for juvenile nephronophthisis have been identified and one gene for infantile NPH has been identified. *NPHP1*, the most common gene for juvenile NPH, is found in 20% to 40% of cases. *NPHP1* encodes a protein called nephrocystin-1. Nephrocystin-1 and the other *NPHP* gene products are expressed in the primary cilia and are believed to modulate the cytoskeleton and maintain epithelial cell polarity.

18. **What extrarenal findings have been associated with NPH?**
    Of patients with NPH, 10% to 20% have extrarenal symptoms including retinitis pigmentosa (Senior-Loken syndrome), cerebellar ataxia (Joubert syndrome), developmental delay, skeletal anomalies, and hepatic fibrosis.

19. **What are the ultrasound findings in NPH?**
    The renal ultrasound of patients with NPH shows small, hyperechoic kidneys with small, 1- to 2-mm corticomedullary cysts. Absence of medullary cysts does not rule out the diagnosis of NPH.

20. **What are the renal biopsy findings in NPH?**
    Renal biopsy findings in NPH show tubular basement membrane disruption, tubulointerstitial nephropathy, interstitial fibrosis, and corticomedullary cysts.

21. **What is the treatment for NPH?**
    There is currently no definitive treatment for NPH. Treatment is focused on supportive therapy for progressive kidney dysfunction, control of hypertension, and early identification of affected family members. Renal transplantation is successful, and recurrent disease in the renal allograft has not been reported.

22. **What is medullary cystic kidney disease?**
    Medullary cystic kidney disease (MCKD) is a rare inherited kidney disease with a similar clinical phenotype as NPH. However, MCKD is distinct from NPH in that it is inherited in an autosomal-dominant fashion, leads to ESRD between 40 and 70 years of age, and is in general not associated with extrarenal disease.

23. **What is the genetic basis of MCKD?**
    MCKD is inherited in an autosomal-dominant fashion; therefore, the diagnosis must be considered in any adult with chronic kidney disease unrelated to hypertension and diabetes, a bland urinalysis, and positive family history of ESRD. Two forms of MCKD have been identified: MCKD-1 and MCKD-2. MCKD-1 is caused by an abnormality on chromosome 19,

although the exact gene has not been identified. MCKD-2 is associated with an abnormality in the UMOD gene, which expresses uromodulin (Tamm-Horsfall protein). A cardinal feature of MCKD-2 is hyperuricemia and gout. MCKD is felt to be closely related to another uromodulin-related kidney disease called familial juvenile hyperuricemic nephropathy (FJHN).

KEY POINTS: OTHER HEREDITARY RENAL DISEASES

1. The major forms of familial hematuria are Alport syndrome and thin basement membrane nephropathy (TBMN).

2. X-linked Alport syndrome results from mutations in the gene for the alpha-5 chain of type IV collagen (*COL4A5*) on the X chromosome.

3. Alport syndrome is associated with microscopic hematuria, proteinuria, sensorineural hearing loss, and progressive loss of kidney function.

4. TBMN is a benign autosomal-dominant condition associated with microscopic hematuria without proteinuria, hearing loss, or progressive kidney failure.

5. Nephronophthisis (NPH) is an autosomal recessive cystic kidney disease characterized by chronic tubulointerstitial nephritis and progression to end-stage kidney disease.

6. Medullary cystic kidney disease is a rare autosomal-dominant cystic kidney disease seen in adults with clinical features similar to NPH.

24. **What is the treatment for MCKD?**
    There is no definitive treatment for MCKD. Treatment remains supportive in nature and should include blood pressure control and management of the complications of chronic kidney disease when indicated. In patients with MCKD-2, allopurinol may be used to control hyperuricemia, although its effectiveness at slowing the progression of kidney disease is uncertain.

BIBLIOGRAPHY

1. Hildebrandt F, Zhou W. Nephronophthisis-associated ciliopathies. *J Am Soc Nephrol* 2007;18:1855–1871.
2. Kashtan CE. Familial hematuria. *Pediatr Nephrol* 2009;24:1951–1958.
3. Salomon R, Saunier S, Niaudet P. Nephronophthisis. *Pediatr Nephrol* 2009;24:2333–2344.
4. Thorner PS. Alport syndrome and thin basement membrane nephropathy. *Nephron Clin Pract* 2007;106:c82–88.
5. Tryggvason K, Patrakka J. Thin basement membrane nephropathy. *J Am Soc Nephrol* 2006;17:813–822.

TUBULOINTERSTITIAL DISEASES

Edgar V. Lerma, MD

CHAPTER 46

ACUTE TUBULOINTERSTITIAL NEPHRITIS

1. **What is acute tubulointerstitial nephritis?**

   Acute tubulointerstitial nephritis (ATIN) is one of the common causes of acute kidney injury (AKI), accounting for 15% to 27% of cases. Clinically, it is characterized by an acute decline in renal function, manifested by an acute elevation of blood urea nitrogen (BUN) and serum creatinine. Histopathologically, it is characterized by the presence of inflammatory infiltrates and edema in the tubulointerstitium.

   Its true incidence, however, is unknown because of the nonspecificity of usual clinical symptomatology, thereby leading to underdiagnosis. Definitive diagnosis is only determined via a renal biopsy. A great majority of the patients are subjected to empiric therapy, including withdrawal of the suspected etiologic agent.

2. **What are the most common causes of ATIN?**

   The most common causes of ATIN are classified according to the following:
   - Drug induced: The most common cause is antibiotics.
   - Infection related: The most common cause is ascending or hematogenous bacterial pyelonephritis
   - Systemic disease related
   - Idiopathic

   The majority of cases are immune mediated and are related to either drug or drug-induced antigens. It must be noted that drug-induced ATIN is not dose dependent. Also, a repeat exposure to the same drug or closely related agent can potentially lead to recurrence of the disease process (Table 46-1).

3. **Describe the pathogenesis of ATIN.**

   The initiating event in ATIN starts with the expression of endogenous and/or exogenous antigens that are nephritogenic. The following antigens have been implicated in the pathogenesis of ATIN:
   - Endogenous renal antigens and proteins
     - Tamm-Horsfall protein
     - Anti-tubular basement membrane (TBM)
   - Nonrenal antigens
     - Microbial antigens
     T cells are also believed to have a pathogenetic role in ATIN.

4. **What are the characteristic histopathologic findings in ATIN?**

   - Presence of inflammatory cell infiltrate (CD4+ T cells, macrophages, eosinophils, and plasma cells) in a diffuse or patchy distribution
   - Interstitial edema
   - Normal glomeruli and vessels: This, in particular, distinguishes this disease process from inflammatory glomerular diseases (e.g., glomerulonephritides)

TABLE 46-1. DRUGS CAUSING ACUTE TUBULOINTERSTITIAL NEPHRITIS

ANTIMICROBIAL AGENTS
Acyclovir
AMPICILLIN*
Amoxicillin
Aztreonam
Carbenicillin
Cefaclor
Cefamandole
Cefazolin
Cephalexin
Cephaloridine
Cephalothin
Cephapirin
Cephradine
Cefoxitin
Cefotetan
Cefotaxime
CIPROFLOXACIN
Cloxacillin
Colistin
Cotrimoxazole*
Erythromycin
Ethambutol
Foscarnet
Gentamicin
Indinavir
Interferon
Isoniazid
Lincomycin
METHICILLIN*
Mezlocillin
Minocycline
Nafcillin
Nitrofurantoin*
Norfloxacin
Oxacillin*
PENICILLIN G*
Piperacillin
Piromidic acid
Polymyxin acid*
Quinine
RIFAMPICIN*
Spiramycin*
SULFONAMIDES
Teicoplanin
Tetracycline
Vancomycin

NSAIDs, INCLUDING SALICYLATES
Alclofenac
Azapropazone
ASPIRIN
Benoxaprofen
Diclofenac
Diflunisal*
Fenclofenac
FENOPROFEN
Flurbiprofen
IBUPROFEN
INDOMETHACIN
Ketoprofen
Mefenamic acid
Meloxicam
Mesalazine (5-ASA)
NAPROXEN
Niflumic acid
Phenazone
PHENYLBUTAZONE
PIROXICAM
Pirprofen
Sulfasalazine
Sulindac
Suprofen
TOLEMETIN
ZOMEPIRAC

ANALGESICS
Aminopyrine
Antipyrine
Antrafenin
Clometacin*
Floctafenin*
Glafenin*
Metamizol
Noramidopyrine

ANTICONVULSANTS
Carbamazepine
Phenobarbital
PHENYTOIN*
Valproate sodium

DIURETICS
Chlorthalidone
Ethacrynic acid
FUROSEMIDE*
Hydrochlorothiazide*
Indapamide
Tienilic acid*
Triamterene*

OTHERS
ALLOPURINOL*
Alpha-methyldopa
Azathioprine
Bismuth salts
Captopril*
Carbimazole
Chlorpropamide*
Cyclosporine
CIMETIDINE
Clofibrate
Clozapine
D-penicillamine
Fenofibrate*
Gold salts
Griseofulvin
Interferon
Interleukin-2
OMEPRAZOLE
PHENINDIONE*
Phenothiazine
Phenylpropanolamine
Probenecid
Propranolol
Propylthiouracil
Ranitidine
Streptokinase
Sulphinpyrazone
Warfarin

Drugs most commonly involved are shown in capital letters.
*Drugs that can induce granulomatous acute interstitial nephritis.

- Granulomas located in the interstitium
- Immunofluorescence: linear deposition of immunoglobulin G (IgG) along the TBM
- Electron microscopy: diffuse effacement of the foot processes
- Interstitial fibrosis and tubular atrophy

5. **What are the clinical manifestations of ATIN?**

Depending on the etiologic agent, there is usually a delay between the initial insult (exposure to offending drug or infectious agent) and the onset of decline in renal function. This latent period can vary from as short as 1 day to as long as several weeks to months.

Most commonly, patients remain asymptomatic or present with nonspecific symptoms (e.g., nausea, vomiting, generalized weakness). The classical triad of fever, maculopapular rash, and peripheral eosinophilia (suggestive of an allergic-type reaction), which was originally described with methicillin-induced ATIN, is seen in only a minority of cases.

6. **What are the laboratory manifestations of ATIN?**

- Azotemia (elevated BUN and serum creatinine)
- Peripheral eosinophilia
- Eosinophiluria
- Sterile pyuria (occasionally, white blood cell [WBC] casts)
- Microscopic hematuria (very rarely, red blood cell [RBC] casts)
- Proteinuria (usually in the non-nephrotic range)
- Renal tubular acidosis (RTA; varies depending on which particular segment of the renal tubule is involved)

7. **What is the importance of eosinophiluria in ATIN?**

In analyzing the urine sample, the presence of >1% eosinophils is considered significant. Hansel's stain, commonly used to stain the cytoplasmic granules in eosinophils, is believed to be more sensitive than Wright's stain or Giemsa stain. However, eosinophiluria is a nonspecific finding that can be seen in a variety of conditions (e.g., acute pyelonephritis, acute glomerulonephritis, acute cystitis and prostatitis).

Eosinophiluria has a sensitivity of 63% to 85% and a specificity of 91% to 93% in identifying ATIN. Therefore, in cases whereby the index of suspicion for ATIN is very high (on the basis of other clinical and laboratory studies and historical features), the presence of eosinophiluria should help in the diagnosis. Its absence, however, does not necessarily exclude the diagnosis of ATIN.

8. **How does a typical patient with ATIN present?**

As in most other cases of AKI, patients usually present with either an acute elevation in BUN and serum creatinine or an incidentally discovered asymptomatic urinary abnormality, such as sterile pyuria, microscopic hematuria, or proteinuria. At times, a temporal relation can be established between the offending agent or drug and the onset of clinical and laboratory manifestations.

At times, the urinary sediment can be helpful in excluding other causes of AKI. For instance, RBC casts are usually seen in acute glomerulonephritis and muddy-brown granular casts are seen in acute tubular necrosis (ATN).

However, it must be remembered that whenever the index of suspicion is high, a normal urinalysis should not be used to exclude the diagnosis of ATIN.

9. **What is unique about rifampin-induced ATIN?**

Among the various antibiotics that can cause ATIN, rifampin is unique in that the interstitial nephritis can occur after re-exposure after a period of latency. It is not characteristically known to be associated with peripheral eosinophilia and in some case reports have been demonstrated to manifest as casts containing immunoglobulin light chains in the tubular lumina. In other case reports, circulating anti-rifampin antibodies and immunoglobulin G (IgG) deposits along the tubular basement membranes have been reported.

Although the prognosis for renal recovery is generally favorable, it does carry significant morbidity and mortality. Screening for microscopic hematuria has been suggested for patients who will require re-exposure to the medication.

Schubert C, Bates WD, Moosa MR. Acute tubulointerstitial nephritis related to antituberculous drug therapy. *Clin Nephrol* 2010;73(6):413-419.

Muthukumar T, Jayakumar M, Fernando EM, Muthusethupathi MA. Acute renal failure due to rifampicin: a study of 25 patients. *Am J Kidney Dis* 2002;40(4):690-696.

10. What is the role of gallium scanning in the diagnosis of ATIN?

The presence of active interstitial inflammatory infiltrate in ATIN leads to a diffuse, intense uptake of the gallium67 radioisotope in the kidneys. This finding is nonspecific, as can be seen in most other causes of AKI, especially those characterized by inflammation. However, one of the most common differential diagnoses of ATIN is ATN, whereby there is usually decreased uptake of gallium67.

Therefore, the results of a gallium scan should always be interpreted in the context of the accompanying clinical and laboratory findings.

11. What is the most definitive means to diagnose ATIN?

The only definitive and confirmatory diagnostic procedure is a renal biopsy. Because it is common practice to simply withdraw the suspected etiologic agent and carefully observe the renal function in the ensuing days, renal biopsies are not typically performed in suspected cases of ATIN.

The most common indications for doing a renal biopsy in suspected ATIN are as follows:

- AKI, whereby the diagnosis remains uncertain despite extensive laboratory testing, especially if it is progressively worsening
- Absence of any signs of improvement after withdrawal of suspected offending agent
- In suspected ATIN cases, where immunosuppressive therapy is being considered

12. What are the treatment options for ATIN?

- Conservative measures (withdrawal of offending agent and avoidance of exposure to other potential nephrotoxic agents)
- Corticosteroid therapy
- Immunosuppressive therapy

To date, the optimal treatment for ATIN remains speculative because there have been no randomized controlled trials. The current literature consists only of uncontrolled reports and retrospective studies.

A typical candidate for corticosteroid therapy is a patient with features suggestive of ATIN in whom there is prolonged and progressive renal dysfunction despite the conservative measures noted earlier. The optimal dose and duration of corticosteroid therapy remain elusive. Most patients improve within the first 1 to 2 weeks of administration of prednisone at a dose of 40 to 60 mg/kg/day (maximum of 60 mg/day) for a total duration of 2 to 3 months. Typical steroid taper is done as soon as the serum creatinine has declined to baseline or near-baseline values. Some have advocated the initiation of the use of intravenous methylprednisolone at a dose of 0.5 to 1.0 g/day for 3 days, followed by a prednisone course.

Preddie et al. reported the use of mycophenolate mofetil (MMF) for 13 to 34 months in a group of patients who were steroid dependent for up to 6 months.

For now, one may consider the use of MMF for those who have biopsy-proven ATIN, who are either dependent or resistant to corticosteroids, or who are intolerant to it.

The option of initiating empirical corticosteroid therapy in patients suspected of having ATIN (not biopsy proven) remains controversial.

13. What is the typical course of ATIN?

The majority of suspected cases of ATIN, whether treated primarily with withdrawal of the suspected offending agent alone or with initiation of corticosteroid therapy, lead to eventual recovery of renal function in a few days to weeks. Certain features, however, are considered as negative prognosticators such as prolonged renal dysfunction (>3 weeks) and the presence of interstitial fibrosis and tubular atrophy on histopathology.

KEY POINTS: ACUTE TUBULOINTERSTITIAL NEPHRITIS

1. Acute tubulointerstitial nephritis (ATIN) is one of the common causes of acute kidney injury, accounting for 15% to 27% of cases.

2. The classical triad of fever, maculopapular rash, and peripheral eosinophilia is seen in only a minority of cases (<10%) of ATIN.

3. In cases whereby the index of suspicion for ATIN is very high, the presence of eosinophiluria should help in the diagnosis. Its absence, however, does not necessarily exclude the diagnosis of ATIN.

4. Drug-induced ATIN is not dose-dependent. A repeat exposure to the same drug can potentially lead to recurrence of the disease process.

5. Majority of suspected cases of ATIN lead to eventual recovery of renal function in a few days to weeks.

6. The option of initiating empirical corticosteroid therapy in patients suspected of having ATIN (not biopsy proven) remains controversial.

CHRONIC TUBULOINTERSTITIAL NEPHRITIS

14. **What is chronic tubulointerstitial nephritis?**
Chronic tubulointerstitial nephritis is, by definition, tubulointerstitial nephritis that has failed to resolve on its own, or has been resistant to whatever treatment was rendered, after several months or years. It can also arise de novo as a consequence of chronic, low-grade, or injurious exposures of the tubulointerstitium to the culprit agent (e.g., medication, physical factors, infectious agents) (Table 46-2). Such exposures may be intermittent or persistent. Histopathologically, it is characterized by the presence of chronic interstitial inflammation, interstitial fibrosis, and tubular atrophy.

    Depending on the culprit agent, the disease may have a particular predilection for either the proximal tubules or the distal tubules or both. The functional abnormalities usually depend on the tubular site of involvement (i.e., distal tubule). Dysfunction may be characterized by acidosis and hyperkalemia, as seen in obstructive uropathies, whereas injury involving the renal medulla is characterized by impaired ability to concentrate urine, as seen in sickle cell nephropathy (Table 46-3).

    As chronic tubulointerstitial nephritis progress, there may be concomitant glomerular abnormalities, probably secondary to maladaptive alterations in the glomeruli or as a result of the tubulointerstitial processes. At that time, patients may present with nephrotic-range proteinuria, which can cloud the primary underlying disease process.

15. **Do viral infections cause chronic tubulointerstitial nephritis?**
The localization of Epstein-Barr virus (EBV) DNA in the proximal tubule cells in those with chronic interstitial nephritis of unknown etiology has suggested a causative role for the Epstein-Barr virus. Further studies, however, need to be done to demonstrate if a true cause and effect of EBV renal scarring truly exists.

    In individuals who are immunosuppressed, such as transplant recipients, BK polyomavirus infection has been shown to cause interstitial nephritis.

16. **What common infections cause chronic tubulointerstitial nephritis?**
- Acute pyelonephritis is classified under the category of complicated.
  - Urinary tract infections. Patients clinically present with a combination of symptoms that include fever and chills, dysuria, urgency, and increased frequency. They

TABLE 46-2. CAUSES OF CHRONIC TUBULOINTERSTITIAL NEPHRITIS

PRIMARY or IDIOPATHIC

Epstein-Barr virus

SECONDARY

Infections

Polyomavirus
Pyelonephritis (acute and chronic)

Drugs

Analgesic abuse nephropathy
Lithium-induced renal disease
Acyclic nucleoside inhibitors
Calcineurin inhibitors
Aristolochic acid/Chinese herb nephropathy
Chemotherapeutic agents: cisplatin,
    ifosfamide, carmustine

Heavy Metals

Lead nephropathy
Cadmium

Hematologic Diseases

Multiple myeloma
Lymphoproliferative disorders
Light chain disease
Sickle cell nephropathy

Obstructive Uropathy

Reflux nephropathy

Immune-Mediated Diseases

Sarcoidosis
Primary Sjögren's syndrome
Tubulointerstitial nephritis with uveitis
Idiopathic hypocomplementemic
    interstitial nephritis

Metabolic Disorders

Hyperoxaluria
Hyperuricemia/hyperuricosuria
Hypercalcemia/hypercalciuria
Hypokalemic nephropathy

Genetic Disorders

Cystinosis
Dent disease

Miscellaneous

Endemic (Balkan) nephropathy
Radiation nephritis

---

  commonly complain of flank discomfort with a physical correlate of costovertebral
  angle tenderness.
- Urine microscopy usually reveals an active urinary sediment consisting of leukocytes
  and leukocyte casts and even RBCs on occasion.
- Histopathologically, there is infiltration of polymorphonuclear cells and lymphocytes and
  edema grossly distorting normal tubulointerstitial architecture.
- Most cases respond to appropriate antibiotic therapy targeting the causative organism,
  which is most commonly a gram-negative *Escherichia coli*. In those who do not respond
  to antimicrobial therapy readily or who develop recurrent infections, there may be renal
  scarring and possible progression to chronic pyelonephritis.
- Chronic pyelonephritis
  - Chronic bacterial infections of the urinary tract are among the most common causes of
    chronic tubulointerstitial nephritis. The majority of these cases are associated with vesi-
    coureteral reflux (VUR)—hence the term "reflux nephropathy." For those not associated
    with VUR, however, the disease is termed "chronic pyelonephritis."
  - Clinically, patients with chronic pyelonephritis present with symptoms consisting of
    fever and chills, dysuria, vague flank or back pain, and hypertension. Some patients
    may present with tubular abnormalities such as impaired urinary concentrating ability,
    hyperkalemia, and salt wasting, all of which reflect distal tubular dysfunction. Chronic or
    repeated urinary tract infections are predisposing risk factors.
  - Examination of the urine often reveals an active urinary sediment consisting of WBCs
    and WBC casts.
  - Grossly, the kidneys may appear contracted.

TABLE 46-3. CLINICAL FEATURES OF CHRONIC TUBULOINTERSTITIAL NEPHRITIS

ELECTROLYTE AND ACID–BASE DISORDERS

Proximal RTA or Fanconi Syndrome

Myeloma
Dent disease
Cystinosis
Sjögren syndrome

Distal RTA

Bacterial pyelonephritis
Reflux nephropathy
Lithium
Lead
Myeloma
Light chain disease
Lupus nephritis
Hypercalcemia

Hyperkalemia (Type 4) RTA

Reflux nephropathy
Lead
Lupus nephritis
Sickle cell nephropathy
Sodium wasting

CLINICAL SYNDROMES

Kidney Stones

Hypercalcemia
Hyperoxaluria
Uric acid nephropathy
Dent disease
Sarcoidosis

Nephrogenic Diabetes Insipidus

Lithium
Cisplatin
Hypokalemia
Hypercalcemia
Dent disease

Acute Renal Failure

Pyelonephritis
Analgesic nephropathy
Lithium
Calcineurin inhibitors
Cisplatin
Myeloma
Lymphoma
Lupus nephritis
Hypercalcemia
Uric acid nephropathy
Radiation nephritis

Papillary Necrosis

Acute pyelonephritis
Analgesic nephropathy
Sickle cell nephropathy

RTA = renal tubular acidosis.

- Histopathologically, findings are similar to other forms of chronic tubulointerstitial nephritis, with tubular atrophy and interstitial fibrosis. Lymphocytes and mononuclear cells predominate the chronic inflammatory infiltrative population.
- Xanthogranulomatous pyelonephritis
  - Persistent chronic pyelonephritis can progress to a localized infection called "xanthogranulomatous pyelonephritis." Its exact pathogenesis is unknown. Typically, there is an underlying urinary tract obstruction (e.g., nephrolithiasis), which is complicated by the infection, leading to ischemia and destruction of renal parenchymal tissue, with granuloma formation subsequent accumulation of lipid deposits. These lipid deposits are actually lipid-laden macrophages called foam cells.
  - Symptoms are similar to those of chronic pyelonephritis, including hypertension. Characteristically, a distinct mass may be palpable over the affected "nonfunctioning" kidney.
  - Urine cultures are usually positive for *E. coli* and other gram-negative bacilli or *Staphylococcus aureus*.

- Computed tomography (CT) is the imaging modality of choice, which demonstrates the kidney to be significantly enlarged. Other findings include the predisposing renal calculus and low-density masses or xanthomatous tissues. One must exclude neoplastic renal disease among the differentials.
- On intravenous pyelography (IVP), the involved kidney may contain a localized "abscess-looking" area, which may look like a complex cyst or tumor. This is usually distinguished by doing either a magnetic resonance imaging or CT scan.
- Current treatment recommendations consist of appropriate coverage with broad-spectrum intravenous antibiotics combined with total or partial nephrectomy.

17. **What medications are commonly associated with chronic tubulointerstitial nephritis?**

Analgesics, lithium, calcineurin inhibitors, Chinese herbs, chemotherapeutic agents, and heavy metals are commonly associated with chronic tubulointerstitial nephritis.

18. **What is analgesic abuse nephropathy?**

Analgesic abuse nephropathy (AAN) is the most common cause of chronic tubulointerstitial nephritis. There has been a positive correlation between the incidence of renal disease secondary to analgesic nephropathy and the daily consumption of analgesics—in particular, phenacetin and other analgesic mixtures.

In the past it was believed that only phenacetin-containing analgesics were responsible for the disease, but it has been reported in numerous occasions that all analgesics including acetaminophen and aspirin can cause the same disease process.

The main site of renal injury in analgesic nephropathy is the renal medulla (area of the medullary loops of Henle, the vasa recta, and collecting ducts), primarily because of its inherent low oxygen tension. This is also the region where toxic metabolites of various analgesic compounds build up as a result of the countercurrent mechanism. As the vasoconstrictive effects on the renal medulla predominate, ischemic injury continues, leading to cortical atrophy and eventual interstitial changes.

It is most commonly seen in females in their 60s or 70s who have chronic pain syndromes, (e.g., headaches, joint pains, back pains). Ingestion of 1 g of analgesic preparations daily for more than 2 years is considered the minimum dosage and time required to produce clinical analgesic nephropathy.

Peptic ulcer disease and gastrointestinal symptoms are a common occurrence.

Renal dysfunction is manifested by isosthenuria (impaired urinary concentration) and impaired sodium conservation that may predispose to intravascular volume depletion. Renal tubular acidification defects are also seen. Urinalysis may show evidence of sterile pyuria, urinary tract infection, microscopic or macroscopic hematuria, and mild proteinuria.

Occasionally, patients present with flank pain or gross hematuria associated with papillary necrosis. Such papillae can slough off and cause obstructive manifestations. These are usually demonstrated on IVP or ultrasonography. Papillary calcification and characteristic "bumpy" renal contours are usually demonstrated on CT. In some instances, the kidneys can appear bilaterally atrophic or asymmetric in size.

Patients with analgesic nephropathy are also at increased risk for transitional cell carcinoma of the uroepithelium.

The oxidative effects of phenacetin are believed to be responsible for the increased formation of atherogenic low-density lipoprotein, thereby predisposing to increased risk of premature atherosclerosis with attendant cardiovascular morbidity and mortality.

Management is primarily supportive, including discontinuation of the culprit analgesic agent. Even after cessation of the analgesic, close monitoring, especially for development of new symptoms such as gross hematuria, is recommended because of increased risk of uroepithelial tumors.

19. **How is lithium associated with chronic tubulointerstitial nephritis?**
Lithium has been commonly used in patients treated for bipolar disorders. Chronic lithium ingestion is a known cause of nephrogenic diabetes insipidus (NDI). Lithium enters the collecting tubule cells via the Na channels and, by inhibiting adenylate cyclase and subsequent cyclic adenosine monophosphate (cAMP) production, it interferes with the ability of antidiuretic hormone (ADH) to increase water reabsorption. Likewise, it decreases the expression of the water channels (aquaporin 2) in the collecting tubules. A positive correlation has been described between the length of duration of treatment (average 6.5 to 10 years) with lithium and such impairment of urinary-concentrating ability manifested by polyuria (and polydipsia). An incomplete distal (type 1) RTA, secondary to a lithium-induced decreased H ATPase pump activity in the distal tubule, has been described.

Lithium has also been associated with hypercalcemia. It has been suggested that it induces morphologic changes in the parathyroid glands, resulting in increased parathyroid volume and parathyroid hormone (PTH) secretion (hyperparathyroidism), which consequently promotes bone resorption and subsequent release of calcium into the bloodstream, leading to hypercalcemia.

Pathologically, lithium-induced nephropathy is characterized by formation of microcysts (cortical and medullary tubular cysts) in the distal convoluted tubules and collecting ducts. Such distal tubular involvement is clinically correlated with NDI, manifested by polyuria and polydipsia.

Typically, renal dysfunction secondary to chronic lithium use is mild to moderate. However, those with serum creatinine levels greater than 2.5 mg/dL at the time of presentation progress to end-stage renal disease (ESRD) even after cessation of lithium. In those with less severe renal dysfunction, however, such discontinuation of lithium usually leads to stabilization of kidney function.

Amiloride, a potassium-sparing diuretic, has been shown to reduce polyuria and has been shown to block lithium uptake in the sodium channels of the collecting duct. In contrast, although thiazide diuretics can reduce lithium-induced polyuria, they can also cause intravascular volume depletion, which can lead to increased sodium and lithium reabsorption in the proximal tubule, thereby aggravating acute lithium toxicity.

For those patients receiving chronic maintenance therapy with lithium, a regular follow-up of serum creatinine, estimated glomerular filtration rate (GFR), and 24-hour urine volume is recommended. Elevations in creatinine should lead to either appropriate dose reduction or complete withdrawal of the drug.

The average latent period between initiation of lithium therapy and onset of ESRD is 20 years.

20. **How are calcineurin inhibitors associated with chronic tubulointerstitial nephritis?**
Cyclosporine and tacrolimus belong to a class of immunosuppressive agents primarily called calcineurin inhibitors and are commonly used in solid organ transplantation. Cyclosporine has also been used commonly in the treatment of various autoimmune diseases. These agents have been described to cause acute and chronic renal failure. The pathogenesis can be attributed to the drugs' predominantly vasoconstrictive effect on the afferent arteriole, thereby causing glomerular ischemia.

Pathologically, the tubulointerstitial damage occurs in a bandlike pattern, referred to as "striped interstitial fibrosis," and involve the cortex and medulla.

Tubular injury secondary to calcineurin inhibitors can lead to hyperkalemia and a nonanion gap metabolic acidosis. Other electrolyte abnormalities include hypomagnesemia, hypophosphatemia, and hyperuricemia.

Treatment of renal dysfunction requires a significant dose reduction of the offending agent, which often translates to an improvement in GFR. Mycophenolate mofetil and rapamycin are alternative immunosuppressive agents commonly used in transplant recipients.

Of note, calcineurin inhibitor–induced nephropathy is rare in recipients of bone marrow transplant, and this has been attributed to the shorter duration and lower doses of usual treatment regimens.

21. **How are Chinese herbs associated with chronic tubulointerstitial nephritis?**

   Typical changes of chronic tubulointerstitial nephritis have been described in mostly middle-aged women in Belgium who were using Chinese herb pills as part of a weight loss regimen in 1992. It was discovered that the culprit active ingredient was that of aristolochic acid, which was not only nephrotoxic, but also carcinogenic.

   Of note, affected patients have normal blood pressure readings. There is a positive correlation between the total dose of aristolochic acid consumption and the decline in GFR.

   If untreated, patients usually rapidly progress to ESRD. Histopathologically, a hypocellular interstitial fibrosis with marked tubular atrophy is seen. A short course of oral steroids has been shown to slow progression of renal failure.

22. **Describe the association between chemotherapeutic agents and chronic tubulointerstitial nephritis.**

   Chronic tubulointerstitial nephritis changes have been associated with chemotherapeutic agents, especially those with predominant renal routes of excretion. Cisplatin-induced chronic tubulointerstitial nephritis appears to be mediated by increased production of tumor necrosis factor-alpha (TNF-α). Pentoxyphyllin (a known TNF-α inhibitor) has been shown by Ramesh and Reeves to prevent such cisplatin-induced injury. Damage to the tubulointerstitial areas leads to salt wasting (may be complicated by orthostatic hypotension, hypomagnesemia, and hypocalcemia). Other chronic tubulointerstitial nephritis lesion–producing chemotherapeutic agents include ifosfamide and carmustine.

   Findings of interstitial fibrosis and chronic inflammatory changes are common.

   Treatment entails discontinuation of the culprit agent and avoiding coadministration of other agents with potential nephrotoxicities.

23. **Describe the association between heavy metals and chronic tubulointerstitial nephritis.**

   Years of prolonged environmental or occupational exposure to cadmium also leads to chronic tubulointerstitial nephritis and eventual progression to renal failure. Proximal tubular dysfunction, presenting as Fanconi syndrome, characterized by glucosuria, aminoaciduria, and tubular proteinuria, is common.

   Increased urinary cadmium excretion is characteristic. At present, treatment for cadmium nephrotoxicity is primarily supportive.

   Similar to cadmium, the proximal tubule cells tend to be the site of accumulation for lead, thereby leading to a Fanconi-type picture. Chronic tubulointerstitial nephritis secondary to lead exposure for several years is characterized histopathologically by progressive tubular atrophy and widespread fibrosis, which clinically translates into significant GFR decline. There seems to be an inverse relationship between the serum lead measurement and renal function as estimated by GFR. Hypertension is also common.

   Lead nephropathy also reduces urinary excretion of uric acid, thereby leading to hyperuricemia and gout.

   In contrast, acute exposure to high levels of lead usually is characterized by acute onset of abdominal discomfort, encephalopathic manifestations, and anemia.

   The diagnosis of lead nephropathy is established by increased urinary excretion of chelated lead (that is, after administration of ethylenediamine tetraacetic acid [EDTA]). Cumulative body stores of lead are estimated by doing the EDTA mobilization test or by doing the x-ray fluorescence, which determines bone lead content. In the EDTA mobilization test, 2 g of EDTA are administered either by the intravenous or intramuscular route, and 24-hour urine lead excretion is measured subsequently. Urinary lead >0.6 g/day is considered abnormal. One major limitation of the EDTA mobilization test is that it cannot mobilize lead deposits in bone. Reduced levels of erythrocyte aminolevulinate dehydrase (ALAD) compared with levels of ALAD "restored" by the addition of dithiothreitol may be even more efficient in detecting increased body lead burden in patients with chronic renal failure.

Note that serum levels of lead, although elevated during acute exposure, are not very helpful in the chronically exposed. The explanation for this is that, during acute exposure, lead is concentrated in the RBCs, which later die and extract lead into the bones and other tissues. Renal biopsy shows nonspecific findings seen in chronic tubulointerstitial nephritis.

The treatment of choice is EDTA chelation therapy or oral succimer, which has been shown to slow the progression of CKD.

KEY POINTS: CHRONIC TUBULOINTERSTITIAL NEPHRITIS

1. In chronic tubulointerstitial nephritis, depending on the culprit agent, the disease may have a particular predilection for either the proximal tubules or the distal tubules or both; the consequent functional abnormalities usually depend on the tubular site of involvement.

2. As CIN progresses, there may be concomitant glomerular abnormalities probably secondary to maladaptive alterations in the glomeruli or as a result of the tubulointerstitial processes. At that time, patients may present with nephrotic-range proteinuria, which can cloud the primary underlying disease process.

3. Lithium-induced nephropathy is characterized by formation of microcysts (cortical and medullary tubular cysts) in the distal convoluted tubules and collecting ducts.

24. **What are immune-mediated causes of chronic tubulointerstitial nephritis?**
    - Sarcoidosis
        - Renal involvement in sarcoidosis can occur in a variety of ways. Most commonly, patients have hypercalcemia secondary to increased production of 1, 25-dihydroxyvitamin D_3 by the activated macrophages in the characteristic granulomatous tissues. Such hypercalcemia can lead to other renal manifestations such as nephrogenic diabetes insipidus; hypercalciuria-related nephrolithiasis; and, in some cases, renal failure.
        - Sarcoidosis can also present as a form of interstitial nephritis with associated "noncaseating granulomas."
        - Typical tubular manifestations include mild proteinuria, sterile pyuria, and impaired ability to concentrate urine.
        - Treatment is with corticosteroids 1 mg/kg/day, which has been reported to lead to improved renal function. More commonly, however, because the renal involvement is longstanding, recovery is usually incomplete, even in those treated with steroids.
    - **Sjögren's syndrome:** Sjögren's syndrome–associated chronic interstitial nephritis characteristically presents as type 1 RTA with hypokalemia and a normal anion gap metabolic acidosis. Although the mechanism for this is incompletely understood, it is believed to be related to autoantibodies against carbonic anhydrase II. Treatment with high-dose corticosteroids has resulted in dramatic improvement of renal function.
    - **Tubulointerstitial nephritis with uveitis syndrome:** Tubulointerstitial nephritis with uveitis (TINU) was first described by Dobrin et al. in 1975. It usually is seen in adolescents and young adults, with a female preponderance and no particular racial predilection.
        - The exact pathogenesis remains unclear, but the predominance of T lymphocytes in the tissues and possible association with chlamydia and EBV suggest that delayed-type hypersensitivity and suppressed cell-mediated immunity may play major roles.
        - Clinically, patients present with nonspecific signs and symptoms (i.e., fever, generalized malaise, anemia, asthenia). Typically, uveitis of the anterior chamber is seen bilaterally, presenting as redness and pain over the eyes. Occasionally, patients complain of accompanying blurring of vision and photophobia. Uveitis has been described to occur as short as 2 months prior to, simultaneously, or up to 14 months since the onset of interstitial nephritis, presenting as acute renal failure.

- Renal manifestations include both proximal and distal tubular dysfunction (i.e., tubular proteinuria). Increased urine $\beta 2$ microglobulin (a marker of tubulointerstitial disease) has been noted. Ultrasonography may reveal enlarged swollen kidneys.
- Definitive diagnosis is established by demonstrating typical findings of interstitial nephritis (i.e., tubulointerstitial edema with infiltration of lymphocytes, plasma cells, and histiocytes). Predominance of CD4 and CD8 T lymphocytes, monocytes, and macrophages has been described. Eosinophils and noncaseating granulomas may also be seen.
- The aforementioned findings combined with their temporal relation to the concomitant uveitis make the diagnosis likely.
- Other common causes of tubulointerstitial disease process with uveitis include sarcoidosis and Sjögren's syndrome.
- Renal disease frequently resolves spontaneously over the course of 12 months without steroid therapy. However, for those with moderately advanced chronic kidney disease, prednisone 1 mg/kg/day (usually 40–60 mg PO daily) can be given for 3 to 6 months depending on the response and then tapered subsequently. Note that this steroid regimen is somewhat similar to that given for patients with persistent acute tubulointerstitial nephritis, except that duration of therapy is slightly more prolonged because of more frequent relapses noted with TINU. Although the renal manifestations may resolve spontaneously and respond well to a course of systemic steroids, the uveitis often has a chronic or relapsing course that may require more aggressive therapy. For uveitis, topical or systemic corticosteroids have been used.
- As in other chronic tubulointerstitial diseases, there is a positive correlation between prognosis and the degree of interstitial fibrosis.

- **Idiopathic hypocomplementemic interstitial nephritis:** This disease entity is usually seen in older men and, as the name implies, is characterized by decreased levels of C3 and C4 (hypocomplementemia) in the absence of evidence of SLE or Sjögren's syndrome. Histopathology reveals extensive tubulointerstitial infiltration with lymphocytes and Ig and complement deposits, which suggest local immune complex formation as the pathogenetic mechanism. Treatment consists of glucocorticoids and cyclophosphamide.

25. **What are the metabolic causes of chronic tubulointerstitial nephritis?**
    - Hyperoxaluria
      - Oxalate is normally excreted via renal means. However, when combined with calcium it becomes highly insoluble. The calcium oxalate product can cause nephrolithiasis and chronic tubulointerstitial nephritis. The diagnosis is established by demonstrating birefringent positive crystals (using polarized light microscopy) not only in the interstitial spaces, but also in the tubular lumens with surrounding inflammation and interstitial fibrosis.
      - Commonly seen in those with autosomal-recessive, primary hyperoxalurias, affected individuals may present with gross hematuria and renal colic secondary to oxalate stones. The majority of patients progress to ESRD by the second decade of life. Treatment recommended for those with recurrent nephrolithiasis and/or ESRD is combined liver and kidney transplantation.
      - Ingestion of ethylene glycol (antifreeze) or inhalation of methoxyflurane (anesthetic agent commonly used in the past) are other sources of oxalate. They both cause severe renal failure and residual tubulointerstitial damage in those who recover.
      - Of note, ingestion of a sour "star fruit," which is noted for its very high oxalate content, is another cause of acute interstitial oxalate deposition leading to interstitial nephritis and eventual renal failure.
      - In enteric hyperoxaluria, because of chronic diarrhea there is less calcium available in the intestines able to bind oxalate. Because of this, much of the unbound oxalate is reabsorbed and excreted in the urinary tract, thereby increasing urinary oxalate levels. In addition to severe hyperoxaluria, patients may have secondary hypocalciuria and hypocitraturia. This is commonly seen in those who underwent extensive small bowel resections or jejuno-ileal bypass procedures. Individuals who consume excessive

amounts of ascorbic acid can also develop oxalate stones and chronic tubulointerstitial nephritis, as ascorbic acid is metabolized to glyoxylate and oxalate.

- **Hyperuricemia/hyperuricosuria:** In tumor lysis syndrome (see Chapter 13), there is massive release of uric acid, thereby accounting for occurrence of hyperuricemia and hyperuricosuria. Histopathologically, urine uric acid and crystals deposit in the interstitium, leading to tubular atrophy, predominance of interstitial inflammatory infiltrates, and eventual fibrosis.
- **Hypercalcemia/hypercalciuria:** Hypercalcemia (resulting from hyperparathyroidism, sarcoidosis, multiple myeloma, etc.) causes renal vasoconstriction and a decrease in glomerular filtration rate.
  - Pathologically, the collecting ducts, distal convoluted tubules, and the loops of Henle are commonly involved. Calcium salts can be precipitated and deposited in the tubulointerstitium (nephrocalcinosis). Impaired renal concentration ability and resistance to antidiuretic hormone (leading to impaired urinary-concentrating ability and increased free water diuresis or nephrogenic diabetes insipidus) manifested as polyuria and polydipsia are the most common abnormalities associated with hypercalcemic nephropathy
- **Hypokalemia:** In patients with eating disorders causing them to abuse laxatives and diuretics, chronically low levels of potassium have been described. Chronic hypokalemia has had histopathologic correlates consisting of proximal tubular cell vacuolization, dilated intercellular spaces, and medullary cysts; which clinically correlate with impaired ability to concentrate urine (nephrogenic diabetes insipidus), conserve salt, and hypertension. It remains unclear, however, how often chronic tubulointerstitial nephritis occurs secondary to chronic hypokalemia.

26. **What is Balkan (endemic) nephropathy?**
As the name implies, this disease is particularly endemic in the so-called Balkan states or the former Yugoslavia, Bulgaria, and Romania. No specific etiologic cause has yet been identified, but as a result of its specific geographic distribution, environmental factors have long been suspect. Genetic and immune-related factors have also been identified.

Balkan nephropathy is a slow yet progressive form of chronic tubulointerstitial nephritis that eventually leads to ESRD.

One publication has linked dietary consumption of aristolochic acid (see previous discussion above on Chinese herb nephropathy) with this disease and its attendant risk of transitional cell cancer.

Clinically, a characteristic early feature is that of normochromic normocytic anemia, the degree of which is significantly disproportionate to the stage of chronic kidney disease. Urinalysis usually shows mild proteinuria (increased urine β2 microglobulin has been noted) with few RBCs and WBCs. Patients tend to be normotensive in the earlier stages of the disease with eventual progression to hypertension toward more advanced stages.

Grossly, the kidneys may appear symmetrically reduced in size.

An important complication of this disease is the development of uroepithelial carcinoma involving the urinary bladder or one or both ureters and renal pelvis.

Treatment is primarily supportive.

27. **What is radiation nephritis?**
Radiation nephritis is classified into two categories based on the onset of symptom presentation: (1) acute radiation nephritis and (2) chronic radiation nephritis.

Acute radiation nephritis usually presents after 6 to 12 months of exposure to radiation. Patients usually have edema, hypertension (occasionally accelerated hypertension), and marked proteinuria. Normochromic normocytic anemia secondary to intravascular hemolysis (microangiopathic hemolytic anemia) accompanying acute renal failure is common.

Chronic radiation nephritis, however, usually presents after more than 18 months of radiation exposure and also is characterized by proteinuria, hypertension, and progression of chronic kidney disease toward ESRD.

Although the exact pathogenesis remains elusive, it is believed that exposure of the kidneys to >1500 to 2500 rads leads to endothelial cell injury and eventual swelling, which leads to vascular occlusion and congestion and chronic ischemic injury. Radiation can also cause direct injury to the tubular epithelial cells. Furthermore, patients receiving radiation therapy for some underlying malignancy also receive concomitant chemotherapy. The latter may potentiate radiation's toxic effects to the kidneys.

Histopathologically, aside from the common findings of tubular atrophy and interstitial fibrosis, there is characteristic thickening of the capillary walls, which may also demonstrate "splitting." Interposition of deposits between the split layers of the glomerular basement membrane, is noticeably similar to that seen in hemolytic uremic syndrome and thrombotic thrombocytopenic purpura, thereby supporting the postulated possible role of endothelial cell injury, leading to intravascular congestion and chronic ischemic injury, as alluded to earlier.

In recipients of bone marrow transplant treated with radiotherapy followed by chemotherapy (i.e., cyclosporine) pathologic findings similar to thrombotic microangiopathies are similarly found, as opposed to when only chemotherapy is used.

Prevention is the only means to approach radiation nephritis. Proper shielding of the kidneys, especially in those with underlying chronic kidney disease to begin with, should be emphasized. Fractionizing the total irradiation dose into several small doses over several days may also have some merit. Likewise, minimizing the total irradiation dose is also suggested.

For those with radiation nephritis who develop hypertension, the antihypertensive agent recommended is an angiotensin-converting enzyme (ACE) inhibitor.

28. **What is acute phosphate nephropathy?**
Acute phosphate nephropathy is a newly described entity commonly seen in patients after exposure to oral sodium phosphate solutions (OSPS), which is used as a bowel cleanser, in preparation for colonoscopy. This is characterized by low-grade proteinuria and hyperphosphatemia. Histopathologically, there is evidence of acute and chronic tubular injury with interstitial edema, accompanied by tubular atrophy and interstitial fibrosis. The distinctive feature of this entity is the presence of abundant calcium phosphate deposits in the distal tubules and collecting ducts. The following factors are considered to predispose patients to acute renal failure: volume depletion, advanced age, hypertension, concurrent treatment with ACE inhibitors or angiotensin receptor blockers (ARBs), diuretics and NSAIDs, baseline creatinine elevation, or inappropriate use of OSPS in those with underlying chronic kidney disease.

Preventive measures include adequate hydration and possibly withholding ACE inhibitors, ARBs, diuretics, and NSAIDs on the day prior to and on the day of colonoscopy. OSPS should be used cautiously in elderly individuals.

BIBLIOGRAPHY

1. Appel GB, Bhat P. Tubulointerstitial diseases. In: Dale DC (ed.). *ACP Medicine* Philadelphia: American College of Physicians, 2007.
2. Appel GB. The treatment of acute interstitial nephritis: More data at last. *Kidney Int* 2008;73:905.
3. Baker RJ, Pusey CD. The changing profile of acute tubulointerstitial nephritis. *Nephrol Dial Transplant* 2004;19:8.
4. Bossini N, Savoldi S, Franceschini F, et al. Clinical and morphological features of kidney involvement in primary Sjögren's syndrome. *Nephrol Dial Transplant* 2000;16:2328.
5. Boton R, Gaviria M, Batlle DC. Prevalence, pathogenesis, and treatment of renal dysfunction associated with chronic lithium therapy. *Am J Kidney Dis* 1987;10:329.
6. Braden GL, O'Shea MH, Mulhern JG. Core curriculum in nephrology: Tubulointerstitial diseases. *Am J Kidney Dis* 2005;46:560–572.
7. Clarkson MR, Giblin L, O'Connell FP, et al. Acute interstitial nephritis: Clinical features and response to corticosteroid therapy. *Nephrol Dial Transplant* 2004;19:2778.
8. Dobrin RS, Vernier RL, Fish AL. Acute eosinophilic interstitial nephritis and renal failure with bone marrow-lymph node granulomas and anterior uveitis. A new syndrome. *Am J Med* 1975;59(3):325–333.
9. Fontanellas A, Navarro S, Moran-Jimenez M-J, et al. Erythrocyte aminolevulinate dehydrase activity as a lead marker in patients with chronic renal failure. *Am J Kidney Dis* 2002;40:43–50.

10. Gonzalez, E, Gutierrez, E, Galeano, C, et al. Early steroid treatment improves the recovery of renal function in patients with drug-induced acute interstitial nephritis. *Kidney Int* 2008;73:940.
11. Grollman AP, Shibutani S, Moriya M, et al. Aristolochic acid and the etiology of Balkan (endemic) nephropathy. *Proc Natl Acad Sci USA* 2007;104(29):12129–12134.
12. Kambham N, Markowitz GS, Tanji N, et al. Idiopathic hypocomplementemic interstitial nephritis with extensive tubulointerstitial deposits. *Am J Kidney Dis* 2001;37:388–399.
13. Mandeville JT, Levinson RD, Hollnad GN. The tubulointerstitial nephritis and uveitis syndrome. *Surv Ophthalmol* 2001;46:195.
14. Markowitz GS, Radhakrishnan J, Kambham N, et al. Lithium nephrotoxicity: A progressive combined glomerular and tubulointerstitial nephropathy. *J Am Soc Nephrol* 2000;11:1439.
15. Markowitz GS, Stokes MB, Radhakrishnan J, et al. Acute phosphate nephropathy following oral sodium phosphate bowel purgative: An underrecognized cause of chronic renal failure. *J Am Soc Nephrol* 2005;16:3389–3396.
16. Martinez M-CM, Nortier J, Vereerstrateten P, et al. Progression rate of Chinese herb nephropathy: Impact of Aristolochia fungchi ingested dose. *Nephrol Dial Transplant* 2002;17:408–412.
17. Michel DM, Kelly CJ. Acute interstitial nephritis. *J Am Soc Nephrol* 1998;9:506.
18. Muntner P, He J, Vupputuri S, et al. Blood lead and chronic kidney disease in the general US population: Results from NHANES III. *Kidney Int* 2003;63:1044.
19. Preddie, DC, Markowitz, GS, Radhakrishnan J, et al. Mycophenolate mofetil for the treatment of interstitial nephritis. *Clin J Am Soc Nephrol* 2006;1:718.
20. Presne C, Fakhouri F, Nöel LH, et al. Lithium-induced nephropathy: Rate of progression and prognostic factors. *Kidney Int* 2003;64:585–592.
21. Ramesh G, Reeves WB. Salicylate reduces cisplatin nephrotoxicity by inhibition of tumor necrosis factor-alpha. 2004 Feb. *Kidney Int* 65(2):490–499.
22. Walker R. Chronic interstitial nephritis. In: Johnson RJ, Feehally J (eds.). *Comprehensive Clinical Nephrology* Philadelphia: Mosby, 2005, pp. 793–807.

CHAPTER 47

URINARY TRACT INFECTION

Lindsay E. Nicolle, MD

1. **What is a urinary tract infection?**

   Urinary tract infection (UTI) is the presence of micro-organisms in the urine or tissues of the normally sterile genitourinary tract. Infection may be localized to the bladder alone or the kidneys or, in men, the prostate. Acute uncomplicated urinary tract infection occurs in women with a normal genitourinary tract and usually manifests as acute cystitis (bladder infection or lower tract infection). These same women experience, less frequently, kidney (upper tract or renal) infection, referred to as acute uncomplicated or acute nonobstructive pyelonephritis. Complicated urinary tract infection occurs in individuals with structural or functional abnormalities of the genitourinary tract, including those with indwelling devices such as urethral catheters. Recurrent urinary infection may be reinfection with a new organism or relapse, when the same organism is isolated post-therapy.

2. **Who gets urinary tract infections?**

   UTI occurs primarily in two groups of individuals. The first is healthy girls and women with normal genitourinary tracts. About 10% of all women experience at least one episode of infection in a given year, and 20% to 45% of young women will have a recurrence within 1 year following a first infection. The second group at risk for UTI are individuals with underlying functional or structural abnormalities of the genitourinary tract, such as obstruction, diverticula, ureteric reflux, or indwelling devices. This group includes urinary infection in infants, men, and many older women.

3. **What is the pathogenesis of UTI?**

   Urinary infection usually occurs following colonization of the periurethral area by organisms from the normal gut flora and subsequent ascension of these bacteria into the bladder. This is facilitated by sexual intercourse in women, by urologic procedures including catheter insertion, or by turbulent urine flow in men with prostate hypertrophy. Vesicoureteral reflux, if present, facilitates the ascension of organisms from the bladder to the kidneys. Rarely, UTI follows hematogenous spread from another source, which usually presents with renal abscesses.

   Healthy women and girls have both genetic and behavioral risks for UTI. Genetic variables, such as being a nonsecretor of the blood group substances, are most important for girls and postmenopausal women. For premenopausal women, 75% to 90% of episodes of infection are attributable to sexual intercourse. Other risk factors include use of spermicides, which disrupt the normal vaginal flora and promote colonization by potential uropathogens, or a new sexual partner within 1 year, which is associated with colonization with new organisms. A wide variety of genitourinary abnormalities contribute to complicated urinary infection, either through increased access of bacteria to the bladder or by interfering with normal voiding to allow organisms to persist. Indwelling urethral catheters and other urologic devices uniformly acquire a surface biofilm composed of microorganisms and extracellular polysaccharide material, which incorporates urine components such as magnesium and calcium ions and Tamm Horsfall protein. Organisms persist and multiply within the protected environment provided by this biofilm, where there is restricted diffusion of antibiotics and impaired access of host defenses such as neutrophils.

4. **What are the common infecting organisms in UTI?**

   Escherichia coli is isolated in from 80% to 85% of episodes of acute cystitis and 85% to 90% of episodes of acute pyelonephritis. Uropathogenic *E. coli* are characterized by expression of diverse virulence factors including adhesins, iron sequestration systems, and toxins. Pyelonephritis, but not cystitis, is consistently associated with expression of the P pilus, a Gal ($\propto$ 1-4), Gal-β disaccharide galabiose adhesin. *Staphylococcus saprophyticus,* a coagulase negative staphylococcus, is isolated from 5% to 10% of cystitis episodes and is virtually unique to this clinical presentation. A greater variety of bacteria and yeast are isolated from complicated urinary infection. *E. coli* remains an important pathogen, and *Klebsiella pneumoniae, Citrobacter* spp, *Proteus mirabilis, Pseudomonas aeruginosa,* and *Enterococcus* spp. are frequently isolated. These bacteria are more likely to be resistant to antimicrobials as a result of prior antimicrobial therapy or nosocomial acquisition with repeated exposures to health care interventions. Urease producing organisms such as *P. mirabilis, Morganella morganii,* and *Providencia stuartii* and yeast are more common in biofilm on indwelling devices.

5. **What are the usual symptoms of UTI?**

   Bladder infection presents with one or more of acute dysuria, frequency, urgency, stranguria, hematuria, and suprapubic discomfort. Women with recurrent cystitis are more than 90% accurate for self-diagnosis based on symptoms. Kidney infection presents with costovertebral angle pain or tenderness with or without fever, usually accompanied by lower tract symptoms. Patients with complicated UTI may present with symptoms of either bladder or kidney infection. Urinary infection in infants is more common in boys and presents as fever and failure to thrive. Patients with an indwelling urethral catheter also usually present with fever without localizing genitourinary findings, although hematuria, catheter obstruction, or costovertebral angle pain and tenderness may be present. Nonlocalizing or nonspecific signs or symptoms in elderly individuals are often attributed to urinary infection. However, in the absence of an indwelling catheter, a clinical diagnosis of urinary infection in an elderly person should be made only if localizing genitourinary symptoms are present. Acute prostatitis is a severe systemic illness characterized by high fever; bacteremia; and, often, acute urinary obstruction. Chronic bacterial prostatitis frequently presents as relapsing acute cystitis in older men.

6. **How do you make a laboratory diagnosis of UTI?**

   A urine specimen for culture should be obtained prior to initiating antimicrobial therapy for all presentations of symptomatic urinary infection other than women with acute uncomplicated cystitis. These women, however, should have a urine culture obtained if presenting symptoms are not characteristic or with recurrence of infection within 1 month. The culture confirms the diagnosis and identifies the specific infecting organism and susceptibilities. A voided urine specimen, collected using a method to minimize contamination, is usually appropriate. If a voided specimen cannot be obtained, an in-and-out catheter specimen is recommended. Patients with a short-term indwelling urinary catheter have the urine specimen obtained by puncture through the catheter port. When a long-term indwelling catheter is present, the catheter should be replaced and a specimen should be obtained through the replacement catheter to obtain a sample of bladder urine not contaminated by microorganisms present in the biofilm.

   Isolation of $\geq 10^5$ CFU/mL of an organism distinguishes bacteria causing infection from contaminants. However, 25% to 30% of young women with acute cystitis have organisms isolated in quantitative counts $< 10^5$ CFU/mL; any gram-negative organism isolated in counts $\geq 10^2$ CFU/mL is considered relevant for this presentation. Lower quantitative counts are also occasionally isolated from patients with other clinical presentations of urinary infection. In these cases, the diagnosis should be critically reassessed, considering the specimen collection method (i.e., likelihood of contamination) and the number and species of organisms grown. Multiple organisms and gram-positive organisms are more likely to be contaminants.

Specimens obtained by in-and-out catheter, including intermittent catheterization, are less subject to contamination, and any quantitative count $\geq 10^2$ CFU/mL is considered diagnostic of infection.

Pyuria has low specificity for identification of symptomatic infection in older individuals or in patients with underlying genitourinary abnormalities or with indwelling devices and is not by itself diagnostic of urinary infection. However, the absence of pyuria in a symptomatic patient effectively excludes urinary infection.

7. How should acute uncomplicated urinary infection be treated?

Acute cystitis is a mucosal infection effectively treated with relatively short courses of antimicrobial agents that achieve high urinary concentrations. First-line empiric regimens include nitrofurantoin macrocrystals/monohydrate 100 mg bid for 5 days, trimethoprim/sulfamethoxazole (TMP/SMX) 160/800 mg bid for 3 days, or trimethoprim 100 mg bid for 3 days. Fosfomycin trometamol as a single dose or pivmecillinam as a 5- to 7-day course are also effective but are not widely available. The fluoroquinolones, norfloxacin, ciprofloxacin, and levofloxacin, are effective given as a 3-day course but are not recommended for first-line therapy because of concerns of resistance emergence. They are contraindicated in children because of adverse effects on cartilage development. The beta-lactam antimicrobials such as amoxicillin, cephalosporins, and amoxicillin/clavulanic acid are all 10% to 20% less effective for susceptible organisms than first-line agents and must be given for 7 days.

8. How do you prevent acute uncomplicated UTI?

Prophylactic antimicrobial therapy given as a long-term, low-dose regimen or as a single dose postintercourse prevents up to 95% of episodes of recurrent cystitis. This approach is recommended for women who experience two infections within 6 months or three infections within 1 year. Long-term regimens include ½ tablet TMP/SMX daily or every other day or nitrofurantoin 50 or 100 mg daily at bedtime. For postintercourse prophylaxis, nitrofurantoin 50 or 100 mg or ½ tablet of TMP/SMX are recommended. Patient self-treatment with a 3-day course of TMP/SMX, norfloxacin, or ciprofloxacin is also effective and is a useful approach for women who are traveling or who experience severe but less frequent episodes.

Women with recurrent urinary infection should be advised not to use spermicides. Other behavioral interventions such as changing type of underwear, showering rather than bathing, postintercourse voiding, and postvoiding hygiene are not helpful. The use of probiotics, including yogurt, to re-establish normal vaginal flora is not effective. Daily cranberry tablets or juice decreases the risk of recurrent symptomatic infection by about one third. The mechanism of action is thought to be by blocking of *E. coli* adhesins by proanthocyandins in cranberry juice. The role of topical vaginal estrogen to prevent recurrent infection in postmenopausal women is controversial; vaginal estrogen is not currently recommended solely for the prevention of recurrent urinary infection.

9. How is uncomplicated pyelonephritis treated?

Acute nonobstructive pyelonephritis is a serious infection requiring prompt investigation and treatment. If the patient is clinically stable and can tolerate oral therapy, ciprofloxacin 500 mg twice a day for 7 days or levofloxacin 750 mg once a day for 5 days are recommended empiric regimens. Two regular-strength tablets of TMP/SMX twice a day for 14 days is also effective for susceptible organisms, but it is not recommended for empiric therapy because TMP/SMX resistance of *E. coli* exceeds 20% in many geographic areas. Effective parenteral antimicrobial regimens include ceftriaxone 1 to 2 g daily, or gentamicin or tobramycin 3 to 5 mg/kg daily. The clinical status and urine culture results should be reviewed at 48 to 72 hours following initiation of antimicrobial therapy to confirm a satisfactory clinical response and the efficacy of the antimicrobial for the infecting organism. Patients receiving parenteral therapy can usually be switched to oral therapy to complete a 10-day course. If the clinical response is not satisfactory and the infecting organism is susceptible to the antimicrobial given, underlying abnormalities requiring urologic intervention should be excluded by ultrasound or CT scan.

10. **How is UTI in pregnant women managed?**

Women with asymptomatic bacteriuria identified in early pregnancy who are not treated have a 20% to 30% risk of developing pyelonephritis in later pregnancy, when the risk of premature labor and delivery with any febrile illness is greatest. The high risk of pyelonephritis is attributed to urine stasis from hormone-induced dilation of the smooth muscle of the urinary tract and ureteric obstruction by the fetal head. All pregnant women are screened for bacteriuria by urine culture in early pregnancy. Asymptomatic women with a positive urine culture ($\geq 10^5$ CFU/mL of a single gram-negative organism) or women with symptomatic infection at any time are treated and subsequently screened for bacteriuria, usually monthly, for the duration of the pregnancy. If a second episode of urinary infection occurs, prophylactic antimicrobial therapy is given until the end of the pregnancy. The preferred regimen is a beta-lactam antibiotic because these antimicrobials are safe for the fetus. Nitrofurantoin is also safe and effective. For prophylactic therapy, either cephalexin 500 mg or nitrofurantoin 50 or 100 mg daily are recommended. TMP/SMX is avoided because of a small but well-documented association with fetal abnormalities when given in the first trimester, and fluoroquinolone antimicrobials are contraindicated because of potential detrimental effects on fetal cartilage. A pregnant woman who presents with pyelonephritis should be hospitalized for initial management. The recommended empiric regimen is ceftriaxone 1 to 2 g once daily. An aminoglycoside, usually gentamicin, may be used if there is antimicrobial resistance or patient intolerance to ceftriaxone.

11. **What is the management of complicated UTI?**

The treatment of complicated UTI requires consideration of the underlying abnormality and an appreciation of the wide spectrum of potential infecting organisms and increased likelihood of antimicrobial resistance. When symptoms are mild, antimicrobial therapy should be delayed pending urine culture results so specific therapy can be prescribed. Empiric antimicrobial therapy is chosen considering recent antimicrobial therapy, any previous urine culture results, and patient tolerance. An antimicrobial with good urinary excretion should be selected, based on the likely infecting organism. A fluoroquinolone is often prescribed for empiric therapy. When parenteral therapy is indicated, aminoglycosides (gentamicin, tobramycin) are effective for patients without renal failure because most gram-negative organisms remain susceptible to these agents. If aminoglycosides cannot be used, an extended spectrum cephalosporin (cefotaxime, ceftriaxone, ceftazidime), penicillin (piperacillin/tazobactam), or carbapenem (meropenem, ertapenem) are other options.

An unusual presentation is emphysematous pyelonephritis, an acute necrotizing renal infection characterized by gas formation in renal tissue and the perinephric space. Patients with this presentation usually have diabetes and often obstruction. Management requires antimicrobial therapy together with glucose control, correction of obstruction, and percutaneous or open drainage of abscesses. Percutaneous drainage is the recommended initial approach, if possible, but delayed elective nephrectomy may subsequently be required for some patients.

12. **How is complicated UTI prevented?**

The most important intervention to prevent complicated UTI is to characterize and correct the underlying genitourinary abnormality. If the underlying abnormality persists, such as in a patient with spinal cord injury, the goal of management is to optimize voiding and limit use of indwelling devices. Prophylactic antimicrobial therapy is not effective to prevent recurrence because there is rapid reinfection with resistant organisms. Cranberry juice or capsules are also not effective in preventing reinfection. Limiting use of indwelling urethral catheters will prevent some infections, so catheters should be used only when essential and removed promptly once no longer needed. Optimal practices for catheter care and maintenance should be followed. Replacement of a chronic indwelling catheter immediately prior to initiating antimicrobial therapy decreases the frequency of early post-therapy symptomatic relapse and leads to more rapid defervescence.

13. **What is suppressive antimicrobial therapy, and when should this be used?**

Suppressive antimicrobial therapy is long-term antimicrobial therapy given to prevent symptomatic relapsing infection in selected patients with recurrent complicated UTI in whom infection cannot be eradicated. Some examples include use in men with frequent recurrent cystitis from a prostate source, in patients who have undergone renal transplant with recurrent symptomatic infection from an infected native kidney, or in an individual with an inoperable infection stone to prevent further stone enlargement and preserve renal function. Antimicrobial therapy is selected based on the organism isolated from urine culture and considering patient tolerance. Initial treatment is for 2 to 4 weeks at the full therapeutic dose. If this is effective and well tolerated, therapy is usually continued indefinitely at one half the dose or until the underlying abnormality is corrected.

14. **When should you treat asymptomatic urinary infection?**

Asymptomatic bacteriuria or funguria is isolation of bacteria or yeast from the urine culture in quantitative counts consistent with infection but with no signs or symptoms referable to the urinary tract. Asymptomatic bacteriuria may be transient or persistent and is common in women, the elderly, and individuals with complicated UTI. From 25% to 50% of long-term care facility residents and 50% of patients with spinal cord injury managed with intermittent catheters have positive urine cultures at any time. Screening for and treatment of asymptomatic bacteriuria is indicated only for pregnant women, as previously discussed, and to prevent bacteremia and sepsis in individuals following invasive genitourinary procedures associated with mucosal trauma and bleeding. For these procedures, antimicrobial therapy is initiated immediately prior to the intervention. Screening for and treatment of asymptomatic bacteriuria or funguria is not recommended for other individuals because this strategy will not decrease subsequent episodes of symptomatic infection or other morbidity but is associated with increased adverse drug reactions and reinfection with more resistant bacteria.

15. **How do you manage urinary infection in the elderly patient who resides in a nursing home?**

For elderly individuals without an indwelling catheter, ascertainment of clinical signs and symptoms may be difficult because of dementia or impaired communication. However, localizing genitourinary symptoms such as frequency, urgency, hematuria, or costovertebral angle pain or tenderness should be present before making a diagnosis of urinary infection. For the 30% to 50% of male or female nursing home residents with bacteriuria at any time, 90% will also have pyuria. The presence of pyuria, "foul smelling urine," or other urinalysis findings such as bacteria or hematuria without localizing signs or symptoms is not an indication for antimicrobial therapy irrespective of whether bacteria or fungi are isolated. For the elderly resident with an indwelling Foley catheter, fever by itself may be a manifestation of symptomatic infection. These residents with chronic catheters uniformly have bacteriuria and pyuria. Urinalysis abnormalities such as pyuria, smell, or cloudy urine are not sufficient for diagnosis of symptomatic urinary infection in a resident with an indwelling catheter, for either bacteriuria or funguria. If symptoms attributed to urinary infection are present, the indwelling Foley catheter should be replaced and a urine specimen for culture should be obtained through the new catheter before initiating antimicrobial therapy.

16. **How do you diagnose and treat bacterial prostatitis?**

Acute bacterial prostatitis is a urologic emergency. Patients are severely ill with high fever and prominent voiding symptoms. Broad-spectrum parenteral antimicrobial treatment is initiated following collection of urine and blood cultures. Any obstruction to voiding must be corrected promptly. Chronic bacterial prostatitis is diagnosed when bacterial growth and pyuria are documented in expressed prostate secretions and the voided urine culture is negative. However, chronic pelvic pain syndrome/chronic prostatitis symptoms are attributable to chronic bacterial prostatitis for only 10% of men with this complaint. The most common clinical presentation in older men is recurrent cystitis when bacteria that persist in the prostate re-enter the urine. Treatment for documented chronic bacterial prostatitis is 4 weeks of ciprofloxacin or levofloxacin. This regimen is 70% to 80% effective for long-term cure.

KEY POINTS: URINARY TRACT INFECTIONS

1. Acute uncomplicated urinary tract infection is common in women of any age. These women have a normal genitourinary tract and can usually be effectively treated with short courses of antimicrobial therapy.

2. Complicated urinary tract infection occurs in individuals with structural or functional abnormalities of the genitourinary tract. A principal goal of therapy in these patients is the characterization and correction of abnormalities that promote infection.

3. *Escherichia coli* is the single most common cause of urinary tract infection. *E. coli* isolated from women with acute uncomplicated urinary infection express diverse virulence factors. *E. coli* strains isolated from individuals with complicated urinary tract infection or asymptomatic bacteriuria less frequently express virulence factors.

4. Pyuria is not, by itself, diagnostic of urinary tract infection or an indication for antimicrobial therapy. However, the absence of pyuria has a high negative predictive value to exclude urinary tract infection.

5. Asymptomatic bacteriuria should be screened for and treated only in pregnant women or individuals who are to undergo an invasive genitourinary procedure likely to be associated with mucosal bleeding.

17. **How do you diagnose and treat fungal UTI?**
    Risk factors for fungal UTI include exposure to broad-spectrum antimicrobial therapy, diabetes, and the presence of chronic indwelling catheters. *Candida albicans* is the most common organism, but other *Candida* spp. may also be isolated. Patients are usually asymptomatic, and asymptomatic funguria should not be treated. Fluconazole has good urinary excretion and is the treatment of choice for symptomatic infection. Some species, such as *C. glabrata,* are resistant to fluconazole, and the recommended alternate treatment is amphotericin B deoxycholate. 5-flucytocine may also be effective but has substantial side effects and requires careful monitoring when used. Other azoles and echinocandins do not achieve therapeutic concentrations in the urine and are not recommended for treatment of urinary infection. Patients with an inadequate therapeutic response to appropriate antifungal therapy should have imaging studies to exclude a fungus ball, which will require surgical intervention if present.

BIBLIOGRAPHY

1. Benway BM, Moon TD. Bacterial prostatitis. *Urol Clin N Am* 2008;35:23–32.
2. Hooton TM, Bradley SF, Cardenas DD, et al. 2009. International clinical practice guidelines for the diagnosis, prevention, and treatment of catheter-associated urinary tract infection in adults. *Clin Infect Dis* 2010;50:625–663.
3. Hooton TM. The current management strategies for community-acquired urinary tract infection. *Infect Dis Clin N Am* 2003;17:303–332.
4. Nicolle LE, Bradley S, Colgan R, et al. IDSA guideline for the diagnosis and treatment of asymptomatic bacteriuria in adults. *Clin Infect Dis* 2005;40:643–654.
5. Nicolle LE. Urinary tract infections in the elderly. *Clin Geriatr Med* 2009;25:423–436.
6. Schlager TA. Urinary tract infections in infants and children. *Infect Dis Clin N Am* 2003;17:353–366.

CHAPTER 48

RENAL NEOPLASIAS

Sumanta Kumar Pal, MD, and Robert A. Figlin, MD

1. **Describe the demographics of renal cell carcinoma (RCC). How many cases of RCC are diagnosed annually, and how many deaths are attributable to this disease? Is RCC more common in males or females? What is the median age at diagnosis of RCC?**

   In 2009 an estimated 57,650 cases of RCC were diagnosed and 12,980 deaths were attributable to the disease. Approximately 61% and 71% of diagnoses and deaths, respectively, occurred in males. The median age at diagnosis is 65.

   Jemal A, Siegel R, Ward E, et al. Cancer statistics, 2009. *CA Cancer J Clin* 2009;59:225–249.

2. **What are the three most common histologic subtypes of RCC, and what proportion of RCC cases do they account for?**

   Clear cell RCC accounts for approximately 80% of cases, whereas papillary and chromophobe histologies represent 10% and 5% of cases, respectively.

   Karumanchi SA, Merchan J, Sukhatme VP. Renal cancer: molecular mechanisms and newer therapeutic options. *Curr Opin Nephrol Hypertens* 2002;11:37–42.

3. **What are the clinical features of collecting duct (Bellini duct) carcinoma? What clinical disorder is associated with the medullary variant of collecting duct carcinoma?**

   Collecting duct carcinoma comprises less than 1% of RCC cases and has a particularly aggressive phenotype. Medullary RCC represents a variant of collecting duct carcinoma and was first noted to occur among patients with sickle-cell trait.

   National Comprehensive Cancer Network Clinical Practice Guidelines: Renal Cell Carcinoma. Available at http://www.nccn.org; last accessed November 29, 2009.

4. **What are common presenting signs of RCC?**

   Often, RCC presents as an incidental finding on radiographic imaging of the abdomen. With respect to symptoms, common complaints include hematuria and flank pain. In the setting of metastatic disease, patients may note bone pain, palpable adenopathy, or pulmonary complaints (i.e., shortness of breath secondary to bulky lung disease or pleural effusions).

   National Comprehensive Cancer Network Clinical Practice Guidelines: Renal Cell Carcinoma. Available at http://www.nccn.org; last accessed November 29, 2009.

5. **What paraneoplastic syndromes are associated with RCC? What is Stauffer's syndrome?**

   Nearly 40% of patients with RCC develop paraneoplastic syndromes. RCC produces a range of ectopic hormones, including parathyroid-like hormone, erythropoietin, insulin, gonadotropins, renin, and placental lactogen. Clinically, this may manifest in a range of symptoms and laboratory abnormalities, including but not limited to hypertension (24%), hypercalcemia (10% to 15%), and erythrocytosis (4%). Stauffer's syndrome, which occurs in roughly 6% of patients, implies liver function test abnormalities but absent hepatic metastases. This reversible hepatorenal syndrome is pathognomonic for RCC.

Bostwick DG. Chapter 18C: Renal cell carcinoma. In: Lenhard RE (ed.). *The American Cancer Society's Clinical Oncology*. Atlanta: American Cancer Society, 2001.

6. **What gene is disrupted in the majority of sporadic cases of clear cell RCC?**
    The von Hippel-Lindau (VHL) gene is disrupted in up to 70% of sporadic cases of clear cell RCC. In approximately 50% of cases, somatic mutations occur, and in 10% to 20% of cases, the gene is hypermethylated. A consequence of VHL mutation is upregulation of hypoxia-induced genes, leading to increased production of moieties such as vascular endothelial growth factor (VEGF). This, in turn, causes increased tumor angiogenesis.

    Kim WY, Kaelin WG. Role of VHL gene mutation in human cancer. *J Clin Oncol* 2004;22:4991–5004.

7. **Describe the features of (1) hereditary papillary renal cell carcinoma, (2) Birt-Hogg-Dubé syndrome, and (3) hereditary leiomyomatosis/renal cell carcinoma (HLRCC).**
    Hereditary papillary renal cell carcinoma is characterized by mutations in the *MET* proto-oncogene, located at 7q31. The mutations are highly penetrant and autosomal dominant. The resulting tumors are classified as papillary type 1 and are often multifocal and bilateral.

    Birt-Hogg-Dubé syndrome is characterized by the triad of hair follicle hamartomas, lung cysts, and renal neoplasia. The disorder is caused by mutations in the *BHD* gene, located at 17p11.2. Although the disorder is highly penetrant with respect to lung and skin findings (>85%), renal neoplasia only occurs in 25% to 35% of patients.

    HLRCC is characterized by mutations in the gene encoding fumarate hydratase (FH, located at 1q24-43). The resulting phenotype includes type 2 papillary RCC, along with cutaneous and uterine leiomyomas.

    Schmidt LE, Linehan WM. When should genetic syndromes be considered? In: American Society of Clinical Oncology. *2009 Genitourinary Cancers Symposium Abstract Book*. Alexandria, VA: American Society of Clinical Oncology, 2009, p. 62.

8. **What is the staging workup for RCC?**
    Guidelines from the National Comprehensive Cancer Network (NCCN) suggest that the initial workup for RCC should include a complete history and physical examination, comprehensive laboratories (including an lactate dehydrogenase [LDH] and urinalysis), and abdominal/pelvic computed tomography (CT) or magnetic resonance imaging (MRI). If clinically indicated, an MRI of the brain and bone scan should be ordered. If urothelial carcinoma is suspected, urine cytology or ureteroscopy should be considered. Finally, in patients with small lesions, needle biopsy may be performed to confirm malignancy and guide surveillance strategies.

    National Comprehensive Cancer Network Clinical Practice Guidelines: Renal Cell Carcinoma. Available at http://www.nccn.org; last accessed November 29, 2009.

9. **For patients with localized RCC (stage I–III), what treatment is recommended after surgical resection of the tumor? What follow-up examinations are recommended after surgical resection?**
    At present, no adjuvant therapy is recommended for patients with resected RCC. Follow-up (per NCCN guidelines) is guided by risk stratification according to the UCLA Integrated Staging System. This staging system incorporates tumor stage (by standard TNM criteria), Fuhrman grade (a histologic grading schema), and functionality of the patient (based on the Eastern Cooperative Oncology Group performance status scale). Based on categorization with low, intermediate, or high-risk disease (or positive nodal status), patients are assigned to receive a history and physical examination, laboratory studies, chest CT, and abdominal CT at set intervals.

    Lam JS, Shvarts O, Leppert JT, et al. Postoperative surveillance protocol for patients with localized and locally advanced renal cell carcinoma based on a validated prognostic nomogram and risk group stratification. *J Urol* 2005;174:466–472.

10. **In which patients is nephron-sparing surgery appropriate?**
Nephron-sparing surgery is appropriate in selected patients who have multiple primaries, a uninephric state, or renal insufficiency. Nephron-sparing techniques may also be used in selected patients with small unilateral tumors.

National Comprehensive Cancer Network Clinical Practice Guidelines: Renal Cell Carcinoma. Available at http://www.nccn.org; last accessed November 29, 2009.

11. **What are common sites of metastasis of RCC?**
RCC classically spreads to the lung, bone, brain, liver, and adrenal gland.

Bostwick DG. Chapter 18C: Renal cell carcinoma. In: Lenhard RE (ed.). *The American Cancer Society's Clinical Oncology.* Atlanta: American Cancer Society, 2001.

12. **What are the three classes of agents used to treat metastatic RCC?**
The three classes of agents used to treat metastatic RCC include (1) immunotherapy, (2) VEGF-directed therapy, and (3) inhibitors of the mammalian target of rapamycin (mTOR). Classically, RCC has been approached with immunotherapeutic agents, such as interleukin-2 (IL-2) or interferon-α (IFN-α). However, a greater understanding of angiogenic pathways integral to RCC biology has led to implementation of mTOR inhibitors and VEGF-directed therapy.

13. **What proportion of patients respond to therapy with IFN-α? What are some of the side effects of IFN-α therapy?**
In a cohort of 463 patients who received IFN-α as first-line therapy, an overall response rate (RR) of 11% was noted. In this study, median time to progression (TTP) and overall survival (OS) were 4.7 and 13 months, respectively. Common side effects associated with IFN-α include flulike symptoms, including fevers, chills, myalgias, and arthralgias. IFN-α therapy can also result in hepatotoxicity and neuropsychiatric symptoms.

Motzer RJ, Bacik J, Murphy BA, et al. Interferon-alfa as a comparative treatment for clinical trials of new therapies against advanced renal cell carcinoma. *J Clin Oncol* 2002;20:289–296.

14. **What proportion of patients respond to therapy with high-dose IL-2? What are some of the side effects of therapy?**
In a series of 259 patients treated at the National Institutes of Health between 1986 and 2006, an overall response rate of 20% was noted with IL-2 therapy. All patients who experienced a partial response (12%) were noted to relapse, with a median duration of response of 15.5 months. In contrast, 19 of 23 patients who experienced a complete response remained disease free with a median follow-up ranging between 24 and 221 months. This experience is representative of others, suggesting that although the complete response rate associated with high-dose IL-2 is relatively low, those patients who do develop a complete response may experience a durable remission. The side effects of high-dose IL-2 weigh heavily in the risk–benefit discussion with the patient. High-dose IL-2 causes vasodilatation, diarrhea, and a capillary leak syndrome, all of which can contribute to hypotension and oliguria. Hematologic and hepatic laboratory abnormalities are also frequently seen with IL-2 therapy.

Klapper JA, Downey SG, Smith FO, et al. High-dose interleukin-2 for the treatment of metastatic renal cell carcinoma. *Cancer* 2008;113:293–301.

15. **What are the three VEGF-tyrosine kinase inhibitors (VEGF-TKIs) approved by the U.S. Food and Drug Administration for the treatment of metastatic RCC?**
Presently, three VEGF-TKIs are approved for the treatment of metastatic RCC: sunitinib, sorafenib, and pazopanib. Notably, the pivotal trial leading to the approval of sunitinib demonstrated an overall survival benefit in treatment-naïve patients with metastatic clear cell RCC as compared to IFN-α. Sorafenib, in contrast, demonstrated a statistically significant improvement in progression-free survival (PFS) as compared to placebo in a landmark study including a largely cytokine-refractory population. Most recently, phase III data for pazopanib

demonstrated a PFS benefit as compared to placebo. Roughly half of these patients were treatment-naïve, and the remainder had received prior cytokine therapy.

Escudier B, Eisen T, Stadler WM, et al. Sorafenib in advanced clear-cell renal-cell carcinoma. *N Engl J Med* 2007;356:125–134.

Motzer RJ, Hutson TE, Tomczak P, et al. Overall survival and updated results for sunitinib compared with interferon alfa in patients with metastatic renal cell carcinoma. *J Clin Oncol* 2009;27:3584–3590.

Sternberg CN, Szczylik C, Lee E, et al. A randomized, double-blind phase III study of pazopanib in treatment-naïve and cytokine-pretreated patients with advanced renal cell carcinoma (RCC). *J Clin Oncol* (Meeting Abstracts) 2009;27:5021.

16. **What are common side effects associated with sunitinib, sorafenib, and pazopanib?**

The most commonly reported moderate to severe side effects in the pivotal trial of sunitinib were hypertension, fatigue, diarrhea, and hand-foot syndrome. Similarly, diarrhea, rash, fatigue, and hand-foot skin reactions were the most frequently reported adverse events in the pivotal trial of sorafenib. Early results from the phase III randomized trial comparing pazopanib and placebo suggested the most frequent adverse events with pazopanib were diarrhea, hypertension, hair color change, nausea, and anorexia. Liver enzymes were also abnormally elevated in a large proportion of patients.

KEY POINTS: RENAL NEOPLASIAS

1. Three principal histologic subtypes of renal cell carcinoma (RCC) exist: (1) clear cell, (2) papillary, and (3) chromophobe. Clear cell RCC accounts for roughly 80% of cases.

2. Initial workup of RCC should include a complete history and physical examination, comprehensive laboratories (including a lactate dehydrogenase and urinalysis), and abdominal/pelvic radiographic imaging, along with magnetic resonance imaging of the brain as clinically indicated.

3. For localized RCC, no adjuvant therapy is recommended. Rather, risk-stratification tools such as the UCLA Integrated Staging System should be applied to determine the appropriate intervals for clinical and radiographic follow-up.

4. Up to 70% of patients with clear cell RCC carry somatic mutations in the VHL gene. As a consequence, hypoxia-induced genes such as vascular endothelial growth factor (VEGF) are upregulated. This provides rationale for the success of VEGF-directed therapy in metastatic RCC.

5. Three broad classes of agents are used in the treatment of metastatic RCC: (1) immunotherapeutic agents, including interferon-α and interleukin-2; (2) VEGF-directed therapies, including sunitinib, sorafenib, bevacizumab and pazopanib; and (3) mammalian target of rapamycin (mTOR) inhibitors, including everolimus and temsirolimus.

17. **What monoclonal antibody directed at VEGF is approved for the first-line therapy of metastatic RCC? What side effects are associated with this treatment?**

Bevacizumab with IFN-α has been approved for the first-line therapy of metastatic RCC on the basis of two randomized, phase III trials showing a benefit in PFS as compared to IFN-α alone. In these studies, patients receiving bevacizumab had a higher incidence of hypertension, anorexia, fatigue and proteinuria.

Escudier BJ, Bellmunt J, Negrier S, et al. Final results of the phase III, randomized, double-blind AVOREN trial of first-line bevacizumab (BEV) + interferon-α 2a (IFN) in metastatic renal cell carcinoma (mRCC). *J Clin Oncol* (Meeting Abstracts) 2009;27:5020.

Rini BI, Halabi S, Rosenberg J, et al. Bevacizumab plus interferon-alpha versus interferon-alpha monotherapy in patients with metastatic renal cell carcinoma: Results of overall survival for CALGB 90206. *J Clin Oncol* (Meeting Abstracts) 2009;27:LBA5019.

18. **How are mTOR inhibitors applied in metastatic RCC?**

    Two mTOR inhibitors, everolimus and temsirolimus, have been approved for use in metastatic RCC. Everolimus was compared to placebo in a phase III study including patients who were refractory to sunitinib and/or sorafenib. In this study, everolimus therapy was associated with an improvement in PFS. As such, everolimus has been approved for use after failure of VEGF-TKI therapy. In contrast, temsirolimus was approved on the basis of a study comparing temsirolimus, IFN-α, and the combination of agents in patients with poor-risk metastatic RCC. In the context of this study, poor risk was defined as having three or more of the following predictors of short survival: (1) LDH >1.5 times the upper limit of normal, (2) hemoglobin below the lower limit of normal, (3) corrected serum calcium >10 mg/dL, (4) interval of <1 year from original diagnosis to the start of systemic therapy, (5) Karnofsky performance score <70, and (6) two or more sites of organ metastases. Among the three treatment arms, temsirolimus was associated with improved overall survival. In light of these data, temsirolimus has been approved for the first-line treatment of poor-risk metastatic RCC.

    Hudes G, Carducci M, Tomczak P, et al. Temsirolimus, interferon alfa, or both for advanced renal-cell carcinoma. *N Engl J Med* 2007;356:2271–2281.

    Motzer RJ, Escudier B, Oudard S, et al. Efficacy of everolimus in advanced renal cell carcinoma: a double-blind, randomised, placebo-controlled phase III trial. *Lancet* 2008;372:449–456.

19. **What side effects are associated with everolimus and temsirolimus?**

    Class effects of the mTOR inhibitors include stomatitis, rash, fatigue, hyperglycemia, and hypertriglyceridemia. Pneumonitis (potentially severe) has also been noted with use of these agents.

    Hudes G, Carducci M, Tomczak P, et al. Temsirolimus, interferon alfa, or both for advanced renal-cell carcinoma. *N Engl J Med* 2007;356:2271–2281.

    Motzer RJ, Escudier B, Oudard S, et al. Efficacy of everolimus in advanced renal cell carcinoma: a double-blind, randomised, placebo-controlled phase III trial. *Lancet* 2008;372:449–456.

20. **What is the role of standard cytotoxic chemotherapy in treating metastatic RCC?**

    Outcomes with standard cytotoxic chemotherapy in metastatic RCC appear to be inferior to those with immunotherapy or newer targeted agents. Nonetheless, the clinician may consider use of cytotoxic therapy in patients with sarcomatoid variant RCC or in the setting of collecting duct carcinoma. The latter appears to bear molecular and genetic similarities to urothelial carcinoma.

    Haas N, Manola J, Pins M, et al. ECOG 8802: Phase II trial of doxorubicin (Dox) and gemcitabine (Gem) in metastatic renal cell carcinoma (RCC) with sarcomatoid features. *J Clin Oncol* (Meeting Abstracts) 2009;27:5038.

    Milowsky MI, Rosmarin A, Tickoo SK, et al. Active chemotherapy for collecting duct carcinoma of the kidney. *Cancer* 2002;94:111–116.

RENAL DISEASE AND HYPERTENSION IN PREGNANCY

Susan Hou, MD

CHAPTER 49

1. **What changes take place in the kidney during pregnancy?**

   The kidney undergoes anatomic and physiologic changes during normal pregnancy. The length of the kidney increases by 1 to 1.5 cm and there is hormonally mediated dilatation of the collecting system to a volume of about 300 cc. The resulting physiologic hydronephrosis makes it difficult to diagnose obstruction by ultrasound. The glomerular filtration rate (GFR) increases by 50% during the first trimester so that the serum creatinine is expected to be 0.5 to 0.7 mg/dL. Pregnancy is also characterized by a reset osmostat where the serum sodium is normally in the range of 134 mEq/L, but a water load can be excreted normally.

2. **How often do urinary tract infections occur during pregnancy?**

   Urinary stasis from the dilated collecting system predisposes to urinary tract infections (UTI). Asymptomatic bacteriuria occurs in 5% of pregnancies. Untreated, 30% of asymptomatic bacteriuria leads to pyelonephritis, which in pregnancy is frequently complicated by decreased renal function/acute renal failure, sepsis, and even acute respiratory distress syndrome (ARDS). Only 2% of women with a negative urine culture on the first screening will develop a UTI later in pregnancy, but women with pre-existing renal disease should be screened monthly.

3. **What is the importance of preeclampsia?**

   Preeclampsia is the most common and important of the hypertensive disorders of pregnancy, affecting between 5% and 7% of pregnancies. Although we recognize it when we see the development of hypertension and proteinuria in a woman beyond the 20th week of gestation, preeclampsia is a multisystem disease. Severe preeclampsia is denoted by its most common symptoms: microangiopathic Hemolytic anemia, Elevated Liver enzymes, and Low Platelets (HELLP syndrome). It can be accompanied by severe manifestations in other organs including acute renal failure, stroke, blindness from vasoconstriction in the occipital lobe or retinal detachment, disseminated intravascular coagulation, or pulmonary edema. Preeclampsia may progress to seizures, a progression that changes the designation to eclampsia. The hypertension in preeclampsia is identified relative to prepregnancy blood pressure. An increase in systolic blood pressure of 30 mm Hg or an increase in diastolic blood pressure of 15 mm Hg raises the possibility of preeclampsia. The definitive treatment of preeclampsia is delivery of the baby, but depending on the severity of the preeclampsia, efforts may be made to postpone delivery if it occurs in the second trimester or early in the third trimester. Anticonvulsants, most commonly magnesium in the United States, and antihypertensive drugs are usually required while preparing the mother for delivery.

4. **What is the pathophysiology of preeclampsia?**

   Preeclampsia is associated with high levels of the antiangiogenic factors soluble Fms-like tyrosine kinase (sFlt1) and soluble endoglin, and low levels of PIGF (placental growth factor) and VEGF (vascular endothelial growth factor). sFlt1 antagonizes the angiogenic activity of VEGF and PIGF, leading to placental ischemia, diffuse vasoconstriction, glomerular endotheliosis, and proteinuria.

5. **What are the other hypertensive disorders of pregnancy?**

Women with preexisting hypertension may become pregnant, so essential hypertension is seen during pregnancy. These women are at increased risk for preeclampsia giving rise to essential hypertension with superimposed preeclampsia. Gestational hypertension occurs late in pregnancy and is not accompanied by proteinuria. It resolves postpartum but is a predictor of long-term hypertension.

6. **What antihypertensive medications can be used to treat hypertension in pregnancy?**

The use of antihypertensive medications during pregnancy has to begin with an admonition against the use of angiotensin-converting enzyme (ACE) inhibitors. Used in the second and third trimester, ACE inhibitors have been associated with renal dysplasia, oligohydramnios, and neonatal death from hypoplastic lungs. The evidence against using ACE inhibitors in the first trimester is not as strong as it is for the latter half of pregnancy, but one report describes an increase in cardiac anomalies in the neonate. There are less data on angiotensin receptor blockers, but they are avoided because of concern that their effects will be similar to that of ACE inhibitors.

7. **What antihypertensive medications can we use in pregnant women?**

Alpha methyldopa has been used for more than 50 years to treat hypertension in pregnant women, and careful follow-up on children supports its safety. Labetalol, hydralazine, and calcium channel blockers are safe. Calcium channel blockers may cause severe hypotension when used with magnesium. Hydralazine is ineffective as a single oral agent but may be effective when used with a sympatholytic drug. Beta blockers and diuretics have been reported to have adverse effects on fetal growth but may be necessary in women with underlying renal disease. Intravenous hydralazine and labetalol are the drugs most commonly used for hypertensive emergencies.

8. **What are the causes of acute renal failure in pregnancy?**

In poor countries sepsis from illegal abortion and from preeclampsia are the most common causes of acute renal failure. With improved health care systems, pregnancy-associated renal failure becomes rare, on the order of 1 in 10,000 to 20,000 pregnancies. Preeclampsia is occasionally associated with acute renal failure, especially in the setting of the HELLP syndrome. Pregnancy can be complicated by hemolytic uremic syndrome (HUS), which presents in a manner similar to HUS in other settings. It can be distinguished from preeclampsia by the elevated transaminases and abnormal clotting parameters seen in preeclampsia. Acute renal failure can complicate acute fatty liver of pregnancy, but acute fatty liver is diagnosed as primarily a liver disease accompanied by renal dysfunction. Despite the rarity of acute renal failure in pregnancy, pregnancy makes the kidney more susceptible to cortical necrosis when acute renal failure occurs in the setting of an obstetric catastrophe such as abruptio placentae, amniotic fluid embolus, or hemorrhage from other causes.

9. **What is the effect of preexisting renal disease on fertility and pregnancy?**

For a woman with renal disease and normal renal function, pregnancy is associated with an increased risk of hypertension and premature delivery. Distinguishing between preeclampsia and other forms of hypertension is difficult in the setting of renal disease because hypertension and proteinuria occur commonly in pregnant women with renal disease. If proteinuria is present before pregnancy, it can be expected to increase during pregnancy and by itself does not necessarily signal a poor prognosis. If a woman has preexisting renal insufficiency, there is a risk of worsening renal function with pregnancy. The level of renal function is more important than the specific disease, except in lupus nephritis. All the studies that have been done have used serum creatinine as a marker of renal function rather than estimated GFR. The Modification of Diet in Renal Disease (MDRD) equation has not been validated in pregnancy. In a woman with a serum creatinine

≤1.4 mg/dL, the risk of accelerating the progression of renal disease by becoming pregnant is very low. When serum creatinine is 2 mg/dL or greater, there is a 30% to 50% chance that renal disease will progress more rapidly if a woman becomes pregnant than without pregnancy. With serum creatinine levels between 1.5 mg/dL and 1.9 mg/dL, the risk is variable. There is a risk of prematurity in women with renal insufficiency, but most infants survive.

10. **Is successful pregnancy possible in patients receiving dialysis?**
Fertility is markedly decreased in patients receiving dialysis, with conception rates ranging from 0.3% to 1.5% per person per year. The only exception is a 15% conception rate among patients receiving dialysis nocturnally in Toronto. Historically, pregnancy outcomes for patients receiving dialysis have been among the worst of any group of women with renal disease. In the past, only about 50% of pregnancies in women undergoing dialysis resulted in surviving infants. Recent series in women receiving extremely intensive dialysis (20–48 hours/week) success rates have been as high as 75% to 100%. Pregnancy is accompanied by a risk of life-threatening hypertension up to 6 weeks postpartum and markedly increased requirements for erythropoietin. Fewer than 20% of infants are born at term. There are no firm data on when to start dialysis in a pregnant woman, but fetal loss appears to increase when dialysis is not initiated in a woman with a serum creatinine level between 3 and 4 mg/dL.

11. **Can erythropoiesis stimulating agents be used during pregnancy?**
Erythropoiesis stimulating agents (ESAs) are continued in patients receiving dialysis during pregnancy, and the dose has to be increased to achieve the same hemoglobin level. They can be started in patients not receiving dialysis if the hemoglobin drops to 8 g/dL.

12. **Should a woman with a kidney transplant become pregnant?**
Fertility is usually restored by kidney transplant. Three broad areas of concern are as follows: (1) the effect of pregnancy on the renal allograft, (2) the effect of immunosuppressive medication on the fetus, and (3) the risk of opportunistic infection. Women are advised to wait a year after transplant and to become pregnant only if they have stable renal function with a serum creatinine of <2 mg/dL. As in other renal diseases, the most important risk factor for worsening renal function is poor renal function prior to pregnancy. Statins and ACE inhibitors are stopped before conception. Of immunosuppressive drugs, only mycophenolate mofetil is believed to be associated with increased congenital anomalies. Cyclosporine and tacrolimus have been associated with babies who are small for gestational age. Prednisone and azathioprine have been the most widely used without major problems. There is no information on sirolimus. Infectious diseases such as cytomegalovirus, toxoplasmosis, herpes simplex, and Listeria, which are seen in transplant recipients, pose a risk for the fetus.

13. **What is the effect of lupus nephritis on pregnancy and vice versa?**
Lupus occurs most frequently in women of childbearing age and may be diagnosed during pregnancy. When the onset of lupus nephritis occurs during pregnancy, the renal histology is often World Health Organization class IV, which requires prompt treatment. New-onset lupus is one of the indications for a renal biopsy in a pregnant woman because the drugs most commonly used for severe lupus nephritis, such as cyclophosphamide, should not be used in early pregnancy. In a woman with diffuse proliferative lupus nephritis, high-dose steroids can be used initially. Oral cyclophosphamide has been used in women beyond 20 weeks of gestation, but long-term follow-up is limited. Lupus nephritis, including membranous lupus nephritis, carries the risk of relapse during pregnancy, but the greatest risks may come from extrarenal lupus. Even women in remission for more than 6 months have a one in three risk of a flare during pregnancy and during the first 6 weeks postpartum. Many antibodies associated with lupus are immunoglobulin G and cross the placenta. They may cause rash and thrombocytopenia in the infant during the first 6 months of life. Anti-SSA antibody is associated with congenital heart block.

14. **What are the indications for and risks of renal biopsy during pregnancy?**
Renal blood flow is increased during pregnancy, which increases the bleeding risk associated with biopsy except in the hands of the rare practitioner with extensive experience. Late in pregnancy, biopsy can be done either in the lateral position or seated and leaning forward on a table for support. The indications for biopsy include new-onset lupus, unexplained acute renal failure (including in transplanted kidneys), and nephritic syndrome. Biopsy is indicated for nephrotic syndrome only when it is severe enough that treatment is warranted and there is a need to know whether there is a responsive lesion in the kidney. One of the most frequent diagnostic dilemmas in pregnancy is distinguishing between preeclampsia and other renal problems, but severe hypertension or thrombocytopenia usually precludes doing a biopsy.

15. **What is diabetes insipidus of pregnancy?**
Diabetes insipidus of pregnancy is a rare disorder that occurs in the third trimester and resolves within a few weeks postpartum. It is characterized by polyuria; polydipsia; and, if inadequate free water is provided, hypernatremia. It is resistant to exogenous vasopressin and vasopressin levels may be normal or high. A second problem with urinary concentration may occur in women with partial central diabetes insipidus. The placenta makes vasopressinase, which breaks down endogenous vasopressin and exogenous vasopressin but not DDAVP (Desmopressin acetate) so that the DDAVP dose may need to be increased to offset accelerated breakdown of residual native antidiuretic hormone (ADH).

16. **How does pregnancy affect nephrolithiasis?**
Nephrolithiasis is the most common nonobstetric cause of abdominal pain during pregnancy. Pregnancy is characterized by factors that promote (increased urinary calcium and uric acid, decreased peristalsis of the ureter and dilatation of the collecting system) and prevent (increased urinary magnesium, citrate and acid glycoproteins) stone formation. Stones may be difficult to diagnose because hydronephrosis is normal in pregnancy and because radio-opaque stones can be obscured by the fetal skeleton, especially in the third trimester when stones are most common. Indications for intervention include intractable pain, infection, complete obstruction, or obstruction of a solitary kidney. Treatments include extraction of the stone by a skilled urologist or placement of percutaneous nephrostomy tubes. Pregnancy is considered a contraindication to lithotripsy.

KEY POINTS: RENAL DISEASE AND HYPERTENSION IN PREGNANCY

1. The major physiologic change in the kidney during pregnancy is a 50% increase in glomerular filtration rate.

2. The most recent explanation of the pathogenesis of preeclampsia is increased levels of antiangiogenic factors and low levels of angiogenic growth factors.

3. The most important predictor of maternal and fetal problems including prematurity, fetal loss, and loss of renal function is prepregnancy renal function.

4. There is a high rate of fetal loss among pregnant women undergoing dialysis, but the outcome of pregnancy in transplant recipients with stable, well-preserved renal function is good despite immunosuppressive medication.

17. **How do we distinguish among different causes of acute renal failure in pregnancy?**
See Table 49-1.

TABLE 49-1. DISTINGUISHING CAUSES OF ACUTE RENAL FAILURE IN PREGNANCY

	HUS	HELLP	Lupus Nephritis	AFLP	Cortical Necrosis
Creatinine	↑	↑ or nl	↑ or nl	↑ or nl	↑
Platelets	↓	↑	↓ or nl	↓ or nl	nl
Transaminases	nl	↑↑	nl	↑	nl
Lactate dehydrogenase	↑	↑	nl	↑	nl
PT/PTT	nl	↑ or nl	nl	↑	nl
Schistocytes	Yes	Yes	No	No	No
Blood pressure	↑	↑	↑ or nl	↓ or nl	↓, ↑, or nl
Progression	Frequent	Rare	Variable	No	Frequent

HUS = hemolytic uremic syndrome; HELLP = Hemolytic anemia, Elevated Liver enzymes, and Low Platelets; AFLP = acute fatty liver of pregnancy; PT/PTT = prothrombin time/partial thromboplastin time.
↑ = increased; ↓ = decreased; nl = normal.

BIBLIOGRAPHY

1. Armenti VT, Radomski JS, Moritz MJ, et al. Report from the National Transplantation Pregnancy registry: Outcomes of pregnancy after transplantation. In: Cecka JM, Terasaki PI (eds.). *Clinical Transplants 2001.* Los Angeles: UCLA Immunogenetics Center, 2002, pp. 97–105.
2. Barron WM, Cohen LH, Ulland LA, et al. Transient vasopressin resistant diabetes insipidus of pregnancy. *N Engl J Med* 1984;310:442–444.
3. Barua M, Hladunewick M, Keunen J, et al. Successful pregnancies on nocturnal home hemodialysis. *CJASN* 2008;3:392–396.
4. Hou S. Lupus in pregnancy. In: Lewis EJ, Schwartz MM, Korbet SM (eds.). *Lupus Nephritis.* Oxford: Oxford University Press, 1999.
5. Jones DC, Hayslett JP. Outcome of pregnancy in women with moderate or severe renal insufficiency. *N Engl J Med* 1996;335:226–232.
6. Matnard SE, Min JY, Merchan J, et al. Excess placental fms-like tyrosine kinase 1(sFlt1) may contribute to endothelial dysfunction, hypertension and proteinuria in preeclampsia. *J Clin Invest* 2003;111:649–658.
7. McKay DB, Josephson MA, Armenti VT, et al.; Women's Health Committee of the American Society of Transplantation. Reproduction and transplantation: Report of the AST Consensus Conference on Reproductive Issues and Transplantation. *Am J Transplant* 2005;5:1592–1599.
8. Okundaye IB, Abrinko P, Hou SH. A registry for pregnancy in dialysis patients. *Am J Kidney Dis* 1998;31:766–773.
9. Sibai BM. Drug therapy: Treatment of hypertension in pregnant women. *N Engl J Med* 1996;335:257–265.
10. Sibai BM, Ramadan MK, Chari RS, et al. Pregnancies complicated by HELLP syndrome (hemolysis, elevated liver enzymes and low platelets): Subsequent pregnancy outcome and long term prognosis. *Am J Obstet Gynecol* 1995;172:125–129.

CHAPTER 50

SICKLE CELL NEPHROPATHY

Edgar V. Lerma, MD

1. Discuss the pathophysiology of sickle cell disease.

Vaso-occlusive phenomena and hemolysis are the clinical hallmarks of sickle cell disease. The polymerization of deoxy hemoglobin S results in distortion of the red blood cell into the classic sickle shape and a marked decrease in red cell deformability and is the primary cause of vaso-occlusive phenomena. Subsequent changes in red cell membrane structure and function, disordered cell volume control, and increased adherence to vascular endothelium also play an important role.

Vaso-occlusion results in recurrent painful episodes and a variety of serious organ system complications that can lead to lifelong disabilities and even death. The renal manifestations of sickle cell disease will be reviewed in this chapter. The other manifestations, diagnosis, and management of this disorder and other sickle cell syndromes are discussed separately.

2. Discuss the pathophysiology of sickle cell nephropathy.

The primary event appears to be sickling of erythrocytes in the vasa recta capillaries in the medulla, leading to microthrombotic infarction and extravasation of blood in the medulla. Sickling is promoted by the normal medullary environment: low oxygen tension, low pH, and high osmolality (which pulls water out of the red cells, thereby increasing the concentration of hemoglobin S). The increased blood viscosity contributes to ischemia and infarction in the renal microcirculation. More severe occlusions can lead to renal infarcts and papillary necrosis.

Glomerular ischemia appears to promote increased renal blood flow and glomerular filtration rate (GFR). This is thought to be mediated primarily by vasodilator prostaglandins released presumably to reverse the medullary ischemia. It is this "hyperfiltration" phenomenon that makes creatinine-based equations to calculate GFR rather inaccurate.

There appears to be a positive correlation between glomerular hyperfiltration and chronic hemolysis. It has been suggested that this results from increased cardiac output and a hemolysis-mediated increase in vascular tone.

Progressive renal failure (glomerulosclerosis) occurs as a result of a combination of continued glomerular ischemia (leading to hypoperfusion), hypertrophy, and other undefined causes. Microangiopathic studies have demonstrated that the vasa recta are almost completely lost in older patients with sickle cell disease. Endothelin-1 (ET-1), stimulated by glomerular hypoxia, may also play a role.

Additional contributors include secondary hemodynamic injury induced by the intraglomerular hypertension and hypertrophy that drive the initial hyperfiltration and additional insults such as analgesic nephropathy secondary to consumption of large doses of analgesics.

3. What are the common presentations of patients with sickle cell nephropathy?

The structural consequences of sickled red blood cells in the renal circulation lead to the myriad renal manifestations seen in this disorder. Such manifestations are generally less common or less severe in patients with sickle cell trait, with the exception of renal medullary carcinoma, which appears to be more frequent among patients with sickle cell trait. The age at presentation of the various manifestations of renal disease varies widely.

- **Hematuria:** Painless microscopic or gross hematuria (resulting from papillary infarcts) is a common complaint that is also seen in patients with sickle cell trait. The renal bleeding is typically mild, unilateral (and predominantly left-sided), and self-limited. The predominant left-sided origin of the hematuria has been attributed to the greater length of the left renal vein and the "nutcracker phenomenon." The compression of the left renal vein between the aorta and superior mesenteric artery leads to increased blood pressure in the vein, thereby further increasing relative anoxia in the renal medulla, which promotes sickling.

- **Renal infarction and papillary necrosis:** More severe ischemia can lead to renal infarcts and papillary necrosis. Papillary necrosis commonly presents as painless gross hematuria and may be complicated by urinary tract infection (UTI) or obstruction. Acute segmental or total renal infarcts may present with nausea, vomiting, flank or abdominal pain, fever, and presumably renin-mediated hypertension.

- **Diminished concentrating ability:** An impairment in concentrating ability (hyposthenuria), leading to nocturia and polyuria, is an early and universal finding in sickle cell disease and is less severe and occurs later in the course of patients with sickle cell trait and sickle cell disease. Sickling in the vasa rectae presumably interferes with countercurrent exchange in the inner medulla, thereby leading to impairment of free water reabsorption.
  - However, both antidiuretic hormone generation and urinary-diluting capacity remain un-perturbed in patients with sickle cell disease. The preservation of normal urinary-diluting capacity is a result of intact reabsorptive function of the superficial loops of Henle of the cortical nephrons, which are supplied by peritubular capillaries and not the maximally affected vasa rectae.

- **Renal tubular acidosis:** Impaired distal hydrogen and potassium secretion can lead to an incomplete form of distal renal tubular acidosis, which can be associated with aldosterone-independent hyperkalemia. Although the exact mechanism is not clear, medullary blood flow disturbance and hypoxia may lead to insufficient energy to maintain the hydrogen ion and electrochemical gradients along the collecting ducts. However, these impairments are usually mild and can become clinically apparent only if there is a complicating factor such as potassium or acid loading or intravascular volume depletion or during rhabdomyolysis.

- **Abnormal proximal tubular function:** For reasons that are unclear, proximal tubular function is supranormal in sickle cell disease. This may be manifested by an elevated creatinine clearance (from enhanced creatinine secretion) in relation to the true GFR. This can also lead to increased secretion of uric acid in patients with sickle cell disease.

- **Acute kidney injury:** There are a number of potential etiologies for acute renal failure (ARF) among patients with sickle cell disease. As a result of impaired concentrating ability, they are predisposed to prerenal failure secondary to intravascular volume depletion. Intrinsic renal causes of ARF include rhabdomyolysis, sepsis, drug nephrotoxicity, renal vein thrombosis, and even hepatorenal syndrome (hemosiderosis-induced hepatic failure). Postrenal causes include urinary tract obstruction secondary to blood clots and, less commonly, papillary necrosis.

- **Progressive renal failure and proteinuria:** In patients with renal disease resulting from sickle cell disease, the GFR and renal blood flow are greater than normal in young patients and below normal in patients older than age 30 and may progressively fall thereafter, leading to end-stage renal failure.
  - Such progressive decline in GFR is often associated with increasing proteinuria. This course is different from the acute onset of the nephrotic syndrome typically seen in idiopathic primary focal glomerulosclerosis and minimal change disease. Thus, acute onset of nephrosis suggests that sickle cell disease is not the cause.
  - Less often, patients with sickle cell disease develop the nephrotic syndrome as a result of membranoproliferative glomerulonephritis. This may be related to a direct effect of sickled red blood cells, but patients may also have membranoproliferative glomerulonephritis (MPGN) associated with hepatitis C infection acquired from multiple blood transfusions.

- In addition to the nephropathy associated with sickle cell disease, it is also possible that the medullary ischemia induced by sickling can exacerbate the course of other underlying renal diseases.
- **Renal medullary carcinoma:** Renal medullary carcinoma is a highly aggressive malignancy found almost exclusively in young African American patients with sickle cell trait and, less commonly, sickle cell disease. Most patients are younger than 20 years of age at presentation, and there appears to be a male predominance.
  - Affected patients typically present with gross hematuria, urinary tract infection, flank pain, an abdominal mass, and/or involuntary weight loss. Metastatic disease is commonly present at the time of diagnosis; thus surgical resection is often not curative. There is very limited experience treating disseminated disease, and the prognosis is dismal; survival after diagnosis is usually less than 6 to 12 months.
- **Urinary tract infection:** Impaired immunity secondary to autosplenectomy, and consequent opsonic antibody deficiency, predisposes patients with sickle cell disease to infections by encapsulated organisms, including urinary tract infections. An additional predisposing factor to UTI is papillary necrosis.
- **Hypertension:** The incidence of hypertension among patients with sickle cell disease is markedly lower than observed in the general African American population, and some patients may have lower than normal blood pressure. Proposed mechanisms for this relative hypotension include sodium and water wasting as a result of the medullary defect, systemic vasodilatation compensating for microcirculatory flow disturbances, increased production of prostaglandins and nitric oxide, and reduced vascular reactivity. Therefore, relatively "normal" blood pressure levels in these patients may actually represent significant hypertension with attendant risks of adverse cardiovascular outcomes and severe hypotension may ensue with the use antihypertensive agents.

4. **What are the risk factors associated with progression of chronic kidney disease (CKD) to end-stage renal disease in patients with sickle cell nephropathy?**
   The following are considered as negative prognosticators:
   - Underlying hypertension
   - Nephrotic-range proteinuria
   - Hematuria
   - Severe anemia
   - Certain genetic factors, such as the Central African Republic globin gene cluster haplotype

5. **What tests are needed to diagnose sickle cell nephropathy?**
   The diagnosis of renal disease as a result of sickle cell disease is based on clinical manifestations and is largely a diagnosis of exclusion. We recommend that all patients suspected of having sickle cell disease–associated renal disease have the following tests performed:
   - Urinalysis with microscopy and quantitation of proteinuria
   - Estimation of kidney function
   - Renal ultrasound (For patients with hematuria, a computed tomography scan and intravenous pyelography should also be obtained)
   - Testing for hepatitis C and HIV
     A percutaneous renal biopsy may be in order but only if the urinalysis or course of renal failure and proteinuria suggest a glomerulonephritis.

6. **What are typical radiographic findings in sickle cell nephropathy?**
   - Increased echodensity and "garland" shadowing pattern of calcification in the medullary pyramids
   - Calyceal clubbing (seen in papillary necrosis)

7. **What is the mechanism by which hyperphosphatemia develops in patients with sickle cell nephropathy?**
There are two possible mechanisms by which hyperphosphatemia develops in these patients:
- Hemolysis commonly leads to an increased phosphate load, and
- The absorption of phosphate in the proximal tubules is increased as it parallels increased sodium reabsorption.

8. **What glomerular disorders are commonly seen in patients with sickle cell nephropathy?**
- **Focal segmental glomerulosclerosis:** In patients who progress to end-stage renal disease as a result of sickle cell disease, renal biopsy shows glomerular enlargement and focal segmental glomerulosclerosis (FSGS). A collapsing form of FSGS has been reported in literature.
- **Membranoproliferative glomerulonephritis:** MPGN with mesangial expansion and basement membrane duplication may be seen, either as an isolated finding or in association with focal segmental glomerulosclerosis. It has been suggested that this 'rare' form of MPGN is caused by fragmented red blood cells lodged in isolated capillary loops and phagocytosed by mesangial cells, stimulating expansion of the mesangium and new basement membrane deposition. The particular absence of immune complexes and electron-dense deposits differentiates this from idiopathic MPGN.
- HIV nephropathy has also been reported in earlier reports.

KEY POINTS: SICKLE CELL NEPHROPATHY

1. Vaso-occlusive phenomena and hemolysis are the clinical hallmarks of sickle cell disease. The primary event leading to renal involvement appears to be sickling of erythrocytes in the vasa recta capillaries leading to microthrombotic infarction and extravasation of blood in the medulla.

2. Renal failure may ensue in more than 10% of affected patients, but other clinically significant renal manifestations occur much more frequently.

3. Patients with sickle cell nephropathy may be particularly vulnerable to develop acute tubular necrosis as a result of hemodynamic insults or toxins, acute pyelonephritis, and urinary tract obstruction.

9. **What are the treatment approaches to patients with sickle cell nephropathy?**
- **Hematuria:** Because of its self-limited nature, conservative measures such as bed rest are recommended to avoid dislodging blood clots. There are case reports and case series of treatment of more severe cases via one or more of the following:
  - Hydration using alkaline fluids, with diuretics as needed to increase urine flow rate. This would help clear blood clots from the bladder, and the resulting diuresis may also help reduce medullary osmolality, thereby alleviating sickling in the vasa recta.
  - Blood transfusion to lower the concentration of hemoglobin S.
  - Some patients have been treated with oral urea in doses high enough to raise the blood urea nitrogen to 100 mg/dL (36 mmol/L) or higher. Urea presumably, acts by inhibiting the gelation of deoxygenated sickle hemoglobin. Although treatment with urea is commonly seen in these patients, the most likely rationale is to inhibit normal Hb S synthesis, allowing increased percentage of Hb E rather than the above.
  - In patients with hyperactive fibrinolysis who have severe, prolonged hematuria, administration of epsilon-aminocaproic acid (EACA) can diminish hematuria. There is, however, a risk of urinary tract obstruction as a result of the formation of blood clots within the collecting system. As a result, antifibrinolytic therapy should be considered only when all other modalities have failed.

- Angiographic localization followed by embolization of the involved renal vessel or balloon tamponade for bleeding due to papillary necrosis has been considered in some special situations.
- Unilateral nephrectomy has been performed, but it is not generally recommended because bleeding can recur in the contralateral kidney.
- Progression of CKD and hypertension.
  - Although not well established, it is theoretically probable that modalities aimed at lowering the intraglomerular pressure may be beneficial in patients with progressive renal disease. At present, there is little evidence to support the use of angiotensin-converting enzyme (ACE) inhibitors (or angiotensin II receptor blockers [ARB]) in these patients.
  - If the patient has hypertension, this should be controlled to recommended goals (<130/80 mm Hg). If an ACE or ARB is insufficient for blood pressure control, agents other than diuretics should be added because diuretics can cause intravascular volume depletion that may precipitate sickle cell crises.
  - The addition of hydroxyurea to an ACE or ARB may lead to further reduction of proteinuria.
  - Nonsteroidal anti-inflammatory drugs (NSAIDs) also prevent hyperfiltration. However, they are not recommended because they also reduce renal plasma flow and glomerular filtration rate in patients with sickle cell disease.
- **Anemia:** The optimal hemoglobin for patients with sickle cell anemia is lower than that for patients with anemia related only to chronic kidney disease. One recommendation is to maintain a hemoglobin concentration not higher than 10 g/dL (hematocrit 30%) with blood transfusions and/or erythropoietin and avoid a hematocrit rise of greater than 1% to 2% per week. Higher hemoglobin levels or a faster rise in hematocrit can precipitate a vaso-occlusive crisis.
  - The role of exogenously administered erythropoietin stimulating agents (ESAs) in the routine management of anemia in patients with sickle cell disease and kidney failure is uncertain. Some patients benefit from blood transfusions to increase the proportion of HbA, whereas ESAs, if used, may not have this beneficial effect. If used, standard doses of ESAs, as in patients with CKD, may be used (target hemoglobin 10 g/dL), although patients receiving hydroxyurea may require higher doses given the bone marrow–suppressive effect of this agent.
- **End-stage renal disease:** Among the various modes of renal replacement therapy available, most patients with end-stage renal disease resulting from sickle cell disease appear to be treated with some form of renal replacement therapy.

10. **What treatment options are available for patients with sickle cell nephropathy who progress to end-stage renal disease?**
    - **Dialysis:** The incidence of hemodialysis-related complications does not appear to be different in patients with sickle cell disease when compared to the general population, although survival appears to be diminished. However, patients with sickle cell disease tend to be substantially younger at initiation of dialysis (mean age 40 versus 60 years). Despite the lack of definitive survival benefit over hemodialysis, patients should receive full explanation of the potential risks and benefits to facilitate an informed decision.
    - **Renal transplantation:** There appears to be a lower rate of wait-listing for transplantation (7 versus 11 per 100 patient years) and of transplantation (2.6 versus 6.8 per 100 patient years) among patients with sickle cell disease compared to patients without sickle cell disease. Potential explanations for lower rates of transplantation, other than possible racial bias as in the general population, include high levels of panel reactive antibody as a result of numerous blood transfusions, concerns about a higher infection risk given their already immunocompromised state (autosplenectomy), increased risk of avascular necrosis as a result of steroids, and contributing to sickle cell crisis (attributed to the partial correction of anemia). Recurrent disease is relatively common because the underlying pathogenetic processes are still present; however, graft loss resulting from recurrent disease appears to be rare.

11. **What is the prognosis of patients with sickle cell nephropathy?**
Survival is decreased in patients with sickle cell disease who develop renal failure. Median survival among patients with and without renal failure was 29 and 51 years, respectively. The mortality risk of patients with renal failure was similar to those who had had a stroke.

Compared to patients with renal failure who do not have sickle cell disease, survival is substantially decreased among patients with renal failure and sickle cell disease, whether treated with dialysis or transplantation.

BIBLIOGRAPHY

1. Abbott KC, Hypolite IO, Agodoa LY. Sickle cell nephropathy at end-stage renal disease in the United States: Patient characteristics and survival. *Clin Nephrol* 2002;58:9.
2. Alvarez O, Lopez-Mitnik G, Zilleruelo G. Short-term follow-up of patients with sickle cell disease and albuminuria. *Pediatr Blood Cancer* 2008;50:1236.
3. Bleyer AJ, Donaldson LA, McIntosh M, et al. Relationship between underlying renal disease and renal transplantation outcome. *Am J Kidney Dis* 2001;37:1152.
4. Bruno D, Wigfall DR, Zimmerman SA, et al. Genitourinary complications of sickle cell disease. *J Urol* 2001;166:803.
5. Bunn HF. Pathogenesis and treatment of sickle cell disease. *N Engl J Med* 1997;337:762.
6. Chatterjee SN. National study in natural history of renal allografts in sickle cell disease or trait: A second report. *Transplant Proc* 1987;19:33.
7. Guasch A, Navarrete J, Nass K, et al. Glomerular involvement in adults with sickle cell hemoglobinopathies: Prevalence and clinical correlates of progressive renal failure. *J Am Soc Nephrol* 2006;17:2228.
8. Hakimi AA, Koi PT, Milhoua PM, et al. Renal medullary carcinoma: The Bronx experience. *Urology* 2007;70:878.
9. Halsey C, Roberts IA. The role of hydroxyurea in sickle cell disease. *Br J Haematol* 2003;120:177.
10. Haymann J-P, Stankovic K, Levy P, et al. Glomerular hyperfiltration in adult sickle cell anemia: a frequent hemolysis associated feature. *Clin J Am Soc Nephrol* 2010.
11. Lerma EV. Renal manifestations of sickle cell disease. *UpToDate* 2010.
12. Locatelli F, Aljama P, Barany P, et al. Revised European best practice guidelines for the management of anaemia in patients with chronic renal failure. *Nephrol Dial Transplant* 2004;19 Suppl 2:ii1.
13. Nasr SH, Markowitz GS, Sentman RL, et al. Sickle cell disease, nephrotic syndrome, and renal failure. *Kidney Int* 2006;69:1276.
14. Scheinman J. Sickle cell nephropathy. In: Lerma EV, Berns JS, Nissenson AR (eds.). *Current Diagnosis and Treatment in Nephrology and Hypertension.* New York: McGraw-Hill, 2008.
15. Scheinman JI. Tools to detect and modify sickle cell nephropathy. *Kidney Int* 2006;69:1927.
16. ter Maaten JC, Gans ROB, De Jong PE. Sickle cell nephropathy. In: Johnson RJ, Feehally J (eds.). *Comphrehensive Clinical Nephrology* Philadelphia: Elsevier, 2003, p. 665.
17. Tharaux PL, Hagege I, Placier S, et al. Urinary endothelin-1 as a marker of renal damage in sickle cell disease. *Nephrol Dial Transplant* 2005;20:2408.
18. Wesson DE. The initiation and progression of sickle cell nephropathy. *Kidney Int* 2002;61:2277.

CHAPTER 51

RENAL DISEASES IN THE ELDERLY

Meryem Tuncel, MD; Moshe Levi, MD; and Devasmita Choudhury, MD

1. **What is the prevalence of chronic kidney disease in the elderly?**
   Approximately 11% of patients older than age 65 years are noted to have chronic kidney disease (CKD) as estimated by using the Modification of Diet in Renal Disease (MDRD) study equation in those participating in National Health and Nutrition Examination Survey III. As the proportion of elderly increases in the population as a whole, the number of elderly patients with CKD is also expected to increase.

   Campbell KH, O'Hare AM. Kidney disease in the elderly: Update on recent literature. *Curr Opin Nephrol Hypertens* 2008;17(3):298–303.

   Coresh J, Astor BC, Greene T, et al. Prevalence of chronic kidney disease and decreased kidney function in the adult US population: Third National Health and Nutrition Examination Survey. *Am J Kidney Dis* 2003;41(1):1–12.

   Knickman JR, Snell EK. The 2030 problem: caring for aging baby boomers. *Health Serv Res* 2002;37(4):849–884.

2. **What structural changes occur in the kidney with age?**
   A progressive decrease in kidney weight and size occurs with increasing age as the glomeruli and the interstitium undergo fibrosis and sclerosis, tubules atrophy with drop in number and size, and vasculature scleroses and simplifies (Fig. 51-1). Individual rates of renal senescence may vary as various factors that are known to mediate fibrosis such as angiotensin II, transforming growth factor, nitric oxide, advanced glycosylated end products, oxidative stress, and factors associated with reducing sclerosis such as calorie restriction, Klotho (antiaging transmembrane protein) are altered as the kidney ages.

   Takazakura E, Sawabu N, Handa A, et al. Intrarenal vascular changes with age and disease. *Kidney Int* 1972;2(4):224–230.

3. **How does age affect kidney function?**
   Functional changes in the kidney occur in parallel to changes in structure.
   - **Decreased effective renal plasma flow (ERPF):** ERPF decreases approximately 10% per decade with age in relation to progressive vascular sclerosis and loss of nephron number. Both changes in the number of functioning glomeruli and altered intrarenal signal and response to vasodilatory and vasoconstrictive mediators may affect renal plasma flow in the elderly.
   - **Decrease in glomerular filtration rate (GFR):** An estimated drop of 0.8 to 1.0 mL/min/1.73 m^2 per year in GFR is noted with progressive age depending on methodology used to measure clearance. Decreases in GFR with age may also be affected by race and underlying comorbidities including hypertension, diabetes, and cardiovascular disease.
   - **Decreased ability to conserve filtered sodium:** An increase in solute load per nephron in the face of decreased nephron number and increased medullary flow, and lower levels of plasma renin and aldosterone with age, likely contribute to individuals 60 years and older taking nearly twice the number of hours (31 versus 18 hours) compared to those 30 years and younger to reach appropriate distal tubular sodium reabsorption when sodium restriction is imposed.

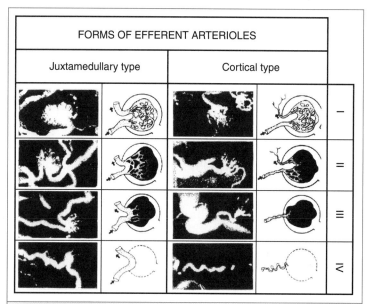

Figure 51-1. Stages of progressive vascular simplification and glomerular degeneration of cortical and juxtamedullary glomeruli and arterioles with associated microangiograms. (From Takazakura E, Sawabu N, Handa A, et al. Intravascular changes with age and disease. *Kidney Int* 1972;2:224. Reprinted by permission from Macmillan Publishers Ltd.)

- **Decreased natriuretic ability:** Individuals older than 40 years also handle a salt load less efficiently, as seen by taking a longer time to excrete 2 L of saline than those younger than 40 years. Although levels of the natriuretic hormone atrial natriuretic peptide appropriately increase, an incremental increase in urine sodium excretion is not evident in older compared to younger subjects, suggesting a possible decreased tubular sensitivity to natriuretic stimuli.
- **Abnormal tubular concentrating and diluting capacity:** The older individual may not be able to reach maximal urinary concentration despite 12 hours of overnight water deprivation. As vascular simplification occurs in parallel to glomerular and tubular senescence leading to decreased cortical blood flow but maintained medullary blood flow, there is suspected "medullary washout" with increased solute and osmolar clearance. In addition, studies in aged animals indicate decrease in tubular transporters, Na-K-2CL, and ENaC beta and gamma subunits and intrarenal resistance to arginine vasopressin. Similarly, maximally dilute urine is also not found with increasing age given that appropriate solute extraction, suppression of arginine vasopressin, and distal delivery of the filtered load is necessary.
- **Decreased net acid excretion:** A diminished capacity for net acid excretion is found in older adults as both renal mass and GFR decrease are particularly noted when there is increased acid generation or acid load.
- **Changes in potassium handling:** Although total body potassium is lower given a decrease in muscle mass in older individuals, lower plasma renin and aldosterone levels in the elderly predispose to decreased tubular excretion of potassium. In the face of sudden potassium load, older individuals may have a decreased ability to shift potassium into cells because Na-K-ATPase activity is found to be decreased with increasing age.

- **Decreased renal phosphate reabsorption:** With phosphate restriction, older kidneys display evidence for decreased tubular phosphate absorption.
- **Tubular calcium excretion:** Remains unchanged in the kidney with increasing age.

Adler S, Lindeman RD, Yiengst MJ, et al. Effect of acute acid loading on urinary acid excretion by the aging human kidney. *J Lab Clin Med* 1968;72(2):278–289.

Armbrecht HJ, Zenser TV, Gross CJ, et al. Adaptation to dietary calcium and phosphorus restriction changes with age in the rat. *Am J Physiol* 1980;239(5):E322–327.

Back SE, Ljungberg B, Nilsson-Ehle I, et al. Age dependence of renal function: clearance of iohexol and p-amino hippurate in healthy males. *Scand J Clin Lab Invest* 1989;49(7):641–646.

Bauer JH. Age-related changes in the renin-aldosterone system. Physiological effects and clinical implications. *Drugs Aging* 1993;3(3):238–245.

Berg UB. Differences in decline in GFR with age between males and females. Reference data on clearances of inulin and PAH in potential kidney donors. *Nephrol Dial Transplant* 2006;21(9):2577–2582.

Crowe MJ, Forsling ML, Rolls BJ, et al. Altered water excretion in healthy elderly men. *Age Ageing* 1987;16(5):285–293.

Epstein M, Hollenberg NK. Age as a determinant of renal sodium conservation in normal man. *J Lab Clin Med* 1976;87(3):411–417.

Fliser D, Franek E, Joest M, et al. Renal function in the elderly: impact of hypertension and cardiac function. *Kidney Int* 1997;51(4):1196–1204.

Ford GA, Blaschke TF, Wiswell R, et al. Effect of aging on changes in plasma potassium during exercise. *J Gerontol* 1993;48(4):M140–145.

Frassetto LA, Morris RC Jr, Sebastian A. Effect of age on blood acid-base composition in adult humans: role of age-related renal functional decline. *Am J Physiol* 1996;271(6 Pt 2):F1114–1122.

Levi M, Jameson DM, van der Meer BW. Role of BBM lipid composition and fluidity in impaired renal Pi transport in aged rat. *Am J Physiol* 1989;256(1 Pt 2):F85–94.

Luft FC, Fineberg NS, Miller JZ, et al. The effects of age, race and heredity on glomerular filtration rate following volume expansion and contraction in normal man. *Am J Med Sci* 1980;279(1):15–24.

Luft FC, Grim CE, Fineberg N, et al. Effects of volume expansion and contraction in normotensive whites, blacks, and subjects of different ages. *Circulation* 1979;59(4):643–650.

Ohashi M, Fujio N, Nawata H, et al. High plasma concentrations of human atrial natriuretic polypeptide in aged men. *J Clin Endocrinol Metab* 1987;64(1):81–85.

Ribstein J, Du Cailar G, Mimran A. Glucose tolerance and age-associated decline in renal function of hypertensive patients. *J Hypertens* 2001;19(12):2257–2264.

Rowe JW, Shock NW, DeFronzo RA. The influence of age on the renal response to water deprivation in man. *Nephron* 1976;17(4):270–278.

Tajima F, Sagawa S, Iwamoto J, et al. Renal and endocrine responses in the elderly during head-out water immersion. *Am J Physiol* 1988;254(6 Pt 2):R977–983.

Tauchi H, Tsuboi K, Okutomi J. Age changes in the human kidney of the different races. *Gerontologia* 1971;17(2):87–97.

Tian Y, Riazi S, Khan O, et al. Renal ENaC subunit, Na-K-2Cl and Na-Cl cotransporter abundances in aged, water-restricted F344 x Brown Norway rats. *Kidney Int* 2006;69(2):304–312.

Weidmann P, De Myttenaere-Bursztein S, Maxwell MH, et al. Effect on aging on plasma renin and aldosterone in normal man. *Kidney Int* 1975;8(5):325–333.

4. **Why are the elderly more susceptible to osmolar disorders such as hyponatremia and hypernatremia?**

   With inability to maximally dilute urine, the elderly face a greater likelihood for hyponatremia when situations lead to increased arginine vasopressin (AVP) secretion or response. Medications such as morphine (high dose), nicotine, vincristine, and cyclophosphamide can enhance, whereas chlorpropamide, tolbutamide, nonsteroidal agents, and lamotrigine may promote AVP action. Hyponatremia with thiazide-type diuretics, commonly used to treat hypertension, is more common in the elderly. Similarly the presence of a decreased thirst response in addition to a urinary-concentrating defect can predispose older individuals to hypernatremia. Medications associated with decreased AVP secretion such as morphine (low dose), fluphenazine, promethazine, carbamazepine, and Haldol or decreased AVP response including propoxyphene, demeclocycline, glyburide, and lithium may increase likelihood of developing hypernatremia in older patients.

5. **What makes older kidneys susceptible to kidney injury?**

Acute kidney injury occurs with 3.5 times greater prevalence in those older than 70 years, with nearly one third unable to regain kidney function after an acute insult. Loss of nephron number and function and decreased vascular response to vasodilation in aging contributes to decreased renal reserve. Thus any process that further compromises renal perfusion or loss of nephron function including prerenal, intrinsic, or postrenal increases susceptibility to renal injury. Volume loss, marked vasoconstriction, or decreased cardiac output are frequent prerenal processes in the elderly with numerous comorbidities such as hypertension, diabetes, heart failure, malignancy, or atherosclerosis. Medications, including angiotensin-converting enzyme inhibitors or angiotensin receptor blockers, and nonsteroidal agents or contrast infusion, can exacerbate the prerenal process, thereby requiring careful volume assessment before use. Intrinsic renal processes such as toxin-associated tubular dysfunction (i.e., aminoglycosides), interstitial inflammation (i.e., antibiotic or other drug mediated), or manipulation of the arterial tree leading to cholesterol embolization are often evident in the older individuals undergoing diagnoses and treatment for comorbid illnesses. Urinary tract obstruction can present with acute decline in renal function in the elderly given laxity or overgrowth of pelvic structures with age and enlarged or prolapsed uterus in females and prostatic hypertrophy in male patients.

Xue JL, Daniels F, Star RA, et al. Incidence and mortality of acute renal failure in Medicare beneficiaries, 1992 to 2001. *J Am Soc Nephrol* 2006;17(4):1135–1142.

6. **What are the best ways to estimate renal clearance in the elderly?**

Given loss of muscle mass with age, serum creatinine may not be the most useful marker for estimating renal clearance. When appropriately collected, 24-hour urine creatinine clearances can be useful to measure steady-state clearances in the elderly. Formulas derived from 24-hour urine collections of populations of elderly with and without renal disease are frequently used to estimate GFR at the bedside (Table 51-1), minimizing frequent cumbersome 24-hour urine clearances in the elderly. Radioisotopes including iothalamate or iohexol x-ray fluorescence can be accurate; however, expense, radioactivity exposure, and availability limit these procedures for routine GFR measurements.

7. **How does age affect blood pressure?**

Data from the National Health and Nutrition Examination Survey (NHANES) report 67% of adults ≥60 years have hypertension. Changes in vascular elasticity with altered extracellular matrix cross-linking, fibrosis, and calcium deposition with age lead to stiffness and decreased capacity in the larger elastic vasculature. Older adults are thus noted to have high systolic blood pressure (SBP) and low diastolic blood pressure (DBP) with subsequent widened pulse pressure. Isolated systolic hypertension (ISH), defined as SBP >160 mm Hg and DBP <90 mm Hg, can be found in 75% of elderly patients with hypertension.

Franklin SS, Jacobs MJ, Wong ND, et al. Predominance of isolated systolic hypertension among middle-aged and elderly US hypertensives: Analysis based on National Health and Nutrition Examination Survey (NHANES) III. *Hypertension* 2001;37(3):869–874.

Ostchega Y, Dillon CF, Hughes JP, et al. Trends in hypertension prevalence, awareness, treatment, and control in older U.S. adults: data from the National Health and Nutrition Examination Survey 1988 to 2004. *J Am Geriatr Soc* 2007;55(7):1056–1065.

8. **What is the importance of isolated systolic hypertension in the elderly?**

ISH is associated with a twofold to fourfold increase in the risk of myocardial infarction, left ventricular hypertrophy, renal dysfunction, stroke, and cardiovascular mortality. Even in patients who also have diastolic hypertension, the cardiovascular risk correlates more closely with the systolic than the diastolic BP. Among elderly patients, coronary heart disease risk varies directly with the systolic and pulse pressures and inversely with the diastolic pressure.

TABLE 51-1. EQUATIONS FOR ESTIMATING GFR IN THE ELDERLY

COCKCROFT-GAULT EQUATION

$$\text{Creatinine clearance (mL/min)} = \frac{(140 - age) \times weight\,(kg)}{72 \times serum\,creatinine\,(mg\,/\,DL)^{*}}$$

MODIFICATION OF DIET IN RENAL DISEASE EQUATION (MDRD)

GFR (mL/min) = 170 × (pcr) − 0.999 × (age) − 0.0176 × (0.762 if female) × (1.180 if African American) × (SUN) − 0.0170 × (albumin)

CKD-EPI GFR ESTIMATE ON THE NATURAL SCALE

African American

Female	≤62 (≤0.7)	GFR = $166 \times (scr/0.7)^{-0.329} \times (0.993)^{age}$
	>62 (>0.7)	GFR = $166 \times (scr/0.7)^{-0.209} \times (0.993)^{age}$
Male	≤80 (≤0.9)	GFR = $163 \times (scr/0.9)^{-0.411} \times (0.993)^{age}$
	>80 (>0.9)	GFR = $163 \times (scr/0.9)^{-0.209} \times (0.993)^{age}$

White or Other

Female	≤62 (≤0.7)	GFR = $144 \times (scr/0.7)^{-0.329} \times (0.993)^{age}$
	>62 (>0.7)	GFR = $144 \times (scr/0.7)^{-0.209} \times (0.993)^{age}$
Male	≤80 (≤0.9)	GFR = $141 \times (scr/0.9)^{-0.411} \times (0.993)^{age}$
	>80 (>0.9)	GFR = $141 \times (scr/0.9)^{-0.209} \times (0.993)^{age}$

*15% less in females.
GFR = glomerular filtration rate; Pcr = plasma creatinine; SUN = serum urea nitrogen; Scr = serum creatinine (mg/dl or μmol/L).
Equations obtained from Cockcroft DW, Gault MH. Prediction of creatinine clearance from serum creatinine. *Nephron* 1976;16(1):31–41; Levey AS, Bosch JP, Lewis JB, et al. A more accurate method to estimate glomerular filtration rate from serum creatinine: A new prediction equation. Modification of Diet in Renal Disease Study Group. *Ann Intern Med* 1999;130(6):461–470; and Levey AS, Stevens LA, Schmid CH, et al. A new equation to estimate glomerular filtration rate. *Ann Intern Med* 2009;150(9):604–612.

9. **Should target blood pressure in the elderly be the same as in younger patients?**
Although treatment of elevated blood pressure in the elderly, including those older than 80 years of age, is clearly beneficial, goals of SBP <140 mm Hg for the general population may need to be adjusted for those with ISH and for patients age 80 years and older. When treating elderly patients with isolated systolic hypertension, no clear data provide guidance related to the minimum diastolic BP that can be tolerated. An analysis from the SHEP trial found significant increases in cardiovascular events in the active treatment group when the diastolic BP was ≤60 mm Hg. Among patients being treated for ISH, the post-treatment diastolic blood pressure should be >60 mm Hg overall or, in patients with known coronary artery disease, >65 mm Hg unless symptoms that could be attributable to hypoperfusion occur at higher pressures. SBP goals should not be reached at the expense of excessive DBP reduction.

Beckett NS, Peters R, Fletcher AE, et al. Treatment of hypertension in patients 80 years of age or older. *N Engl J Med* 2008;358(18):1887–1898.

Chobanian AV, Bakris GL, Black HR, et al. The Seventh Report of the Joint National Committee on Prevention, Detection, Evaluation, and Treatment of High Blood Pressure: The JNC 7 report. *JAMA* 2003;289(19):2560–2572.

Staessen JA, Gasowski J, Wang JG, et al. Risks of untreated and treated isolated systolic hypertension in the elderly: Meta-analysis of outcome trials. *Lancet* 2000;355(9207):865–872.

10. **What are important considerations in treating hypertension in the elderly?**
    BP reduction should always be gradual in elderly patients. All patients should receive nonpharmacologic therapy, particularly dietary salt restriction and weight loss in patients who are obese. Drug therapy should be started if lifestyle changes are not sufficient. A potential limiting factor to the use of antihypertensive drugs is that orthostatic (postural) and/or postprandial hypotension is common among elderly patients with hypertension. A long-acting dihydropyridine or a thiazide diuretic is generally preferred in elderly patients because of increased efficacy in blood pressure lowering.

11. **Does revascularization in atherosclerotic renovascular disease improve outcomes in comparison to medical therapy alone?**
    With age, vascular changes, and as part of generalized atherosclerosis, atherosclerotic renovascular disease (ARVD) prevalence is estimated at 6.8% in community-dwelling patients older than age 65. Heightened suspicion for ARVD in older patients should occur when sudden increase in blood pressure or worsening of renal function is noted. Screening methodologies including duplex ultrasonography, computed tomographic angiography, or magnetic resonance angiography in conjunction with functional significance for underlying stenotic lesions should be utilized based on patient tolerance and test availability. Medical therapy with antihypertensives, particularly agents blocking the renin-angiotensin system, are useful, although careful follow-up is necessary in the face of high-grade bilateral stenotic lesions given an associated drop in GFR. Although concern for loss of renal mass or poorly controlled hypertension with risk for increased cardiovascular events endorses need for a revascularization procedure either percutaneous or surgical, a recent randomized trial showed no evidence for increased clinical benefit in the initial years after revascularization in patients with atherosclerotic renal-artery stenosis when compared to medical therapy. No significant improvements in blood pressure or reductions in renal or cardiovascular events or mortality were seen.

Mailloux LU, Napolitano B, Bellucci AG, Vernace M, Wilkes BM, Mossey RT. Renal vascular disease causing end-stage renal disease, incidence, clinical correlates, and outcomes: A 20-year clinical experience. *Am J Kidney Dis* 1994;24(4):622–629.

Wheatley K, Ives N, Gray R, et al. Revascularization versus medical therapy for renal-artery stenosis. *N Engl J Med* 2009;361(20):1953–1962.

12. **What glomerular diseases are common in the elderly?**
    Elderly patients presenting with nephritic sediment and acute or rapidly progressive kidney failure often have pauci-immune glomerulonephritis, although antiglomerular basement membrane and postinfectious glomerulonephritis should also be considered.

    A nephrotic presentation, particularly not diabetes related, is commonly associated with membranous glomerulopathy. Although minimal change disease is most common in children, it can be seen in 1 out of 10 older adults with nephrosis. Amyloidosis should also be suspected in older adults with marked proteinuria. Secondary etiologies such as malignancy for these presentations should also be investigated in the older adults given increased association of solid tumors with membranous renal lesions, Hodgkin's and non-Hodgkin's lymphoma with minimal change disease, and the presence of paraproteinemia with amyloidosis.

Davison AM, Johnston PA. Glomerulonephritis in the elderly. *Nephrol Dial Transplant* 1996;11(Suppl 9):34–37.

13. **What is the most common cause for mortality the elderly with chronic kidney disease?**
    The presence of CKD adds further burden to underlying cardiovascular risks and disease noted with age. As prevalence of hypertension increases with age, lipid abnormalities are also

seen with aging and CKD. Dyslipidemia in the elderly is characterized by increased triglyceride levels, small high-dense low-density lipoprotein (LDL), and a low concentration of high-density lipoprotein (HDL), characteristics similar to CKD. Therefore it is not unusual that mortality in elderly with CKD results more from cardiovascular causes than in the progression of kidney disease and kidney failure. Cardiovascular risk management in elderly with CKD becomes particularly important.

Choudhury D, Tuncel M, Levi M. Disorders of lipid metabolism and chronic kidney disease in the elderly. *Semin Nephrol* 2009;29(6):610–620.

O'Hare AM, Choi AI, Bertenthal D, et al. Age affects outcomes in chronic kidney disease. *J Am Soc Nephrol* 2007;18(10):2758–2765.

14. **Does modality of renal replacement affect outcome in the elderly?**
Neither hemodialysis nor peritoneal dialysis in the elderly is clearly associated with a survival advantage, although some epidemiologic studies suggest a higher mortality for elderly patients, particularly with diabetes, undergoing peritoneal dialysis. At this time, modality choice in the elderly should be individualized based on the ability to reach adequate clearance and tolerability of the procedure, considering both medical and psychosocial factors for each person.

15. **What is the best hemodialysis access in elderly patients with end-stage renal disease (ESRD)?**
If the patient does not have severe peripheral vascular disease, the initial attempt at vascular access surgery should be an arteriovenous fistula resulting from a lower incidence of infectious complications.

16. **What are considered major contraindications to dialysis in the elderly?**
The major contraindications to dialysis are advanced malignancy, irreversible dementia, or advanced liver disease.

17. **Does transplant have advantages over dialysis in the elderly?**
Specific data evaluating relative mortality for dialysis versus transplantation or comparing quality of life for the elderly patient with ESRD is lacking. Thus, currently it remains unclear whether the possible benefits with transplantation are sufficiently great for the clinician to advocate transplantation over dialysis in the elderly patient with ESRD.

18. **What is the major cause of renal transplant graft loss in the elderly?**
Renal transplant graft loss in the elderly is related primarily to patient death. Two main causes of morbidity and mortality in the elderly following renal transplantation are cardiovascular disease and infection.

19. **What are the important considerations for immunosuppression in the elderly?**
Immunosuppressive therapy must be modified in the elderly transplant recipient because immune-competence lessens, thereby resulting in a decreased likelihood of immunologic rejection but increasing the risk of infection. The other important consideration is altered pharmacokinetics and effects of drugs in the elderly. Some studies suggest that lower levels of immunosuppression may be sufficient in elderly patients to achieve adequate patient and graft survival.

Martins PN, Pratschke J, Pascher A, et al. Age and immune response in organ transplantation. *Transplantation* 2005;79(2):127–132.

20. **What is the patient and graft survival in the elderly renal transplant recipient?**
Recipient survival is affected by allograft type. Recipient survival at 1, 3, and 5 years from 2007 registry data are reported to be 99%, 96%, and 79%, respectively, for living donor recipients ≥65 years; 97%, 92%, and 67%, respectively, for deceased nonextended criteria donor; and 95%, 88%, and 58%, respectively, for deceased extended criteria donor grafts.

Registry data of 2007 also note excellent allograft survival for recipients ≥65 years after 1, 3, and 5 years with living donor allografts having better outcome with 97%, 94%, and 73%, respectively, followed by deceased nonextended criteria donor graft survival of 94%, 86%, and 60%, respectively, and 91%, 81%, and 49% for deceased extended criteria donors, respectively.

The 2007 Annual Report of the OPTN and SRTR: Transplant Data 1997–2006. The 2007 Annual Report of the OPTN and SRTR: Transplant Data 1997–2006. Available at www.ustransplant.org/annual_reports/ accessed August 2009. 2009.

21. **What is the prevalence of simple cysts in older people?**

The prevalence of simple cysts increases with age. Presence of at least one or more simple cysts is found in approximately 11.5% of those aged 50 to 70 years. The prevalence appears to double to 22.1% in those older than age 70 years and has been reported as high as 36.1% in those older than age 80 years, with a 2:1 frequency in men compared to women.

Terada N, Ichioka K, Matsuta Y, et al. The natural history of simple renal cysts. *J Urol* 2002;167(1):21–23.

Yahalom G, Schwartz R, Schwammenthal Y, et al. Chronic kidney disease and clinical outcome in patients with acute stroke. *Stroke* 2009;40(4):1296–1303.

KEY POINTS: RENAL DISEASES IN THE ELDERLY

1. Both effective renal plasma flow and glomerular filtration rate decrease in parallel to progressive sclerotic changes seen in glomeruli, interstitium, and vasculature of the aging kidney.

2. A decrease in both concentrating and diluting ability can predispose elderly patients to osmolar disorders of hyponatremia and hypernatremia.

3. Decreased renal reserve with aging increases susceptibility for acute kidney injury.

4. Isolated systolic hypertension is most common in the elderly.

5. Blood pressure reduction should always be gradual in older patients.

6. Membranous nephropathy is common in older patients presenting with nephrotic syndrome, and pauci-immune glomerulonephritis can be a common presentation of rapidly progressive glomerulonephritis in older patients.

7. Revascularization for atherosclerotic renal artery lesions may not add benefit to treatment with medical therapy alone.

8. Elderly patients with chronic kidney disease die primarily from cardiovascular disease.

9. Renal transplant graft loss in the elderly is primarily from patient death.

10. The prevalence of simple cysts increases with age.

HEMODIALYSIS

Michael V. Rocco, MD

CHAPTER 52

TECHNICAL ASPECTS OF HEMODIALYSIS

1. **What are the components used during a dialysis procedure?**

   To conduct dialysis, it is required to have a dialysis machine, a method to access the patient's arterial and/or venous system, and a supply of treated water. The dialysis machine consists of two major components: (1) a blood pump and associated safety equipment for the blood pump to monitor pressures in the system and to ensure that air does not enter the blood circuit and (2) a dialysate pump, with associated safety devices to ensure that the dialysate is at the correct temperature, has the correct concentration of electrolytes, and has not been exposed to blood from a leak in the dialyzer membrane. The dialysis machine uses the blood pump to move blood through the dialysis circuit, from the patient, through the dialyzer, and back to the patient. The patient needs to have some type of access to allow for the rapid removal and replacement of blood during the dialysis procedure. Treated water is needed to make the dialysate used during the dialysis procedure.

2. **What is a dialysis access?**

   A dialysis access allows blood to be removed from the patient, sent to the dialyzer, and then returned to the patient. The minimum blood flow rate that should be delivered is 300 mL/min; thus, peripheral intravenous (IV) lines, Hickman catheters, and peripherally inserted central catheter (PICC) lines cannot be used for this purpose because none of these devices can deliver a high blood flow rate. There are three different types of vascular access that can be used for hemodialysis: an arteriovenous fistula, a GORE-TEX graft, or a catheter. The preferred type of vascular access is an arteriovenous (AV) fistula. The AV fistula is created by making a surgical anastomosis between an artery in the forearm or upper arm with an adjacent vein. Over a period of 4 to 8 weeks, the increased pressure that the vein is exposed to from the arterial bed causes the vein to dilate and develop a thicker vessel wall. Once the fistula has matured, defined as a blood flow rate of at least 600 mL/min and a diameter of at least 6 mm, the fistula can be cannulated with dialysis needles to allow for the removal and return of blood. Typically, 15-gauge needles are used as dialysis needles, although smaller needles may be used at first if the fistula is not fully mature. A GORE-TEX graft is created by the surgical interposition of a synthetic blood vessel between an artery and a vein. Both the AV fistula and the GORE-TEX graft are below the skin. An AV fistula is preferred over a GORE-TEX graft because the AV fistula has fewer complications and a longer primary and secondary patency rate. Specifically, there is a much higher rate in grafts versus fistulas of intimal hyperplasia at the vein anastomosis, resulting in stenosis and ultimately obstruction with thrombosis and a higher infection rates with grafts versus fistulas as a result of the presence of a foreign body. A catheter is used for hemodialysis access when a patient requires dialysis and does not have a mature AV fistula or GORE-TEX graft. This circumstance can occur if either the patient needs dialysis acutely and does not have a functional AV fistula or GORE-TEX graft in place or if the patient has no suitable site to place an AV fistula or GORE-TEX graft and thus uses the catheter for permanent hemodialysis access. Catheters are least desirable because patients with this access have a higher rate of morbidity and mortality than patients with either AV grafts or AV fistulas. More permanent catheters are usually placed into the superior vena cava through the internal jugular vein using a subcutaneous tunnel to decrease the risk of infection. Temporary catheters can be placed without a subcutaneous tunnel into an internal jugular vein or into a femoral vein.

3. **What is a dialyzer?**
A dialyzer consists of a container that contains a semipermeable membrane that separates the dialysate from the blood that has been removed from the patient. A hollow fiber dialyzer, the type most commonly used today, consists of a cylinder that contains more than 10,000 hollow fibers that are made of a semipermeable material. To maximize the diffusion that takes place between the blood and dialysate, blood travels through the hollow fibers and dialysate flows around the outside of these hollow fibers in a countercurrent direction from the blood. The size of the dialyzer is measured by the surface area of the semipermeable membrane and is expressed in square meters. Most adult hemodialysis membranes have a surface area between 1.5 and 2.5 m^2; pediatric dialyzers are often less than 1 meter squared. A number of different materials are used for the semipermeable membranes. These materials vary in the degree to which small and middle molecules can pass through the membrane, which in turn is determined by the number and size of the pores in the dialyzer membrane. In the United States, most membranes are composed of either semisynthetic or synthetic materials that allow for the removal of larger molecules to some degree. Typical dialyzer membranes consist of polysulfone, polyethersulfone, cellulose acetate, biacetate or triacetate, or polyamides.

4. **What is dialysate?**
Dialysate is a physiologic solution that consists of inorganic ions found in the body and glucose. The dialysate concentration of sodium and chloride is usually physiologic, whereas the concentration of magnesium and phosphorus is usually less than physiologic to allow for removal of these substances on dialysis. The bicarbonate concentration is usually higher than the physiologic concentration to allow for the treatment of metabolic acidosis that is common in patients undergoing dialysis. Typically, several different potassium and calcium concentrations are available so that the rate of removal of these ions can be varied as clinical circumstances dictate. The dialysate flows through the dialyzer in a countercurrent direction, preferably at a rate that is at least 100 mL/min higher than the blood flow rate to maximize diffusion. The temperature of the dialysate is usually set at just below the patient's body temperature because this will allow for vasoconstriction and thus minimize the risk of hypotension with volume removal on dialysis. The dialysate temperature can be adjusted by 1°C to 2°C to assist with volume removal.

5. **What occurs during the dialysis procedure?**
The two processes that occur during a hemodialysis session are diffusion and ultrafiltration. Diffusion refers to a process by which small and middle molecules move, based on concentration gradients, between the blood and dialysate compartments of a dialyzer via a semipermeable membrane. Molecules can move through the semipermeable membrane by both diffusion and ultrafiltration. Small molecules move across the semipermeable membrane from an area of higher concentration (usually the blood) to an area of lower concentration (usually the dialysate). The overall effect is to remove small molecules that are likely to be toxins in high concentrations (such as potassium, phosphorus, and urea) while repleting those small molecules that are likely to be deficient (such as calcium or bicarbonate). Larger molecules do not move as readily across the membrane, and molecules that are bound to protein are unlikely to be removed by dialysis. In addition, fluid can be removed during the dialysis procedure via the process of ultrafiltration (see Question 7).

6. **What determines the rate of toxin removal?**
   The rate of toxin removal is traditionally measured by the removal of urea. The removal of urea during the hemodialysis session is increased by any of these factors:
   - **Higher blood flow rate and dialysis flow rate:** The higher the blood flow rate, the more urea diffusion that will occur per unit time. The limiting factor is the dialysis access, with a fistula usually being able to deliver the highest flow rates (up to about 550 mL/min) and a catheter usually being able to deliver the lowest flow rates (300–350 mL/min).
   - **Higher efficiency of the dialyzer:** A higher-efficiency dialyzer typically has a large surface area, a thin membrane, and increased porosity. This efficiency is expressed as the dialyzer mass transfer area coefficient or KoA of the dialyzer.
   - **Longer time on dialysis:** The longer the time for a single dialysis treatment, the more urea diffusion will occur. However, the urea removal per hour diminishes with each additional hour of dialysis provided. Alternatively, more urea can be removed by performing hemodialysis more than three times per week.

7. **How does fluid removal occur during the dialysis procedure?**
   The removal of water during the dialysis treatment is referred to as ultrafiltration. During a hemodialysis treatment, a transmembrane hydrostatic pressure gradient develops between the blood and dialysate compartments. The total pressure difference between these two compartments determines the rate of ultrafiltration. The removal of fluid during the hemodialysis session is increased by any of these factors:
   - **Higher transmembrane hydrostatic pressure:** In most modern dialysis machines, the amount of fluid to be removed during the dialysis session is set on the dialysis machine and the machine will automatically adjust the pressures to allow for the appropriate amount of fluid to be removed. A higher transmembrane pressure results in more fluid being removed per unit time.
   - **Higher ultrafiltration coefficient (K_{uf}) of the dialysis membrane:** The value of this coefficient is dependent on the dialyzer surface area, composition, thickness, and porosity.
   - **Longer duration of a dialysis session.**

8. **How does one determine the amount of fluid to remove during a hemodialysis session?**
   Typically, a patient will gain between 1% and 5% of their body weight from fluid accumulation between dialysis sessions. Patients receiving chronic hemodialysis are assigned a dry weight by their nephrologist. A common definition of dry weight is the weight below which patients become hypotensive on dialysis. A more precise physiologic definition of dry weight is the body weight at a physiologic extracellular volume (ECV) state. Practically speaking, the dry weight is the weight at which the patient is euvolemic on a minimal number of blood pressure medications. The dry weight is set based on clinical findings and by patient response to removing additional fluid. The patient's dry weight will vary over time as a result of changes in appetite, the presence of diarrhea, and the like; thus, the patient's dry weight should be reassessed on a regular basis.

9. **How does one prevent clotting of blood in the blood circuit system during hemodialysis?**
   Heparin is routinely given during the hemodialysis treatment to prevent thrombosis in the extracorporeal circuit. Heparin is usually given as a bolus at the initiation of dialysis, followed by a constant infusion of heparin. The initial dose of heparin required is weight based but over time is individualized for each patient receiving dialysis to prevent complications. The appropriate dose of heparin is generally the amount that prevents clotting in the extracorporeal circuit but, at the same time, does not lead to bleeding from the needle puncture sites for more than 10 minutes after the needles are removed at the end of the hemodialysis treatment. In patients who are at high risk for bleeding, such as in postoperative patients or those with gastrointestinal bleeding, no heparin is given and instead the dialyzer is flushed with normal saline every 20 to 30 minutes to help minimize clotting.

10. **What are the differences between conventional in-center hemodialysis and home hemodialysis?**
Home hemodialysis is performed by about 1% of patients receiving chronic hemodialysis in the United States. Patients performing home hemodialysis need a partner to assist with the dialysis procedure (or at a minimum to assist with emergencies) and will need about 4 to 8 weeks of training to learn the home hemodialysis procedure. Patients can perform dialysis with a catheter or by self-cannulation using a fistula. Several different hemodialysis modalities can be performed at home, including conventional three times per week dialysis, short (1–3 hours per session) daily (six times per week) hemodialysis, and overnight or nocturnal (6–8 hours per session) hemodialysis performed three to six times per week. The Frequent Hemodialysis Network trials will assess if more frequent hemodialysis therapies are associated with improved secondary outcomes.

ASSESSING THE DOSE OF DIALYSIS

11. **How is the dose of dialysis determined?**
The dose of dialysis is determined by measuring the urea concentration in the blood at the start and end of the dialysis procedure to determine the amount of urea that is removed during the dialysis session and concurrently determining the amount of fluid removed during a single hemodialysis session. Once these values are available, a variety of techniques can be used to determine the dose of dialysis provided to the patient.

12. **What are the methods for measuring dose of dialysis?**
The dose of dialysis can be expressed as the urea reduction ratio, the single pool Kt/V, the double pool or equilibrated Kt/V, or the weekly or standard Kt/V. The first three expressions can be used only for patients who receive hemodialysis three times per week, whereas the standard or weekly Kt/V can be used to estimate the dose of dialysis regardless of the number of times per week that the patient receives hemodialysis.
1. The **urea reduction ratio** (URR) is expressed as follows:

$$URR = 100\% \times [1 - (C_t/C_o)]$$

where C_t and C_o represent postdialysis and predialysis serum urea levels. Because the URR equation does not account for volume removal during a dialysis treatment, it is considered less accurate than any of the Kt/V formulas.
2. **Single pool Kt/Vurea** (spKt/Vurea) is a unitless parameter that can be used to estimate the dose of dialysis provided to the patient, where K is the dialyzer blood water urea clearance (L/hour), t is the dialysis session length (hours), and V is the volume of distribution of urea (L). Because both K and V are difficult to measure accurately in vivo, several regression equations have been developed to estimate Kt/V. The most commonly used equation is the Daugirdas II equation:

$$Kt/V = -Ln [(R - 0.008) \times t] + [(4 - 3.5 R) (UF/W)]$$

where R is the postdialysis over predialysis serum urea level (C_t/C_o), t is the time of dialysis (in hours), UF is ultrafiltration volume in liters (amount of fluid removed by dialysis), and W is patient's postdialysis weight in kilograms. The first part of the equation represents the effects of urea generation during dialysis, whereas the second part of the equation represents the additional urea removed with volume removal during dialysis.
3. **Equilibrated Kt/Vurea** (eKt/Vurea) values accounts for urea release from sequestered tissue sites into the blood that occurs in the first 30 to 60 minutes after dialysis. The eKt/V is usually about 0.2 units less than the spKt/V. The formula for eKt/V depends on whether the patient is using a catheter for hemodialysis access:

$$Arterial\ access:\ eKt/V = spKt/V - 0.6 \times (spKt/V)/t + 0.03$$

$$Venous\ access:\ eKt/V = spKt/V - 0.47 \times (spKt/V)/t + 0.02$$

4. **Standard or weekly Kt/V** can be used to estimate the dose of dialysis regardless of the number of days per week that the patient receives dialysis. The formula for the weekly Kt/V is complex; calculators are available that can provide the value for the weekly Kt/V (including http://www.hdcn.com/ukm/).

13. **How often should the dose of dialysis be measured?**
The National Kidney Foundation's (NKF) Kidney Outcomes Quality Improvement Initiative (KDOQI) guidelines for hemodialysis adequacy recommend that the dose of dialysis be measured on a monthly basis in patients receiving chronic hemodialysis. Note that if residual renal function is being included in calculating the dose of dialysis (see Question 16), then this residual renal function should be measured at least every 2 months and also any time that an event has occurred that could have reduced the patient's residual renal function (e.g., contrast load, prolonged hypotension).

14. **What technical factors should be considered when measuring the dose of dialysis?**
The method by which the predialysis and postdialysis blood samples are obtained is important in ensuring accurate results. Blood urea nitrogen (BUN) levels are subject to rebound of three different types, including access recirculation, cardiopulmonary recirculation, and remote compartment rebound. By following a specific technique for blood drawing, the effect of access recirculation on the postdialysis BUN sample is minimized. Both the predialysis and postdialysis samples should be drawn during the same dialysis session. The postdialysis BUN samples should be obtained using either the slow flow or stop flow technique. With the slow flow technique, the dialysate flow is turned off and the blood pump is slowed to about 100 mL/min for about 15 seconds prior to obtaining the sample from the sampling port. Alternatively, with the stop flow technique, after the aforementioned procedures are performed, the blood pump is stopped and the arterial and venous blood lines are clamped prior to obtaining the sample.

15. **What factors can cause for differences between the prescribed and delivered Kt/V?**
The factors that can cause a discrepancy between the prescribed and delivered dose of dialysis can be categorized into factors resulting from compromised urea clearance (Table 52-1) and factors resulting from a decrease in the effective dialysis session length (Table 52-2).

16. **What dose of dialysis is considered adequate?**
Two major studies that have addressed dialysis adequacy include the National Cooperative Dialysis study (NCDS) and the HEMO Study. The NCDS study results suggest that there is an increase in patient mortality and morbidity when the spKt/V is <1.0. Based on the results from these and other studies, the NKF-KDOQI Hemodialysis Adequacy guidelines recommend that the minimum dose of dialysis for a patient with anuria is a single pool Kt/V of 1.2 per session, which is equivalent to a weekly Kt/V of 2.0. If the patient has substantial residual renal function, the renal urea clearance, as measured by a 24 hour urine collection, can also be included in the Kt/V equation. The NKF-KDOQI recommended minimal doses for patients undergoing chronic hemodialysis are shown in Table 52-3.

The HEMO study results demonstrated that in patients receiving hemodialysis three times per week, increasing the single pool Kt/V from 1.25 to 1.65 did not result in an improvement in mortality or major cardiovascular or infectious mortality or morbidity. The NKF-KDOQI guidelines do acknowledge, however, that certain subgroups of patients may benefit from a higher dose of dialysis including women, patients of smaller body size, and patients who are malnourished.

Two ongoing trials are assessing whether more frequent hemodialysis (six times per week versus three times per week) will improve secondary outcomes in patients who receive chronic hemodialysis. In the Frequent Hemodialysis Network daily trial, where patients receive

TABLE 52-1. REASONS FOR COMPROMISED UREA CLEARANCE

Patient-Related Reasons	Staff-Related Reasons	Mechanical Problems
Decreased effective time on dialysis ■ Decreased BFR ■ Access clotting ■ Use of intravenous catheters (instead of arteriovenous graft or fistula) ■ Inadequate flow through vascular access **Recirculation** ■ Use of catheters ■ Inadequate access for prescribed BFR ■ Stenosis, clotting of access	**Decreased effective time** **Decreased BFR** ■ Less than prescribed ■ Difficult cannulation **Decreased dialysate flow rate** ■ Less than prescribed ■ Inappropriately set **Dialyzer** ■ Inadequate quality control of "reuse"	**Dialyzer clotting during reuse** ■ Blood pump calibration error **Dialysate pump calibration error** **Inaccurate estimation of dialyzer performance by the manufacturer** **Variability in blood tubing**

BFR = blood flow rate.
Adapted from Parker TF. Trends and concepts in the prescription and delivery of dialysis in the United States. *Semin Nephrol* 1992;12:267–275.

TABLE 52-2. REASONS FOR DECREASED EFFECTIVE TIME ON DIALYSIS

Patient-Related Reasons	Staff-Related Reasons	Mechanical Reasons
Late start (patient tardy) ■ Early sign off ■ With consent (i.e., symptoms) ■ Against advice (i.e., social) **Medical complications (e.g., hypotension)** **No show**	**Late start (staff tardy)** **Wrong patient taken off** **Time calculated incorrectly** **Time on/off read incorrectly** **Clinical deficiencies (i.e., no time registered)** **Premature discontinuation for unit convenience** ■ Scheduling conflicts ■ Emergencies **Incorrect assumptions of continuous treatment time (e.g., failure to account for interruptions of treatment such as repositioning needles or accidental removal)** **Inaccurate assessment of effective time by using variable timepieces**	**Clotting of dialyzer** **Dialyzer leaks** **Machine malfunction**

Adapted from Parker TF. Trends and concepts in the prescription and delivery of dialysis in the United States. *Semin Nephrol* 1992;12:267–275.

TABLE 52-3. MINIMUM s/pKt/V VALUES CORRESPONDING TO A WEEKLY Kt/V OF ABOUT 2.0		
Schedule	$K_r < 2$ mL/min/1.73 m^2	$K_r > 2$ mL/min/1.73 m^2
2 times/week	Not recommended	2.0*
3 times/week	1.2	0.9
4 times/week	0.8	0.6
6 times/week (short daily)	0.5	0.4

*Not recommended unless $K_r > 3$.

hemodialysis for 1.5 to 2.75 hours six times per week, the estimated weekly Kt/V is 3.8. In the Frequent Hemodialysis Network nocturnal trial, where patients receive hemodialysis for 6 to 7 hours overnight six times per week, the estimated weekly Kt/V is 5.6.

Note that the optimal dose of dialysis has not been defined. Some have suggested that optimal dialysis occurs when patients do not need therapy for anemia or secondary hyperparathyroidism. The only current hemodialysis therapy that may provide this level of dialysis is nocturnal hemodialysis 6 nights per week.

17. **How does one achieve an adequate dose of dialysis in an individual patient?**
The actual delivered dose of dialysis is usually less than the predicted dose of dialysis. Thus, to achieve a delivered (measured) dose of dialysis with a single pool Kt/V of 1.2, the NKF-KDOQI guidelines recommend that the prescribed dialysis prescription should provide a single pool Kt/V of 1.4. A variety of calculators can be used to estimate the dose of dialysis once the patient's size, dialyzer type, and patient size are inputted into the program. Factors that influence the dose of dialysis that can be adjusted include the size of the dialyzer, the blood and dialysate flow rates, and the time per dialysis session. Increasing any of these parameters should increase the delivered dose of dialysis.

18. **Are there other uremic toxins that are present in patients with end-stage renal disease?**
Yes. There are literally hundreds of toxins that accumulate in renal failure. Some of them are middle or large molecules, some are charged particles, and others are protein bound. Many of these compounds are not well removed by conventional hemodialysis. Urea is thus a surrogate marker for uremic toxins, although the removal of urea on dialysis is often dissimilar to that of most other uremic toxins. Additional research is needed in this area to determine the extent and effects of these other uremic toxins on morbidity and mortality of patients with ESRD. A database of uremic toxins may be found on this website: http://www.nephro-leipzig.de/eutoxdb/index.php.

COMPLICATIONS OF HEMODIALYSIS

19. **What are some of the common complications that are seen during a hemodialysis session?**
Hypotension is the most common complication of the dialysis procedure, seen in 10% to 50% of treatments, depending on the patient population and the definition of hypotension used. Other common complications include cramping (5%–30%), nausea and vomiting (5%–10%), headache (5%–10%), pruritus (1%–5%), chest pain (1%–5%), back pain (1%–5%), and fever and chills (<1%).

20. **What are the symptoms associated with intradialytic hypotension?**
Intradialytic hypotension is often accompanied by lightheadedness, dizziness, cramping, and nausea. At times, there may be no symptoms until the patient's blood pressure has dropped to very low and potentially dangerous levels. To help monitor for hypotension, blood pressure is monitored during the dialysis treatment on a regular basis, usually every 30 to 60 minutes.

21. **What is the etiology of hypotension during hemodialysis?**
The causes of intradialytic hypotension can be divided into four broad categories, including volume-related issues, inadequate vasoconstriction, cardiac factors, and other causes. Volume-related issues center around a high ultrafiltration rate, an incorrectly low dry weight, or a low sodium level in the dialysate. Vasoconstrictive factors include the use of antihypertensive medications just prior to dialysis, autonomic neuropathy, a dialysate temperature higher than the patient's body temperature, and eating during dialysis. Cardiac factors include cardiac ischemia, heart failure, and arrhythmias. Other less common causes include a number of complications of dialysis that are described in more detail later, including dialyzer reactions, hemolysis, and air embolism, septicemia, myocardial infarction, pericardial tamponade, and severe anemia.

22. **What are some of the treatments used to help minimize intradialytic hypotension?**
The incidence of hypotension can be minimized by assessing dry weight on a regular basis and counseling the patient on avoiding large fluid gains between dialysis treatments, using a combination of a fluid-restricted and low-salt diet. Additional measures that may be beneficial include increasing the dialysis treatment time so as to decrease the hourly ultrafiltration rate, decreasing the dialysate temperature by 0.5°C to 2.0°C, changing the dialysate sodium concentration over time (sodium modeling), avoiding intradialytic food ingestion, and using midodrine (an alpha-adrenergic agonist) in patients who do not have active cardiac ischemia. Midodrine is ineffective if the patient is prescribed alpha-adrenergic blockers.

23. **What is the dialysis dysequilibrium syndrome and how can it be prevented?**
The dialysis dysequilibrium syndrome can occur when patients who are acutely uremic and have a high (>150 mg/dL) BUN level are subjected to a prolonged hemodialysis session. It is thought that the syndrome develops as a result of an acute increase in brain water content from an abrupt decrease in plasma hypotonicity leading to the movement of water from the plasma to brain tissue. Mild manifestations of the dialysis dysequilibrium syndrome are nonspecific and include restlessness, headache, nausea and vomiting; severe cases result in seizures, obtundation, or coma. For severe dysequilibrium, the dialysis session should be stopped, consideration should be given to prescribing IV mannitol, and the airway should be controlled if needed. The risk of dysequilibrium syndrome can be minimized by performing short (2- to 2.5-hour) hemodialysis sessions initially and by prescribing mannitol during these initial sessions.

KEY POINTS: HEMODIALYSIS

1. The dose of dialysis can be expressed as the urea reduction ratio, the single pool Kt/V, the double pool or equilibrated Kt/V, or the weekly or standard Kt/V.

2. Hypotension is the most common complication of the dialysis procedure, seen in 10% to 50% of treatments.

3. Dialysis dysequilibrium syndrome occurs when patients who are acutely uremic and have a high (>150 mg/dL) blood urea nitrogen level are subjected to a prolonged hemodialysis session. It is thought that the syndrome develops as a result of an acute increase in brain water content from an abrupt decrease in plasma hypotonicity leading to the movement of water from the plasma to brain tissue.

24. **What are some of the life-threatening complications that can occur during a hemodialysis session?**
See Table 52-4.

25. **What are the two main types of dialyzer reactions?**
There are type A or anaphylactic reactions and type B or nonspecific dialyzer reactions. Anaphylactic reactions are medical emergencies and are commonly manifested by dyspnea, a feeling of warmth, and a sense of impending catastrophe and can be followed by cardiac arrest and death. Milder symptoms include watery eyes, sneezing, cough, abdominal cramping, diarrhea, itching, and urticaria. Symptoms usually develop during the first several minutes of dialysis, although the symptoms can be delayed for more than 30 minutes. There is a diverse etiology of anaphylactic reactions including an allergy to ethylene oxide (used to sterile dialyzers), AN-69 dialysis membranes, contaminated dialysis solutions, and heparin or dialyzer reuse. Management is to stop dialysis immediately, clamp the blood lines, disconnect the patient from the dialysis circuit, and discharge the blood lines and dialyzer without returning the blood to the patient. The patient may need emergency treatment for anaphylaxis if the reaction is severe. Avoidance of the offending agent is needed to prevent recurrent reactions. Type B reactions are usually much less severe than type A reactions and are usually manifested by chest or back pain, with an onset 20 to 60 minutes after the start of dialysis. Management of type B reactions is supportive; consideration should be given to using a different dialyzer to prevent in the future.

26. **How does hemolysis occur during a hemodialysis session?**
Acute hemolysis is a medical emergency and can result from either problems with the blood tubing or needles or problems with the dialysate. Any obstruction or narrowing of the blood line, as a result of kinks, manufacturing defects, or the use of small-gauge needles in the presence of high blood flow rates, can cause hemolysis. Likewise, dialysate that has an incorrect electrolyte concentration, is too hot, or is contaminated with chemicals also can cause hemolysis. Contaminants include chloramine added to the city water supply; formaldehyde or bleach used to reuse dialyzers; or inadequate water treatment resulting in the presence of fluoride, nitrate, zinc, or copper. Hemolysis may be suspected if the blood in the venous line is port wine in color or if plasma is pink in centrifuged samples or with a marked drop in hemoglobin without an obvious source of bleeding. If hemolysis is suspected, the dialysis session should be stopped immediately and the blood in the dialyzer and blood tubing

TABLE 52-4. LIFE-THREATENING REACTIONS	
Reaction	Risk Factors
Dialyzer reaction	See Question 25
Arrhythmias	Pre-existing cardiovascular disease, hypotension, electrolyte imbalances, acidosis
Myocardial infarction	Pre-existing cardiovascular disease, hypotension
Cardiac tamponade	Recurrent or unexpected hypotension
Seizures	Severe hypertension, markedly elevated blood urea nitrogen levels
Intracranial bleeding	Pre-existing vascular disease, hypertension
Hemolysis	Blood-line obstruction/narrowing, problem with dialysate
Air embolism	Inadvertent air entry into the blood circuit

should be discarded because it may have a markedly elevated potassium level as a result of potassium release from hemolyzed erythrocytes. Patients will need to be hospitalized to monitor the extent of hemolysis and to treat hyperkalemia.

27. **How is an air embolism detected and treated?**
Air embolism is a medical emergency that can lead to death if it is not recognized and promptly treated. The manifestations of air embolism depend on the positioning of the patient and thus where the air embolism travels to. In seated patients, air enters the cerebral circulation, leading to central nervous system events, including loss of consciousness and death. In recumbent patients, air enters the cardiopulmonary system, leading to dyspnea, cough, arrhythmias, chest tightness, and acute cardiac and neurologic events. This emergency should be managed by immediately clamping the blood line, stopping the blood pump, placing the patient in a recumbent position on the left side with the head and chest tilted downward, and administering 100% oxygen by mask or endotracheal tube.

BIBLIOGRAPHY

Technical Aspects of Hemodialysis

1. Beathard GA, Arnold P, Jackson J, et al. Aggressive treatment of early fistula failure. *Kidney Int* 2003;64:1487–1494.
2. Chelamcharla M, Leypoldt JK, Cheung AK. Dialyzer membranes as determinants of the adequacy of dialysis. *Semin Nephrol* 2005;25(2):81–89.
3. Hakim RM, Himmelfarb J. Hemodialysis access failure: A call to action—Revisited. *Kidney Int* 2009;76(10): 1040–1048.
4. Inrig JK. Intradialytic hypertension: A less-recognized cardiovascular complication of hemodialysis. *Am J Kidney Dis* 2009;55(3):580–589.
5. Leypoldt JK, Cheung AK. Increases in mass transfer-area coefficients and urea Kt/V with increasing dialysate flow rate are greater for high-flux dialyzers. *Am J Kidney Dis* 2001;38(3):575–579.
6. National Kidney Foundation. KDOQI Clinical Practice Guidelines and Clinical Practice Recommendations for 2006 Updates: Vascular access. *Am J Kidney Dis* 2006;48(suppl 1):S176–S307.
7. Pastan S, Soucie JM, McClellan WM. Vascular access and increased risk of death among hemodialysis patients. *Kidney Int* 2002;62:620–626.
8. Raimann J, Liu L, Tyagi S, et al. A fresh look at dry weight. *Hemodial Int* 2008;12(4):395–405.
9. Suri RS, Garg AX, Chertow GM, et al.; for the Frequent Hemodialysis Network (FHN) Trial Group. Frequent Hemodialysis Network (FHN) randomized trials: Study design. *Kidney Int* 2007;72:349–359.

Assessing the Dose of Dialysis

10. Daugirdas JT, Depner TA, Greene T, et al. Standard Kt/V(urea): A method of calculation that includes effects of fluid removal and residual kidney clearance. *Kidney Int* 2010;77(7):637–644.
11. Daugirdas JT, Depner TA, Greene T, et al. Solute-solver: A web-based tool for modeling urea kinetics for a broad range of hemodialysis schedules in multiple patients. *Am J Kidney Dis* 2009;54(5):798–809.
12. Daugirdas JT. Prescribing and monitoring hemodialysis in a 3-4 x/week setting. *Hemodial Int* 2008;12(2):215–220.
13. Daugirdas JT, Greene T, Depner TA, et al.; Hemodialysis Study Group. Factors that affect postdialysis rebound in serum urea concentration, including the rate of dialysis: Results from the HEMO Study. *J Am Soc Nephrol* 2004;15(1):194–203.
14. Depner T, Daugirdas J, Greene T, et al.; Hemodialysis Study Group. Dialysis dose and the effect of gender and body size on outcome in the HEMO Study. *Kidney Int* 2004;65(4):1386–1394.
15. Depner T, Beck G, Daugirdas J, et al. Lessons from the Hemodialysis (HEMO) Study: An improved measure of the actual hemodialysis dose. *Am J Kidney Dis* 1999;33(1):142–149.
16. Eknoyan G, Beck GJ, Cheung AK, et al.; Hemodialysis (HEMO) Study Group. Effect of dialysis dose and membrane flux in maintenance hemodialysis. *N Engl J Med* 2002;347(25):2010–2019.

17. Gotch FA, Sargent JA. A mechanistic analysis of the National Cooperative Dialysis Study (NCDS). *Kidney Int* 1985;28(3):526–534.

18. National Kidney Foundation. KDOQI clinical practice guidelines for hemodialysis adequacy, Update 2006. *Am J Kidney Dis* 2006;48(suppl 1):S2–S90.

Complications of Hemodialysis

19. Brummelhuis WJ, van Geest RJ, van Schelven LJ, et al. Sodium profiling, but not cool dialysate, increases the absolute plasma refill rate during hemodialysis. *ASAIO J* 2009;55(6):575–580.

20. Ebo DG, Bosmans JL, Couttenye MM, et al. Haemodialysis-associated anaphylactic and anaphylactoid reactions. *Allergy* 2006;61(2):211–220.

21. Hoeben H, Abu-Alfa AK, Mahnensmith R, et al. Hemodynamics in patients with intradialytic hypotension treated with cool dialysate or midodrine. *Am J Kidney Dis* 2002;39(1):102–107

22. Hoenich NA, Levin R. Water treatment for dialysis: Technology and clinical implications. *Contrib Nephrol* 2008;161:1–6.

23. Polaschegg HD. Red blood cell damage from extracorporeal circulation in hemodialysis. *Semin Dial* 2009;22(5):524–531.

24. Silver SM, Sterns RH, Halperin ML. Brain swelling after dialysis: old urea or new osmoles? *Am J Kidney Dis* 1996;28(1):1–13

25. Ward DM. Hemodialysis water: An update on safety issues, monitoring, and adverse clinical events. *ASAIO J* 2004;50(6):xiii–xviii.

26. Yu AS, Levy E. Paradoxical cerebral air embolism from a hemodialysis catheter. *Am J Kidney Dis* 1997;29(3):453–455.

CHAPTER 53

PERITONEAL DIALYSIS

James A. Sloand, MD, and Sarah Prichard, MD

TECHNICAL ASPECTS OF PERITONEAL DIALYSIS

1. **What is peritoneal dialysis, and how does it work?**
   Peritoneal dialysis (PD) is a means of removing waste (such as urea, creatinine, and phosphate), solutes, and excess fluid from the body when the kidneys have failed. A sterile solution (PD fluid) containing a balanced concentration of electrolytes and an osmotically active agent is introduced into the patient's own peritoneal cavity by a surgically or laparoscopically placed catheter or tube. The introduced PD fluid bathes the capillaries covering the expansive surface area of the peritoneum. As the PD fluid is devoid of any waste, solutes move down concentration gradients across peritoneal capillaries into the PD fluid over time until equilibrium is reached, at which point, the PD fluid ("effluent") is drained and replaced with fresh solution. The osmotically active agent present in the PD fluid works by osmosis to draw fluid across the peritoneal capillaries into the PD fluid. Wastes and excess fluid are removed when "spent" PD fluid effluent is drained. The cycle of infusion of PD fluid, followed by its dwell in the peritoneum, and subsequent drainage from the patient is referred to as an "exchange."

2. **What are the indications for and clinical benefits of peritoneal dialysis?**
   PD can be performed in any patient who has end-stage renal disease (ESRD) and has intact peritoneal anatomy and function. Specific contraindications are discussed later (see Question 6).

   The main clinical benefit of PD is that it allows patients the flexibility and lifestyle choices inherent in a home-based kidney replacement therapy. It also has an advantage in providing continuous removal of waste and fluid, similar to the continuous function provided by one's own kidneys. The resulting physiologically gentle means of dialysis is thought to contribute to better preservation of existing residual kidney function (RKF). Maintenance of RKF has been shown to provide survival advantage for patients with ESRD. Initiating renal replacement therapy (RRT) with PD also helps preserve vascular access as part of an "integrated therapy" strategy for patients anticipated to require multiple RRTs (PD, transplant, hemodialysis) over their lifetime. As such, an RRT strategy of "PD first" is one advocated by an increasing number of clinicians when a pre-emptive kidney transplant is not available. This approach could also reduce the need for and affect complications associated with central venous catheters in patients needing an unplanned dialysis start.

   Perl J, Bargman JM. The importance of residual kidney function for patients on dialysis: A critical review. *Am J Kidney Dis* 2009;53:1068–1081.

3. **What are the different methods of peritoneal dialysis catheter placement?**
   There are currently three techniques for catheter placement. The dissective technique involves surgical placement of the catheter by mini-laparotomy, usually under general anesthesia. The modified Seldinger technique involves "blind" insertion of a needle into the abdomen, placement of a guidewire, dilation of a tract, and insertion of the catheter through a sheath, all without visualization of the peritoneal cavity. Last, PD catheters can be inserted via

laparoscopic insertion using a small optical peritoneoscope for direct inspection of the peritoneal cavity. The latter can be performed as an outpatient procedure under local anesthesia with air insufflation.

The advantage of the Seldinger approach is that it can be placed acutely at the bedside or in the interventional radiology/nephrology suite without the need for general anesthesia. Conversely, superior results have been demonstrated using the advanced laparoscopic technique. This may be operator dependent, but it may also be attributable to rectus sheath tunneling; direct visualization of the PD catheter into the pelvic cavity; and the ability to address other abdominal peritoneal issues such as occult hernias, adhesions, redundant omentum, and epiploic appendices that may influence short- and long-term catheter success.

4. Can elderly, obese, diabetic, and pediatric patients receive PD?

PD can be used successfully in the majority of patients with renal disease requiring dialysis. PD has been shown to be effective for patients with large body size or obesity, polycystic kidney disease, advanced age, diabetes, or other comorbidities (e.g., liver failure, ascites) and in patients without clinically significant kidney function (called anuria; see Question 5). PD is also the preferred form of dialysis for most pediatric patients with ESRD, including neonates and infants. Benefits for this population include absence of the need for a vascular access or venous puncture, association with good blood pressure control, few hospital visits for dialysis and associated care, facilitation of full-time school attendance, and better psychosocial adjustment for both patients and caregivers.

Brown EA, Davies SJ, Rutherford P, et al. Survival of functionally anuric patients on automated peritoneal dialysis: The European APD Outcome Study. *J Am Soc Nephrol* 2003;14:2948–2957.

De Vecchi AF, Maccario M, Braga M, et al. Peritoneal dialysis in nondiabetic patients older than 70 years: Comparison with patients aged 40 to 60 years. *Am J Kidney Dis* 1998;31:479–490.

Snyder JJ, Foley RN, Gilbertson DT, et al. Body size and outcomes on peritoneal dialysis in the United States. *Kidney Int* 2003;64:1838–1844.

5. Can patients continue receiving PD after they are anuric?

Although maintenance of even a minimal amount of kidney function has been demonstrated to have a survival benefit in patients treated with either PD or hemodialysis (HD), patients with anuria have been demonstrated to do well on PD. Adequate nutritional intake and ultrafiltration appear to be key elements to good outcome in patients who are anuric and receiving PD.

Brown EA, Davies SJ, Rutherford P, et al. Survival of functionally anuric patients on automated peritoneal dialysis: The European APD Outcome Study. *J Am Soc Nephrol* 2003;14:2948–2957.

6. What are the contraindications to peritoneal dialysis?

The definition of absolute contraindication is the presence of a clinical condition that makes a treatment either unsafe or unlikely to be effective. There are very few absolute contraindications for PD. PD is contraindicated in patients with diaphragmatic defects (e.g., pleuroperitoneal abnormalities), abdominal defects (e.g., unfixable hernia) or intra-abdominal processes (e.g., acute diverticulitis) that prevent effective PD or increase the risk of infection. PD is also contraindicated in situations where the patient and/or caregiver are unable or unwilling to learn the therapy.

7. Why would a patient want to do PD?

PD provides patients an active role in their own care, a greater level of independence, and more flexibility in dialysis prescription that can be tailored to accommodate and facilitate travel, recreation, and work. Unlike standard hemodialysis, which requires insertion of two large-bore needles to be inserted into the arm at least three times a week, PD is a needleless form of RRT.

8. Which is better: peritoneal dialysis or hemodialysis?

PD, HD, and kidney transplant offer alternative and complementary means to treat ESRD. Most comparative analyses of observational registry studies have demonstrated overall similar outcomes for PD and HD in patients, with an early survival benefit for patients who are able to start on PD. A recent propensity-matched mortality comparison of U.S. patients incident to ESRD in 2003 treated initially with either HD or PD demonstrated a significant 4-year overall survival advantage for those patients able to initiate dialysis (analysis done from day 0) with PD. Alternatively, although overall survival analysis from day 90 after initiation of dialysis in this study demonstrated no significant difference in outcome, cumulative survival probabilities still favored PD at 1 year with no difference between modalities out to 4 years after this. Patient subsets defined by age, cardiovascular disease (CVD), and diabetes showed that 4-year survival was equal or better for PD compared to HD in analysis from day 0. Conversely, in day 90 analysis, whereas 1 year survival in all subsets was equal or better with PD, 4-year survival in patients >65 with diabetes and CVD was better with HD.

When possible, initial treatment with PD has the potential benefit of improving early survival outcome, improving renal transplant results, preserving vascular access, and maintaining more downstream renal replacement options.

9. **What do CAPD, APD, CCPD, and NIPD stand for?**
CAPD is the abbreviation for continuous ambulatory peritoneal dialysis. Typically, patients manually infuse and drain 2 to 3 liters of PD fluid three to four times a day. The PD fluid is allowed to dwell in the peritoneal cavity for a period of 4 to 6 hours per each of three daytime exchanges and 8 to 10 hours during the overnight exchange. Patients will usually carry PD fluid in the peritoneum *continuously,* 24 hours a day. Depending on the individual circumstance, a dry period may be allowed for reasons of patient comfort or convenience.

APD is the abbreviated term for automated peritoneal dialysis. This refers to use of a cycler (see Question 11) to assist in administration and drainage of PD. Typically, this is utilized to administer several dialysis exchanges at night while the patient is sleeping, with a final filling of the abdomen in the morning before the patient disconnects from the device. When APD is programmed to provide dialysis cycles both at night and for a "last fill" of fresh PD fluid that will remain in the peritoneal cavity during the day, it is called continuous cyclic peritoneal dialysis, or CCPD. When a "last fill" is not programmed and the cycler only provides nocturnal dialysis exchanges, the APD is termed nocturnal intermittent peritoneal dialysis, or NIPD.

Use of APD does not preclude additional manual exchanges from being done during the daytime hours, if needed.

10. **What is acute peritoneal dialysis?**
Many patients need urgent or emergent dialysis. This occurs in patients who are not previously known to have chronic kidney disease (CKD) or when dialysis is started in situations of progressively deteriorating but known CKD without a permanent access (i.e., a fistula or a PD catheter). Urgent or emergent dialysis also occurs in situations of acute kidney injury. In the United States, Canada, and Europe, these patients usually start hemodialysis after placement of a central venous catheter.

Peritoneal dialysis can be used in many patients who have an unplanned start for dialysis, and it offers theoretical advantages in reducing the need for tunneled catheters and improving overall outcomes. In a recent retrospective analysis comparing the outcomes of a group of patients started acutely on PD and a nonmatched group of patients with a planned start on chronic PD, there was no difference in infectious complications or technique survival rate, although mechanical complications were significantly more common in the acute group. In another small study in France where patients were nonrandomly selected to unplanned start with either PD or HD, the 1-year survival adjusted for comorbidity (79% survival on HD compared with 83% on PD) and the rehospitalization rate were similar. It should be noted that these are single-center studies where the norm is HD. One would anticipate that increasing experience using PD for unplanned starts would improve outcomes.

Published experience with PD for acute kidney injury is limited. However, in a prospective randomized experience of 120 patients comparing high-volume PD to six times per week HD, outcomes were similar for both survival (58% and 53%) and recovery of kidney function (28% and 26%). Although results here are encouraging, experience with acute placement of PD catheters and PD therapy itself is a critical factor for success. Acute abdominal processes would be a contraindication to using acute PD.

Gabriel DP, Caramori JT, Martim LC, et al. High volume peritoneal dialysis versus daily hemodialysis: A randomized controlled trial in patients with acute kidney injury. *Kidney Int* 2008;108(Suppl):S89–93.

Lobbedez T, Lecouf A, Ficheux M, et al. Is rapid initiation of peritoneal dialysis feasible in unplanned dialysis patients? A single-centre experience. *Nephrol Dial Transplant* 2008;23:3290–3294.

Povlsen JV, Ivarsen P. How to start the late referred ESRD patient urgently on chronic APD. *Nephrol Dial Transplant* 2006; 1(suppl 2):56–59.

11. **What is a cycler, and who can or should use it?**
A cycler is a mechanized device made to assist in the administration and drainage of PD fluid. Use of the cycler to administer part or all of the PD prescription is termed APD. Although the cycler is primarily used by patients to administer their PD prescription at home, it can also be used in settings outside the home such as acute care, chronic care, or rehabilitation facilities to provide dialysis. The automation provided by APD reduces the number of manual connections the patient or care provider needs to perform, improving overall convenience. Ideally, this should also reduce touch contamination and risk of infection.

12. **What are the contents of PD solutions?**
All PD solutions are sterile fluids containing physiologically balanced amounts of electrolytes and an osmotically active agent. The latter is needed to draw fluid across the peritoneal capillaries into the PD fluid (ultrafiltration). There is a portfolio of PD solutions commercially available, with the main differences related to one of two things: the base buffer (and accompanying solution pH) or the osmotically active agent (Table 53-1).

PD solutions all have the following approximate electrolyte composition: sodium 132 meq/L; chloride 95 to 105 meq/L; calcium 2.5 to 3.5 meq/L; and magnesium 0.5 meq/L. Potassium is not in any PD fluid, but it can be manually added using sterile technique if necessary. Standard PD solutions contain lactate as the base buffer so that precipitation of calcium and magnesium in the PD solution is precluded from occurring. The usual concentration of lactate is approximately 40 meq/L and the resulting pH is 5.2 to 5.5. The pH rises rapidly to a physiologic level above 7.0 within about 15 minutes of infusion into the peritoneal cavity. Lactate absorbed from the PD fluid is converted to bicarbonate by a healthy liver.

Alternatively, bicarbonate can be used as the primary base buffer, enabling a final solution pH of 7.4. This can be done by separating bicarbonate from calcium and magnesium using a dual-chambered PD bag with the separation maintained until just before infusion into the peritoneum. This has the real advantage of reducing or eliminating pain during infusion of PD fluid into the peritoneum experienced by some patients. It also has other theoretical advantages based on the more physiologic nature of the solution.

Both standard PD solutions and dual-chambered bicarbonate-buffered PD solutions utilize dextrose as an osmotic agent. Dextrose-containing solutions are usually available in three concentrations: 1.5 g/dL, 2.5 g/dL, and 4.25 g/dL (concentrations based on dextrose in its monohydrous, rather than anhydrous, form*), although manufacturers of some brands of dual-chambered solutions contain 10% more dextrose. Increasing the glucose content of PD solutions increases their osmolality, thus augmenting their ability to enhance fluid removal (called ultrafiltration). The osmolalities associated with the above standard dextrose

---

*The same dextrose content of solutions is used in Europe, but dextrose is referred to in its anhydrous form. Respective dextrose concentrations are therefore 1.36%, 2.27%, and 3.86%.

TABLE 53-1. CONTENTS OF PERITONEAL DIALYSIS SOLUTIONS

	Dianeal PD1	Dianeal PD2	Dianeal PD4	Physioneal 35	Physioneal 40	Extraneal	Nutrineal	Plasma (Adult)
ELECTROLYTES (mmol/L)								
Sodium	132	132	132	132	132	133	132	136-145
Calcium	1.75	1.75	1.25	1.75	1.25	1.75	1.25	1.12-1.32
Magnesium	0.75	0.25	0.25	0.25	0.25	0.25	0.25	0.65-1.05
Chloride	102	96	95	101	95	96	105	98-107
BUFFER (mmol/L)								
Lactate	35	40	40	10	15	40	40	0.6-1.7
Bicarbonate				25	25			21-30
pH	5.5	5.5	5.5	7.4	7.4	5.5	6.7	7.4
OSMOTIC AGENT, OSMOLARITY (mOsm/L)								
1.36% glucose	347	345	344	345	344			
2.27% glucose	398	396	395	396	395			
3.86% glucose	486	484	483	484	483			
7.5% icodextrin						284		
1.1% amino acids							365	

concentrations are 346, 396, and 478 mOsm/kg, respectively. The osmotic gradient generated by dextrose-containing PD solutions dissipates over time as the dextrose is absorbed by the peritoneal capillaries. This gradient will dissipate more rapidly when lower concentrations of dextrose are used (e.g., 1.36 g/dL) and in patients who have a larger peritoneal capillary network (e.g., fast membrane transport). Long exchange dwell times (e.g., >6 hours) can result in poor fluid removal or even net negative fluid balance because lymphatic absorption of PD fluid occurs at a constant rate and can exceed transcapillary ultrafiltration toward the end of a long exchange.

Both icodextrin and amino acids have been used as alternative osmotic agents to dextrose. Icodextrin (Extraneal) is a polyglucose molecule having a very large molecular weight, a property that increases colloid osmosis (oncotic pressure) of the containing PD solution (as opposed to crystalloid osmotic pressure generated by dextrose-containing solutions). Extraneal does not contain any dextrose, has an osmolality of 282 mOsm/kg, and has a pH of 5.2. The fluid-removing capacity of this novel solution is not attenuated over time, making it ideal for long daytime (APD) or night-time (CAPD) exchanges. Nutrineal also has the benefit of being glucose free, utilizing 1.1 g/dL of amino acids as an osmotic agent. It has a pH of 6.4 and an osmolality of 365 mOsm/L.

13. **What is the peritoneal equilibration test?**
The peritoneal equilibration test (PET) is a standardized procedure for assessing the permeability and efficiency of a patient's membrane. The PET uses a series of dialysate (D) and plasma (P) samples obtained over a 4-hour period to measure solute equilibration (D/P creatinine), rate of glucose absorption, and net fluid removal or "ultrafiltration" (Fig. 53-1). After determining these values, the patient's peritoneal membrane is categorized into one of the four membrane transport classifications. Each membrane classification (low, low average, high average, high) has specific characteristics that guide the clinician in tailoring the patient's dialysis prescription. In general, patients found to have high to high average membrane transport characteristics should be prescribed shorter dialysis dwell times to enhance fluid and small solute removal. Rapid equilibration of waste between dialysate and plasma along with absorption of the osmotic agent (dextrose) by abundant peritoneal capillaries are the reason for this.

The standard PET is usually done with a 2.36% dextrose PD solution, but a 3.86% dextrose solution can be used as an alternative. The benefit of using the latter is that it produces near-identical diffusive results to a 2.36% solution and provides additional information about maximal ultrafiltration capacity of the peritoneal membrane being tested. Reproducible and accurate results have been demonstrated with either solution.

Twardowski ZJ, Nolph KD, Khanna R, et al. Peritoneal equilibration test. *Perit Dial Bull* 1987;7:138–147.

14. **What are the elements of a peritoneal dialysis prescription, and how is it determined?**
Elements of a PD prescription include the total number of exchanges per day and the duration, dwell volume, and PD fluid content (dextrose, icodextrin, amino acid) of each exchange. The means by which the prescription is delivered, whether by CAPD or by cycler (APD) and whether the peritoneum is dry for any part of the day is also included in the prescription.

The PD prescription is individualized for each patient based on his or her physiologic needs and desired lifestyle. The former is determined by the size of the patient (volume of distribution of urea), their peritoneal membrane diffusion characteristics, and their residual kidney function. Further adjustment can be made based on dietary and fluid intake of the patient. The prescription can then be modified to accommodate their work, school, or social schedule using either CAPD or APD. In general, patients with fast peritoneal membrane transport require shorter dwell times, whereas those with slower membrane transport require longer dwell times. Although minor differences can be identified, icodextrin is handled similarly irrespective of membrane transport type.

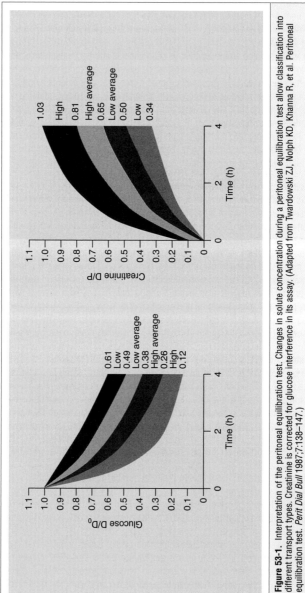

Figure 53-1. Interpretation of the peritoneal equilibration test. Changes in solute concentration during a peritoneal equilibration test allow classification into different transport types. Creatinine is corrected for glucose interference in its assay. (Adapted from Twardowski ZJ, Nolph KD, Khanna R, et al. Peritoneal equilibration test. *Perit Dial Bull* 1987;7:138–147.)

15. **What is pericatheter leakage?**

Pericatheter leakage describes a complication of peritoneal dialysis where administered dialysis fluid and ultrafiltrate is not confined to the peritoneal cavity, but rather escapes or leaks around the entrance site or across the abdominal wall tissue planes crossed by the PD catheter. Leakage around the PD catheter exit site commonly presents as moisture or drainage of clear fluid. Alternatively, leakage can occur around the rectus muscle sheath or Scarpa's fascia resulting in pericatheter edema. The technique of PD catheter placement (median as opposed to paramedian location), factors related to initiation of PD (excessive volume of peritoneal dialysis fluid relative to timing of the PD catheter placement), or intrinsic abdominal wall weakness (excessive physical straining, obesity, or long-term therapy with steroids) are the three main causative factors associated with peri-catheter leak.

PD fluid can also leak into fluid spaces outside of the peritoneum related to intrinsic peritoneal, abdominal wall, or diaphragmatic defects. A patent processes vaginalis; inguinal or periumbilical hernias can result in edema in genital and other respective areas. Conversely, tendinous defects in the diaphragm can result in collection of fluid within the thoracic cavity. Positive abdominal and negative intrathoracic pressure contributes to the collection of fluid in the chest cavity in the setting of a diaphragmatic defect. Leak or extravasation of fluid outside the peritoneum can present with decreased ultrafiltration, increased weight, localized swelling, or shortness of breath. The latter is particularly true in the case of transthoracic infiltration of fluid, which, if sizeable, can result in a unilateral decrease in breath sounds, dullness to percussion on the involved side, and a pleural effusion on chest imaging. An increased glucose content of fluid leaking from the area around the PD catheter or obtained by thoracentesis (in the case of a presumed diaphragmatic defect) relative to the blood glucose level provides a helpful diagnostic clue. Suspicion of internal leakage of PD fluid into tissue planes can be confirmed with imaging studies. If magnetic resonance imaging (MRI) is used, it should be done without gadolinium. The PD fluid itself can serve as the "contrast" for MRI diagnosis of internal leaks.

Peritoneal dialysis should usually be interrupted, if possible, for 1 to 2 weeks when early external or subcutaneous leaks develop to allow more time for healing around the catheter. An alternative is to reduce the dwell volume coupled with use of supine dialysis, leaving the abdomen dry when the patient is sitting, upright, or ambulatory. Antibiotics should be strongly considered in the presence of an external leak to reduce the risk of a tunnel infection or peritonitis. Recurrence of a leak after a several week period of peritoneal rest or modified, supine PD should prompt strong consideration of surgical intervention. Temporary transfer to hemodialysis to allow for primary healing or after correction of an abdominal wall defect may be necessary depending on presence and the amount of residual kidney function in addition to the clinical scenario. Late leaks, defined as those occurring more than 30 days after catheter insertion, are more likely to require surgical correction of the defect to achieve resolution. It is notable that successful continuation of PD using a regimen of supine-attenuated PD has been described.

Discontinuation of PD is appropriate in the case of PD-related hydrothorax. Successful surgical correction of the diaphragmatic defect after surgical repair or pleurodesis may allow the patient to return to PD after a judicious interval to allow for complete healing.

Prischl FC, Muhr T, Seiringer EM, et al. MRI of the peritoneal cavity among PD patients, using the dialysate as "contrast medium." *J Am Soc Nephrol* 2002;13:197–203.

16. **What is inflow/outflow pain?**

Occasionally, patients complain of pain upon infusion or drainage of PD fluid. Infusion pain can result from infusion of an inappropriately cool or warm PD solution, peritoneal sensitivity to the lower than physiologic pH of PD solution (i.e., 5.2–6.4), visceral sensitivity to a directed jet stream of PD fluid from the PD catheter, or a malposition of the PD catheter against the viscera. Discomfort during drainage of PD effluent usually relates to a siphoning effect on the viscera or peritoneum and may therefore also relate to catheter positioning. The effect of constipation on expansion of intestinal diameter and resultant crowding of the viscera around the catheter should not be minimized as a cause of either fill or drain pain.

Timing and duration of the pain usually provide the diagnostic clues as to which of the aforementioned issues are causative and therefore are crucial to discerning appropriate treatment. Transient pain related to inappropriate temperature can be adequately managed with proper patient instruction. Pain related to the lower pH of the PD solution is also transient in nature given the rapid increase in the PD fluid pH to physiologic levels. Use of some neutral pH PD solutions can address this issue if available. Although addition of bicarbonate to the PD solution prior to peritoneal infusion can also help reduce pain, introduction of any exogenous substance to the PD fluid theoretically may increase infection risks. Alternatively, patients can leave a small residual volume of PD fluid in the abdomen at the end of the drain phase of the exchange. This residual volume serves as a buffer to the inflowing dialysate and reduces the tugging sensation associated with the last phase of the drain. However, caution should be taken not to leave a large volume in as residual volume so as to avoid a total intraperitoneal volume that is too large and may cause clinical problems. Effective treatment of constipation should always be undertaken as a simpler means to relieve either fill or drain pain prior to considering leaving a residual volume after each exchange.

17. **What is poor or slow inflow/outflow?**

Poor or slow inflow or outflow of PD fluid is a problem that more frequently occurs during the initial break-in period of a PD catheter but can occur at any time in the course of treatment. The most common cause is constipation, and the first step is to effectively clear the bowel of excessive stool. If this is not effective at resolving the problem, then other causes need to be investigated.

Discernment as to whether the flow problem is bidirectional or unidirectional (only poor outflow) helps determine the cause of the problem. Bidirectional flow problems usually indicate obstruction of the catheter lumen by clot, fibrin, or a kink or bend in the catheter. Conversely, unidirectional poor outflow suggests either of the following:

1. Malposition of the PD catheter in a place where the PD fluid cannot be drained (i.e., migration of the catheter out of the true pelvis) or
2. Encumbrance of catheter drainage pores by tissue or viscera. Although the force of PD fluid inflow can more easily push bowels engorged with stool, epiploic appendices, omental wraps, or adhesions aside, the negative pressure of outflow results in collapse of these organs and tissues on the draining catheter.

Plain-film roentgenographic imaging of the abdomen provides diagnostic assistance in determining the presence of constipation or malposition or kinking of the PD catheter. Catheters can be repositioned by trocar or laparoscopy. By exclusion, outflow occlusion not related to constipation is most likely related to adhesions, omental wrapping, or epiploic appendices and would require surgical or laparoscopic intervention and correction. Injection of catheters with sterile contrast by radiology can facilitate diagnosis. Inability to resolve these issues would be an indication for transfer to hemodialysis.

The presence of fibrin or blood occluding a PD catheter at times can be signaled by the appearance of either in the PD catheter or effluent. Heparin should be added in a concentration of 500 to 2000 U/L to each dialysate exchange in this situation and used for at least 24 to 48 hours after the effluent is clear.

A catheter obstructed with blood or fibrin can be treated with push–pull infusion of dialysate or sterile saline under moderate pressure with a 50-mL syringe. The procedure should be discontinued if the patient has any pain or cramping. Alternatively, there are several anecdotal reports of success utilizing different regimens of tissue plasminogen activator (tPA) infused with sterile saline or sterile water into the PD catheter. No controlled studies demonstrate the safety or efficacy of this methodology, however.

Zorzanello MM, Fleming WJ, Prowant BE. Use of tissue plasminogen activator in peritoneal dialysis catheters: a literature review and one center's experience. *Nephrol Nurs J* 2004;31:534–537.

ASSESSING THE DOSE OF DIALYSIS

18. **What is dialysis adequacy, how is it measured in PD, and what are the current targets in PD?**

Accumulation of uremic waste not removed by the failing kidneys contributes to poor outcome in patients with ESRD. Ideally, removal of a threshold or *adequate* amount of waste with dialysis would result in improved outcome, with any incremental amount removed above this amount having little impact on improving clinical outcome. Previous and more recent studies have focused on the relationship between clearance of small solutes, in particular urea and creatinine, and outcome. Based on the results of randomized controlled interventional trials, both the National Kidney Foundation Kidney Disease Outcomes Quality Initiative and the International Society of Peritoneal Dialysis guidelines for PD recommend that *adequacy* be assessed by total (peritoneal and kidney) clearance of urea (termed "Kt") normalized to its volume of distribution (V_{urea}). Assessment of this requires collection and measurement of urea present in 24-hour collections of both drained peritoneal dialysis effluent and urine. Although the current weekly Kt/V_{urea} target recommended by both Kidney Disease Outcome Quality Initiative (KDOQI) and International Society for Peritoneal Dialysis (ISPD) is 1.7, both guidelines recognize the importance of clinical assessment of the individual patient in determining need for more dialysis. Other factors possibly important in patient outcome include volume, phosphate, and middle molecule (e.g., beta-2-microglobulin) removal. These are currently being considered as additional measures of adequacy that can be managed with the dialysis prescription.

Lo W-K, Wu Y-W, Li C-S, et al. Effect of Kt/V on survival and clinical outcome in CAPD patients in a randomized prospective study. *Kidney Int* 2003;64:649–656.

Paniagua R, Amato D, Vonesh E, et al. Effects of increasing peritoneal clearances on mortality rates in peritoneal dialysis: ADEMEX, a prospective, randomized, controlled trial. *J Am Soc Nephrol* 2002;13:1307–1320.

19. **Why is residual renal function (RRF) important in patients with PD?**

Residual kidney function is strongly associated with survival advantage for patients receiving both peritoneal and hemodialysis. Improved salt and water balance, better removal of middle molecular wastes, and an association with reduced inflammation and inflammatory mediators are postulated reasons for this association. Therefore it is important to protect residual kidney function in all patients receiving dialysis. It should be noted that the weight of data demonstrates PD to be superior to HD in preserving residual kidney function.

Based on its survival advantage, it is important to protect residual kidney function in patients irrespective of their chosen form of kidney replacement therapy. This includes use of agents to block the renin-angiotensin-aldosterone system, judicious avoidance of nonsteroidal inflammatory drugs and radiocontrast agents (barring absolute need), volume depletion, and sodium phosphate bowel preparations. Although temporary decreases in kidney function can be seen, long-term renal risks of contrast can be reduced with appropriate precontrast hydration, N-acetyl cystine, and use of low-osmolar radiocontrast agents. Alternatively, other imaging techniques that avoid use of contrast should be sought. Prolonged use of aminoglycosides should also be avoided to attenuate risks of both vestibular toxicity and renal functional loss. Conversely, published experience has demonstrated safety of short-term use of aminoglycosides in patients with ESRD. Initial, short-term use of aminoglycoside antibiotics pending identification and sensitivity of organisms causing peritonitis with subsequent change to an alternative nonaminoglycoside agent can thus be safely advocated.

Vilar E, Wellsted D, Chandna SM, et al. Residual renal function improves outcome in incremental haemodialysis despite reduced dialysis dose. *Nephrol Dial Transplant* 2009;24:2502–2510.

COMPLICATIONS OF PERITONEAL DIALYSIS

20. **What are the risks of infection with PD compared with HD?**

The overall incidence of infection among patients with PD is no greater than among patients with HD. According to data collected by USRDS, patients on PD are significantly less likely to have dialysis-associated bacteremia or sepsis, a complication almost completely associated with HD. This undoubtedly relates to the intrinsic need of HD to use a vascular access to carry out the therapy. Conversely, the most serious infection and one almost exclusively occurring in patients on PD is peritonitis. Technical advances in the past decade around "patient-to-dialysate connectology" and infection control strategies have reduced the peritonitis infection rates markedly. As a result, hospitalization for infection related to dialysis has progressively fallen for PD over the past decade and has been lower than that for HD since 2001.

Ishani A, Collins AJ, Herzog CA, et al. Septicemia, access and cardiovascular disease in dialysis patients: The USRDS Wave 2 study. *Kidney Int* 2005;68:311–318.

National Institute of Diabetes, Digestive, and Kidney Disease. Renal Data System: USRDS 2009 Annual Data Report, Bethesda, MD.

21. **What are an exit site infection and a tunnel infection?**

The presence of purulent drainage, with or without erythema on the skin around the catheter exit site, indicates the existence of an exit site infection. Redness around the catheter may be an early heralding sign of infection or simply local irritation. The latter is more likely if it occurs shortly after catheter placement, trauma, or traction about the catheter exit site. A positive culture in the absence of abnormal exit site appearance is suggestive of colonization, not infection.

The presence of catheter tunnel infection can occur in the setting of an exit site infection. This is suggested by erythema, edema, and tenderness over the subcutaneous course of the PD catheter. A fluid collection demonstrated by ultrasound can facilitate diagnosis (and adequate duration of treatment) of a tunnel infection.

22. **How is an exit site infection prevented and treated?**

Prevention of exit site infections (and peritonitis, described later) starts with proper placement of the PD catheter. The exit site of the catheter should be in a location that can be clearly seen by the patient, downward or laterally facing to preclude funneling of dirt or cellular debris into the catheter exit site, and not buried in a panniculus or abdominal skinfold. Prophylactic antibiotics given prior to PD catheter placement have been shown to have additional value in preventing subsequent peritonitis. Avoidance of anchoring sutures at the PD exit site and allowing the PD catheter to remain covered, clean, dry, and undisturbed until well healed are additional key factors in preventing an infectious nidus from being seeded about the catheter exit site or tunnel. Consistent, steadfast training of the patient and staff regarding sterile technique, observation of meticulous hand washing, and daily exit site care is then required. Clear advantages of daily application of either mupirocin or gentamycin cream to the exit site have been demonstrated.

If an exit site infection is present, antimicrobial therapy should be initiated. Antibiotics can be started immediately on diagnosis, or treatment can be deferred until identification of the offending agent is made from the exit site culture. *Staphylococcus aureus* should always be covered if treatment is empiric, however. Consideration should be given to using two antibiotics having different mechanisms of action when treating exit site infections caused by *Pseudomonas aeruginosa,* given the tenacity of these organisms. Irrespective of the organism causing an exit site infection, treatment should be continued for at least 2 weeks or more with the goal of restoring a normal exit site appearance. Failure to adequately eradicate the infection should prompt replacement of the PD catheter. The ISPD has published guidelines for the prevention, diagnosis, and treatment of exit site and tunnel infection.

Li PK-T, Szeto CC, Piraino B et al. Peritoneal dialysis-related infections recommendations: 2010 update. *Perit Dial Int* 2010;30:393-423.

23. **What is the appropriate initial empiric antibiotic therapy for PD catheter exit site infection?**
   Staphylococcus aureus, coagulase-negative *staphylococcus,* and other gram-positive organisms have been found to be the most frequent causes of exit site infection, followed in frequency by *Pseudomonas aeruginosa* and other gram-negative organisms. As with peritonitis, however, knowledge of both the epidemiology of exit site/tunnel infections and the local antibiotic sensitivities in each PD unit is imperative to guide therapy in that unit. After identification of an exit site or tunnel infection, empiric antibiotic therapy may be initiated immediately, or therapy can be deferred until the results of the culture of the exit site drainage can guide the choice of agent. Empiric therapy should always cover *S. aureus* and consider *P. aeruginosa* because these are common causes of infection and have the strongest association with peritonitis. An oral *Penicillinase*-resistant penicillin (i.e., dicloxacillin 250–500 mg twice a day) or a first-generation cephalosporin (i.e., cephalexin 500 mg twice a day) provide good gram-positive coverage, whereas oral quinolones can provide gram-negative (including antipseudomonal) and some gram-positive coverage. Documented *P. aeruginosa* may require two antipseudomonal drugs given its relative resistance to therapy. Antimicrobial agents should be continued for 2 weeks or until the exit site appears normal, whichever is longer. Ultrasound may be helpful in determining the presence, response, and duration of therapy in the case of a tunnel infection. Dosing recommendations of other commonly used antibiotics and details useful in the treatment of exit site and tunnel infection can be found at www.ISPD.org.

24. **What is peritonitis?**
   Peritonitis is inflammation of the peritoneal membrane. Although this most often results from infection, peritonitis can also result from noninfectious cause. Entry of infectious organisms into the peritoneum can occur from touch contamination by the patient because of improper technique, extension of infection from around the PD catheter, transluminal migration of bacteria across the bowel wall, or hematogenous seeding in the case of bacteremia or sepsis from another source. Patients usually present with symptoms of abdominal pain and cloudy peritoneal dialysis effluent.

25. **What is the appropriate diagnostic workup of peritonitis in a patient undergoing peritoneal dialysis?**
   Upon presentation by any patient with PD with symptoms of either abdominal pain or cloudy effluent, a diagnosis of peritonitis should be entertained and ruled out. However, the clinician should also be mindful of other non-PD-related causes of these symptoms such as a ruptured viscus, diverticulitis, cholecystitis, ischemic bowel, or pancreatitis. Prompt diagnosis and treatment are imperative for best outcomes in PD-related peritonitis and any of the other conditions.

   A sample of PD effluent that has ideally been dwelling in the peritoneum for at least 1-2 hours should be obtained by the patient or health care provider. The effluent fluid is sent to the laboratory for cell count, gram stain, and microbial culture. The diagnosis of peritonitis requires at least two of the following three features: (1) peritoneal fluid leukocytosis ($>100/mm^3$ and at least 50% polymorphonuclear cells), (2) abdominal pain, and (3) positive culture of the dialysis effluent.

   Li PK-T, Szeto CC, Piraino B et al. Peritoneal dialysis-related infections recommendations: 2010 update. *Perit Dial Int* 2010;30:393-423.

26. **How should peritonitis be prevented and treated?**
   A number of peritonitis episodes are the result of direct extension of an infection associated with the exit site, in particular when the infecting organism at the exit site is either *Staphylococcus aureus* or *Pseudomonas aeruginosa*. All best demonstrated practices in reducing exit site infections will have a positive impact on decreasing peritonitis episodes. Another measure to reduce peritonitis is "flush before fill" connectology, a technology that washes any bacteria introduced at the tubing-catheter interface during an exchange into the

drainage bag rather than into the patient's peritoneum. Avoidance of constipation has also been demonstrated to reduce the risk of peritonitis by attenuating transmigration of enteric bacteria across the bowel wall. Although not evidence based, observational studies have suggested benefit in draining the peritoneum dry and providing appropriate prophylactic antibiotics prior to dental, gastrointestinal, and genitourinary procedures.

Once a presumptive diagnosis of peritonitis is made, prompt treatment with antibiotics capable of covering both gram-negative and gram-positive organisms is implemented. Although antibiotics can be given orally or intravenously, intraperitoneal administration has the benefit of providing immediate delivery of bacteriocidal concentrations of antibiotics. PD fluid culture results should then help narrow the spectrum and guide the duration of antimicrobial therapy. Attention to achieving a consistent mean inhibitory concentration (MIC) of antibiotics in the PD fluid, particularly if the patient is receiving APD or if intermittent antibiotic therapy is being used, is critical to successful treatment.

The signs and symptoms of peritonitis usually resolve within 48 hours after appropriate antimicrobial therapy. Persistent pain, cloudy fluid, and elevation of peritoneal fluid WBC count should prompt re-evaluation of the infectious cause and whether antibiotic therapy is suitable. Peritonitis refractory to treatment, defined as failure of the effluent to clear within 5 days of appropriate antibiotic therapy, should result in removal of the catheter. The ISPD has published guidelines for the prevention, diagnosis, and treatment of peritonitis.

Li PK-T, Szeto CC, Piraino B et al. Peritoneal dialysis-related infections recommendations: 2010 update. *Perit Dial Int* 2010;30:393-423.

27. **What is the appropriate initial empiric antibiotic therapy for suspected PD-related peritonitis?**

Initial empiric therapy should reflect knowledge of both the epidemiology of peritonitis and the antibiotic sensitivities in the local PD unit. In general, ISPD recommends initial coverage of both gram-positive and gram-negative microorganisms. Use of a third-generation cephalosporin or an aminoglycoside for Gram-negative coverage AND vancomycin or a first-generation cephalosporin for Gram-positive coverage would accomplish these goals. This should provide coverage against the majority of organisms that cause peritonitis including *Pseudomonas* and *Staphylococcus aureus*. Initial and subsequent doses of antibiotics for intraperitoneal administration can be found at www.ISPD.org.

28. **How do you approach fungal peritonitis?**

Fungal peritonitis is a very serious disease that can lead to death in up to 25% of patients affected. Diagnosis either by microscopy or culture usually requires removal of the PD catheter along with initiation of dual therapy with intravenous amphotericin B (dose adjusted to weight) and oral flucytosine 1000 mg/day. Given poor peritoneal penetration with intravenous use and chemical peritonitis with intraperitoneal use, amphotericin should be replaced with another antifungal agent after fungal susceptibilities are determined. Most peritoneal fungal infections are a result of either *Candida albicans* or *Candida parapsilosis* but can result from an assortment of fungi.

Recent antibiotic treatment has been shown to be a predisposing factor associated with subsequent development of fungal peritonitis. Consideration should be given to providing antifungal coverage to patients treated with antibiotics, especially in programs with high rates of fungal peritonitis, as per ISPD guidelines. Oral nystatin at a dose of 50,000U QID coprescribed with antibiotic treatment was used in one study.

Miles R, Hawley CM, McDonald SP, et al. Predictors and outcomes of fungal peritonitis in peritoneal dialysis patients. *Kidney Int* 2009;76:622–628.

29. **What are the indications for removal of a PD catheter?**

Removal of the PD catheter should be strongly considered in cases of the following:
- Refractory peritonitis, defined as failure of the peritoneal effluent to clear after 5 days of appropriate antibiotics

- Relapsing peritonitis, defined as redevelopment of peritonitis with the same organism or after an episode of sterile peritonitis occurring within 4 weeks of completion of therapy of the previous episode
- An exit site and/or tunnel infection failing to respond to recommended treatment with appropriate antibiotics
- Fungal peritonitis
- Peritonitis associated with the growth of multiple enteric organisms, particularly anaerobic organisms; the risk of intra-abdominal pathology is raised in the latter setting.

30. **How long can patients stay on PD?**
There is no time limit to a patient being able to stay on peritoneal dialysis. Patients have been reported in the literature to have been on PD for 10 to 17 years. Adequate nutritional intake, maintenance of a normal volume status, and avoidance of infection are key elements to successful longevity (technique survival) on PD, however.

Maitra S, Burkart J, Fine A, et al. Patients on chronic peritoneal dialysis for ten years or more in North America. *Perit Dial Int* 2000;20 (Suppl 2):S127–S133.

31. **What dietary restrictions are required for PD?**
In general, there are fewer dietary restrictions for patients on PD than there are for those on thrice-weekly HD because of the continuous nature of PD as a renal replacement therapy. Patients on PD can be allowed a reasonably liberal intake of potassium with relative impunity from hyperkalemia. Conversely, unrestricted sodium and water intake should be discouraged unless the patient has an excellent urine output and little need for high-concentration dextrose PD solutions. Chronic exposure to consistently high dextrose–containing PD solutions may result in adverse changes in the peritoneal membrane and weight gain by the patient.

KDOQI recommendations suggest that all patients with ESRD on renal replacement therapy be encouraged to ingest a diet high in protein, particularly protein with high biologic value. This helps to offset catabolic effects of dialysis related to HD and amino acids and/or protein lost in the spent hemodialysis or peritoneal dialysate. Approximately 5 to 15 g of protein can be lost in PD effluent over a 24-hour period, highlighting the importance of a recommended intake of 1.0 to 1.2 g/kg/day of dietary protein.

National Kidney Foundation. Clinical practice guidelines for nutrition in chronic renal failure. Available at: http://www.kidney.org/professionals/kdoqi/guidelines_updates/doqi_nut.html. Accessed May 17, 2007.

32. **How important is volume control in patients treated with PD, and how is it best managed?**
Attainment of euvolemia has been demonstrated to be important in patients with ESRD, whether treated with PD or HD. Although determination of dry weight is challenging for any patient, observational analyses have demonstrated that enhanced ultrafiltration in patients treated with PD is associated with improved survival.

Conservative management is the cornerstone of volume management and includes renal protective measures, sodium restriction, and optimal use of diuretics. Peritoneal ultrafiltration using icodextrin (Extraneal) has been shown to be clearly superior compared to dextrose-based solutions in randomized controlled trials. Use of icodextrin also helps reduce peritoneal glucose exposure and systemic glucose absorption.

Brown EA, Davies SJ, Rutherford P, et al. Survival of functionally anuric patients on automated peritoneal dialysis: the European APD Outcome Study. *J Am Soc Nephrol* 2003;14:2948–2957.

Finkelstein F, Healy H, Abu-Alfa A, et al. Superiority of icodextrin compared with 4.25% dextrose for peritoneal ultrafiltration. *J Am Soc Nephrol* 2005;16:546–554.

Perl J, Bargman JM. The importance of residual kidney function for patients on dialysis: A critical review. *Am J Kidney Dis* 2009;53:1068–1081.

KEY POINTS: PERITONEAL DIALYSIS

1. The main clinical benefit of peritoneal dialysis (PD) is that it allows patients the flexibility and lifestyle choices inherent in a home-based kidney replacement therapy. It also has an advantage in providing continuous removal of waste and fluid, similar to the continuous function provided by one's own kidneys. The renal replacement therapy strategy of "PD first" is an approach that could reduce need for, and affect complications associated with, central venous catheters in patients needing an unplanned dialysis start.

2. When possible, initial treatment with PD has the potential benefit of improving early survival outcome and renal transplant results, preserving vascular access, and maintaining more downstream renal replacement options.

3. According to data collected by U.S. Renal Data System, patients on PD are significantly less likely to have dialysis-associated bacteremia or sepsis, a complication almost completely associated with hemodialysis. Conversely, the most serious infection and one almost exclusively occurring in patients on PD is peritonitis. Technical advances in the past decade around "patient-to-dialysate connectology" and infection control strategies have reduced the peritonitis infection rates markedly.

4. Although determination of dry weight is challenging for any patient, observational analyses have demonstrated that enhanced ultrafiltration in patients treated with PD is associated with improved survival. Peritoneal ultrafiltration using icodextrin (Extraneal) has been shown to be clearly superior compared to dextrose-based solutions in randomized controlled trials.

33. **Why is hypokalemia common in patients with PD?**
Potassium homeostasis in patients with ESRD is facilitated on peritoneal dialysis given the continuous nature of the therapy resulting in ongoing potassium removal related to the maintenance of a diffusion gradient between dialysate and plasma. This gives patients on PD therapy greater dietary flexibility and clinicians treating these patients greater flexibility in prescription of medications that influence potassium balance (i.e., angiotensin-converting enzyme inhibitors, angiotensin receptor antagonists, or aldosterone antagonists) compared to treatment with hemodialysis. Conversely, when dietary intake is suboptimal, hypokalemia can develop. This can be treated with a more liberal diet for potassium or oral potassium supplements. If necessary, intraperitoneal potassium sterilely administered at a concentration of up to 4 meq/L of PD fluid. Careful monitoring of serum potassium levels is important in these situations.

34. **Why is hypoalbuminemia common in patients with PD?**
Hypoalbuminemia is a frequent finding in patients treated with either peritoneal and hemodialysis. Serum albumin levels in patients with PD are a function of synthesis, catabolism, volume of distribution, and loss, usually in urine or the peritoneal effluent. As such, all should be considered in evaluation of patients with hypoalbuminemia.

Low albumin levels can be related to poor nutritional intake, an etiology that can be determined by subjective global assessment. When nutritional intake is deemed inadequate, attempts should be made to embellish oral intake of protein in these patients. Depression and medications should always be considered as potential contributing causes to poor dietary intake and should be appropriately addressed.

An expanded intravascular volume relating to failure to achieve dry weight can be another cause of low serum albumin levels. Therefore, in evaluating hypoalbuminemia, the clinician should look for and treat volume overload

Albumin is a negative acute-phase reactant, decreasing with any infectious or inflammatory processes. Patients should be evaluated for any source of inflammation and treatment should be initiated for this as appropriate. In PD, there can be significant loss of protein across the peritoneal membrane. This has been reported to be as high as 1 gram per liter of PD effluent. This can be even higher during episodes of peritonitis, when the peritoneal membrane becomes both inflamed and generally more "leaky."

35. **Does PD affect kidney transplantation?**
Patients receiving PD as their means of RRT are much more likely to receive a kidney transplant. Although this may be explained by demographics of the PD population, there may be other contributing factors. Infectious and cardiovascular challenges inherent to intermittent HD related to risks associated with central venous catheters and interdialytic fluid gains, respectively, could potentially result in removal of prospective transplant patients from an "active" transplant list, delaying transplantation.

Patients receiving PD as their pretransplant means of RRT have a lower incidence of delayed graft dysfunction, but long-term outcomes are equivalent for patients on PD and HD. Of note, whereas graft and patient survival appear to be unaffected by the modality of pretransplant RRT, recent data have shown that patient survival is negatively influenced by immediate transplant nonfunction.

REFERENCES

1. Krishnan RG, Moghal NE. TPA for blocked PD catheters. *Ped Nephrol* 2006;21:300.
2. Weinhandl ED, Foley RN, Gilbertson DT, et al. Propensity-matched mortality comparison of incident hemodialysis and peritoneal dialysis patients. *J Am Soc Nephrol* 2010;21:449–506.

CHAPTER 54

THERAPEUTIC PLASMA EXCHANGE (PLASMAPHERESIS)

Ernesto Sabath, MD, and Bradley M. Denker, MD

1. **What is the definition of plasmapheresis and when is it indicated?**
   The term "apheresis" is Greek for "taking away" and refers to a procedure where the therapeutic removal of macromolecules from the plasma is done for therapeutic reasons. It is indicated for conditions where substances that are not removable with conventional dialysis must be removed from the blood.

2. **Define the possible mechanisms of action for plasmapheresis leading to clinical improvement.**
   Two general mechanisms may lead to improvement: (1) removal of pathologic substances or (2) replacement of a missing or abnormal plasma component. The pathologic factors that can be removed by plasmapheresis are autoantibodies, immune complexes, cryoglobulins, complement products, lipoproteins, and protein-bound toxins. The success of plasmapheresis depends on the rate of production of the abnormal protein or antibody and the efficiency of removal with plasmapheresis. Plasmapheresis is most often utilized with other immunosuppressive strategies to decrease production and reduce inflammation. Other additional benefits include reversal of impaired splenic function to remove immune complexes and replacement of plasma factors (such as ADAMTS-13 in TTP).

3. **Describe the techniques for plasma separation during the plasmapheresis procedure.**
   The two major modalities to separate the plasma from the blood during a plasmapheresis procedure are by centrifugation and membrane filtration. The centrifugation method uses centrifugal force to separate whole blood into plasma and cellular fractions according to their density. The membrane filtration technique is based on a synthetic membrane filter composed of different pore sizes. This filter is similar to a hemodialysis filter, composed of many hollow fiber tubes with relatively large pore sizes (0.2–0.6 μm in diameter), and arranged in parallel.

4. **What type of venous access may I use for plasmapheresis?**
   The clinical scenario, especially the possibility for long-term venous access, and the type of plasmapheresis being used are important factors to consider when deciding on peripheral or central venous access. A peripheral vein allows a maximum flow of up to about 90 mL/min, so a single venous access is adequate for intermittent centrifugation. Continuous centrifugation techniques will require two venous access sites or a central venous catheter. If long-term (more than 1 to 2 weeks) plasmapheresis is planned, a central venous catheter is required.

5. **List the anticoagulants commonly used during the plasmapheresis procedure.**
   Citrate, unfractionated heparin, and hirudin are commonly used.

6. **What types of replacement fluid replacement are used during the plasmapheresis procedure?**
   The choice of replacement fluids include 5% albumin, fresh-frozen plasma (FFP; or other plasma derivatives like cryosupernatant), crystalloids (e.g., 0.9% saline, Ringer's lactate), and

synthetic plasma expanders like hydroxyethyl starch. Albumin is the most commonly used replacement solution in plasmapheresis. It is generally combined 1:1 with 0.9% saline, does not contain calcium or potassium, and lacks coagulation factors and immunoglobulins. It is safe and has never been associated with transmission of hepatitis or HIV viruses. FFP contains complement and coagulation factors and is the replacement fluid of choice in patients with thrombotic thrombocytopenic purpura (TTP) because the infusion of normal plasma may contribute to the replacement of the deficient plasma factor, ADAMTS-13. Plasma may also be preferable in patients at risk of bleeding (e.g., those with liver disease or disseminated intravascular coagulation, after a renal biopsy), or those requiring intensive therapy (e.g., daily exchanges for several weeks) because frequent replacements with albumin solution will eventually result in postplasmapheresis coagulopathy and a net loss of immunoglobulins.

7. **How do I estimate how much plasma to remove?**
   Each plasmapheresis session should remove 1.0 to 1.5 times the plasma volume, and this can be calculated from the following formula:

   Estimated plasma volume (in liters) = 0.07 weight (in kg) (1 − hematocrit [Hct])

8. **Describe the main complications of plasmapheresis and how often they occur.**
   Plasmapheresis is a relatively (but not entirely) safe procedure. Some registries reported a 4.2% incidence of adverse events, and just 1% of all apheresis procedures had to be interrupted because of an adverse event. The most common adverse effects reported are paresthesias (0.52%), hypotension (0.5%), urticaria (0.34%), shivering, and nausea. Paresthesias are often related to hypocalcemia caused by the citrate infusion as anticoagulant for the extracorporeal system or in the FFP administered as a replacement fluid. Citrate binds to free calcium to form soluble calcium citrate, thereby lowering the free, but not the total, serum calcium concentration. Death is rare, occurring in less than 0.1% of all the procedures.

9. **What are the main clinical indications of plasmapheresis for renal diseases?**
   Table 54-1 summarizes the most important clinical indications for renal diseases according to category.

10. **What is the role of plasmapheresis in anti-glomerular basement membrane disease?**
    In anti-glomerular basement membrane (GBM) disease, the role of plasmapheresis is the rapid removal of the pathogenic antibodies, in combination with cyclophosphamide and corticosteroids, that are essential to prevent additional antibody synthesis and reduce inflammation. All patients with anti-GBM antibody disease and severe renal failure who do not require immediate dialysis should be treated with aggressive immunosuppression and intensive plasmapheresis. Because pulmonary hemorrhage is associated with high mortality, plasmapheresis should be initiated in this group of patients regardless of the severity of the renal failure. However, patients presenting with dialysis dependence only had 8% renal survival, and if the renal biopsy showed crescentic lesions in all glomeruli, renal survival was 0%. Plasmapheresis is usually done for 14 days or until the anti-GBM antibody is no longer detectable.

11. **What is the evidence for the use of plasmapheresis in rapidly progressive glomerulonephritis (RPGN)?**
    There is a beneficial role for plasmapheresis in patients with severe renal involvement (creatinine > 500 μmol/L or 5.7 mg/dL) and antineutrophil cytoplasmic antibodies (ANCA)-associated vasculitis. In contrast to anti-GBM disease, the addition of plasmapheresis to treatments including cyclophosphamide, azathioprine, and steroids was associated with better renal survival. In patients with ANCA and anti-GBM associated disease, and in any patient with diffuse pulmonary alveolar hemorrhage, plasmapheresis is beneficial for the recovery and reduction of risk progression to dialysis. The use of plasmapheresis for less severe renal disease remains unresolved.

TABLE 54-1. CLINICAL INDICATORS FOR RENAL DISEASE	
Disease	**Category***
Anti-GBM disease	I
TTP	I
Rapidly progressive glomerulonephritis	II
Cryoglobulinemia	II
Hemolytic uremic syndrome	III
Desensitization for renal transplantation	II
Recurrent FSGS	III
Renal transplant rejection	IV
Systemic lupus erythematosus	III

GBM = glomerular basement membrane; TTP = thrombotic thrombocytopenia purpura; FSGS, Focal and segmentary glomerulosclerosis.
*Category I, standard primary therapy; Category II, supportive therapy; Category III, when the evidence of benefit is unclear; Category IV, when there is no current evidence of benefit or for research protocols.

12. **Is there any evidence for a role of plasmapheresis in lupus nephritis?**
    The current literature does not support a benefit for the addition of plasmapheresis to immunosuppressive therapy for lupus nephritis. However, there are individual patients who are refractory for whom there is anecdotal evidence that it may provide some benefit.

13. **Is plasmapheresis indicated as treatment in patients with multiple myeloma and cast nephropathy?**
    The role of plasmapheresis in myeloma cast nephropathy is debated. Although early studies demonstrated improvement in renal function and patient survival, the largest study to date of 104 patients with multiple myeloma and acute renal failure randomly assigned to conventional therapy plus plasma exchanges or conventional therapy alone did not show differences in composite outcome of death, dialysis dependence, or severely reduced renal function. The findings of this study do not support the routine use of plasmapheresis in patients with myeloma, but it can be considered in patients with unusually high paraprotein burdens or Waldenström's macroglobulinemia and hyperviscosity syndromes.

14. **What is the efficacy of plasma exchange in the treatment of TTP?**
    Plasmapheresis may replenish the levels of ADAMTS-13 protease that is deficient in some cases of TTP. Duration of daily therapeutic plasma exchange to achieve a durable remission (e.g., platelet count greater than 150,000 for 3 days and lactase dehydrogenase near normal and no neurologic deficit, if initially present) is extremely variable, depending on the condition. There is no evidence for a beneficial role of plasmapheresis in patients with TTP secondary to cancer, chemotherapy, or bone marrow transplantation.

15. **Can plasmapheresis be used to remove toxic substances?**
    Plasmapheresis can be considered for the removal of protein-bound toxins that are not readily removed with dialysis or hemoperfusion. Plasmapheresis is effective in removing highly protein-bound toxins from the blood but not from other fluid compartments. Reports of the

successful use of plasmapheresis in the treatment of various drug overdoses and poisonings are generally anecdotal. Amanita poisoning (mushrooms) is the most frequent clinical diagnosis where plasmapheresis has been utilized with success, perhaps showing decreased mortality, especially in children.

16. **Is there any indication for plasmapheresis in the treatment of dyslipidemia?**
Low-density lipoprotein apheresis should be the treatment of choice for patients who are homozygotic for familial hypercholesterolemia (FH). Therapy is initiated from age 7 unless their serum cholesterol can be reduced by more than 50% (or decreased to <9 mmol/L) with drug therapy. It is also indicated in individual patients with either heterozygous FH or a family history of premature cardiac death or progressive coronary disease and for whom low-density lipoprotein cholesterol remains higher than 5.0 mmol/L or is decreased less than 40% with maximal drug therapy.

17. **Is there a role for plasmapheresis in recurrent focal and segmental glomerulosclerosis?**
Yes, the mechanisms of recurrent focal and segmental glomerulosclerosis (FSGS) and early detection of proteinuria after renal transplantation are unclear, but the early reappearance of proteinuria suggests that a nondialyzable circulating factor that alters glomerular permeability may be present. Removal of a circulating factor by immunoadsorption or plasma exchange may account for the remission of the disease in some patients.

18. **Describe the role of plasmapheresis in renal transplantation.**
In addition to reducing the risk of recurrent FSGS in some patients, plasmapheresis is now widely utilized for ABO blood group-incompatible transplants, positive T-cell cross-match, and acute humoral rejection.

19. **List some indications for plasmapheresis in nonrenal diseases that are supported by clinical trials (Category I).**
- Guillain-Barré syndrome
- Myasthenia gravis
- Chronic inflammatory demyelinating polyneuropathy
- Hyperviscosity in monoclonal gammopathies (Waldenström macroglobulinemia)
- Cutaneous T-cell lymphoma (photopheresis)

20. **Is there any indication for plasmapheresis in pregnancy?**
Plasmapheresis can be safely performed during pregnancy, and introduction of plasmapheresis for specific indications has improved maternal and fetal survival rates. Plasmapheresis has been safely carried out in myasthenic crisis, Guillain-Barré syndrome, anti-GBM disease, acute fatty liver of pregnancy, and TTP. Some complications of plasmapheresis are premature delivery as a result of the removal of essential hormones maintaining pregnancy, hypovolemic reaction, allergy, transitory cardiac arrhythmias, and nausea.

During the exchanges, hypotension must be carefully monitored and corrected, and in the second or third trimester, it is preferable to place the patient on her left side to avoid compression of the inferior vena cava by the gravid uterus.

KEY POINTS: PLASMAPHERESIS

1. All patients with anti-glomerular basement membrane antibody disease and severe renal failure (but not yet requiring dialysis) or with hemoptysis should be treated with aggressive immunosuppression and intensive plasmapheresis.

2. Evidence suggests a beneficial role for plasmapheresis in patients with severe renal involvement (creatinine >500 μmol/L or 5.7 mg/dL) and antineutrophil cytoplasmic antibodies–associated vasculitis.

3. In patients with multiple myeloma and cast nephropathy, there is no support for the routine use of plasmapheresis.

4. In patients with thrombotic thrombocytopenia purpura secondary to cancer, chemotherapy, or bone marrow transplantation there is no evidence for a beneficial role of plasmapheresis.

BIBLIOGRAPHY

1. Byrnes JJ, Khurana M. Treatment of thrombotic thrombocytopenic purpura with plasma. *N Engl J Med* 1977;297:1386–1389.
2. Clark WF, Stewart AK, Rock GA, et al. Plasma exchange when myeloma presents as acute renal failure: A randomized, controlled trial. *Ann Intern Med* 2005;143:777–784.
3. Deegens JK, Andresdottir MB, Croockewit S, et al. Plasma exchange improves graft survival in patients with recurrent focal glomerulosclerosis after renal transplant. *Transpl Int* 2004;17:151–157.
4. De Lind van Wijngaarden RA, Hauer HA, Wolterbeek R, et al.; EUVAS. Chances of renal recovery for dialysis dependent ANCA associated glomerulonephritis. *J Am Soc Nephrol* 2007;18:2189–2197.
5. Jayne DR, Gaskin G, Rasmussen N, et al. Randomized trial of plasma exchange or high dosage methylprednisolone as adjunctive therapy for severe renal vasculitis. *J Am Soc Nephrol* 2007;18:2180–2188.
6. Kambic HE, Nose Y. Historical perspective on plasmapheresis. *Ther Apher* 1997;1:83–108.
7. Levy JB, Turner AN, Rees AJ, et al. Long-term outcome of anti-glomerular basement membrane antibody disease treated with plasma exchange and immunosuppression. *Ann Intern Med* 2001;134:1033–1042.
8. Madore F. Plasmapheresis. Technical aspects and indications. *Crit Care Clin* 2002;18:375–392.
9. Montgomery RA, Locke JE, King KE, et al. ABO Incompatible renal transplantation: A paradigm ready for broad implementation. *Transplantation* 2009;87:1246–1255.
10. Szczepiorkowski ZM, Bandarenko N, Kim HC, et al. Guidelines on the use of therapeutic apheresis in clinical practice—Evidence-based approach from the Apheresis Applications Committee of the American Society for Apheresis. *J Clin Apher* 2007;22:106–175.

EPIDEMIOLOGY AND OUTCOMES

Michael R. Lattanzio, DO, and Matthew R. Weir, MD

CHAPTER 55

1. **What is UNOS?**

   UNOS stands for the **U**nited **N**etwork of **O**rgan **S**haring. UNOS is a nonprofit, scientific, and educational organization that administers the Organ Procurement and Transplantation Network (OPTN), established by the U.S. Congress in 1984. The main objectives of OPTN include collection and management of data about every transplant event occurring in the United States, facilitation of the organ matching and placement process, and development of organ transplantation policy. Annual data collection for renal transplants across the United States is compiled in the Scientific Registry of Transplant Recipients (SRTR). These data are available online at www.ustransplant.org.

2. **What is involved in kidney donor procurement?**

   When kidneys are donated, an intricate process ensues. The procuring organization accesses the national transplant computer system, UNet^{sm}, through the Internet or contacts the UNOS Organ Center directly. In either situation, information about the kidney donor is entered into UNet^{sm} and a donor/recipient match is determined for each donated kidney.

   The resulting match list of potential recipients is ranked according to objective medical criteria (blood type, tissue type, size of the organ, medical urgency of the recipient, time accrued on the waiting list, and distance between donor and recipient).

   Using the match of potential recipients, the local organ procurement coordinator or an organ placement specialist contacts the transplant center of the highest-ranked patient, based on policy criteria, and offers the kidney. If the kidney is rejected, the next potential recipient's transplant center on the match list is contacted. Calls are made to multiple recipients' transplant centers in succession to expedite the organ placement process until the kidney is placed. Once the kidney is accepted for a patient, transportation arrangements are made and the transplant surgery team is notified.

3. **What are the most recent trends in renal transplant survival?**

   The most recent data provided from UNOS has demonstrated small improvements in both living and deceased renal transplant survival from 2005 to 2006. The data from 2005 to 2006 are consistent with a decade-long trend of improved renal allograft survival for both living and deceased renal transplants. The improvements in allograft survival over the last decade have been attributed to a reduction in acute/chronic rejection episodes, shortened cold-ischemia times, and lower plasma reactive antibody levels among recipients.

4. **What donor type confers the best outcomes in regard to kidney recipient survival?**

   Living donor kidney transplants have the best recipient survival, followed by standard-criteria donors, then extended criteria donors (Fig. 55-1).

5. **What donor type confers the best outcomes in regard to kidney graft survival?**

   Living donor kidney transplants have the best allograft survival, followed by standard-criteria donors, then extended criteria donors (Fig. 55-2).

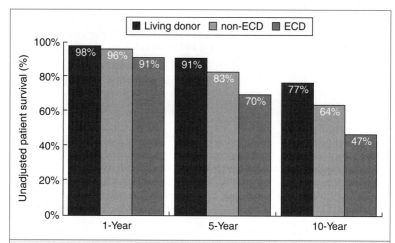

Figure 55-1. Unadjusted 1-year (2005–2006), 5-year (2001–2006), and 10-year (1996–2006) kidney recipient survival by donor type. (From Annual Report of the US Procurement and Transplantation Network and the Scientific Registry of Transplant Recipients: Transplant Data 1998–2007. US Department of Health and Human Services, Health Resources and Services Administration, Health Care Systems Bureau, Division of Transplantation, Rockville, MD.)

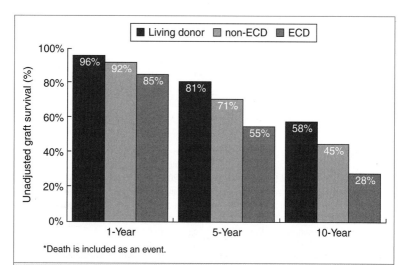

*Death is included as an event.

Figure 55-2. Unadjusted 1-year (2005–2006), 5-year (2001–2006), and 10-year (1996–2006) kidney graft survival by donor type. (From Annual Report of the US Procurement and Transplantation Network and the Scientific Registry of Transplant Recipients: Transplant Data 1998–2007. US Department of Health and Human Services, Health Resources and Services Administration, Health Care Systems Bureau, Division of Transplantation, Rockville, MD.)

6. **What is the current trend in actual number and types of kidney tranplants performed?**
   In 2007 there were 7729 standard criteria donors (SCD), 1828 extended criteria donors (ECD), and 1029 donation after cardiac death (DCD) transplants performed (Fig. 55-3). The greatest numeric increment compared with 2002 has been in DCD transplants, with a total gain of 765. SCD increased by 739, and ECD (includes ECD/DCD) increased by 543. There were 73 fewer total transplants in 2007 (10,586) than in 2006 (10,659); this change represented 239 fewer SCD, 11 more ECD (includes ECD/DCD), and 155 more DCD transplants.

7. **Is the waiting list for kidney transplant growing?**
   Yes. Over the past 10 years, the total number of candidates listed for a kidney-alone transplant at any time during the calendar year increased by 78%, from 53,315 to 94,741, whereas the total number of candidates wait-listed for a kidney-alone transplant at year's end rose by 86%, from 38,690 to 71,862. To meet this demand, the annual number of kidney transplants performed nationally grew by 31%, from 12,318 transplants in 1998 to 16,119 transplants in 2007. Unfortunately, the growth in the number of wait-listed patients has been accompanied by a similar increase of 76% in deaths on the waiting list, from 2,528 in 1998 to 4,452 in 2007. However, although the absolute number of deaths has increased, the annual death rate for candidates on the wait-list has decreased from a high of 84 deaths per 1000 patient-years at risk in 1999 to 65 deaths per 1000 patient-years at risk in 2007.

8. **Has the age of patients on the waiting list changed over the last few years?**
   Yes. The proportion of candidates on the active kidney transplant waiting list older than age 50 years has increased during the past decade from 44% to 58%. The absolute number of candidates aged 50 years or older more than doubled, from 8704 in 1998 to 18,436 in 2007. This shift in the age distribution of the wait-list reflects, in part, lengthier wait-listing periods. By comparison, the proportion of younger candidates has decreased over time. New policies have been proposed that would favor the allocation of kidney transplants from younger donors to younger recipients. This allocation schema would increase allocation of kidneys to patients more likely to benefit from transplantation, resulting in many thousands of additional life-years

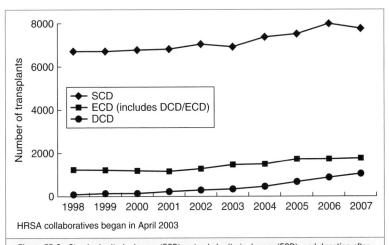

HRSA collaboratives began in April 2003

Figure 55-3. Standard criteria donors (SCD), extended criteria donors (ECD), and donation after cardiac death (DCD) kidney transplants, 1998–2007. (From Annual Report of the US Procurement and Transplantation Network and the Scientific Registry of Transplant Recipients: Transplant Data 1998–2007. US Department of Health and Human Services, Health Resources and Services Administration, Health Care Systems Bureau, Division of Transplantation, Rockville, MD.)

saved. This allocation schema has generated great controversy because it would preferentially divert good kidneys away from older recipients on the wait-list.

9. **What is the distribution of race among individuals on the kidney wait-list?**
During the past decade, the distribution of race among candidates on the kidney wait-list has shifted. The number of white and African American active candidates grew from 15,113 and 12,493, respectively, in 1998 to 18,467 and 16,632 in 2007. At the same time, however, the percentage of white candidates on the active wait-list declined from 44% to 38% and the percentage of African American candidates decreased slightly from 36% to 34%. The total number of active Hispanic/Latino candidates more than doubled, from 4320 in 1998 to 8827 in 2007; Asian candidates also increased over the same time, from 2154 to 4148. These changes parallel the proportionate increase in the percentage representation of Hispanic/Latino and Asian candidates in both active and inactive status on the kidney wait-list.

10. **What is the most common cause of kidney disease in patients on the wait-list?**
Diabetes is the most common cause of kidney disease for those waiting for a kidney. Overall, the percentage of active candidates with diabetes has increased from 24% to 28% over the past 10 years. Hypertension closely follows diabetes as the etiology of renal disease in patients on the wait-list. Glomerular disease as the cause of renal disease in patients on the wait-list has declined over the last decade.

11. **What are recent trends in waiting lists for kidney transplants?**
There is a very large gap between the number of patients waiting for a transplant and the number receiving a transplant. This gap has widened over the past decade, meaning that the waiting times from listing to transplant continues to increase. Projections based on the most recent 5-year data suggest that the total wait-list will grow at a rate of 4138 registrations per year, whereas the active wait-list will grow by 663 registrations per year. Fortunately, there has been some growth in the total number of kidneys transplanted. Most of this growth has resulted from the use of expanded-criteria donors and donation after cardiac death.

12. **What is "status 7"?**
"Status 7" is defined as a transplant candidiate who is considered temporarily unsuitable for kidney transplantation. These patients usually have a medical condition that temporarily makes them unable to receive a kidney transplant. Patients accrue waiting time points while in status 7. Once the condition is resolved, the patient is reinstated to the active wait-list and is eligible for kidney transplant allocation.

13. **What is the median time to transplantation for individuals on the wait-list?**
In 2004 the median time until any type of kidney transplant was 1219 days or approximately 3.3 years. The length of time until kidney transplantation has changed little between 1998 and 2004.

14. **Does a candidate's blood type affect their time on the waiting list?**
Yes. Blood groups AB, A, O, and B have mean wait times of 2, 3, 5, and 6 years, respectively.

15. **Is the access to renal transplantation equitable among all persons?**
Equal access to renal transplantation for all who could benefit is a major problem. Disparities exist in patient education, geography, race, and level of pretransplantation nephrology care. UNOS is attempting to make the process of organ accessibility and allocation equitable among all different patient populations.

16. **What are the major factors that determine a potential recipient's UNOS score for kidney allocation?**
   - **Time on the wait-list:** Priority to individuals with longest wait-time
   - **Age:** Priority to individuals younger than 18 years old, particularly younger than 11 years old

- **Human leukocyte antigen mismatch**: Priority to zero antigen mismatch
- **Degree of panel reactivity antibody:** Priority to higher percentages
- **Medical urgency:** Only considered in local kidney allocation
  Potential recipients with the highest score have the most immediate chance of kidney allocation.

KEY POINTS: TRANSPLANT EPIDEMIOLOGY AND OUTCOMES

1. Improvements in allograft survival over the past decade have been attributed to a reduction in acute/chronic rejection episodes, shortened cold-ischemia times, and lower plasma reactive antibody levels among recipients.

2. New policies have been proposed that would favor the allocation of kidney transplants from younger donors to younger recipients. This allocation schema would increase allocation of kidneys to patients more likely to benefit from transplantation, resulting in many thousands of additional life-years saved.

3. In 2004 the median time until any type of kidney transplant was 1219 days or approximately 3.3 years. The length of time until kidney transplantation has changed little between 1998 and 2004.

4. The United Network of Organ Sharing is attempting to make the process of organ accessibility and allocation equitable among all different patient populations.

17. **What is the kidney allocation score?**
    The kidney allocation score (KAS) is an allocation schema recently proposed by UNOS that would focus on three main criteria:
    - **Life years from transplant (LYFT):** The estimated survival that a recipient of a specific donor kidney may expect to receive versus survival on dialysis
    - **Dialysis time (DT):** Time spent on dialysis
    - **Donor profile index (DPI):** A continuous measure of organ quality based on clinical information
      LYFT, DPI, and DT are incorporated so that kidneys are matched to candidates based on the expected survival of both the kidney and the recipient.

18. **What are the major causes of long-term kidney allograft failure?**
    The major causes of long-term kidney allograft failure are chronic rejection and death with a functioning kidney.

19. **What are the most common causes of death after kidney transplantation?**
    - The most common cause of death after kidney transplantation is cardiovascular disease, followed by infections and malignancy.

BIBLIOGRAPHY

1. Annual Report of the US Procurement and Transplantation Network and the Scientific Registry of Transplant Recipients: Transplant Data 1998–2007. US Department of Health and Human Services, Health Resources and Services Administration, Health Care Systems Bureau, Division of Transplantation, Rockville, MD.

2. Arend SM, Mallat MJ, Westendorp RJ, et al. Patient survival after renal transplantation; more than 25 years follow-up. *Nephrol Dial Transplant* 1997;12:1672–1679.

3. Gaston RS, Danovitch GM, Adams PL, et al. The report of a national conference on the wait list for kidney transplantation. *Am J Transplant* 2003;3:775–785.

4. Hariharan S, Johnson CP, Bresnahan BA, et al. Improved graft survival after renal transplantation in the United States, 1988 to 1996. *N Engl J Med* 2000;342:605–612.

5. Leichtman AB, Cohen D, Keith D, et al. Kidney and pancreas transplantation in the United States, 1997–2006: The HRSA Breakthrough Collaboratives and the 58 DSA Challenge. *Am J Transplant* 2008;8:946–957.

6. Ojo AO, Hanson JA, Wolfe RA, et al. Long-term survival in renal transplant recipients with graft function. *Kidney Int* 2000;57:307–313.

7. Schweitzer EJ, Matas AJ, Gillingham KJ, et al. Causes of renal allograft loss. Progress in the 1980s, challenges for the 1990s. *Ann Surg* 1991;214:679–688.

DONOR AND RECIPIENT EVALUATION

Michael R. Lattanzio, DO, and Matthew R. Weir, MD

CHAPTER 56

1. **What are the various categories of living-donor transplants?**
   - **Related donors:** Donor and recipient are biologically related.
   - **Unrelated donors:** Donor is not biologically related, but an emotional relationship exists between the donor and recipient (e.g., coworkers, classmates, friends).
   - **Directed anonymous donors:** Donor has no relationship to the recipient; the donor learned of the recipient's situation and decided to donate altruistically.
   - **Undirected anonymous donors:** Donor decides donate his or her kidney to the waiting list.
   - **Paired exchange donors:** A pair of donor–recipient candidates (from the related or unrelated categories) enters into a scheme in which the donor is exchanged with another donor–recipient candidate pair so as to achieve donor–recipient biologic compatibility of the ABO blood group system and/or negative cross-match reactivity.
   - **Multiple paired exchange donors:** A paired exchange donation as described in the preceding section and involves more than two donor–recipient candidate pairs.

2. **What do SCD, ECD, DCD, and DBD stand for?**
   - SCD = standard criteria donor
   - ECD = expanded criteria donor
   - DCD = donation after cardiac death
   - DBD = donation after brain death

3. **What is an expanded criteria donor?**
   An expanded criteria donor is >60 years old or age 50 to 59 years old and has two of the following: cerebrovascular accident as the cause of death, pre-existing hypertension, or terminal serum creatinine greater than or equal to 1.5 mg/dL. Expanded criteria donors have a 70% increased risk of graft failure over standard criteria donors.

   Metzger RA, Delmonico FL, Feng S, et al. Expanded criteria donors for kidney transplantation. *Am J Transplant* 2003;3(Suppl 4):114–125.

4. **What is the difference in graft survival among living donor transplants, standard criteria donor transplants, and expanded criteria donor transplants?**
   See Figure 56-1.

5. **What are some general contraindications for kidney donation?**
   - Chronic kidney disease (glomerular filtration rate <80 mL/min/1.73 m^2)
   - Proteinuria
   - Hematuria
   - Active infection
   - Chronic, active viral infections (e.g., HIV, hepatitis B/C)
   - Active malignancy
   - Family history of renal cell carcinoma
   - Hypertension
   - Diabetes

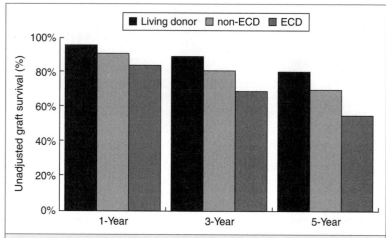

Figure 56-1. Unadjusted 1-year, 3-year, and 5-year graft survival of living, standard criteria, and expanded criteria donor transplants. (From Annual Report of the US Procurement and Transplantation Network and the Scientific Registry of Transplant Recipients: Transplant Data 1998–2007. US Department of Health and Human Services, Health Resources and Services Administration, Health Care Systems Bureau, Division of Transplantation, Rockville, MD.)

- Urologic abnormalities, including nephrolithiasis
- Substance abuse
- Obesity (body mass index >35 kg/m²)
- Age younger than 18 years

Kasiske BL, Ravenscraft M, Ramos EL, et al. The evaluation of living renal transplant donors: Clinical practice guidelines. Ad Hoc Clinical Practice Guidelines Subcommittee of the Patient Care and Education Committee of the American Society of Transplant Physicians. *J Am Soc Nephrol* 1996;7:2288–2313.

Screening of donor and recipient prior to solid organ transplantation. *Am J Transplant* 2004;4(Suppl 10):10–20.

6. **How is a living kidney donor evaluated to determine suitability?**
   The evaluation of a potential living kidney generally begins with an assessment of the donor and recipient blood groups and a cross-match. When a potential donor is identified, a cross-match is performed prior to transplantation to evaluate for any evidence of preformed antibodies against the specific donor (human leukocyte antigens [HLA]) that could result in hyperacute and/or acute humoral rejection. A final cross-match using fresh serum is performed in all cases immediately preceding transplantation to ensure compatibility between the donor and recipient. The methods available for cross-match testing include: enzyme-linked immunosorbent assay (ELISA), flow cytometry, complement-dependent cytotoxicity, and single antigen bead assay.

   The donor and recipient generally must be ABO compatible. This can occur under one of the following circumstances: the donor and recipient are ABO identical, the donor has blood type O (universal donor), or the recipient is blood type AB (universal recipient). Given the distribution of blood group antigens in the United States, the waiting time on the deceased donor list is prolonged for patients with blood group O and B. The practice of donor swapping in the case of ABO mismatches with a willing acceptable donor has gained some favor in the United States. ABO-incompatible transplantations following desensitization strategies have been performed successfully at some institutions.

   Rh antigens are not expressed in kidney tissue; therefore Rh mismatches are not considered to play a substantial role in allograft rejection. Female Rh-negative recipients of childbearing age are at risk for sensitization when the donor is Rh-positive and should receive anti-Rh immunoglobulin (RhoGAM) at the time of transplantation.

The major histocompatibility complex (MHC) antigens measured routinely in HLA laboratories include the class I antigens (A, B, and C) and class II antigens (DP, DQ, DR). HLA matching is an important predictor of survival of deceased donor allografts. However, with the use of better immunosuppressive agents, the use of HLA matching in allocation policies has come under considerable debate. A recent study demonstrated that with each successive year from 1994 to 1998, ever-increasing degrees of HLA mismatching was required to have a statistically significant adverse effect on graft failure. It also appears that not all HLA mismatches confer the same risk. HLA-DR matches have been associated with the most beneficial effect on long-term allograft survival. As a result, some centers advocate matching schemes to include kidneys without DR mismatches even if mismatched at the A and B loci. Given the scarcity of kidneys, the reliance on the number of HLA mismatches to determine the compatibility of a particular donor/recipient pairing is likely to be replaced by a determination of the significance of each mismatch on future graft survival.

2007 OPTN/SRTR Annual Report: Transplant Data 1997–2006. Rockville, MD: U.S. Department of Health and Human Services, Health Resources and Services Administration, Healthcare Systems Bureau, Division of Transplantation, 2007.

Beimler J, Zeier M. ABO-incompatible transplantation—A safe way to perform renal transplantation? *Nephrol Dial Transplant* 2007;22:25–27.

Hata Y, Cecka JM, Takemoto S, et al. Effects of changes in the criteria for nationally shared kidney transplants for HLA-matched patients. *Transplantation* 1998;65:208–212.

Leffell MS, Zachary AA. The national impact of the 1995 changes to the UNOS renal allocation system. United Network for Organ Sharing. *Clin Transplant* 1999;13:287–295.

Morris PJ, Johnson RJ, Fuggle SV, et al. Analysis of factors that affect outcome of primary cadaveric renal transplantation in the UK. HLA Task Force of the Kidney Advisory Group of the United Kingdom Transplant Support Service Authority (UKTSSA). *Lancet* 1999;354:1147–1152.

Su X, Zenios SA, Chakkera H, et al. Diminishing significance of HLA matching in kidney transplantation. *Am J Transplant* 2004;4:1501–1508.

7. **Why are renal imaging tests performed in living kidney donors prior to transplantation?**
   - To ensure the presence of two kidneys
   - To exclude malignancy involving the urinary tract
   - To exclude anatomic abnormalities of the urinary tract
   - To assess the vascular supply to the donor kidney

8. **What are some common imaging tests performed to evaluate the donor kidney?**
   - Helical computed tomography (CT)
   - CT angiogram
   - Magnetic resonance angiogram

9. **What are the surgical risks to the donor?**
   Laparoscopic surgical techniques have resulted in shorter hospital stays, reduced incisional pain, and an earlier return to work for living donors when compared to open nephrectomies. Conversion to open nephrectomy occurs in approximately 2% of the procedures. The perioperative mortality reported for living kidney donation is approximately 0.03%. Bleeding and reoperation are more common in laparoscopic techniques, although they are still relatively rare (0.45% and 1%, respectively).

Jacobs SC, Cho E, Foster C, et al. Laparoscopic donor nephrectomy: The University of Maryland 6-year experience. *J Urol* 2004;171:47–51.

Jacobs SC, Ramey JR, Sklar GN, et al. Laparoscopic kidney donation from patients older than 60 years. *J Am Coll Surg* 2004;198:892–897.

Matas AJ, Bartlett ST, Leichtman AB, et al. Morbidity and mortality after living kidney donation, 1999–2001: Survey of United States transplant centers. *Am J Transplant* 2003;3:830–834.

Ratner LE, Montgomery RA, Kavoussi LR. Laparoscopic live donor nephrectomy. A review of the first 5 years. *Urol Clin North Am* 2001;28:709–719.

Schweitzer EJ, Wilson J, Jacobs S, et al. Increased rates of donation with laparoscopic donor nephrectomy. *Ann Surg* 2000;232:392–400.

10. **What are the long-term outcomes for living kidney donors?**
    A major concern for living donors is the long-term impact of having a solitary kidney with risk for developing hypertension, proteinuria, and chronic kidney disease. A recent study that followed 3700 donors over a 12-year period demonstrated that survival of kidney donors was similar to that of control subjects who were matched for age, gender, and ethnicity. Additionally, ESRD developed in 11 donors, a rate of 180 cases per million persons per year, compared with a rate of 268 per million per year in the general population. Last, donors had quality-of-life scores that were better than population norms. In conclusion, it appears that the individual and kidney life span are not adversely affected by kidney donation.

    Ibrahim HN, Foley R, Tan L, et al. Long-term consequences of kidney donation. *N Engl J Med* 2009;360:459–469.

11. **At what level of renal dysfunction is it appropriate to refer a patient for kidney transplant evaluation?**
    If a medically acceptable living donor has been identified, elective renal transplantation ideally is performed just before dialysis is required ("pre-emptive"). If a living donor is not available, patients can be evaluated for transplantation at any time but cannot officially be listed for transplantation until their glomerular filtration rate falls below 20 mL/min.

12. **What are some general contraindications for renal transplantation from a recipient perspective?**
    - Presence of vascular disease that precludes the arterial and venous anastomoses requisite for a technically successful transplant
    - Recent or current malignancy (Table 56-1)
    - Chronic illness with short life expectancy
    - Active substance abuse
    - Active infectious process
    - Coronary artery disease
    - Psychosocial factors that may hinder future medicine adherence

TABLE 56–1. GUIDELINES FOR TRANSPLANTATION IN PATIENTS WITH PREVIOUS MALIGNANCIES
Generally: Advised waiting time is 2 years

No waiting time necessary:
    Incidental renal carcinoma
    In situ carcinoma
    Focal neoplasm (defined as a localized tumor without metastases)
    Low-grade bladder cancer
    Basal cell skin cancer

Waiting time of more than 2 years necessary:
    Melanoma
    Breast carcinoma
    Colorectal carcinoma
    Uterine carcinoma

Data from Penn I. The effect of immunosuppression on pre-existing cancers. *Transplantation* 1993;55:742–747.

13. **What is a "sensitized" potential recipient?**
A "sensitized" potential recipient is an individual that has detectable preformed HLA antibodies that pose considerable future risk to the allograft survival. Patient sensitization is classically reported as the percent panel reactivity antibody (PRA). PRA is defined as the percentage of donors expected to react with a patient's serum based on known antibody activities (i.e., the patient's degree of sensitization). Approximately 17% of the patients currently on the deceased donor waiting list are highly presensitized (defined as >80% percent panel reactivity). Highly "sensitized" patients often cross-match positive to multiple potential donors and require a zero antigen mismatch allograft to increase success. Consequently, these "sensitized" patients are less likely to be transplanted or will spend an extended time on the wait-list pending the availability of a suitable donor.

Akalin E. Posttransplant immunosuppression in highly sensitized patients. *Contrib Nephrol* 2009;162:27–34.

KEY POINTS: DONOR AND RECIPIENT EVALUATION

1. Living donor kidneys provide better long-term graft function than non-expanded criteria donor (ECD) and ECD kidneys.

2. Individual and kidney life span is not affected by kidney donation.

3. Patients who are sensitized are less likely to be transplanted and wait longer on the wait-list than patients who are not sensitized.

14. **What are some ways that potential recipients become sensitized?**
   - Pregnancy
   - Exposure to antigens from previous transplants
   - Exposure to antigens from blood product exposure (e.g., transfusions)

15. **What are some methods to desensitize potential recipients who possess preformed HLA antibodies?**
   - Intravenous immunoglobulin
   - Plasmapheresis
   - Rituximab
   - Splenectomy

BIBLIOGRAPHY

1. Annual Report of the US Procurement and Transplantation Network and the Scientific Registry of Transplant Recipients: Transplant Data 1998–2007. US Department of Health and Human Services, Health Resources and Services Administration, Health Care Systems Bureau, Division of Transplantation, Rockville, MD.

CHAPTER 57

IMMUNOSUPPRESSION

Michael R. Lattanzio, DO, and Matthew R. Weir, MD

1. **What is the goal of immunosuppression?**
   The suppression of allograft rejection through the use of immunosuppressive drugs remains the central goal of immunosuppression. The intensity of immunosuppression must be weighed against the undesired consequences of immunodeficiency (infection or cancer). Close monitoring, knowledge, and expertise are required to balance the efficacy and toxicity of renal transplantation immunosuppression.

2. **What are the classes of immunosuppressive therapies used in renal transplantation?**
   See Table 57-1.

3. **What are the different phases of immunosuppression?**
   Induction involves the use of immunosuppressive agents during the immediate post-transplant time frame until the maintenance levels are achieved. The optimal prophylactic induction immunosuppressive therapy to prevent renal transplantation rejection remains a subject of debate. **Maintenance** involves the use of immunosuppressive agents in the early and extended post-transplant period and is typically maintained for life.
   Kahan BD. Individuality: The barrier to optimal immunosuppression. *Nat Rev Immunol* 2003;3(10):831–838.

4. **What are the methods of induction therapy?**
   In general, induction strategies utilized by transplant centers fall into one of two categories: high-dose conventional agents (calcineurin inhibitors, steroids, antimetabolites) or antibody-depleting, biologic agents (i.e., monoclonal or polyclonal antibodies) with low-dose conventional agents. Several studies from single centers and registries, and meta-analyses, have found that induction with antibodies may be superior to nonantibody-based regiments, even in low-risk groups. Moreover, induction therapy has been associated with reduced incidence of acute rejection and improved allograft survival.
   Banhegyi C, Rockenschaub S, Muhlbacher F, et al. Preliminary results of a prospective randomized clinical trial comparing cyclosporine A to antithymocyte globulin immunosuppressive induction therapy in kidney transplantation. *Transplant Proc* 1991;23(4):2207–2208.

   Belitsky P, MacDonald AS, Cohen AD, et al. Comparison of antilymphocyte globulin and continuous i.v. cyclosporine A as induction immunosuppression for cadaver kidney transplants: A prospective randomized study. *Transplant Proc* 1991;23(1 Pt 2):999–1000.

   Michael HJ, Francos GC, Burke JF, et al. A comparison of the effects of cyclosporine versus antilymphocyte globulin on delayed graft function in cadaver renal transplant recipients. *Transplantation* 1989;48(5):805–808.

   Norman DJ, Kahana L, Stuart FP Jr, et al. A randomized clinical trial of induction therapy with OKT3 in kidney transplantation. *Transplantation* 1993;55(1):44–50.

   Opelz G. Efficacy of rejection prophylaxis with OKT3 in renal transplantation. Collaborative Transplant Study. *Transplantation* 1995;60(11):1220–1224.

   Szczech LA, Berlin JA, Aradhye S, et al. Effect of anti-lymphocyte induction therapy on renal allograft survival: a meta-analysis. *J Am Soc Nephrol* 1997;8(11):1771–1777.

   Szczech LA, Feldman HI. Effect of anti-lymphocyte antibody induction therapy on renal allograft survival. *Transplant Proc* 1999;31(3B Suppl):9S–11S.

TABLE 57-1.   CLASSES OF IMMUNOSUPPRESSIVE DRUGS USED IN RENAL TRANSPLANTATION

A. Glucocorticoids

B. Small molecule drugs

   1. Immunophilin-binding drugs*

      a. Calcineurin inhibitors (cyclosporine, tacrolimus)

      b. Mammalian target of rapamycin (mTOR) inhibitors (sirolimus, everolimus)

   2. Inhibitors of nucleotide synthesis

      a. Purine synthesis (inosine monophosphate dehydrogenase) inhibitors (mycophenolate mofetil [MMF], mycophenolic acid ([MPA])

      b. Pyrimidine synthesis inhibitors (Leflunomide)

   3. Antimetabolites (Azathioprine [AZA])

C. Protein drugs

   1. Antibody-depleting agents against T cells, B cells, or both

      a. Polyclonal antibody (thymoglobulin)

      b. Monoclonal antibody (muromonab)

   2. Nondepleting antibodies (basiliximab)

   3. Fusion drugs

   4. Intravenous immune globulin (IVIG)

*Immunophilin is an intracellular protein that, when bound to calcineurin inhibitors, will engage calcineurin.

---

5. **What are the three mechanisms utilized to achieve immunosuppression?**
   - Lymphocyte depletion
   - Lymphocyte traffic diversion
   - Blockade of lymphocyte response pathways

6. **What is the three-signal model of T cell-mediated rejection?**
   - Signal 1: Antigen triggers T-cell receptors and synapse formation occurs.
   - Signal 2: Signal 1 allows costimulation of antigen-presenting cells to occur.
   - Signal 3: Signal 1 and signal 2 stimulate a cascade of intracellular events culminating in the initiation of the T-cell cycle; stimulation of the T-cell cycle allows T cells to infiltrate the graft.

   Halloran PF. Immunosuppressive drugs for kidney transplantation. *N Engl J Med* 2004;351(26):2715–2729.

7. **What are the classes of antibody agents?**
   - **Depleting antibodies:** Less selective and more potent examples: thymoglobulin, anti-thymocyte gamma-globulin (ATGAM), anti-CD52 (alemtuzumab), rituximab
   - **Nondepleting antibodies:** More selective and less potent examples: anti-interleukin 2 (basiliximab)

8. **What is the frequency of use of various induction agents in the United States?**
   - Thymoglobulin: 42%
   - None: 21%
   - Basiliximab: 18%
   - Daclizumab: 11%
   - Alemtuzumab: 10%

- OKT3: 1%
- ATGAM: 1%

Meier-Kriesche HU, Li S, Gruessner RW, et al. Immunosuppression: evolution in practice and trends, 1994–2004. *Am J Transplant* 2006;6(5 Pt 2):1111–1131.

9. **What are the main drugs used for maintenance therapy?**
   The main medications used are glucocorticoids, calcineurin inhibitors (tacrolimus, cyclosporine), inosine monophosphate dehydrogenase (IMPDH) inhibitors (mycophenolate mofetil and mycophenolic acid), and rapamycin inhibitors.

10. **What are calcineurin inhibitors?**
    Calcineurin inhibitors remain a cornerstone of immunosuppressive regiments in renal transplantation. This class of drugs works by blocking calcineurin, an intricate protein in the signal transduction pathway. The two prototypes of the class are cyclosporine and tacrolimus. The side effects of the calcineurin inhibitors include nephrotoxicity, hemolytic uremic syndrome, and tremor. Cyclosporine use may be complicated by hypertension, post-transplant diabetes mellitus, and/or gingival hyperplasia. Calcineurin inhibitors require trough monitoring to ensure adequate degree of immunosuppression.

11. **What are inosine monophosphate dehydrogenase inhibitors?**
    IMPDH inhibitors are an important class of immunosuppressive agents that work by inhibiting purine synthesis. Two important drugs in this class are mycophenolic acid (MPA) and mycophenolate mofetil (MMF). MPA directly inhibits IMPDH (a key enzyme in purine synthesis), whereas MMF is a prodrug that releases MPA. The principal side effects of these medications are gastrointestinal (nausea, vomiting, diarrhea) and hematologic (anemia, leukopenia).

12. **What are mTOR inhibitors?**
    mTOR inhibitors (mammalian target of rapamycin) block the mammalian target of rapamycin and thus prevent cytokine signals from activating the T-cell cycle (signal 3). Two examples of these medications are sirolimus and everolimus. The principal adverse drug reactions include hyperlipidemia, impaired wound healing, and thrombocytopenia. Additionally, mTOR inhibitors have been linked to mouth ulcers and pneumonitis.

13. **What are the common drug interactions of concern with immunosuppressants?**
    The major drug interactions involve the calcineurin inhibitors (cyclosporine, tacrolimus) with drugs that are metabolized through the cytochrome p450-3A4 system (Table 57-2).

TABLE 57-2. COMMON DRUG IINTERACTIONS	
Increase Metabolism Decrease CNI Levels	**Decrease Metabolism Increase CNI Levels**
Carbamazepine	Ketoconazole
Phenytoin	Erythromycin
Phenobarbital	Clarithromycin
INH	Verapamil
Rifampin	Diltiazem
	Nicardipine
CNI = calcineurin inhibitor.	

14. **When should steroids be withdrawn following renal transplantation?**
The long-term use of steroids is associated with numerous adverse effects, including osteoporosis, new-onset diabetes after transplant, poor wound healing, hypertension, obesity, and dyslipidemia. To minimize these adverse effects, early steroid withdrawal or complete steroid avoidance has been investigated. Patients at lower immunologic risk do well with early steroid withdrawal 3 to 21 days post-transplantation; however, the benefits of early steroid withdrawal may be outweighed in patients at higher immunologic risk. The late withdrawal of steroids has demonstrated conflicting results. Steroid-free protocols are increasingly used, despite some controversy over their efficacy and safety. Data from the Following Rehabilitation, Economics, and Everyday-Dialysis Outcome Measurements (FREEDOM) study group showed a higher rate of acute rejection in the steroid-free group, despite no differences in creatinine, glomerular filtration rate, or graft survival compared to the steroid maintenance arm. It is not surprising that, the steroid-free group had less statin use, weight gain, and hyperglycemic medicine use. The issue of steroid use post-transplantation remains controversial and requires further investigation to identify the optimal strategy. For now, the use of steroids post-transplantation should be individualized, considering a recipient's comorbidities and overall risk of allograft rejection.

Hricik DE, O'Toole MA, Schulak JA, et al. Steroid-free immunosuppression in cyclosporine-treated renal transplant recipients: A meta-analysis. *J Am Soc Nephrol* 1993;4(6):1300–1305.

Opelz G, Dohler B, Laux G. Long-term prospective study of steroid withdrawal in kidney and heart transplant recipients. *Am J Transplant* 2005;5(4 Pt 1):720–728.

Pascual J, Quereda C, Zamora J, et al. Steroid withdrawal in renal transplant patients on triple therapy with a calcineurin inhibitor and mycophenolate mofetil: A meta-analysis of randomized, controlled trials. *Transplantation* 2004;78(10):1548–1556.

Ratcliffe PJ, Dudley CR, Higgins RM, et al. Randomised controlled trial of steroid withdrawal in renal transplant recipients receiving triple immunosuppression. *Lancet* 1996;348(9028):643–648.

Sandrini S, Maiorca R, Scolari F, et al. A prospective randomized trial on azathioprine addition to cyclosporine versus cyclosporine monotherapy at steroid withdrawal, 6 months after renal transplantation. *Transplantation* 2000;69(9):1861–1867.

Vincenti F, Schena FP, Paraskevas S, et al. A randomized, multicenter study of steroid avoidance, early steroid withdrawal or standard steroid therapy in kidney transplant recipients. *Am J Transplant* 2008;8(2):307–316.

KEY POINTS: IMMUNOSUPPRESSION

1. The intensity of immunosuppression must be weighed against the undesired consequences of immunodeficiency (infection or cancer).

2. In general, induction strategies utilized by transplant centers fall into one of two categories: high-dose conventional agents (calcineurin inhibitors, steroids, antimetabolites) or antibody-depleting biologic agents (i.e., monoclonal or polyclonal antibodies) with low-dose conventional agents.

3. Calcineurin inhibitors remain a cornerstone of immunosuppressive regiments in renal transplantation. This class of drugs works by blocking calcineurin, an intricate protein in the signal transduction pathway.

4. Mammalian target of rapamycin (mTOR) inhibitors block the mammalian target of rapamycin and thus prevent cytokine signals from activating the T-cell cycle.

5. The issue of steroid use post-transplantation remains controversial and requires further investigation to identify the optimal strategy. For now, the use of steroids post-transplantation should be individualized, considering a recipient's comorbidities and overall risk of allograft rejection.

CHAPTER 58

REJECTION OF THE RENAL TRANSPLANT

Michael R. Lattanzio, DO, and Matthew R. Weir, MD

1. **What are the various types of rejection?**

   There are three general types of organ rejection: hyperacute, acute, and chronic. Hyperacute rejection is a complement-mediated response by the recipient with pre-existing donor antibodies. Hyperacute rejection occurs almost immediately following organ implantation and necessitates immediate explant of the organ. Hyperacute rejection is uncommon with pretransplantation cross-matches and screening. Acute rejection is associated with a sudden deterioration in allograft function that can occur as early as 1 week post-transplantation. Acute rejection may also be subclinical, associated with a more insidious rise in creatinine. Acute rejection has a major adverse effect on long-term graft survival. Chronic rejection, renamed chronic allograft nephropathy (because a poorly defined multifactorial entity that may not always include rejection) causes an insidious deterioration in renal function that occurs following renal transplantation. Chronic allograft nephropathy is characterized by histologic changes including interstitial fibrosis, tubular atrophy, vascular occlusive changes, and varying degrees of glomerulosclerosis.

   Berczi C, Asztalos L, Kincses Z, et al. Effect of acute rejection episodes on long-term renal graft survival. *Transplant Proc* 1998;30:1775.

   Racusen LC, Solez K, Colvin RB, et al. The Banff 97 working classification of renal allograft pathology. *Kidney Int* 1999;55:713–723.

2. **What are the different types of acute rejection?**
   - T-cell-mediated rejection
   - Antibody-mediated, humoral rejection

3. **What is the Banff criteria for acute T-cell-mediated rejection?**

   The Banff classification of renal allograft rejection grades acute tubulointerstitial rejection (AIR) by severity of tubulitis and acute vascular rejection (AVR) by severity of arteritis. Types of T-cell mediated rejection are as follows:
   - **Type IA:** Cases with significant interstitial infiltration (>25% of parenchyma affected) and foci of *moderate* tubulitis
   - **Type IB:** Cases with significant interstitial infiltration (>25% of parenchyma affected) and foci of *severe* tubulitis
   - **Type IIA:** Cases with *mild-to-moderate* intimal arteritis
   - **Type IIB:** Cases with *severe* intimal arteritis
   - **Type III:** Cases with transmural arteritis and/or arterial fibrinoid change and necrosis of medial smooth muscle cells with accompanying lymphocytic inflammation

   Solez K, Axelsen RA, Benediktsson H, et al. International standardization of criteria for the histologic diagnosis of renal allograft rejection: The Banff working classification of kidney transplant pathology. *Kidney Int* 1993;44:411–422.

4. **What should be considered when acute rejection is diagnosed?**

   The possibility of inadequate immunosuppression should be considered whenever acute rejection is confirmed. This inadequacy may result from noncompliance, underdosing of maintenance immunosuppressants, drug interactions, and/or rapid withdrawal of immunosuppressants post-transplantation. A systematic approach to identify the contributing factors for acute rejection should be instituted to mitigate further graft damage and eventual graft failure.

5. **What are the treatment options for acute cellular rejection?**
   - Pulse corticosteroids
   - Anti-T-cell antibody therapies (e.g., OKT3, thymoglobulin, ATG)
   - Antimetabolites (cyclophosphamide)—rarely used

6. **What are some general principles when treating acute cellular rejection?**
   Pulse corticosteroids, typically methylprednisolone 3 to 5 mg/kg, given intravenously for 3 to 5 days are considered the first-line therapy for Banff class I. The calcineurin inhibitor dose should be adjusted if levels preceding the acute rejection episode were subtherapeutic. If tolerable, the dose of mycophenolate mofetil/mycophenolic acid (MMF/MPA) should be increased. With successful response, the urine output increases and serum creatinine decreases within 5 days after pulse steroids.

   Steroid resistance is defined as a lack of improvement in urine output and/or creatinine concentration within 5 to 7 days. In this scenario, second-line agents (antilymphocyte antibodies) should be considered. The antilymphocyte antibody agents used include polyclonal anti-T-cell antibodies (ATG) and monoclonal antibodies (OKT3).

   In the setting of worsening graft function and biopsy demonstration of Banff class II to III, combined steroid and antilymphocyte therapy may be a reasonable first-line approach. If there is no response to this strategy, the exclusion of acute humoral rejection through measurement of donor-specific antibody and C4d staining of the biopsy specimen are necessary. If there are no contraindications, an alternate antilymphocyte agent, plasmapheresis, and/or intravenous immune globulin may be considered to salvage the allograft. The decision to discontinue therapy should be based on many factors but mainly the recipient's clinical status and degree of damage on repeat allograft biopsy.

   Gray D, Shepherd H, Daar A, et al. Oral versus intravenous high-dose steroid treatment of renal allograft rejection. The big shot or not? *Lancet* 1978;1:117–118.

   Shinn C, Malhotra D, Chan L, et al. Time course of response to pulse methylprednisolone therapy in renal transplant recipients with acute allograft rejection. *Am J Kidney Dis* 1999;34:304–307.

   Vineyard GC, Fadem SZ, Dmochowski J, et al. Evaluation of corticosteroid therapy for acute renal allograft rejection. *Surg Gynecol Obstet* 1974;138:225–229.

7. **What are the Banff criteria for humoral rejection?**
   Acute, antibody-mediated rejection requires documentation of circulating antidonor-specific antibody, C4d, and allograft pathology consistent with this diagnosis. The histologic grades of acute humoral rejection include type I (ATN-like histology with minimal inflammation, C4d positive), type II (a capillary glomerulitis, with margination and/or thrombosis, C4d positive), and type III (arterial-transmural inflammation/fibrinoid changes, C4d positive).

   Chronic, active antibody-mediated rejection results in glomerular double contours and/or multilayering of the peritubular capillary basement membrane and/or interstitial fibrosis/tubular atrophy and/or fibrous intimal thickening in arteries in the setting of C4d positivity.

   Solez K, Colvin RB, Racusen LC, et al. Banff '05 meeting report: Differential diagnosis of chronic allograft injury and elimination of chronic allograft nephropathy ('can'). *Am J Transplant* 2007;7:518–526.

8. **What are PRA, DSA, and C4d?**
   Patient sensitization is classically reported as the percent panel reactive antibody (PRA) and is an estimate of the likelihood of a positive cross-match to a pool of potential donors and their respective human leukocyte antigens (HLA). In simpler terms, it is a method for determining a patient's risk of organ rejection prior to transplantation. PRA greater than 80% is considered highly sensitized.

DSA stands for donor-specific antibody. DSA are immunoglobulin G antibodies targeted against HLAs. DSA may be anticlass I or anticlass II. Antidonor HLA antibodies against either class I or class II antigens are associated with higher frequency of acute and chronic antibody-mediated rejection.

C4d is a degradation product of the classic complement pathway. C4d has a high affinity for endothelial and collagen basement membranes and serves as a method of detecting antibody activation within the glomerulus and tubules. C4d is considered a footprint of antibody-mediated rejection.

Patel AM, Pancoska C, Mulgaonkar S, et al. Renal transplantation in patients with pre-transplant donor-specific antibodies and negative flow cytometry crossmatches. *Am J Transplant* 2007;7:2371–2377.

Terasaki PI, Cai J. Human leukocyte antigen antibodies and chronic rejection: From association to causation. *Transplantation* 2008;86:377–383.

9. **What is the ABCD tetrad of transplant glomerulopathy?**
   Transplant glomerulopathy is a severe, pathophysiologic process that likely represents the end stage of chronic, active humoral rejection. It is often characterized by progressive graft dysfunction and varying degrees of proteinuria. Transplant glomerulopathy can be defined based on the presence of the following:
   - **A** = Circulating anti-HLA **A**lloantibody
   - **B** = Peritubular capillary **B**asement membrane multilayering
   - **C** = Peritubular **C**4d deposition
   - **D** = **D**ouble contouring of the basement membrane

   Sis B, Campbell PM, Mueller T, et al. Transplant glomerulopathy, late antibody-mediated rejection and the ABCD tetrad in kidney allograft biopsies for cause. *Am J Transplant* 2007;7:1743–1752.

10. **What are the postulated stages of antibody-mediated rejection?**
    See Figure 58-1.

    Colvin RB. Antibody-mediated renal allograft rejection: Diagnosis and pathogenesis. *J Am Soc Nephrol* 2007;18:1046–1056.

11. **What are the treatment options for acute humoral rejection?**
    - IVIG
    - Plasmapheresis
    - Rituximab (chimeric anti-CD20 antibody)

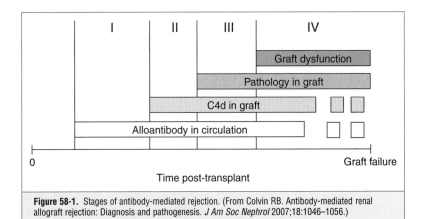

Figure 58-1. Stages of antibody-mediated rejection. (From Colvin RB. Antibody-mediated renal allograft rejection: Diagnosis and pathogenesis. *J Am Soc Nephrol* 2007;18:1046–1056.)

12. **What is chronic allograft nephropathy?**

Chronic allograft nephropathy (CAN) is a major cause of graft failure. CAN is characterized by progressive renal dysfunction accompanied by chronic interstitial fibrosis, tubular atrophy, vascular occlusive changes, and glomerulosclerosis. CAN appears to consist of two distinctive phases of injury occurring at various times after transplantation within different histologic compartments. Early tubulointerstitial damage correlates with immunologic factors, including severe acute rejection or subclinical rejection with the addition of ischemia–reperfusion injury. The later damage is characterized by progressive arteriolar hyalinosis, ischemic glomerulosclerosis, and further interstitial fibrosis associated with long-term calcineurin-inhibitor nephrotoxicity. Multiple factors, both alloantigen-dependent and alloantigen-independent, appear to contribute to the pathogenesis of chronic graft dysfunction.

Nankivell BJ, Borrows RJ, Fung CL, et al. The natural history of chronic allograft nephropathy. *N Engl J Med* 2003;349:2326–2333.

13. **How should maintenance immunosuppression be handled in patients with CAN?**

Given the long-term, detrimental effects of calcineurin inhibitors (CNIs) on graft survival, substitution or withdrawal of CNIs in individuals with CAN is an attractive therapy. The conversion from calcineurin inhibitors to sirolimus maintenance therapy in renal allograft recipients (CONVERT) trial aimed to determine the efficacy and safety of conversion from CNIs to sirolimus in individuals with CAN. The CONVERT study showed improvements in glomerular filtration rate (GFR) only in individuals with GFR >40 mL/min and protein-to-creatinine ratios less than 0.11. Moreover, in individuals with GFR <40 mL/min, excess rates of pneumonia and death were observed. In the "Creeping creatinine" study, patients with discontinuation of cyclosporine and addition of MMF had higher rates of stabilization in serum creatinine than individuals maintained on cyclosporine alone. Additionally, a 2009 systematic review and meta-analysis found that CNI sparing and minimization strategies in which MMF is used as the sole adjunctive immunosuppressant appeared beneficial. Taken together, these studies suggest benefit in minimizing CNIs in individuals with CAN; however, he substitution of CNI with an mammalian target of rapamycin (mTOR) inhibitor may also be beneficial but should be reserved for individuals with better preserved kidney function without proteinuria.

Dudley C, Pohanka E, Riad H, et al. Mycophenolate mofetil substitution for cyclosporine a in renal transplant recipients with chronic progressive allograft dysfunction: The "Creeping creatinine" Study. *Transplantation* 2005;79:466–475.

Moore J, Middleton L, Cockwell P, et al. Calcineurin inhibitor sparing with mycophenolate in kidney transplantation: A systematic review and meta-analysis. *Transplantation* 2009;87:591–605.

Schena FP, Pascoe MD, Alberu J, et al. Conversion from calcineurin inhibitors to sirolimus maintenance therapy in renal allograft recipients: 24-month efficacy and safety results from the convert trial. *Transplantation* 2009;87:233–242.

KEY POINTS: REJECTION OF THE RENAL TRANSPLANT

1. The possibility of inadequate immunosuppression should be considered whenever acute rejection is confirmed.

2. Acute antibody-mediated rejection requires documentation of circulating antidonor specific antibody, C4d staining in the peritubular capillaries, and allograft pathology consistent with this diagnosis.

3. Chronic, active antibody-mediated rejection results in double contours and/or multilayering of the peritubular capillary basement membrane in the glomeruli and/or interstitial fibrosis/tubular atrophy and/or fibrous intimal thickening in arteries in the setting of C4d positivity.

4. Transplant glomerulopathy can be defined based on the presence of the following:
   - **A** = Circulating anti-HLA **A**lloantibody
   - **B** = Peritubular capillary **B**asement membrane multilayering
   - **C** = Peritubular **C**4d deposition
   - **D** = **D**ouble-contouring of the basement membrane

5. Multiple factors, both alloantigen-dependent and alloantigen-independent, appear to contribute to the pathogenesis of chronic graft dysfunction.

6. In 2009 a systematic review and meta-analysis found that calcineurin inhibitor (CNI) sparing and minimization strategies in which MMF is used as the sole adjunctive immunosuppressant appeared beneficial. Substitution of CNI with an mammalian target of rapamycin (mTOR) inhibitor may also be beneficial but should be reserved for individuals with better preserved kidney function without proteinuria.

POST-TRANSPLANTATION MALIGNANCIES

Michael R. Lattanzio, DO, and Matthew R. Weir, MD

1. **Are transplant recipients at greater risk for the development of malignancies?**
   Yes. The chronic exposure to immunosuppressive agents increases the long-term risk of many malignancies, particularly when compared to the general population.

   Dharnidharka VR, Harmon WE. Management of pediatric postrenal transplantation infections. *Semin Nephrol* 2001;21:521–531.

   McDonald RA, Smith JM, Ho M, et al. Incidence of PTLD in pediatric renal transplant recipients receiving basiliximab, calcineurin inhibitor, sirolimus and steroids. *Am J Transplant* 2008;8:984–989.

2. **What is the risk of developing various malignances in transplant recipients compared to the general population?**
   See Figure 59-1.

3. **What is PTLD?**
   Post-transplant lymphoproliferative disorder (PTLD) is the heterogenous group of lymphoproliferative disorders that primarily results from active Epstein-Barr virus infection provocated by chronic immunosuppression. They are predominantly B cell in origin. The incidence of PTLD is approximately 1%, which is 30 to 50 times higher than in the general population, with a recent trend toward increased frequency. The degree of immunosuppression is the major determinant of the development of PTLD.

   Andreone P, Gramenzi A, Lorenzini S, et al. Posttransplantation lymphoproliferative disorders. *Arch Intern Med* 2003;163:1997–2004.

   Caillard S, Agodoa LY, Bohen EM, et al. Myeloma, Hodgkin disease, and lymphoid leukemia after renal transplantation: Characteristics, risk factors and prognosis. *Transplantation* 2006;81:888–895.

   Caillard S, Lelong C, Pessione F, et al. Post-transplant lymphoproliferative disorders occurring after renal transplantation in adults: Report of 230 cases from the French registry. *Am J Transplant* 2006;6:2735–2742.

   Hanto DW. Classification of Epstein-Barr virus-associated posttransplant lymphoproliferative diseases: Implications for understanding their pathogenesis and developing rational treatment strategies. *Annu Rev Med* 1995;46:381–394.

   Patton DF, Wilkowski CW, Hanson CA, et al. Epstein-Barr virus-determined clonality in posttransplant lymphoproliferative disease. *Transplantation* 1990;49:1080–1084.

4. **How common are lymphoproliferative disorders following transplantation?**
   According to the Cincinnati Transplant Tumor Registry, lymphoproliferative disorders are the most common malignancies complicating organ transplantation, excluding nonmelanoma skin cancer and in situ cervical cancer. Lymphoproliferative disorders account for 21% of all malignancies in patients who have received transplant compared to 5% of malignancies in the general population.

   Penn I. Cancers complicating organ transplantation. *N Engl J Med* 1990;323:1767–1769.

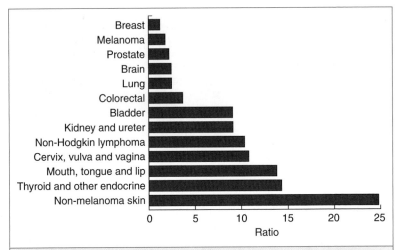

Figure 59-1. Risk of developing malignancies in transplant recipients compared to the general population. (Adapted from Kasiske BL, Vazquez MA, Harmon WE, et al. Recommendations for the outpatient surveillance of renal transplant recipients. American Society of Transplantation. *J Am Soc Nephrol* 2000;11(Suppl 15):S1–86.)

5. **Does PTLD have the same characteristics as lymphoproliferative disease in the general population?**
   Non-Hodgkin's lymphoma accounts for 65% of lymphomas in the general population, compared to 93% in transplant recipients. PTLD is mainly a B-cell-derived, large-cell lymphoma. Extra-nodal involvement is very common.

   Hanson MN, Morrison VA, Peterson BA, et al. Posttransplant T-cell lymphoproliferative disorders—An aggressive, late complication of solid-organ transplantation. *Blood* 1996;88:3626–3633.

   Penn I. Cancers complicating organ transplantation. *N Engl J Med* 1990;323:1767–1769.

6. **What is the clinical presentation of PTLD?**
   The clinical presentation of PTLD is protean. Most patients present with nonspecific complaints, including fatigue, weight loss, and fever. Some patients present with symptoms resembling infectious mononucleosis. Last, patients may present with lymphadenopathy or palpable masses. Given the nonspecific nature of clinical presentation, the diagnosis of PTLD requires a high index of suspicion.

7. **What are the different types of PTLD?**
   - Benign polyclonal lymphoproliferation
   - Polyclonal lymphoproliferation with malignant transformation
   - Monoclonal lymphoproliferation with malignant transformation

8. **What are the treatment options for various PTLDs?**
   The treatment and management of PTLD is varied. Treatment is often dictated by the cell type and stage of the lymphoproliferative process. Treatment strategies are individualized and can include reduction of immunosuppression, antiviral therapy, chemotherapy, IVIG, surgical resection, radiation, interferon therapy, and anti-CD 20 monoclonal antibody therapies. Management and surveillance requires collaboration among hematologists/oncologists, infectious disease specialists, and transplant nephrologists.

9. **Is treatment of Epstein-Barr virus with antiviral therapies beneficial for PTLD?**
Despite their widespread use, there is currently no evidence that any antiviral therapy is efficacious for the treatment of PTLD. Given the lack of evidence-based support for antiviral therapies, they are not recommended as a sole treatment. The use of antivirals to reduce the incidence of PTLD following transplantation has been validated.

Darenkov IA, Marcarelli MA, Basadonna GP, et al. Reduced incidence of Epstein-Barr virus-associated posttransplant lymphoproliferative disorder using preemptive antiviral therapy. *Transplantation* 1997;64:848–852.

Davis CL, Harrison KL, McVicar JP, et al. Antiviral prophylaxis and the Epstein Barr virus-related post-transplant lymphoproliferative disorder. *Clin Transplant* 1995;9:53–59.

Paya CV, Fung JJ, Nalesnik MA, et al. Epstein-Barr virus-induced posttransplant lymphoproliferative disorders. ASTS/ASTP EBV-PTLD Task Force and the Mayo Clinic Organized International Consensus Development Meeting. *Transplantation* 1999;68:1517–1525.

10. **What is the most common form of skin cancer in transplant recipients?**
Squamous cell carcinoma is the most common, occurring 65 to 250 times more frequently in the transplant population than in the general population. In the general population, basal cell carcinoma is more common than squamous cell skin cancer.

Hartevelt MM, Bavinck JN, Kootte AM, et al. Incidence of skin cancer after renal transplantation in the Netherlands. *Transplantation* 1990;49:506–509.

Jensen P, Hansen S, Moller B, et al. Skin cancer in kidney and heart transplant recipients and different long-term immunosuppressive therapy regimens. *J Am Acad Dermatol* 1999;40:177–186.

KEY POINTS: POST-TRANSPLANTATION MALIGNANCIES

1. The chronic exposure to immunosuppressive agents increases the long-term risk of many malignancies, particularly when compared to the general population.

2. Lymphoproliferative disorders are the most common malignancies complicating organ transplantation, excluding nonmelanoma skin cancer and in situ cervical cancer.

3. The clinical presentation of post-transplant lymphoproliferative disorder is protean. Most patients present with nonspecific complaints, including fatigue, weight loss, and fever.

4. Squamous cell carcinoma occurs 65 to 250 times more frequently in the transplant population than in the general population.

11. **How can we reduce the risk of skin cancer in patients who have received renal transplant?**
All kidney transplant recipients, especially those who have fair skin, live in sun-exposed climates, had significant sun exposure as a child, or have a history of skin cancer, should be educated on their high risk of skin cancer. Minimization of sun exposure, the use of sunscreen, and meticulous skin self-examinations should be instituted to reduce the risk of skin cancers in this high-risk population. An annual skin examination by a dermatologist is recommended in most kidney transplant recipients.

12. **How should the transplant recipient be screened for malignancies?**
   - History and physical examination to exclude disseminated or localized organ involvement by PTLD (every 3 months during the first year post-transplant, subsequently annually)
   - Skin examinations by dermatologist (every 6 months in patients at high risk, otherwise yearly)
   - Ultrasound or computed tomography scan of the native kidneys annually

- Gynecologic examinations, including Pap test and ultrasound of genitourinary organs annually
- Prostate-specific antigen and digital rectal examination annually in men older than 50 years old or younger in high-risk groups
- Fecal occult blood test annually in men older than 50 years old or younger in high-risk groups
- Abdominal ultrasound and serum alpha-fetoprotein levels in carriers of hepatitis B or C virus
- Colonoscopy in individuals, as per general population guidelines
- Mammogram in females, as per general population guidelines
- Cystoscopy in individuals with hematuria, particularly with a history of cyclophosphamide therapy

   These guidelines are in accordance with Kasiske et al.

Kasiske BL, Vazquez MA, Harmon WE, et al. Recommendations for the outpatient surveillance of renal transplant recipients. American Society of Transplantation. *J Am Soc Nephrol* 2000;11(Suppl 15):S1–86.

POST-TRANSPLANTATION INFECTIONS

Michael R. Lattanzio, DO, and Matthew R. Weir, MD

CHAPTER 60

1. **What type of infections do kidney transplant recipients develop?**
   - Donor-derived infections
   - Recipient-derived infections
   - Nosocomial-acquired infections
   - Community-acquired infections

2. **Is there any pattern to infections that occur post-transplantation?**
   Yes. Infections occur in a generally predictable pattern after renal transplantation. Nosocomial and surgery-related infections are the predominant infections that occur within the first month post-transplantation. Common infections in the first month include aspiration pneumonia, catheter infections, wound infections, anastomotic leaks, and *Clostridium difficile* colitis. Resistant organisms (methicillin-resistant *Staphylococcus aureus,* vancomycin-resistant *Enterococcus, Candida)* are most common within the first month. Opportunistic infections are usually absent in the first month after transplantation, owing to the delay in complete immunosuppression. In post-transplantation months 1 through 6, the activation of latent infections is most common. Chemoprophylaxis aids in preventing common infections such as *Pneumocystic carinii* pneumonia, fungal infections, and herpes-related disease during this time period. Common infections in months 1 through 6 include BK virus, *C. difficile* colitis, hepatitis C virus, adenovirus, influenza, *Cryptococcus,* and *Mycobacterium* tuberculosis. After 6 months, community-acquired infections are predominant. These infections include community-acquired pneumonia, urinary tract infections, *Nocardia, Aspergillus, Mucor,* and late viral infections (cytomegalovirus, hepatitis B, hepatitis C, herpes simplex virus, JC virus).

3. **What is BK virus?**
   BK virus is a ubiquitous, double-stranded DNA polyomavirus with a 5300-base pair genome that replicates in the host nucleus. The polyoma family includes JC virus (infectious cause of progressive multifocal leukoencephalopathy [PML]), SV 40, and monkey polyomavirus. Although the human polyomaviruses are highly seroprevalent in humans, they appear to cause clinical disease only in immunocompromised hosts.

   Hirsch HH, Brennan DC, Drachenberg CB, et al. Polyomavirus-associated nephropathy in renal transplantation: Interdisciplinary analyses and recommendations. *Transplantation* 2005;79:1277–1286.

   Hirsch HH, Steiger J. Polyomavirus BK. *Lancet Infect Dis* 2003;3:611–623.

4. **What is BK-associated nephropathy?**
   BK virus has been implicated as the causative agent of a particular form of nephropathy that occurs post-transplantation. The prevalence of BK nephropathy ranges from 1% to 10% based on interdisciplinary analyses. BK nephropathy is characterized by a tubulointerstitial disease pattern that closely resembles acute rejection.

   Dharnidharka VR, Cherikh WS, Abbott KC. An OPTN analysis of national registry data on treatment of BK virus allograft nephropathy in the United States. *Transplantation* 2009;87:1019–1026.

   Hirsch HH, Brennan DC, Drachenberg CB, et al. Polyomavirus-associated nephropathy in renal transplantation: Interdisciplinary analyses and recommendations. *Transplantation* 2005;79:1277–1286.

5. **Besides nephropathy, can BK virus cause any other renal problems?**
   Yes. BK virus is associated with ureteral stenosis/strictures, which may lead to obstructive uropathy in a renal transplant recipient. Obstructions associated with BK virus usually occurs 2 to 4 months post-transplant, whereas ischemia-induced stenosis usually occurs 1 to 2 weeks postoperatively.

   Coleman DV, Mackenzie EF, Gardner SD, et al. Human polyomavirus (BK) infection and ureteric stenosis in renal allograft recipients. *J Clin Pathol* 1978;31:338–347.

   Gardner SD, Field AM, Coleman DV, et al. New human papovavirus (B.K.) isolated from urine after renal transplantation. *Lancet* 1971;1:1253–1257.

6. **What are the risk factors for the development of BK-associated nephropathy?**
   - Human leukocyte antigen mismatch
   - Previous acute rejection
   - Use of antilymphocyte therapy
   - Use of steroid pulses
   - Mycophenolate mofetil (MMF) use at baseline
   - Age >55
   - Male gender
   - White race
   - Diabetes

7. **What are the clinical features of BK-associated nephropathy?**
   Patients with BK-associated nephropathy are typically asymptomatic and are detected when they develop renal insufficiency. A high index of suspicion and low threshold to biopsy are required to make a timely diagnosis.

8. **How can you diagnose BK-virus nephropathy?**
   - Cytology
   - Serology
   - Biopsy

   The diagnosis of BK-associated nephropathy requires the presence of sustained and significant BK replication (plasma DNA polymerase chain reaction [PCR] load >10^4 copies/mL) and renal dysfunction. The diagnosis is confirmed by renal biopsy.

   Drachenberg CB, Papadimitriou JC. Polyomavirus-associated nephropathy: Update in diagnosis. *Transpl Infect Dis* 2006;8:68–75.

   Hirsch HH, Brennan DC, Drachenberg CB, et al. Polyomavirus-associated nephropathy in renal transplantation: Interdisciplinary analyses and recommendations. *Transplantation* 2005;79:1277–1286.

9. **What does cytology show in BK-associated nephropathy?**
   Cytologic examination of the urine can detect BK-infected cells ("decoy cells"). These characteristic cells have enlarged nuclei with a single, basophilic, intranuclear inclusion. Identification of decoy cells is sensitive, but not specific, for the diagnosis of BK-associated nephropathy.

   Nickeleit V, Hirsch HH, Binet IF, et al. Polyomavirus infection of renal allograft recipients: From latent infection to manifest disease. *J Am Soc Nephrol* 1999;10:1080–1089.

10. **Is serology helpful in the diagnosis of BK-associated nephropathy?**
    Yes. Quantification of BK virus DNA in plasma by polymerase chain reaction has a sensitivity and specificity of 100% and 88%, respectively; however, not all patients with viremia have nephritis (positive predictive value of 50%).

    Hirsch HH, Knowles W, Dickenmann M, et al. Prospective study of polyomavirus type BK replication and nephropathy in renal-transplant recipients. *N Engl J Med* 2002;347:488–496.

11. **Is the quantification of BK virus in the urine useful?**
    Yes. The detection of BK virus in the urine, particularly at high levels, may predict the development of viremia and clinically overt nephropathy. DNA PCR levels >10^7 in the urine should prompt investigation for overt BK viremia.

12. **What does the renal biopsy show in BK-associated nephropathy?**
    Biopsy remains the gold standard for the diagnosis of BK-associated nephropathy. BK virus can induce a number of characteristic changes on renal biopsy, including intranuclear viral

inclusions, tubular injury/tubulitis, and tubulointerstitial inflammation. Because none of these renal biopsy findings are pathognomonic for BK-associated nephropathy, the diagnosis must be confirmed by demonstrating antibodies against BK with immunohistochemistry.

Drachenberg CB, Papadimitriou JC, Hirsch HH, et al. Histological patterns of polyomavirus nephropathy: correlation with graft outcome and viral load. *Am J Transplant* 2004;4:2082–2092.

13. **What is the treatment for BK-associated nephropathy?**
The goal in treating BK-associated nephropathy is to eradicate the virus while maintaining renal function and preventing acute or chronic rejection. Most treatments of BK-associated nephropathy involve manipulation of immunosuppression to permit native, immune-mediated handling of the BK virus. Possible strategies include discontinuation of a single immunosuppressive agent, reduction in immunosuppression by reducing dosages, and steroid avoidance. Antiviral therapy with leflunomide or cidofovir has been used in conjunction with decreasing immunosuppressants in some instances. Fluoroquinolones possess anti-BK virus activity that may be a therapeutic option.

Araya CE, Lew JF, Fennell RS 3rd, et al. Intermediate-dose cidofovir without probenecid in the treatment of BK virus allograft nephropathy. *Pediatr Transplant* 2006;10:32–37.

Randhawa PS. Anti-BK virus activity of ciprofloxacin and related antibiotics. *Clin Infect Dis* 2005;41: 1366–1367.

Williams JW, Javaid B, Kadambi PV, et al. Leflunomide for polyomavirus type BK nephropathy. *N Engl J Med* 2005;352:1157–1158.

14. **Can patients with graft failure resulting from BK nephropathy be retransplanted?**
Yes. There are case reports of successful retransplantation. However, it is preferable to use well-matched grafts with less intense immunosuppression.

15. **What is cytomegalovirus?**
Cytomegalovirus (CMV) is a member of the genus *Herpesvirus* and belongs to the family *Herpesviridae*. It is composed of a double-stranded DNA genome. Exposure to the virus, as indicated by immunoglobulin G (IgG) anti-CMV antibodies, is present in more than two thirds of donors and recipients prior to transplantation. CMV can be transmitted from the donor either by blood transfusions or by the transplanted kidney. Symptomatic CMV infection occurs in 20% to 60% of all transplant recipients and is a significant cause of increased morbidity and mortality in this population.

Sagedal S, Hartmann A, Nordal KP, et al. Impact of early cytomegalovirus infection and disease on long-term recipient and kidney graft survival. *Kidney Int* 2004;66:329–336.

16. **Are there any risk factors for the development of CMV infections post-transplantation?**
Yes. Antilymphocyte induction therapy, high-dose MMF, and absence of adequate antiviral prophylaxis are all associated with higher incidence of CMV infections following transplantation.

17. **What groups are at highest risk from CMV infections?**
Historically, groups who are CMV donor positive and CMV recipient negative (CMV D+/R−) are at greatest risk for severe "primary" infection during the first 3 months post-transplantation. Recent data, however, demonstrated that the CMV D+/R+ group and not the D+/R− group has a worst graft and patient survival at 3 years.

Schnitzler MA, Woodward RS, Brennan DC, et al. The effects of cytomegalovirus serology on graft and recipient survival in cadaveric renal transplantation: Implications for organ allocation. *Am J Kidney Dis* 1997;29:428–434.

Schnitzler MA, Woodward RS, Brennan DC, et al. Impact of cytomegalovirus serology on graft survival in living related kidney transplantation: Implications for donor selection. *Surgery* 1997;121:563–568.

18. **Besides infection, what other ways does CMV infection affect the transplant recipient?**

CMV has been associated with atherosclerosis and chronic allograft rejection. CMV has been associated with several other vascular injuries, including transplant glomerulopathy, hemolytic uremic syndrome (HUS), thrombotic microangiopathy (TMA), and transplant renal artery stenosis.

19. **How do you diagnose CMV disease in a renal transplant recipient?**

CMV infection implies the mere detection of CMV via culture or polymerase chain reaction. CMV disease, by comparison, requires clinical signs and symptoms, in addition to viral detection. The clinical signs and symptoms of CMV disease include fever, leukopenia, or organ involvement (hepatitis, pneumonitis, colitis, chorioretinitis, etc.). The quantitative assessment of viral load via PCR can help determine the clinical phenotype. CMV DNA levels >500 copies/μg of total DNA in peripheral blood correlates with clinical evident disease.

Toyoda M, Carlos JB, Galera OA, et al. Correlation of cytomegalovirus DNA levels with response to antiviral therapy in cardiac and renal allograft recipients. *Transplantation* 1997;63:957–963.

20. **Is prophylaxis for CMV infection necessary?**

Usually. A meta-analysis of 19 trials involving 1981 solid-organ transplant recipients found that antiviral prophylaxis significantly lowered the risk of CMV disease, CMV infection, and mortality. For prophylaxis, ganciclovir is superior to acyclovir, whereas oral ganciclovir was similarly effective as valganciclovir and intravenous (IV) ganciclovir. CMV prophylaxis is generally continued for 3 months after transplantation. Low-risk recipients (D−/R−) do not require prophylaxis but are generally given antivirals to prevent other herpes-related infections during the early post-transplantation period.

Hodson EM, Barclay PG, Craig JC, et al. Antiviral medications for preventing cytomegalovirus disease in solid organ transplant recipients. *Cochrane Database Syst Rev* CD003774, 2005.

Kalil AC, Levitsky J, Lyden E, et al. Meta-analysis: the efficacy of strategies to prevent organ disease by cytomegalovirus in solid organ transplant recipients. *Ann Intern Med* 2005;143:870–880.

21. **What is the treatment for CMV?**

Ganciclovir and valganciclovir are the most commonly used agents for the prevention of CMV infection and disease in renal transplant recipients. Valganciclovir and ganciclovir are the mainstay of general prophylaxis, but they can also be used as part of preemptive strategies. High-risk recipients (D+/R−) who receive induction therapy or treatment of acute rejection with antilymphocyte agents should be administered IV ganciclovir for 3 weeks, followed by oral valganciclovir or ganciclovir for a total of 12 weeks. Intermediate-risk recipients (D+/R− or D+/R+) who receive induction therapy or treatment of acute rejection with antilymphocyte agents should be administered IV ganciclovir while hospitalized, followed by oral ganciclovir for a total of 12 weeks. Prophylactic therapy with IVIG preparations such as hyperimmune CMV Ig (Cytogam) or standard-pooled Ig has been used to control CMV infection but is associated with variable efficacy and tremendous expense. The concern surrounding the emergence of ganciclovir-resistant CMV has been mitigated by the emergence of valganciclovir, a prodrug of ganciclovir. All patients with serious CMV disease need treatment with IV ganciclovir. Treatment should be continued until CMV is no longer detectable. Reduction of immunosuppression may be necessary in life-threatening CMV disease and in CMV disease that persists despite treatment.

22. **What is EBV and what post-transplantation condition is it associated with?**

Epstein-Barr virus (EBV) is a member of the herpesvirus family and one of the most common human viruses. Most people become infected with EBV some time during their lives. It can flourish in the setting of immunosuppression and is associated with post-transplant lymphoproliferative disorder (PTLD).

KEY POINTS: POST-TRANSPLANTATION INFECTIONS

1. Nosocomial and surgery-related infections are the predominant infections that occur within the first month post-transplantation.

2. Although the human polyomaviruses are highly seroprevalent in humans, they appear to cause clinical disease only in immunocomprised hosts.

3. Quantification of BK virus DNA in plasma by polymerase chain reaction has a sensitivity and specificity of 100% and 88%, respectively; however, not all patients with viremia have nephritis (positive predictive value of 50%).

4. Biospy remains the gold standard for the diagnosis of BK-associated nephropathy.

5. The goal in treating BK-associated nephropathy is to eradicate the virus while maintaining renal function and preventing acute or chronic rejection.

6. Cytomegalovirus (CMV) donor positive and CMV recipient negative (CMV D+/R−) are at greatest risk for severe "primary" infection during the first 3 months post-transplantation. Recent data, however, demonstrated that the CMV D+/R+ group and not the D+/R− group has a worst graft and patient survival at 3 years.

7. Epstein-Barr virus can flourish in the setting of immunosuppression and is associated with post-transplant lymphoproliferative disorder.

---

23. **What central nervous system infections are of particular concern in patients who have undergone solid organ transplant?**
   - Listeria meningitis
   - Herpes simplex virus encephalitis
   - JC virus-induced progressive multifocal leukoencephalopathy
   - *Cryptococcus neoformans* meningitis

CHAPTER 61

PRIMARY CARE OF THE RENAL TRANSPLANT RECIPIENT

Michael R. Lattanzio, DO, and Matthew R. Weir, MD

1. **What are the risk factors for cardiovascular disease (CVD) in patients receiving renal transplant?**
   See Table 61-1.

2. **Are statins beneficial in patients receiving renal transplant?**
   Yes. The Assessment of Lescol in Renal Transplantation (ALERT) study demonstrated that statin use among patients receiving renal transplant conferred significant reductions in cardiovascular mortality. In the extended follow-up of ALERT participants, the incidence of cardiac events was reduced in patients treated with statin. Moreover, post hoc analysis showed that early administration of statin therapy post-transplant was associated with the most benefit. Additionally, statin use is associated with decreased proteinuria, decreased C-reactive protein, and decreased interstitial fibrosis incidence in transplant protocol biopsies, all which may confer additional benefit.

   Holdaas H, Fellstrom B, Cole E, et al. Long-term cardiac outcomes in renal transplant recipients receiving fluvastatin: The ALERT extension study. *Am J Transplant* 2005;5:2929–2936.

   Holdaas H, Fellstrom B, Jardine AG, et al. Effect of fluvastatin on cardiac outcomes in renal transplant recipients: A multicentre, randomised, placebo-controlled trial. *Lancet* 2003;361:2024–2031.

   Holdaas H, Fellstrom B, Jardine AG, et al. Beneficial effect of early initiation of lipid-lowering therapy following renal transplantation. *Nephrol Dial Transplant* 2005;20:974–980.

   Masterson R, Hewitson T, Leikis M, et al. Impact of statin treatment on 1-year functional and histologic renal allograft outcome. *Transplantation* 2005;80:332–338.

   Ridker PM, Cannon CP, Morrow D, et al. C-reactive protein levels and outcomes after statin therapy. *N Engl J Med* 2005;352:20–28.

   Sandhu S, Wiebe N, Fried LF, et al. Statins for improving renal outcomes: A meta-analysis. *J Am Soc Nephrol* 2006;17:2006–2016.

3. **What are the targets for cholesterol therapy in patients receiving renal transplant?**
   - Low-density lipoprotein <100 mg/dL
   - Nonhigh-density lipoprotein-C ≤130 mg/dL
   - Triglycerides <200 mg/day

4. **Are there any risks of statin use in transplant recipients?**
   Yes. Most statins are metabolized by the same cytochrome P450 system (CP3A4) as calcineurin inhibitors (CNIs). As a consequence, calcineurin inhibitors (particularly cyclosporine) may accumulate in plasma and may be associated with a greater frequency of rhabdomyolysis. Data on tacrolimus are sparse, although pharmacokinetic studies on concomitant atorvastatin and tacrolimus therapy did not demonstrate significant interactions. Fluvastatin and pravastatin may be safer because they are metabolized through non-CP3A4 mechanisms. The potential for rhabdomyolysis also increases as the lipophilicity of the compound increases because the more lipid-soluble statins are more likely to deposit in extrahepatic tissues and cause toxicity. Among statins in current use, simvastatin and lovastatin are the most lipophilic compounds, whereas

TABLE 61-1. RISK FACTORS FOR CARDIOVASCULAR DISEASE		
Traditional	Transplant-Related	Conditional
Age	Immunosuppression	Homocysteine
Male sex	CKD	CRP
Family history	Proteinuria	AGEs
Obesity	Anemia	
Diabetes		
Hypertension		
Hyperlipidemia		
Tobacco abuse		

CKD = chronic kidney disease; CRP = C-reactive protein; AGEs = advanced glycosylated end products.

atorvastatin and fluvastatin are less so and pravastatin is hydrophilic. In considering these differences among statins, fluvastatin, pravastatin, and atorvastatin seem to have a more favorable safety profile in renal transplant recipients.

Lemahieu WP, Hermann M, Asberg A, et al. Combined therapy with atorvastatin and calcineurin inhibitors: No interactions with tacrolimus. *Am J Transplant* 2005;5:2236–2243.

Maltz HC, Balog DL, Cheigh JS. Rhabdomyolysis associated with concomitant use of atorvastatin and cyclosporine. *Ann Pharmacother* 1999;33:1176–1179.

Neuvonen PJ, Niemi M, Backman JT. Drug interactions with lipid-lowering drugs: Mechanisms and clinical relevance. *Clin Pharmacol Ther* 2006;80:565–581.

5. **What are the causes of hypertension (HTN) in patients who have undergone renal transplant?**
   - Primary HTN
   - Secondary HTN-related to native kidneys
   - Calcineurin inhibitor use
   - Corticosteroid use
   - Kidney allograft dysfunction
   - Allograft vascular compromise
   - Obstructive sleep apnea

6. **What is the optimal blood pressure medication for renal transplant recipients?**
   Because there is no evidence that a particular class of antihypertensive agents is more effective than other classes, the choice of medications should be individualized and based on various comorbidities. Calcium channel blockers (CCBs) are an attractive first-line agent, mainly because they counteract the vasoconstrictive effects of calcineurin inhibitors. CCB use may cause untoward effects, particularly nondependent edema and worsening proteinuria. Also, calcineurin inhibitor doses may need reduction with the use of nondihydropyridine CCBs.

   The use of angiotensin-converting enzyme (ACE) inhibitors/angiotensin receptor blockers (ARBs) in renal transplant recipients is safe and effective. Additionally, the use of ACE inhibitors/ARBs has been associated with prolonged allograft and patient survival. Because the combination of afferent arteriolar vasoconstriction from CNI and efferent arteriolar vasodilation as a result of renin-angiotensin system (RAS) blockade can predispose to acute kidney injury, we routinely advise our patients to discontinue their ACE inhibitors/ARBs if they are acutely ill and at risk for volume depletion. Additionally, we advise postponing the addition of RAS blockers until 3 months post-transplantation to obviate superfluous renal biopsies.

Beta blockers should be considered in all patients who have received renal transplant with known CVD. Diuretics can be utilized to control volume-mediated hypertension and to enhance the antihypertensive effects of ACE inhibitors/ARBs. Alpha-1 blockers and centrally acting agents may be necessary to achieve blood pressure goals.

Andres A, Morales E, Morales JM, et al. Efficacy and safety of valsartan, an angiotensin ii receptor antagonist, in hypertension after renal transplantation: A randomized multicenter study. *Transplant Proc* 2006;38:2419–2423.

Heinze G, Mitterbauer C, Regele H, et al. Angiotensin-converting enzyme inhibitor or angiotensin II type 1 receptor antagonist therapy is associated with prolonged patient and graft survival after renal transplantation. *J Am Soc Nephrol* 2006;17:889–899.

Stigant CE, Cohen J, Vivera M, et al. Ace inhibitors and angiotensin II antagonists in renal transplantation: An analysis of safety and efficacy. *Am J Kidney Dis* 2000;35:58–63.

7. What is the blood pressure goal for renal transplant recipients?

Kidney Disease Outcomes Quality Initiative (K/DOQI) guidelines suggest goal blood pressure less than 130/80 mm Hg for all renal transplant recipients, with a decreased goal of less than 125/75 mm Hg being considered in patients with significant proteinuria. What is not known is whether it is better to allow higher level of blood pressure post-transplant ($\sim$140/90 mm Hg) to ensure adequate blood flow to the allograft.

K/DOQI clinical practice guidelines on hypertension and antihypertensive agents in chronic kidney disease. *Am J Kidney Dis* 2004;43:S1–290.

8. What is NODAT?

NODAT is an acronym for new-onset diabetes after transplantation. The prevalence of NODAT in the U.S. Renal Data system cohort is estimated at 9.1%, 16.1%, and 24% at 3, 12, and 36 months after transplantation, respectively. Several studies have documented that NODAT is an independent predictor of major cardiovascular events after transplantation. Additionally, NODAT is also a likely contributor to chronic allograft dysfunction and subsequent allograft loss. The International Consensus Guidelines recommend that glycemic control in established diabetes be based on glycosylated hemoglobin (HbA1c) less than 6.5% and fasting plasma glucose 90 to 130 mg/dL.

Chapman JR, O'Connell PJ, Nankivell BJ. Chronic renal allograft dysfunction. *J Am Soc Nephrol* 2005;16: 3015–3026.

Davidson J, Wilkinson A, Dantal J, et al. New-onset diabetes after transplantation: 2003 international consensus guidelines. Proceedings of an international expert panel meeting. Barcelona, Spain, 19 February 2003. *Transplantation* 2003;75:SS3–24.

Kasiske BL, Snyder JJ, Gilbertson D, et al. Diabetes mellitus after kidney transplantation in the United States. *Am J Transplant* 2003;3:178–185.

Wilkinson A, Davidson J, Dotta F, et al. Guidelines for the treatment and management of new-onset diabetes after transplantation. *Clin Transplant* 2005;19:291–298.

9. Should all patients who have received kidney transplant be screened and counseled on tobacco use?

Yes. The same strategies to prevent and treat tobacco use in the general population should be applied to all transplant recipients. Smoking at the time of transplantation is associated with graft failure and death. Additionally, smoking has been associated with post-transplantation malignancies. Renal transplant recipients who stopped smoking more than 5 years before transplantation had a 34% risk reduction in cardiovascular events. There are no interactions between immunosuppressive medications and tobacco cessation medications that would obviate their administration.

Kasiske BL, Klinger D. Cigarette smoking in renal transplant recipients. *J Am Soc Nephrol* 2000;11:753–759.

10. **Should kidney transplant recipients be screened and counseled on obesity?**
Yes. Obesity is independently associated with cardiovascular events and mortality in kidney transplant recipients. Additionally, obesity can predispose to insulin resistance, diabetes, and reduced graft survival. Diet and other behavior modifications are safe and may help reduce weight, eventually improving long-term graft survival. Weight loss guidance and support is necessary in all transplant recipients who are overweight.

el-Agroudy AE, Wafa EW, Gheith OE, et al. Weight gain after renal transplantation is a risk factor for patient and graft outcome. *Transplantation* 2004;77:1381–1385.

Jindal RM, Zawada ET Jr. Obesity and kidney transplantation. *Am J Kidney Dis* 2004;43:943–952.

Kasiske BL, Chakkera HA, Roel J. Explained and unexplained ischemic heart disease risk after renal transplantation. *J Am Soc Nephrol* 2000;11:1735–1743.

11. **What is the role of acetylsalicylic acid prophylaxis in transplant recipients?**
In the general population, daily acetylsalicylic acid (ASA) use resulted in a reduction in cardiovascular events in patients at high risk of CVD. In patients receiving renal transplant, low-dose aspirin therapy is associated with improved allograft function and prolonged allograft survival. The current guidelines recommend the use of aspirin, 65 to 325 mg/day, for primary and secondary prevention in renal transplant recipients with cardiovascular disease, diabetes, and/or other risk factors for CVD. The institution of daily ASA therapy for all patients receiving renal transplant should be weighed against the higher risk of gastrointestinal bleeding in this population.

Grotz W, Siebig S, Olschewski M, et al. Low-dose aspirin therapy is associated with improved allograft function and prolonged allograft survival after kidney transplantation. *Transplantation* 2004;77:1848–1853.

Kasiske BL, Vazquez MA, Harmon WE, et al. Recommendations for the outpatient surveillance of renal transplant recipients. American Society of Transplantation. *J Am Soc Nephrol* 2000;11(Suppl 15):S1–86.

12. **What is the significance of proteinuria in kidney transplant recipients?**
In patients who have received kidney transplant, proteinuria is associated with CVD events and mortality. Proteinuria may also herald recurrent or de novo renal disease in the transplanted kidney. A baseline level of urine protein should be obtained in the first month post-transplantation, every 3 months in the first year post-transplantation, then annually. In general, mammalian target of rapamycin (mTOR) inhibitors should be avoided or substituted because they tend to exacerbate proteinuria. The institution of RAS blockade should be considered to reduce proteinuria to normal levels.

Fernandez-Fresnedo G, Escallada R, Rodrigo E, et al. The risk of cardiovascular disease associated with proteinuria in renal transplant patients. *Transplantation* 2002;73:1345–1348.

Roodnat JI, Mulder PG, Rischen-Vos J, et al. Proteinuria after renal transplantation affects not only graft survival but also patient survival. *Transplantation* 2001;72:438–444.

Roodnat JI, Mulder PG, Rischen-Vos J, et al. Proteinuria and death risk in the renal transplant population. *Transplant Proc* 2001;33:1170–1171.

13. **Is mineral bone disease common in the renal transplant population?**
Yes. Chronic kidney disease-mineral bone disease (CKD-MBD) is common in kidney transplant recipients. The use of corticosteroids as part of the immunosuppressive regiment may further affect CKD-MBD management. Studies have demonstrated a rapid decrease in bone mineral density in the first 6 to 12 months after transplantation. Also, fractures are common in kidney transplant recipients and are associated with substantial morbidity. Monitoring bone mineral density should be routine for all patients taking chronic corticosteroids. Bisphosphonate administration is often necessary to maintain and restore bone mineral density, particularly in the setting of chronic steroid and immunosuppressant use.

Julian BA, Laskow DA, Dubovsky J, et al. Rapid loss of vertebral mineral density after renal transplantation. *N Engl J Med* 1991;325:544–550.

KEY POINTS: PRIMARY CARE OF THE RENAL TRANSPLANT RECIPIENT

1. The ALERT study demonstrated that statin use among patients who have received renal transplant conferred significant reductions in cardiovascular mortality.

2. Fluvastatin, pravastatin, and atorvastatin seem to have a more favorable safety profile in renal transplant recipients.

3. Because there is no evidence that a particular class of antihypertensive agents is more effective than other classes, the choice of medications should be individualized and based on various comorbidities.

4. Kidney Disease Outcomes Quality Initiative (K/DOQI) guidelines suggest goal blood pressure less than 130/80 mm Hg for all renal transplant recipients, with a decreased goal of less than 125/75 mm Hg being considered in patients with significant proteinuria.

5. The prevalence of NODAT (new-onset diabetes after transplantation) in the U.S. Renal Data system cohort is estimated at 9.1%, 16.1%, and 24% at 3, 12, and 36 months after transplantation, respectively.

6. In patients who have received a kidney transplant, proteinuria is associated with cardiovascular events and mortality.

7. Studies have demonstrated a rapid decrease in bone-mineral density in the first 6 to 12 months after transplantation.

14. **Is nutritional vitamin D deficiency prevalent in the renal transplant population?**
It is extremely prevalent. It is estimated that 56% of early renal transplant patients are vitamin D deficient (12–39 nmol/L) and 12% are severely vitamin D deficient (<12 nmol/L). Vitamin D stores should be repleted as per general population guidelines.

Stavroulopoulos A, Cassidy MJ, Porter CJ, et al. Vitamin D status in renal transplant recipients. *Am J Transplant* 2007;7:2546–2552.

15. **When is the best time to vaccinate a transplant recipient?**
Ideally, patients who have received a transplant should receive all vaccinations prior to transplantation to provide the strongest native immunoprotection. If this is not possible, vaccinations should be administered when the immunosuppressant dosages are reduced (usually 6–12 months post-transplantation). Influenza vaccinations should be given to all patients who have undergone transplant and their close contacts. It is recommended that the influenza vaccine be given prior to the onset of the annual influenza season, provided the recipient is at least 1 month post-transplant. If available, H1N1 vaccinations should be administered to all eligible renal transplant recipients.

16. **What vaccinations should not be given to patients who have undergone renal transplant?**
In general, all live vaccines are contradicted in patients on immunosuppression. These include vaccines for varicella zoster, bacille Calmette-Guérin, smallpox, intranasal influenza, measles-mumps-rubella, oral polio, and yellow fever.

PRIMARY HYPERTENSION

Suneel M. Udani, MD, and George L. Bakris, MD

CHAPTER 62

1. **How is hypertension defined and classified?**

   The Seventh Report of the Joint National Committee on Prevention, Detection, Evaluation, and Treatment of High Blood Pressure (JNC 7) updated the definition of hypertension and classified it according to stages (Table 62-1). The measurement must be based on the average of at least two seated measurements on each of two or more office visits. For children, hypertension is defined as systolic or diastolic blood pressure that is, on repeat measurement, greater than the 95th percentile of blood pressure for a given age, height, or gender. The addition of prehypertension is an update from the previous (JNC 6) guidelines.

2. **What is the appropriate means of measuring blood pressure?**

   Measuring blood pressure in the office should be performed with individuals seated for at least 5 minutes in a chair with their feet on the ground and an arm supported at the level of the heart. An appropriate-size cuff with the cuff bladder encircling at least 80% of the arm should be used. The systolic blood pressure is determined at the point where the first sound is auscultated, and the diastolic blood pressure is determined at the point of the disappearance of the sound.

   A common pitfall in blood pressure measurement that occurs in older individuals or individuals with arterial stiffening is the auscultatory gap. The auscultatory gap is where the first Korotkoff sound appears, disappears, and reappears 30 to 40 mm Hg lower. Systolic blood pressure can be underestimated in the presence of the auscultatory gap. If arteriosclerosis is suspected, blood pressure can be confirmed by inflating the blood pressure cuff to the point where the radial artery pulse is no longer detectable prior to deflation.

3. **What is the proper use of self-blood pressure monitoring?**

   Self-blood pressure monitoring in the form of home blood pressure monitoring or ambulatory blood pressure monitoring should be used to evaluate for white-coat hypertension (in the absence of evidence of end-organ damage) or masked hypertension, assess blood pressure during reported symptomatic hypotension, and assess for appropriate diurnal variation in blood pressure.

   Home blood pressure monitoring is useful to improve adherence with medication and provide information about early morning increases in blood pressure, the period most vulnerable for cardiovascular events. It is also useful in cases in which white-coat hypertension is suspected. If suspected, ambulatory blood pressure monitoring (24-hour recorded blood pressures) should be performed to confirm the diagnosis.

4. **What is the prevalence of hypertension in the United States? How well is hypertension controlled among those with a diagnosis of hypertension?**

   Hypertension is the most common diagnosis made in the primary care setting. According to the most recent National Health and Nutrition Examination Survey (NHANES), conducted in 2006, the prevalence of hypertension in the United States for adults is approximately 29%. However, the prevalence of hypertension continues to increase with age. According to the National Health Interview Survey (NHIS), in individuals older than age 55, the prevalence of

TABLE 62-1. CLASSIFICATION FOR ADULTS 18 YEARS OR OLDER WITH ELEVATED BLOOD PRESSURE

Hypertension Stage	Systolic Blood Pressure	Diastolic Blood Pressure
Prehypertension	120–139 mm Hg	Or 80–89 mm Hg
Stage I	140–159 mm Hg	Or 90–99 mm Hg
Stage II	≥160 mm Hg	Or ≥100 mm Hg

hypertension was 47.3%. Defining that group further, in those 55 to 64, the prevalence of hypertension was 40.8% versus 55.7% in those 75 to 84 years old.

Despite the widespread prevalence of hypertension and available medications, hypertension remains poorly controlled in the United States, with only 34% of individuals with hypertension controlled. Individuals with hypertension, 30% remain unaware they have the disease.

5. **What is the appropriate initial evaluation for individuals with hypertension?**
The evaluation of an individual with hypertension should target three objectives:
- Identify lifestyle factors and/or other cardiovascular risk factors that may guide treatment and contribute to prognosis.
- Identify comorbid disease states that contribute to blood pressure elevation.
- Evaluate for the presence of end-organ damage as a result of hypertension.

The appropriate evaluation includes a full history and physical examination, including family history, alcohol or drug use, over-the-counter medication use, and the like.

Initial laboratory evaluation prior to initiating therapy should include a serum potassium, calcium and creatinine (or alternate method of estimating glomerular filtration rate), urinalysis with evaluation for proteinuria or hematuria, glucose, and hematocrit.

The initial evaluation should also include an electrocardiogram to evaluate for the presence of left ventricular hypertrophy or evidence of previous myocardial infarct.

Fasting lipid profile should also be done in these individuals as risk stratification for coronary artery disease.

6. **What is the appropriate initial therapy for individuals with diagnosed hypertension?**
Initial therapy is based on stage of hypertension and comorbid disease, referred to in the JNC 7 guidelines often as "compelling indications."

For all stages of hypertension, lifestyle modification should be recommended including restriction of dietary salt intake, increase in activity with goal of weight loss, moderation of alcohol intake, and adoption of the DASH (Dietary Approaches to Stop Hypertension) diet with increased intake of fruits and vegetables. If lifestyle modifications are not effective enough to reach the blood pressure target (<140/90 in patients with isolated hypertension and <130/80 in patients with hypertension with kidney disease or diabetes), medication should be added.

For those with stage I hypertension, monotherapy with a thiazide-type diuretic is recommended unless there is a compelling indication to use an alternative agent or a second-line agent, such as an angiotensin-converting enzyme (ACE) inhibitor or angiotensin receptor blocker (ARB) for individuals with proteinuria or a β-blocker for individuals with coronary artery disease.

For those with stage II hypertension, dual therapy should be initiated. The agent of choice should be a thiazide-type diuretic with an additional agent—either an ACE inhibitor (or ARB), calcium channel blocker, or β-blocker.

7. **What are the most common side effects of commonly used antihypertensives that patients should be alerted to prior to starting therapy?**
All patients should be notified that with any medication, idiosyncratic drug reactions can occur, ranging in severity from urticaria to anaphylaxis. However, the most common side effects are as follows:

- **Thiazide-type diuretics:** polyuria, hypokalemia, hypercalcemia, hypomagnesemia, hyperuricemia, hyponatremia (especially in the elderly or those with low solute intake), orthostatic hypotension, impaired glucose tolerance
- **ACE inhibitors:** cough, hyperkalemia, orthostatic hypotension, angioedema (rare but life threatening and patients must be aware of possible reaction)
- **Angiotensin receptor blockers:** hyperkalemia, orthostatic hypotension, angioedema (rare; cough does not tend to occur with ARBs)
- **Dihydropyridine calcium channel blockers:** lower-extremity edema, flushing, headache, orthostatic hypotension
- **Nondihydropyridine calcium channel blockers:** bradycardia, constipation, and rash (contraindicated in systolic heart failure)
- **β-blockers:** bronchospasm, bradycardia, negative inotropic effect (acutely), depression, erectile dysfunction, orthostatic hypotension (exceptions are low-dose nebivolol)

8. **What is the pathophysiology of primary hypertension?**
Primary hypertension remains a complex pathophysiologic state linking genetic and behavioral factors. Ultimately, the final common pathway leads to increased vascular resistance. The various pathways leading to increased vascular resistance include increased sympathetic tone, increased total body sodium content, increased activity of the renin-angiotensin-aldosterone axis, and an imbalance between endogenous vasoconstrictors (e.g., endothelin) and vasodilators (e.g., nitric oxide).

Sodium intake and reabsorption likely play a central role in the development and maintenance of essential hypertension as demonstrated by the monogenic disorders of hypertension all being related to excessive renal sodium reabsorption and the dramatic effect of salt restriction on blood pressure control.

9. **Why are thiazide-type diuretics preferred as first-line therapy for stage I primary hypertension?**
There are more than four decades of outcome trials that support the use of not only thiazide-type diuretics, but also, specifically, chlorthalidone. These trials were all randomized and powered for cardiovascular outcomes and include the VA Cooperative studies from the early to mid-1960s, the Multiple Risk Factor Intervention Trial (MRFIT), the Systolic Hypertension in the Elderly (SHEP), and the multicenter Antihypertensive and Lipid-Lowering Treatment to Prevent Heart Attack Trial (ALLHAT) trial. ALLHAT compared initial therapy with thiazide-type diuretics (chlorthalidone) with a dihydropyridine calcium channel blocker (amlodipine), an ACE inhibitor (lisinopril), and an alpha-adrenergic antagonist (doxazosin). Thiazide-type diuretics were found to be as effective at lowering blood pressure and preventing cardiovascular outcomes (e.g., heart failure and stroke) as newer agents such as amlodipine and lisinopril.

Thiazide-type diuretics remain much cheaper than newer agents; thus, given their at least equivalent efficacy and much lower cost, they are preferred as initial therapy for those with primary hypertension. Moreover, failure to achieve blood pressure goals in most patients is accounted for by lack of diuretic use.

ALLHAT included a larger number of African American and elderly individuals, who have traditionally been considered "salt-sensitive." Further, the benefits of chlorthalidone were more pronounced in the African American subgroups than the non-African American subgroups.

The major adverse events associated with chlorthalidone use were increased hypokalemia, increased hyperlipidemia, and development of diabetes. Other studies have demonstrated that the glucose intolerance associated with thiazide-type diuretics (which may be the mediator for the adverse metabolic effects observed) is mediated by the hypokalemia and shifts in adipose tissue from the subcutaneous to visceral area, hence worsening insulin resistance.

10. **Why are blockers of the renin-angiotensin system preferred in individuals with diabetes?**

ACE inhibitors and ARBs lower systemic and intrarenal angiotensin II activity. In patients with diabetes and albuminuria, the angiotensin II-mediated vasoconstrictive effect on the efferent arteriole raises intraglomerular pressure, facilitating increases in glomerular filtration, and contributes to podocyte dysfunction and, hence, albuminuria, thus contributing to the progression of diabetic nephropathy. In both type I and type 2 diabetes with albuminuria, agents that block the renin-angiotensin aldosterone system have been demonstrated to reduce albuminuria and slow the progression of diabetic nephropathy to a greater extent than other agents at similar levels of blood pressure reduction.

An initial increase in serum creatinine with agents that work by blocking the renin-angiotensin axis is expected and suggestive of effective lowering of intraglomerular pressure. One should expect up to a 30% increase in serum creatinine within a month of starting an ACE inhibitor or ARB. This is correlated with a better long-term renal outcome in clinical trials. Thus, in the absence of hyperkalemia (serum potassium = 6 mEq/L), symptomatic hypotension, or other evidence of drug intolerance, an initial increase in serum creatinine by up to 30% is **not** an indication to stop the ACE inhibitor or ARB. Continued increase in serum creatinine, hyperkalemia, or symptomatic hypotension, however, should lead to discontinuation of the ACE inhibitor or ARB and evaluation for volume depletion or possible bilateral renal artery stenosis, especially in smokers.

Although ACE inhibitors and ARBs have been studied in different cohorts, in one study of direct comparison they appear to have equivalent benefits. The primary reason for an individual to select an ACE inhibitor over an ARB is that they are often cheaper than ARBs. Conversely, one may select an ARB primarily if a patient has demonstrated intolerance to ACE inhibitors manifesting a cough. Based on data from trials and U.S. Food and Drug Administration indications, losartan, irbesartan, and telmisartan are all approved for this indication. Angioedema occurring with ACE inhibitor use has also been reported in ARB use, although the incidence is about 10% to that of ACE inhibitors. Thus, ARBs may not be a "totally safe" alternative to ACE inhibitors if someone has experienced angioedema.

11. **What is salt-sensitive hypertension? What is the effect of dietary salt restriction on blood pressure?**

Salt-sensitive hypertension has variable definitions but is conventionally defined as an increase in systolic blood pressure of ≥10 mm Hg in response to dietary salt loading. Salt-sensitive hypertension tends to occur most often in African American and elderly individuals.

Dietary salt restriction has repeatedly been demonstrated to be effective at reducing blood pressure. In the evaluation of the DASH diet, which includes sodium restriction and an increase in dietary potassium intake, there was a significant drop in both systolic and diastolic blood pressure at each level of sodium intake (ranging from a fall in 1.0–2.9 mm Hg diastolic blood pressure and ranging from a fall of 1.7–4.6 mm Hg systolic blood pressure). More recently, salt restriction was demonstrated to be effective at lowering blood pressure in individuals with resistant hypertension (mean decrease in 22.7 mm Hg systolic and 9.1 mm Hg diastolic blood pressure).

Standard recommendations include reduction of sodium intake to 100 mmol/day; however, in the study of salt restriction in resistant hypertension sodium was restricted to 50 mmol/day.

12. **When should a secondary cause of hypertension be suspected and evaluated?**

A secondary cause should be suspected in the presence of resistant hypertension—as defined by the inability to reach target blood pressure despite the use of three antihypertensive agents with complementary pharmacologic mechanisms titrated to the maximum tolerated dose including a diuretic.

- In the presence of the sudden onset of hypertension, especially stage II hypertension or evidence of end-organ damage with previous normal blood pressure
- In the development of hypertension in extremes of age (very young or very old)
- In the presence of stable control of blood pressure with sudden worsening especially in the setting of new symptoms of volume overload are present
- In the presence of symptoms consistent with a secondary cause of hypertension.

The most common cause of these problems includes high sodium ingestion, especially in the presence of underlying kidney disease. If this has been eliminated, the initial evaluation depends on the clinical scenario; however, the routine evaluation should include assessment of any change in renal function including proteinuria, renal ultrasound with assessment of size, echogenicity, and vascular flow. Further, serum electrolytes should be evaluated for evidence suggestive of aldosterone excess (hypokalemia, metabolic alkalosis). Collateral evidence of dietary and medication adherence can be helpful—specifically, family members reporting and 24-hour urine collections for sodium. Finally, screening for symptoms of sleep apnea (daytime somnolence, fatigue, night-time snoring) can identify a potentially reversible cause of resistant hypertension.

13. **What blood pressure should physicians target patients without diabetes but with hypertension and chronic kidney disease (CKD)?**

According to the Modification of Diet in Renal Disease (MDRD) and African-American Study of Kidney Disease and Hypertension (AASK) studies—both studies of blood pressure lowering in individuals with nondiabetic CKD, there appears to be no additional benefit of lowering blood pressure beyond a mean arterial pressure of 92 mm Hg (approximately 120/80 mm Hg) unless the patient has >300 mg/day of proteinuria. Lowering blood pressure beyond 130/80 mm Hg has not consistently demonstrated benefit in preventing progression of CKD or cardiovascular mortality. As noted, certain subgroups may benefit from further blood pressure lowering (i.e., individuals with proteinuria).

14. **What blood pressure is the most important (systolic, diastolic, pulse pressure) mediator of CKD progression?**

Systolic blood pressure appears to be the most important factor in predicting risk of progression of both diabetic and nondiabetic chronic kidney disease. However, excessively lowering the diastolic pressure to achieve a lower systolic pressure has consistently shown to increase cardiovascular events in CKD, especially at levels below a diastolic of 60 mm Hg. People at risk for this problem are those with high pulse pressures.

Arterial stiffness, highly prevalent in individuals with chronic kidney disease, appears to be the mediator between pulse pressure and increased cardiovascular mortality.

15. **How does obesity contribute to hypertension?**

Increasing evidence has suggested a direct role of obesity in the development and maintenance of hypertension mediated by the elevated levels of leptin present in individuals who are obese. Leptin, synthesized and secreted into the circulation by adipocytes, appears to directly stimulate increased sympathetic nervous system activity and increase sympathetic activity via hypothalamic stimulation. Increased sympathetic activity leads to increased urinary sodium retention and resultant increased blood pressure. Further, in healthy subjects (based on animal data), leptin stimulates natriuresis. However, in subjects with hypertension (based on animal data), leptin no longer stimulates increased urinary sodium excretion; combined with the increased sympathetic activity, there is overall decreased urinary sodium excretion and maintenance of hypertension.

Aldosterone also appears to play a role in obesity-mediated hypertension. Human adipocytes produce a mineralocorticoid-releasing factor that stimulates the release of aldosterone from the adrenal cortex. The increased adipocytes in obesity lead to increased aldosterone, with its resultant effect of sodium retention and increased vascular stiffness.

KEY POINTS: PRIMARY HYPERTENSION

1. Reduction in cardiovascular risk and kidney disease progression is achieved by blood pressures substantially <140/90 mm Hg, approaching 130/80 mm Hg.

2. Patients with advanced proteinuric kidney disease and those at high risk for stroke (elderly or those with previous history) should have a blood pressure of <130/80 mm Hg.

3. Indiscriminate sodium (salt) use or intake is a very common cause of resistant hypertension and need for additional blood pressure–lowering medications.

4. In an ideal setting, following lifestyle recommendations will delay development of hypertension by more than a decade in those with a strong family history.

16. **What is the appropriate diurnal variation of blood pressure? What information does the presence or absence of diurnal variation in blood pressure offer?**
Normally mean arterial blood pressure should fall 10 to 20 mm Hg at night-time (defined as midnight to 6 AM or during sleep). Individuals not demonstrating the decrease in blood pressure at night, referred to as "nondippers," have an increased risk of cardiovascular disease compared to individuals demonstrating normal diurnal variation.
 Use of diuretics and nocturnal dosing of blood pressure agents can serve as an effective means of converting "nondippers" to "dippers."

BIBLIOGRAPHY

1. ALLHAT Officers and Coordinators for the ALLHAT Collaborative Research Group. Major outcomes in high-risk hypertensive patients randomized to angiotensin converting enzyme-inhibitor or calcium channel blocker vs. diuretic: The Antihypertensive and Lipid-lowering Treatment to Prevent Heart Attack Trial. *JAMA* 2002;288:2981–2997.

2. Agarwal R. Blood pressure components and the risk for end-stage renal disease and death in chronic kidney disease. *Clin J Am Soc Nephrol* 2009;4:830–837.

3. Bakris GL, Weir MR, Shanifar S, et al.; for the RENAAL Study Group. Effects of blood pressure level on progression of diabetic nephropathy: Results from the RENAAL trial. *Arch Intern Med* 2003;163:1555–1565.

4. Chobanian AV, Bakris GL, Black HR, et al. The Seventh Report of the Joint National Committee on Prevention, Detection, Evaluation, and Treatment of High Blood Pressure: The JNC 7 report. *Hypertension* 2003;42:1206–1252.

5. Bakris GL, Weir MR. Angiotensin-converting enzyme inhibitor-associated elevations in serum creatinine: Is this a cause for concern? *Arch Intern Med* 2000;160(5):685–693.

6. Fagard RH, Thijs L, Staessen JA, et al. Night-day blood pressure ratio and dipping pattern as predictors of death and cardiovascular events in hypertension. *J Hum Hypertens* 2009;23:645–653.

7. Goswami P, Drawz P, Rahman M. Nocturnal dosing and chronic kidney disease progression: New insights. *Curr Opin Nephrol Hypertens* 2009;18:381–385.

8. Johnson RJ, Herrera-Acosta J, Schreiner GF, et al. Subtle-acquired renal injury as a mechanism for salt-sensitive hypertension. *N Engl J Med* 2002;346:913–923.

9. Klahr S, Levey AS, Beck GJ, et al. Modification of Diet in Renal Disease Study Group. The effects of dietary protein restriction and blood-pressure control on the progression of chronic renal disease. *N Engl J Med* 1994;330:877–884.

10. Mallick S, Kanthety R, Rahman M. Home blood pressure monitoring in clinical practice: A review. *Am J Med* 2009;122:803–810.

11. Matthew B, Patel SB, Reams GP, et al. Obesity-hypertension: Emerging concepts in pathophysiology and treatment. *Am J Med Sci* 2007;334:23–30.

12. Natarajan S, Santa EJ, Liao Y, et al. Effect of treatment and adherence on ethnic differences in blood pressure control among adults with hypertension. *Ann Epidemiol* 2009;19:172–179.

13. Ozturk S, Sar F, Bengi-Bozkurt O, et al. Study of ACE-I versus ARB in managing hypertensive overt diabetic nephropathy: A long term analysis. *Kidney Blood Press Res* 2009;32:268–275.

14. Sacks FM, Svetkey LP, Vollmer WM, et al., for the DASH-Sodium Collaborative Research Group. Effects on blood pressure of reduced dietary sodium and the Dietary Approaches to Stop Hypertension (DASH) diet. *New Engl J Med* 2001;344:3–10.

15. Safar ME, Smulyan H. Blood pressure components in clinical hypertension. *J Clin Hypertens* 2006;9:659–666.

16. Sarafidis PA, Bakris GL. Resistant hypertension: An overview of evaluation and treatment. *J Am Coll Cardiol* 2008;52:1749–1757.

17. Schoenborn CA, Heyman KM. Health characteristics of adults aged 55 years and over: United States, 2004–2007. *National Health Statistics Reports*, no. 16. Hyattsville, MD: National Center for Health Statistics, 2009.

18. Shafi T, Appel LJ, Miller ER, et al. Changes in serum potassium mediate thiazide-induced diabetes. *Hypertension* 2008;52:1022–1029.

19. Sowers JR, Whaley-Connell A, Epstein M. Narrative review: The emerging clinical implications of the role of aldosterone in the metabolic syndrome and resistant hypertension. *Ann Intern Med* 2009;150:776–783.

20. Suter PM, Sierro C, Vetter W. Nutritional factors in the control of blood pressure and hypertension. *Nutr Clin Care* 2009;5:9–19.

21. Udani SM, Koyner JL. Effects of blood pressure lowering on markers of kidney disease progression. *Curr Hypertens Rep* 2009;11:368–374.

22. Wright JT, Bakris G, Greene T, et al. Effect of blood pressure lowering and anti-hypertensive drug class on progression of hypertensive kidney disease: Results from the AASK trial. *JAMA* 2002;288:2421–2431.

CHAPTER 63

RENAL PARENCHYMAL HYPERTENSION

Martin J. Andersen, DO, and Rajiv Agarwal, MD

1. **What is the epidemiology of hypertension?**

   National Health and Nutrition Examination Survey (NHANES) data show that 28.7% and 30.5% of American men and women, respectively, are hypertensive, and Framingham data show that even middle-aged patients without hypertension have a 90% residual lifetime risk of becoming hypertensive. Despite improved hypertension treatment over the past two to three decades, demonstrated by left ventricular hypertrophy (LVH) regression, uncontrolled hypertension is becoming more common. More than 30% of Americans are obese, and 8.3% have either diagnosed or undiagnosed diabetes. Both obesity and diabetes make control of hypertension challenging. Among patients with chronic kidney disease (CKD), the prevalence of hypertension is higher than that seen in the general population. NHANES data show that 60% of patients with stage 3 CKD (estimated glomerular filtration rate [GFR] of 30–59 mL/min/1.73m^2) are hypertensive. Patients with stages 4 and 5 CKD (estimated GFR <30 mL/min/1.73m^2) are even more likely to be hypertensive—more than 80% of these patients have elevated blood pressures (BPs). The control of hypertension is even poorer in patients with CKD. Nearly 70% of patients with CKD have uncontrolled hypertension, whereas only ~50% of the hypertensive population without CKD has uncontrolled hypertension.

   Recent epidemiologic studies confirm the association of albuminuria and poor BP control in patients with CKD. In a study of 232 U.S. veterans with CKD, proteinuria, not estimated GFR, was found to be an independent predictor of systolic BP. Among the independent predictors of hypertension (age, race, and number of antihypertensive medications), proteinuria most strongly correlated with hypertension. Compared to estimated GFR, albuminuria (or proteinuria) is a stronger determinant of hypertension; albuminuria is also a stronger determinant of poor control of hypertension.

   Agarwal R, Andersen MJ. Correlates of systolic hypertension in patients with chronic kidney disease. *Hypertension* 2005;46(3):514–520.

   Centers for Disease Control. *2011 National Diabetes Fact Sheet.* http://www.cdc.gov/diabetes/pubs/estimates11.htm#1

   Chobanian AV. Shattuck Lecture. The hypertension paradox—more uncontrolled disease despite improved therapy. *N Engl J Med* 2009;361(9):878–887.

   Mosterd A, D'Agostino RB, Silbershatz H, et al. Trends in the prevalence of hypertension, antihypertensive therapy, and left ventricular hypertrophy from 1950 to 1989. *N Engl J Med* 1999;340(16):1221–1227.

   Ong KL, Cheung BM, Man YB, Lau CP, Lam KS. Prevalence, awareness, treatment, and control of hypertension among United States adults 1999–2004. *Hypertension* 2007;49:69–75.

   Plantinga LC, Miller ER 3rd, Stevens LA, et al. Blood pressure control among persons without and with chronic kidney disease: US trends and risk factors 1999–2006. *Hypertension* 2009;54(1):47–56.

   Vasan RS, Beiser A, Seshadri S, et al. Residual lifetime risk for developing hypertension in middle-aged women and men: The Framingham Heart Study. *JAMA* 2002;287(8):1003–1010.

2. **What is the cardiovascular disease risk?**

   The Prospective Studies Collaboration is a meta-analysis of 1 million patients that evaluated cardiovascular mortality (ischemic heart disease, cerebrovascular disease, and peripheral vascular disease) resulting from hypertension. Risk was noted to begin with BPs as low as

115/75 mm Hg. For patients aged 40 to 69 years, each 20/10 mm Hg increase in BP increased cardiovascular mortality twofold. The risk of cardiovascular disease is elevated when estimated GFR is lower than 45 mL/min/1.73m^2, but the risk of cardiovascular disease is elevated even with small amounts of albuminuria (microalbuminuria). Albuminuria is a stronger risk factor for cardiovascular disease compared to estimated GFR. Data from the Reduction of Endpoints in NIDDM (non-insulin-dependent diabetes mellitus) with the Angiotensin II Antagonist Losartan (RENAAL) Trial show that every 50% reduction in albuminuria translates into an 18% risk reduction in cardiovascular endpoints. However, the risk for cardiovascular disease is most profound when both albuminuria and low estimated GFR coexist. The Action in Diabetes and Vascular Disease: Preterax and Diamicron MR Controlled Evaluation (ADVANCE) trial showed that patients with estimated GFRs <60 mL/min/1.73m^2 and albuminuria have more than a threefold increase in cardiovascular risk compared to patients without CKD and proteinuria.

Anavekar NS, McMurray JJ, Velazquez EJ. Relation between renal dysfunction and cardiovascular outcomes after myocardial infarction. *N Engl J Med* 2004;351(13):1285–1295.

de Zeeuw D, Remuzzi G, Parving HH, et al. Albuminuria, a therapeutic target for cardiovascular protection in type 2 diabetic patients with nephropathy. *Circulation* 2004;110(8):921–927.

Gerstein HC, Mann JF, Yi Q, et al. Albuminuria and risk of cardiovascular events, death, and heart failure in diabetic and nondiabetic individuals. *JAMA* 2001;286(4):421–426.

Lewington S, Clarke R, Qizilbash N, et al. Age-specific relevance of usual blood pressure to vascular mortality: a meta-analysis of individual data for one million adults in 61 prospective studies. *Lancet* 2002;360(9349):1903–1913.

Ninomiya T, Perkovic V, de Galan BE, et al. Albuminuria and kidney function independently predict cardiovascular and renal outcomes in diabetes. *J Am Soc Nephrol* 2009;20(8):1813–1821.

3. **Should diastolic, systolic, or pulse pressure be used as a treatment target?**
   Arterial stiffening seen with increasing age impairs the buffering of the systolic impulse and causes an increase in reflected wave. With increased arterial stiffening, systolic pressure rises and diastolic pressure falls. For younger patients (<50 years), diastolic BPs provide greater information in regards to risk for cardiovascular disease (every 10 mm Hg increase in diastolic BP increases relative cardiovascular risk by 34%). Diastolic and systolic BPs provide equal cardiovascular risk information for patients 50 to 59 years of age. Those patients ≥60 years of age are at greatest risk for arterial stiffening, and pulse pressure gives the most information (24% increase in relative risk for every 10 mm Hg increase in pulse pressure). Patients with CKD, despite being younger, often have increased arterial stiffness and systolic hypertension. Arterial stiffness worsens with higher stages of kidney disease. Therefore, among patients with CKD, systolic hypertension should be the major target for treatment.

Franklin SS, Larson MG, Khan SA, et al. Does the relation of blood pressure to coronary heart disease risk change with aging? The Framingham Heart Study. *Circulation* 2001;103(9):1245–1249.

Groothoff JW, Gruppen MP, Offringa M, et al. Increased arterial stiffness in young adults with end-stage renal disease since childhood. *J Am Soc Nephrol* 2002;13(12):2953–2961.

Wang MC, Tsai WC, Chen JY, Huang JJ. Stepwise increase in arterial stiffness corresponding with the stages of chronic kidney disease. *Am J Kidney Dis* 2005;45(3):494–501.

4. **What are the blood pressure treatment goals?**
   The Seventh Report of the Joint National Committee on Prevention, Detection, Evaluation, and Treatment of High Blood Pressure (JNC 7) guidelines define optimal BPs as <120/80 mm Hg. BPs between 120 and 139/80 to 89 mm Hg are termed prehypertension. Stage I hypertension is defined as 140 to 159/90 to 99 mm Hg, and stage II hypertension ≥160/100 mm Hg. Patients with CKD and diabetes mellitus need tighter BP control, and they are considered hypertensive if their BPs, recorded in the clinic, are ≥130/80 mm Hg. These patients need excellent control of their pressures throughout their lifetime. The United Kingdom Prospective Diabetes Study (UKPDS) trial showed that patients with diabetes initially randomly assigned to tight BPs had less microvascular or macrovascular disease. However, within 2 years after the trial's end, the BP differences between the tight and less-tight groups disappeared, and the microvascular or macrovascular risk were identical during long-term follow-up.

Chobanian AV, Bakris GL, Black HR, et al. The Seventh Report of the Joint National Committee on Prevention, Detection, Evaluation, and Treatment of High Blood Pressure: the JNC 7 report. *JAMA* 2003;289(19):2560–2572.

Holman RR, Paul SK, Bethel MA, Neil HA, Matthews DR. Long-term follow-up after tight control of blood pressure in type 2 diabetes. *N Engl J Med* 2008;359(15):1565–1576.

UK Prospective Diabetes Study Group.Tight blood pressure control and risk of macrovascular and microvascular complications in type 2 diabetes: UKPDS 38. *BMJ* 1998;317(7160):703–713.

5. **Should clinic blood pressures or out-of-office blood pressures be used?**
    Current guidelines are based on BP recorded in the clinic. However, ambulatory BPs, obtained by patients wearing blood pressure cuffs for 24 hours, are superior to clinic BPs for making a diagnosis of hypertension and determining prognosis. Ambulatory BP recordings provide more information about target organ damage (e.g., LVH) and hard cardiovascular endpoints. However, ambulatory BP monitoring is expensive and performed usually in specialty clinics or research settings. Home BPs, self-recorded by the patients, are a good surrogate for ambulatory BPs. As with ambulatory BPs, home BP recordings are obtained in the patients' usual settings. Home BP recordings, compared to clinic BP recordings, provide more information regarding cardiovascular and renal risk. Even patients with limited education can successfully perform home BP monitoring. The American Heart Association has recently published recommendations for home BP monitoring. Goal BPs are <135/85 mm Hg for essential hypertensives and <130/80 mm Hg for patients with diabetes or CKD. When recommending a home BP monitor to patients, it is important to use monitors that are validated. Information has been printed on those home BP monitors that have been validated by the British Hypertension Society or the Association for the Advancement of Medication Instrumentation. An online list of validated monitors appears at www.dableducational.org. A minimum of 12 BP recordings, obtained over 1 week, should be used for clinical decision-making.

Agarwal R, Andersen MJ. Prognostic importance of clinic and home blood pressure recordings in patients with chronic kidney disease. *Kidney Int* 2006;69(2):406–411.

Andersen MJ, Khawandi W, Agarwal R. Home blood pressure monitoring in CKD. *Am J Kidney Dis* 2005;45(6):994–1001.

Bobrie G, Chatellier G, Genes N, et al. Cardiovascular prognosis of "masked hypertension" detected by blood pressure self-measurement in elderly treated hypertensive patients. *JAMA* 2004;291(11):1342–1349.

Clement DL, De Buyzere ML, De Bacquer DA, et al. Prognostic value of ambulatory blood-pressure recordings in patients with treated hypertension. *N Engl J Med* 2003;12;348(24):2407–2415.

Liu JE, Roman MJ, Pini R, Schwartz JE, Pickering TG, Devereux RB. Cardiac and arterial target organ damage in adults with elevated ambulatory and normal office blood pressure. *Ann Intern Med* 1999;131(8):564–572.

O'Brien E, Asmar R, Beilin L, et al. European Society of Hypertension recommendations for conventional, ambulatory and home blood pressure measurement. *J Hypertens* 2003;21(5):821–848.

Pickering TG, Miller NH, Ogedegbe G, et al. Call to action on use and reimbursement for home blood pressure monitoring: a joint scientific statement from the American Heart Association, American Society Of Hypertension, and Preventive Cardiovascular Nurses Association. *Hypertension* 2008;52(1):10–29.

6. **What is the relationship between end-stage renal disease risk and hypertension?**
    Roughly 10% of the American population has kidney disease, and more than 60% of patients with CKD have hypertension. Uncontrolled hypertension predisposes to end-stage renal disease (ESRD). The Multiple Risk Factor Intervention Trial (MRFIT) was a randomized, multicenter trial to prevent coronary artery disease in males by treating hypertension, hyperlipidemia, and tobacco abuse. Investigators followed these patients for several decades. Compared with optimal BPs, those patients with baseline systolic pressures ≥160 mm Hg had at least a sixfold higher risk of progressing to ESRD. Poor African American men were at particularly high risk for developing ESRD. A more recent trial showed that, compared to optimal BPs, patients with prehypertension had 62% to 98% increased relative risk for developing ESRD. Those patients with stage I and II hypertension had a 2.5-fold and nearly

fourfold risk, respectively. Using predialysis BP recordings, patients who undergo long-term hemodialysis are nearly all hypertensive (86%), and only 30% of these patients have controlled BP. However, only one third of patients are found to be hypertensive when ambulatory BP recordings are used to make a diagnosis.

Agarwal R, Andersen MJ, Bishu K, Saha C. Home blood pressure monitoring improves the diagnosis of hypertension in hemodialysis patients. *Kidney Int* 2006;69(5):900–906.

Agarwal R, Nissenson AR, Batlle D, et al. Prevalence, treatment, and control of hypertension in chronic hemodialysis patients in the United States. *Am J Med* 2003;115(4):291–297.

Coresh J, Selvin E, Stevens LA, et al. Prevalence of chronic kidney disease in the United States. *JAMA* 2007;298(17):2038–2047.

Hsu CY, McCulloch CE, Darbinian J, Go AS, Iribarren C. Elevated blood pressure and risk of end-stage renal disease in subjects without baseline kidney disease. *Arch Intern Med* 2005;165(8):923–928.

Klag MJ, Whelton PK, Randall BL, et al. Blood pressure and end-stage renal disease in men. *N Engl J Med* 1996;334(1):13–18.

Klag MJ, Whelton PK, Randall BL, et al. End-stage renal disease in African-American and white men: 16-year MRFIT findings. *JAMA* 1997;277(16):1293–1298.

7. **How does kidney disease cause hypertension?**
   - **Nephron number:** A recent pathologic study noted that middle-aged Caucasians with essential hypertension or LVH had significantly fewer nephrons than age-matched controls. The fewer nephrons that develop during fetal life mean less renal mass for Na and volume homeostasis and may predispose these patients to hypertension.
   - **Salt and volume:** African Americans, patients who are obese, and elderly patients nearly all have salt-sensitive hypertension. Conversely, primitive societies that ingest little salt have no hypertension. Usually, when salt is consumed, a pressure natriuresis occurs that excretes the excess salt and volume. Patients who are salt sensitive need higher BPs to excrete an Na load. One reason for sodium sensitivity could result from renal tubulointerstitial inflammation and ischemia.
   - **The sympathetic nervous system:** The sympathetic nervous system increases renin secretion, decreases urinary Na excretion, and decreases renal blood flow. Increased sympathetic activity may be one of the mechanisms that leads to renal damage and salt-sensitive hypertension. The sympathetic nervous system is overactive in patients with CKD, and renal denervation, nephrectomy, or angiotensin-converting enzyme (ACE) inhibition are possible treatment modalities to decrease sympathetic activation. The recently discovered enzyme renalase, mostly produced in the kidney, inactivates circulating catecholamines and may be important for BP regulation.
   - **The renin-angiotensin-aldosterone system:** Renin, secreted by the juxtaglomerular cells of afferent arteriole, cleaves angiotensinogen to angiotensin I (ATI). ATI is converted to angiotensin II (ATII) by ACE. ATII increases renal Na reabsorption, renal arteriolar vasoconstriction, and aldosterone secretion. With renal damage, increased ACE expression may occur and lead to elevated ATII levels. Pathologic levels of ATII can cause renal damage and salt-sensitive hypertension.
   - **Oxidative stress:** Reactive oxygen species (ROS) are produced in the kidney in the course of oxidative metabolism. An elegant system of enzymes exists in the kidney to neutralize excess ROS. In patients with CKD, this neutralizing system is impaired. Excess ROS can have deleterious consequences. For example, increased ROS can inactivate nitric oxide (NO), a molecule that causes endothelium-dependent vasodilation. Inactivation of NO occurs in oxidative stress (nitrosative stress), and this can lead to hypertension through increased vasoconstriction. Salt-sensitive hypertensives and patients with CKD also have elevated levels of asymmetric dimethylarginine, an inhibitor of NO synthase, which also leads to reduced production of NO.

Andersen MJ, Agarwal R. Etiology and management of hypertension in chronic kidney disease. *Med Clin North Am* 2005 May;89(3):525–547.

Converse RL Jr, Jacobsen TN, Toto RD, et al. Sympathetic overactivity in patients with chronic renal failure. *N Engl J Med* 1992;327(27):1912–1918.

Desir GV. Regulation of blood pressure and cardiovascular function by renalase. *Kidney Int* 2009;76(4):366–370.

Guyton AC, Coleman TG, Young DB, Lohmeier TE, DeClue JW. Salt balance and long-term blood pressure control. *Annu Rev Med* 1980;31:15–27.

Johnson RJ, Herrera-Acosta J, Schreiner GF, Rodriguez-Iturbe B. Subtle acquired renal injury as a mechanism of salt-sensitive hypertension. *N Engl J Med* 2002;346(12):913–923.

Keller G, Zimmer G, Mall G, Ritz E, Amann K. Nephron number in patients with primary hypertension. *N Engl J Med* 2003;348(2):101–108.

Ligtenberg G, Blankestijn PJ, Oey PL, et al. Reduction of sympathetic hyperactivity by enalapril in patients with chronic renal failure. *N Engl J Med* 1999;340(17):1321–1328.

Schlaich MP, Sobotka PA, Krum H, et al. Renal denervation as a therapeutic approach for hypertension: novel implications for an old concept. *Hypertension* 2009;54(6):1195–1201.

Ulrich C, Heine GH, Garcia P, et al. Increased expression of monocytic angiotensin-converting enzyme in dialysis patients with cardiovascular disease. *Nephrol Dial Transplant* 2006;21(6):1596–1602.

Vaziri ND, Rodríguez-Iturbe B. Mechanisms of disease: oxidative stress and inflammation in the pathogenesis of hypertension. *Nat Clin Pract Nephrol* 2006;2(10):582–593.

8. **What is the proper antihypertensive regimen?**
    Clinical trials suggest that tighter BP control reduces cardiovascular risk and kidney disease progression. Which agent should be used first has been debated. With the epidemics of obesity, diabetes mellitus, and CKD, this debate is somewhat moot, because nearly all patients with hypertension will need multiple medications; many will require three or more medications. The trick is finding rational second and third drugs to add to the initial drug choice. For most patients with CKD, an ACE inhibitor or angiotensin receptor blocker (ARB) is an appropriate first choice. Exceptions include pregnant women or women planning to become pregnant and those with hyperkalemia, liver cirrhosis, or volume depletion. A good second drug choice would be a calcium channel blocker (CCB) or diuretic. Recent data comparing a dihydropyridine CCB to a diuretic as a second-line agent show that diuretics may be less appropriate. However, diuretics need be added for adequate BP control in nearly all patients as a second- or a third-line agent. The choices of CCBs and diuretics are more rational because they are more likely to provide better BP control than adding a beta blocker or centrally acting agent like clonidine. Combination therapy is key to successful management, but nonpharmacologic management such as sodium restriction, exercise, smoking cessation, and weight loss should be emphasized. The aforementioned program should be coupled with regular home BP monitoring. ACE inhibitors and ARBs merit special attention. Serum creatinine and potassium should be checked within a week or two of starting either medication or increasing the dose. Labs should be followed periodically thereafter. Patients prone to hyperkalemia (e.g., diabetics) should be given dietary education. Nonsteroidal medications should be discontinued. Creatinine increases of within 30% of baseline levels are acceptable if unaccompanied by volume depletion and symptomatic hypotension. The combination of ACE inhibitors and ARBs has been recommended among patients with proteinuria. Although this combination can reduce proteinuria, whether the combination therapy can prolong time to ESRD or reduce cardiovascular events has never been proven. In fact, a recent trial done largely in patients without CKD (The ONgoing Telmisartan Alone and in combination with Ramipril Global Endpoint [ONTARGET] trial) noted increased renal disease progression and death with combination ACE inhibitor and ARB therapy. These results further raise concerns regarding using proteinuria as a surrogate endpoint for renal protection. Recent studies suggest that spironolactone, in combination with an ARB, may provide more proteinuria reduction, although data on hard endpoints are lacking.

Bakris GL, Weir MR. Angiotensin-converting enzyme inhibitor-associated elevations in serum creatinine: is this a cause for concern? *Arch Intern Med* 2000;160(5):685–663.

Chobanian AV, Bakris GL, Black HR, et al. The Seventh Report of the Joint National Committee on Prevention, Detection, Evaluation, and Treatment of High Blood Pressure: the JNC 7 report. *JAMA* 2003;289(19):2560–2572.

Jamerson K, Weber MA, Bakris GL, et al. Benazepril plus amlodipine or hydrochlorothiazide for hypertension in high-risk patients. *N Engl J Med* 2008 Dec 4;359(23):2417–2428.

Jennings DL, Kalus JS, Coleman CI, Manierski C, Yee J. Combination therapy with an ACE inhibitor and an angiotensin receptor blocker for diabetic nephropathy: a meta-analysis. Diabet Med 2007;24(5):486–493.

Mann JF, Schmieder RE, McQueen M, et al. Renal outcomes with telmisartan, ramipril, or both, in people at high vascular risk (the ONTARGET study): a multicentre, randomised, double-blind, controlled trial. *Lancet* 2008;372(9638):547–553.

Pickering TG, Miller NH, Ogedegbe G, et al. Call to action on use and reimbursement for home blood pressure monitoring: a joint scientific statement from the American Heart Association, American Society Of Hypertension, and Preventive Cardiovascular Nurses Association. *Hypertension* 2008;52(1):10–29.

Saklayen MG, Gyebi LK, Tasosa J, Yap J. Effects of additive therapy with spironolactone on proteinuria in diabetic patients already on ACE inhibitor or ARB therapy: results of a randomized, placebo-controlled, double-blind, crossover trial. *J Investig Med* 2008;56(4):714–719.

Schrier RW, Estacio RO, Esler A, Mehler P. Effects of aggressive blood pressure control in normotensive type 2 diabetic patients on albuminuria, retinopathy and strokes. *Kidney Int* 2002;61(3):1086–1097.

UK Prospective Diabetes Study Group.Tight blood pressure control and risk of macrovascular and microvascular complications in type 2 diabetes: UKPDS 38. *BMJ* 1998;317(7160):703–713.

KEY POINTS: RENAL PARENCHYMAL HYPERTENSION

1. Compared to estimated glomerular filtration rate, albuminuria (or proteinuria) is a stronger determinant of hypertension; albuminuria is also a stronger determinant of poor control of hypertension.

2. Patients with chronic kidney disease (CKD) and diabetes mellitus need tighter blood pressure (BP) control, and they are considered hypertensive if their BPs, recorded in the clinic, are ≥130/80 mm Hg. These patients need excellent control of their BPs throughout their lifetime.

3. Home BP recordings, compared to clinic BP recordings, provide more information regarding cardiovascular and renal risk. Goal BPs are <135/85 mm Hg for essential hypertensives and <130/80 mm Hg for diabetics and patients with CKD.

4. For most patients with CKD, an ACE inhibitor or ARB is an appropriate first choice. With the epidemics of obesity, diabetes mellitus, and CKD, nearly all patients with hypertension will need multiple medications; many will require three or more.

CHAPTER 64

RENOVASCULAR DISEASE

Edward J. Horwitz, MD, and Mahboob Rahman, MD

1. **What clinical syndromes are associated with renal artery stenosis?**
   Renovascular hypertension, progressive loss of kidney function from ischemic nephropathy, and recurrent episodes of flash pulmonary edema (meaning acute/abrupt onset pulmonary edema) are the clinical syndromes typically associated with renal artery stenosis. However, renal artery stenosis can also be completely asymptomatic.

   In the case of renovascular hypertension, hemodynamically significant unilateral or bilateral renal artery stenosis leads to decreased renal perfusion pressure in one or both kidneys. This stimulates activation of the renin-angiotensin-aldosterone system, which increases systemic pressure to restore renal perfusion distal to the stenotic lesion(s). The pathophysiology of ischemic nephropathy is complex and likely relates to activation of multiple pathways triggered by reduced renal perfusion that promote renal injury and fibrosis. Flash pulmonary edema in the context of renal artery stenosis tends to occur only with bilateral stenosis (or renal artery stenosis affecting a solitary kidney). In this situation, patients are felt to be predisposed to episodes of pulmonary edema from enhanced tubular sodium reabsorption and volume expansion from increased renin-angiotensin-aldosterone activity in the absence of a pressure natriuresis phenomenon that would occur within an unaffected kidney.

2. **What are the two main causes of renal artery stenosis?**
   The two important causes of renal artery stenosis are atherosclerosis and fibromuscular dysplasia. Atherosclerotic renal artery stenosis is the more common cause and is often seen in older patients. It occurs in the setting of atherosclerotic disease affecting other vascular beds such as the coronary, cerebral, and peripheral arterial circulation. These patients often have other risk factors for atherosclerosis such as diabetes, hypertension, and smoking. However, fibromuscular dysplasia is typically seen in younger female patients.

3. **How common is renal artery stenosis?**
   It depends on the population examined. Some degree of renal artery stenosis will be found incidentally in 19% to 42% of patients with atherosclerotic vascular disease such as coronary artery disease or peripheral vascular disease. Fibromuscular dysplasia causing renal artery stenosis may be as common as 3% to 5% of healthy patients being evaluated as potential living kidney donors. In studies examining patients with mild to moderate hypertension, renal artery stenosis has been found in the range in 0.6% to 3% of this population. In patients with refractory hypertension, renal artery stenosis may be found in between 10% and 45% of patients.

4. **How often does renal artery stenosis lead to end-stage renal disease?**
   In some series of patients receiving dialysis, atherosclerotic renal artery stenosis may lead to end-stage renal disease in up to 15% of patients. However, in the most recent United States Renal Data Service report (USRDS is a registry that tracks various data on virtually all patients receiving dialysis in the United States) renal artery stenosis or renal artery occlusion is

reported to be the cause of end-stage renal disease in 1.6% of patients between 2003 and 2007, which accounts for 8605 people.

5. **Who is at risk of developing renal artery stenosis?**
Patients with risk factors for atherosclerotic vascular disease, such as hypertension, dyslipidemia, diabetes, tobacco use, and older age, are at increased risk for atherosclerosis affecting the renal arteries causing stenosis.

6. **Who should be screened for renal artery stenosis?**
Features suggestive of renal artery stenosis include abrupt onset of hypertension at a relatively young age (<30 years old) or older age (>50 years old), worsening control of previously well-treated hypertension, recurrent episodes of "flash pulmonary edema," renal failure precipitated by initiation of antihypertensive therapy—especially angiotensin-converting enzyme (ACE) inhibitors or angiotensin receptor blockers (ARBs)—unexplained renal failure, a unilateral atrophic kidney, an abdominal bruit, unexplained hypokalemia, and the presence of atherosclerotic disease in other vascular beds.

7. **What diagnostic tests can you use to identify renal artery stenosis? How do you decide which test to use?**
Screening for suspected renal artery stenosis can be done with duplex ultrasonography of the renal arteries, computed tomographic angiography (CTA), or magnetic resonance angiography (MRA).
   Duplex ultrasonography has the advantage of being noninvasive and does not expose patients to potential toxicities of the contrast agents needed for CTA or MRA. However, accuracy of duplex ultrasound is operator dependent and may be limited in patients who are morbidly obese.
   Computed tomographic angiography is noninvasive and can characterize renal artery stenosis with a high degree of sensitivity (as high as 98%) and specificity (as high as 94%). The main disadvantages of this modality are radiation exposure and the need for iodinated contrast, which is potentially nephrotoxic, particularly in patients with impaired renal function and diabetes.
   Magnetic resonance angiography gives exceptional resolution of lesions causing renal artery stenosis with a very high sensitivity (up to 100%) and specificity (up to 97%), and it has the benefit of not exposing patients to radiation or the risk of contrast nephropathy because gadolinium is used instead of iodinated contrast. However, although gadolinium is generally not considered to be a nephrotoxic, its use is not without risk. In patients with advanced chronic kidney disease, especially those with end-stage renal disease, gadolinium has been associated with a debilitating skin condition known as nephrogenic systemic fibrosis (NSF). In addition, MRA is generally a more expensive noninvasive test to evaluate for renal artery stenosis compared to ultrasound and CTA.
   The gold standard study to diagnose renal artery stenosis is conventional digital subtraction angiography. However, this is an invasive procedure that exposes patients to radiation and iodinated dye in addition to the risk of cholesterol atheroembolic disease (discussed in detail later).

8. **What is the resistance index, and how may it be useful in managing renal artery stenosis?**
The resistance index is a measure of relative blood flow velocity during systole and diastole within the renal arterial supply using Doppler ultrasonography. It is calculated with the following formula:

$$\text{Resistance index} = [1 - (\text{end-diastolic velocity}/\text{maximal systolic velocity})] \times 100$$

   It has been shown to correlate with changes in blood pressure following revascularization. Specifically, a high resistance index of >80 suggests the presence of more extensive atherosclerotic disease in smaller vessels within the arterial network and is associated with a lack of improvement in blood pressure following revascularization.

9. **What is the natural history of renal artery stenosis?**

Atherosclerotic renal artery stenosis often progresses anatomically and is associated with a high mortality. Numerous studies have documented anatomic progression of atherosclerotic lesions over the course of a few years using various imaging methods. For example, in one study angiographic progression was observed in 11% of patients followed an average of about 2.5 years, whereas in another study anatomic progression was seen in 44% of a population followed for slightly longer than an average of 4 years. Patients with fibromuscular dysplasia also may have angiographic progression of their renal artery lesions; 33% of patients with fibromuscular dysplasia in one cohort displayed anatomic progression over an average of about 4 years.

10. **What are the long-term outcomes of patients with renal artery stenosis?**

Far more of these patients with atherosclerotic renal artery stenosis die of cardiovascular disease than will ever live to require dialysis. Mortality at about 2 years ranges between 32% and 45%, whereas the percentage of patients requiring dialysis ranged from 3% to 16% in these cohorts. Renal failure as a result of fibromuscular dysplasia is felt to be very rare.

11. **What treatment options exist for renal artery stenosis caused by atherosclerosis?**

Atherosclerotic renal artery stenosis may be treated by medical management, angioplasty/stent placement, or surgery.

Medical management is based on blood pressure control with appropriate antihypertensive medications along with lifestyle modifications and other medical interventions aimed at reducing the high cardiovascular risk associated with atherosclerotic renal artery stenosis. This includes use of aspirin, statins, smoking cessation, and good glycemic control in patients with diabetes.

In addition to this approach, revascularization, now mainly done with percutaneous interventions (angioplasty and stenting) rather than surgery, can also be used to treat renovascular hypertension and ischemic nephropathy. However, randomized trials to date suggest that revascularization does NOT significantly improve blood pressure control, renal outcomes, or cardiovascular outcomes compared to medical management alone. The largest and most recently published of these studies, the Angioplasty and STenting for Renal Artery Lesions (ASTRAL) trial, involving more than 800 patients randomized to medical management with revascularization or medical management alone, found no statistically significant differences between the two strategies in terms of the rate that renal function declined, renal events, systolic blood pressure control (a greater decrease in diastolic blood pressure was actually observed in the control group), cardiovascular events, and death. In addition, about 9% of patients who underwent revascularization experienced a periprocedural complication.

12. **How should renal artery stenosis caused by fibromuscular dysplasia be managed?**

In contrast to atherosclerotic renal artery stenosis, revascularization of fibromuscular dysplasia generally leads to favorable clinical outcomes and should be considered in many cases. Although there are no randomized trials exclusively involving patients with fibromuscular dysplasia, several case series with these patients have shown that hypertension was improved or even cured in the majority of patients who underwent percutaneous revascularization.

13. **What are the potential benefits and risks associated with percutaneous revascularization of renal artery stenosis?**

Percutaneous revascularization (angioplasty with or without stenting) can potentially correct stenotic lesions in a relatively noninvasive procedure, but it is certainly not without risk.

Patients are at risk for bleeding complications; contrast nephropathy; and even renal artery dissection, occlusion, or perforation. Acute kidney injury associated with any of these events may require renal replacement therapy and is not necessarily reversible.

One other potential complication of conventional angiography and percutaneous revascularization procedures that deserves special mention is cholesterol atheroembolic disease. This disorder occurs when cholesterol fragments from atheromatous plaques embolize to distal arterial blood vessels causing ischemic injury. This embolic event most often occurs in the context of anticoagulation/thrombolytic therapy or some procedure such as vascular surgery or conventional angiography where mechanical trauma to the atherosclerotic vessels with vulnerable plaques may be unavoidable. The clinical manifestations vary depending on where the cholesterol-laden fragments embolize and may include stroke, mesenteric ischemia, acute kidney injury, and ischemic digits. Atheroembolic disease affecting the kidneys should be suspected in patients who have a decline in renal function following a relatively recent vascular procedure or angiography study with or without percutaneous intervention and also demonstrate any of the following examination or laboratory findings: livedo reticularis, ischemic digits, peripheral eosinophilia, and hypocomplementemia. Patients with cholesterol atheroembolic disease may lose kidney function over the course of weeks to months in a stepwise fashion and this may not be reversible. Although treatment is mainly supportive, it is important to avoid anticoagulation if possible because it is believed this may predispose the patient to further embolic events. Cholesterol-lowering agents may also be of some benefit.

14. **Should all patients with hypertension caused by atherosclerotic renal artery stenosis always undergo revascularization?**
No. The randomized trials completed to date have not clearly demonstrated a significant benefit to revascularization compared to medical management alone in regard to renovascular hypertension. The risks and benefits of each option should be discussed with each individual patient, in consultation with a vascular surgeon or interventional radiologist.

15. **Do patients who have chronic kidney disease with significant atherosclerotic renal artery stenosis clearly benefit from revascularization over medical management alone?**
No. The randomized trials completed to date do not clearly show patients with chronic kidney disease who underwent revascularization compared to those with medical management alone had improved renal outcomes, cardiovascular outcomes, or overall mortality.

16. **Does it matter which antihypertensive agents are used to control blood pressure in patients with renal artery stenosis?**
As long as inhibitors of the renin-angiotensin-system (RAS) do not precipitate renal failure, patients with atherosclerotic renal artery stenosis treated with ACE inhibitors seem to have more favorable long-term outcomes compared to those not taking ACE inhibitors. Consequently, this class of medications is preferred in the treatment of hypertension associated with atherosclerotic renal artery stenosis.

Moreover, as long as severe bilateral disease is not present, antagonists of the RAS would not necessarily be expected to precipitate acute renal failure. A rise in serum creatinine of up to 30% from baseline after initiation of an ACE inhibitor or ARB is often observed, particularly in patients with some underlying chronic kidney disease, and should not prompt discontinuation of the medication. In contrast, a more substantial decline in renal function (creatinine increase of >30%) or significant hyperkalemia (potassium >6) after initiation of a RAS inhibitor should raise some suspicion for concurrent states of decreased effective arterial blood volume such as volume depletion or decompensated heart, nonsteroidal anti-inflammatory drug (NSAID) use, bilateral renal artery stenosis, or renal artery stenosis of a solitary kidney. In this situation, the RAS inhibitor should be at least temporarily held and these possibilities should be explored.

17. **In what situations may it be appropriate to consider revascularization for atherosclerotic renal artery stenosis?**

Despite the results of trials that do not suggest patients with ischemic nephropathy or renovascular hypertension benefit from revascularization in general, there still may exist some situations where revascularization is appropriate to attempt. For example, it may be reasonable to try revascularization in patients with recurrent flash pulmonary edema. Moreover, if a patient is intolerant of many antihypertensive medications or their hypertension cannot be adequately controlled with medications, revascularization would be reasonable to attempt. Finally, if a patient were rapidly losing renal function believed to be from atherosclerotic renal artery stenosis, it could be argued that because they will likely require renal replacement therapy very soon if nothing else is done, the potential benefits of an attempted intervention may outweigh the risks.

KEY POINTS: RENOVASCULAR DISEASE

1. Renal artery stenosis is associated with three main clinical syndromes: ischemic nephropathy, renovascular hypertension, and recurrent flash pulmonary edema. However, it may also be completely asymptomatic.

2. Renal artery stenosis should be suspected in patients with resistant hypertension, abrupt onset of hypertension at a relatively young or old age, worsening blood pressure control in someone with previously well-controlled hypertension, recurrent episodes of flash pulmonary edema, unexplained renal dysfunction, unexplained hypokalemia, an atrophic unilateral kidney, renal failure precipitated by initiation of blockers of the renin-angiotensin system, an abdominal bruit, and the presence of atherosclerotic disease in other vascular beds.

3. Screening for suspected renal artery stenosis can be done with duplex ultrasonography, magnetic resonance angiography, or computed tomographic angiography. The gold standard diagnostic study is digital subtraction angiography, but this involves an invasive procedure.

4. Atherosclerotic renal artery stenosis commonly progresses anatomically and is associated with high mortality largely from cardiovascular causes.

5. No randomized trials to date have demonstrated a clear benefit for revascularization over medical management alone in the treatment of atherosclerotic renal artery stenosis.

BIBLIOGRAPHY

1. The ATRAL investigators. Revascularization versus medical therapy for renal artery stenosis. *New Engl J Med* 2009;361:1953–1962.

2. Baboolal K, Evans C, Moore RH. Incidence of ESRD-stage renal disease in medically treated patients with severe bilateral atherosclerotic renovascular disease. *Am J Kidney Dis* 1998; 31(6):971–977.

3. Bakris GL, Weir MR. Angiotensin-converting enzyme inhibitor-associated elevations in serum creatinine: Is this a cause for concern? *Arch Intern Med* 2000;160:685–693.

4. Bax L, Woittiez AJ, Kouwenberg HJ, et al. Stent placement in patients with atherosclerotic renal artery stenosis and impaired renal function: A randomized trial. *Ann Intern Med* 2009;150:840–848.

5. Conlon P, McQuillan R. Secondary hypertension. In: Greenberg A. *Primer on Kidney Diseases*, 5th ed. Philadelphia: Saunders Elsevier 2009, pp. 561–570.

6. Cooper C, Murphey T, Matsumoto A, et al. Stent revascularization for the prevention of cardiovascular and renal events among patients with renal artery stenosis: Rational and design of the CORAL trial. *Am Heart J* 2006;152:59–66.

7. Crowley J, Santos R, Peter R, et al. Progression of renal artery stenosis in patients undergoing cardiac catheterization. *Am Heart J* 1998;136(5)913–918.

8. Dworkin L, Cooper C. Renal artery stenosis. *New Engl J Med* 2009;361:1972–1978.

9. Hackam DG, Duong-Hua M, Mamdani M, et al. Angiotensin inhibition in renovascular disease: A population-based cohort study. *Am Heart J* 2008;156:549–555.

10. Kanso A, Abou Hassan NA, Badr KF. Microvascular and macrovascular diseases of the kidney. In: Brenner BM. *Brenner and Rector's The Kidney*, 8th ed. Philadelphia: W.B. Saunders, 2007, pp. 1147–1173.

11. Mailloux L, Napolitano B, Bellucci A, et al. Renal vascular disease causing end stage renal disease, incidence, clinical correlates, and outcomes. A 20 year clinical experience. *Am J Kidney Dis* 1994;24(4):622–629.

12. Pillay WR, Kan YM, Crinnion JN, et al. Prospective multicentre study of the natural history of atherosclerotic renal artery stenosis in patients with peripheral vascular disease. *Br J Surg* 2002;89:737–740.

13. Pickering TG, Herman L, Devereux RB, et al. Recurrent pulmonary oedema in hypertension due to bilateral renal artery stenosis: Treatment by angioplasty or surgical revascularisation. *Lancet* 1988;2(8610):551.

14. Plouin P, Chatellier, Darne B, et al., for the Essai Multicentrique Medicaments vs Angioplastie (EMMA) Study Group. Blood pressure outcome of angioplasty in atherosclerotic renal artery stenosis: A randomized trial. *Hypertension* 1998;31:823–829.

15. Radermacher J, Chaven A, Bleck J, et al. Use of Doppler ultrasonography to predict the outcome of therapy for renal artery stenosis. *New Engl J Med* 2001;344:410–417.

16. Safian R, Textor S. Renal artery stenosis. *New Engl J Med* 2001;344:431–442.

17. Scoble JE, Maher ER, Hamilton G, et al. Atherosclerotic renovascular disease causing renal impairment—A case for treatment. *Clin Nephrol* 1989;31:119–122.

18. Siddiqui S, MacGregor M, Glynn C, et al. Factors predicting outcome in a cohort of patients with atherosclerotic renal artery disease diagnose by magnetic resonance angiography. *Am J Kidney Dis* 2005;46(6):1065–1073.

19. Slovut D, Olin J. Fibromuscular dysplasia. *New Engl J Med* 2004;350:1862–1871.

20. Textor S. Renovascular hypertension and ischemic nephropathy. In: Brenner BM. *Brenner and Rector's The Kidney*, 8th ed. Philadelphia: W.B. Saunders, 2007, pp. 1528–1562.

21. Webster J, Marshall F, Abdalla M, et al., on behalf of the Scottish and Newcastle Renal Artery Stenosis Collaborative Group. Randomized comparison of percutaneous angioplasty vs continued medical therapy for hypertensive patients with atheromatous renal artery stenosis. *J Human Hypertens.* 1998;12:329–335.

22. Van Jaarsveld BC, Krijnen P, Pieterman H, et al. The effect of balloon angioplasty on hypertension in atherosclerotic renal artery stenosis. *New Engl J Med* 2000;342:1007–1014.

CHAPTER 65

ENDOCRINE HYPERTENSION

William J. Elliott, MD, PhD

HYPERALDOSTERONISM

1. **What is hyperaldosteronism?**
   Hyperaldosteronism is a characteristic set of signs and symptoms resulting from excessive effects of aldosterone or similar mineralocorticoid agent, which typically include hypertension (usually unresponsive to angiotensin-converting enzyme [ACE] inhibitors, angiotensin receptor blockers [ARBs], or direct renin inhibitors), intravascular volume expansion, and hypokalemia.

2. **Describe the most common subtypes or causes of hyperaldosteronism.**
   Hyperaldosteronism as a result of an autonomously functioning adrenal adenoma is historically called Conn's syndrome, after Jerome William Conn (1907–1994), one of seven distinguished physicians of the U.S. Veterans' Administration who detailed his first case in his presidential address to the Central Society for Clinical Research in 1954. More common is bilateral adrenal hyperplasia (sometimes called idiopathic hyperaldosteronism), in which both glands oversecrete aldosterone. More recently, aldosteronism has been linked to obstructive sleep apnea; this is one of the more common causes of resistant hypertension in many series. Glucocorticoid-remediable hyperaldosteronism results from a chimeric gene on chromosome 8 that results from the crossing over of the regulatory sequence for corticotropin of 11β-hydroxylase, which is fused to the enzyme coding sequences for aldosterone synthase. Hyperaldosteronism from an adrenal carcinoma is rare (~30 cases worldwide) and usually presents as a larger tumor.

3. **How common is hyperaldosteronism?**
   The prevalence of hyperaldosteronism depends on where and how one looks and is controversial. Some referral centers report a prevalence of hyperaldosteronism related to sleep apnea at about 20%, similar to the original estimate of aldosterone-secreting adenomas proposed by Conn in 1954. Other population-based studies suggest that such a high prevalence is a result of a lack of specificity of the aldosterone-renin ratio that is most often used to screen for the condition. In a series from the Mayo Clinic, about 10% of community-dwelling hypertensives had an "abnormal" ratio, but no tumors were detected on computed tomographic screening.

4. **What is the most appropriate test to screen for hyperaldosteronism?**
   After total body potassium stores have been repleted, the ratio of plasma aldosterone-renin measured in (optimally, untreated) patients in the seated position at 8 AM is widely recommended. A plasma aldosterone/renin activity ratio >20 ng/dL per ng/mL/hour and a simultaneous plasma aldosterone level >15 ng/dL is suggestive of hyperaldosteronism. The test can be confounded by high-sodium diets, antihypertensive drug therapy, and many other factors.

5. **What additional tests may be useful in identifying patients with hyperaldosteronism?**
   Urinary potassium and aldosterone concentrations in a 24-hour urine were formerly very popular as screening tests.

The Berlin Questionnaire is a useful screening tool for sleep apnea; when used in patients with hypertension and persistent hypokalemia, it can often distinguish those who should have a formal polysomnographic study.

Many different tests have been proposed to distinguish between an aldosterone-producing adenoma and bilateral adrenal hyperplasia, including assay of blood or urine for aldosterone (and/or other mineralocorticoids) before and after infusion of 2 liters of saline after a high-sodium diet, postural change, either an ACE inhibitor or an ARB, or assay of 11-oxo-aldosterone. None of these are perfect discriminators, so many physicians simply image the adrenals after the screening test is positive. A computed tomographic (CT) scan of the abdomen, with thin (5-mm cuts) through the adrenals, is usually done first. If a unilateral hypodense mass >1 cm is found, a surgeon is consulted for laparoscopic removal (see later). Some physicians prefer a magnetic resonance imaging scan, again with thin cuts through the adrenals, but this is probably less sensitive (because of better resolution of the CT scans). A few centers are experienced with iodocholesterol scintigraphic scanning, but most centers use the CT scan first.

Glucocorticoid-remediable hyperaldosteronism can now be detected by genetic testing of leukocyte DNA.

Adrenal venous sampling is a complex undertaking, typically done only at large centers with much experience in the technique, which is useful when bilateral nodules are found or when there are questions about which side is involved.

6. **List treatments for hyperaldosteronism.**
   - **For a Conn's adenoma:** Unilateral adrenalectomy, now often by laparoscopic surgery, is indicated.
   - **For bilateral adrenal hyperplasia:** Chronic therapy with an aldosterone antagonist (originally spironolactone, now more often eplerenone, because it has fewer adverse effects).
   - **For hyperaldosteronism related to sleep apnea:** Spironolactone (or eplerenone) is effective in the vast majority of cases; continuous positive airway pressure is recommended for the signs and symptoms of sleep apnea.
   - **For glucocorticoid-suppressible hyperaldosteronism:** Low-dose glucocorticoid therapy is indicated.

7. **What are the short- and long-term challenges after surgery?**
   Strict attention to eukalemia is important, particularly in the first few days after the operation. Long-term resolution of hypokalemia is common, but most patients remain hypertensive, even after a successful operation.

CUSHING'S SYNDROME AND CONGENITAL ADRENAL HYPERPLASIA

8. **What is Cushing's syndrome?**
   Cushing's syndrome is a characteristic set of signs and symptoms resulting from excessive effects of cortisol, initially attributed to a basophilic pituitary adenoma (Cushing's disease) by Harvey Williams Cushing ("the father of neurosurgery") in 1932.

9. **Describe the most common clinical features of Cushing's syndrome.**
   Cushing's syndrome is characterized by progressive physical changes, often best appreciated in serial photographs. Central (truncal) obesity, moon facies, and a dorsocervical fat pad ("buffalo hump") are classic physical findings. Additional physical findings include purple abdominal striae (said to be the most specific physical sign if >2.5-cm wide), plethora, ecchymoses, hypertrichosis, and muscle weakness and atrophy (typically noted when climbing stairs or arising from a chair). Other features of Cushing's syndrome include emotional and cognitive changes, menstrual irregularity, glucose intolerance, and hypertension. Growth restriction is a universal finding in children with Cushing's syndrome.

10. **How common is hypertension in Cushing's syndrome?**
Although 80% of patients with Cushing's syndrome have hypertension, Cushing's syndrome is a relatively rare cause of hypertension in children and adults.

11. **Explain the mechanism of hypertension in patients with Cushing's syndrome.**
Hypertension in patients with hypercortisolism is multifactorial in origin:
   - Excessive cortisol exposure increases peripheral resistance by the following:
     - Enhancing the effects of catecholamines and angiotensin II
     - Suppressing synthesis of endogenous vasodilatory agents, including nitric oxide and prostaglandins.
   - Cortisol also directly stimulates sodium reabsorption in the distal nephron, while indirectly increasing sodium reabsorption in the proximal nephron by enhancing the activity of various transporters.
   - Synthesis of certain mineralocorticoids is increased in corticotropin– (formerly adrenocorticotropic hormone, or ACTH), dependent types of Cushing's syndrome.

12. **List the most common causes of Cushing's syndrome.**

ACTH-dependent:
   - Pituitary microadenoma (~68% of endogenous cases in large series)
   - Ectopic ACTH production (~12%, from other tumors, typically small-cell lung cancer)
   - Ectopic corticotropin-releasing hormone (CRH) secretion (<1%)

ACTH-independent:
   - Exogenous glucocorticoid administration (iatrogenic causes are the most common in the United States)
   - Adrenal adenoma (~10%)
   - Adrenal adenocarcinoma (~8%)
   - Primary pigmented nodular adrenal hyperplasia (<1%)
   - McCune-Albright syndrome (<1%)
   - Macronodular adrenal disease (<1%)
   - Hyperfunction of adrenal rest tissue (<1%)

13. **What is the difference between Cushing's syndrome and Cushing's disease?**
Cushing's syndrome refers to the condition that includes all patients with hypercortisolism. Cushing's disease refers to that subset of patients with Cushing's syndrome who have a pituitary microadenoma as the cause of their hypercortisolism.

14. **What are the best tests to confirm a diagnosis of Cushing's syndrome?**
Plasma cortisol levels >15 μg/dL in the afternoon or evening (in an unstressed patient) are suggestive of hypercortisolism; British endocrinologists prefer a midnight cortisol level, which can be measured noninvasively in saliva.

Urinary free cortisol values >100 μg/day are abnormal, and values >400 μg/day (>4 times the upper limit of the reference range) are suggestive of Cushing's syndrome.

Many clinicians use the overnight dexamethasone suppression test (which is more convenient than the classical "low-dose" test) as a screen for Cushing's syndrome. Morning (8 AM) plasma cortisol levels >5 μg/dL are suggestive of Cushing's syndrome; patients with levels >1.8 μg/dL are candidates for further testing.

15. **What additional tests may be useful in identifying the cause of Cushing's syndrome?**
Classically, the high-dose dexamethasone suppression test (2 mg every 6 hours for eight doses) suppresses production of cortisol (and its urinary metabolites) in patients with Cushing's disease because these microadenomas retain some of their capacity for negative feedback as a result of circulating corticosteroids. This test does not distinguish well between Cushing's disease and ectopic corticotropin secretion, however.

To distinguish between these two possibilities, simultaneous measurement of plasma corticotropin and cortisol is now available in a few laboratories, but it is expensive.

Naloxone, insulin-induced hypoglycemia, and CRH (after eight doses of low-dose dexamethasone) can help distinguish Cushing's syndrome from depression or alcohol-associated illness (pseudo-Cushing's). Petrosal venous sinus sampling or, rarely, the metyrapone test (blocks conversion of 11-deoxycortisol to cortisol) may help distinguish the origin of excessive corticosteroid effect.

Head and abdominal CT scans may identify a pituitary or adrenal tumor; the magnetic resonance imaging (MRI) is slightly less sensitive for adrenal tumors than a CT with thin cuts (5 mm) through the adrenals. Sometimes a chest x-ray and/or a chest CT is done because the most common source of ectopic corticotropin secretion is a lung tumor (usually small cell).

16. **List treatments for Cushing's syndrome.**
   - Pituitary adenoma resection (for Cushing's disease)
   - Adrenalectomy (particularly unilateral adrenalectomy, but occasionally bilateral adrenalectomy is performed if the pituitary tumor cannot be resected).
   - Resection of the tumor that is secreting ectopic corticotropin.

17. **Is there a role for medical therapy?**
   Agents that modulate corticotropin release (cyproheptadine, bromocriptine, valproic acid) **or** inhibit cortisol synthesis and/or production (mitotane, trilostane, ketoconazole, aminoglutethimide, and metyrapone) may be useful preoperatively or for patients who are not surgical candidates.

18. **Should all patients with hypertension who are obese be evaluated for Cushing's syndrome?**
   No. Testing should be considered for patients with hypertension who present with the characteristic clinical features of Cushing's syndrome.

19. **Define congenital adrenal hyperplasia.**
   Congenital adrenal hyperplasia (CAH) is a diverse family of autosomal-recessive disorders characterized by deficient function of one of the enzymes necessary for cortisol synthesis (Fig. 65-1).

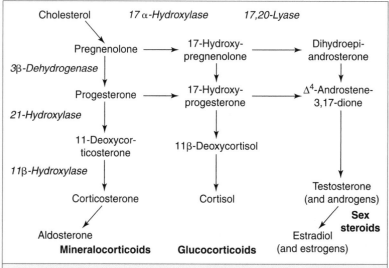

Figure 65-1. Simplified biochemical pathways for steroid biosynthesis (enzymes are given in italics).

The reduction in cortisol synthesis leads to a loss of feedback inhibition of the hypothalamic-pituitary-adrenal axis, with excessive production of corticotropin. Exposure to excessive corticotropin leads to adrenal hyperplasia, overproduction of adrenal steroids that do not require the deficient enzyme, and deficiency of steroids distal to the deficient enzyme.

20. **List the typical clinical manifestations of CAH.**
    - Abnormal fetal genital development: disturbance in sodium and potassium homeostasis (salt wasting or volume overload)
    - Abnormal blood pressure regulation: postnatal consequences of sex-steroid imbalance, including abnormal patterns of growth and maturation and impaired fertility
      The specific clinical features depend on the deficient enzyme involved.

21. **What is the most common cause of CAH?**
    Deficiency of 21-hydroxylase activity, which makes up >90% of cases (1:14,000 live births), is the most common cause of CAH.

22. **What are other causes of CAH?**
    Deficiency of 11β-hydroxylase activity (5% to 8% of cases) is the second most common cause of CAH. Rare causes include 3β-hydroxysteroid dehydrogenase deficiency, 17α-hydroxylase deficiency, and lipoid CAH.

23. **Which forms of CAH are associated with hypertension?**
    11β-hydroxylase deficiency and 17α-hydroxylase deficiency are associated with hypertension.

24. **What about 21-hydroxylase deficiency?**
    Patients with classic 21-hydroxylase deficiency do not have hypertension, but instead have severe salt wasting with dehydration, hyponatremia, and hyperkalemia related to aldosterone deficiency.

25. **Describe the pathophysiology of 11β-hydroxylase deficiency.**
    11β-hydroxylase (P450c11) is the mitochondrial enzyme responsible for the biosynthetic step immediately before cortisol production. More than 30 mutations have been identified on *CYP11B1*, the gene on chromosome 8, which encodes 11β-hydroxylase synthesis. Inadequate 11β-hydroxylation leads to inadequate cortisol production, excessive effect of corticotropin, and increased levels of the precursor deoxycorticosterone (DOC). Steroid biosynthesis is largely diverted to androgen production.

26. **What are the typical clinical features of 11β-hydroxylase deficiency (Bongiovanni's syndrome)?**
    - 11β-Hydroxylase deficiency occurs in about 1:100,000 births.
    - All affected females are born with some degree of masculinization of the external genitalia, including clitoromegaly and partial or complete fusion of the labioscrotal folds. Internal genitalia are normal.
    - Other symptoms of androgen excess that occur postnatally include rapid somatic growth with accelerated skeletal maturation, leading to premature closure of the epiphyses and short adult stature.
    - Mineralocorticoid excess leads to hypokalemic metabolic alkalosis in many patients.
    - About 67% of these patients have stage 1 (or occasionally 2) low-renin hypertension beginning early in life (e.g., ages 1–2 years).

27. **Explain the mechanism of hypertension in patients with 11β-hydroxylase deficiency.**
    Hypertension is the result of volume expansion mediated by increased levels of DOC, a potent mineralocorticoid. Although relatively weak compared to aldosterone, high levels of DOC produce significant sodium and water retention. Serum levels of DOC do not correlate entirely with the degree of hypertension, however, suggesting that other factors may be involved.

28. **Describe the pathophysiology of 17α-hydroxylase deficiency.**
17α-Hydroxylase (P450c17) is the enzyme responsible for the biosynthetic step that converts mineralocorticoids to glucocorticoids (17α-hydroxylase activity) and glucocorticoids to sex steroids (17,20-lyase activity). More than 20 mutations have been identified on *CYP17*, the gene on chromosome 10 that encodes 17α-hydroxylase synthesis. Abnormal enzyme activity can be manifested as isolated 17α-hydroxylase deficiency, 17,20-lyase deficiency, or a combined 17α-hydroxylase/17,20-lyase deficiency. Inadequate 17α-hydroxylase activity leads to inadequate cortisol production, excessive effects of corticotropin, and increased levels of DOC. In contrast to 11β-hydroxylase deficiency, sex-steroid production is decreased.

29. **What are the typical clinical features of 17α-hydroxylase deficiency (Biglieri's syndrome)?**
   - Because patients with 17α-hydroxylase deficiency do not have excessive androgen synthesis, they tend to present later than patients with 11β-hydroxylase deficiency.
   - Males may present with incomplete virilization, and females may present with primary amenorrhea and sexual infantilism at the time of puberty.
   - Occasionally, genetic males with a female phenotype may present for evaluation of a hernia or inguinal mass.
   - Mineralocorticoid excess leads to hypokalemic metabolic alkalosis and Stage 1 low-renin hypertension.

30. **Explain the mechanism of hypertension in patients with 17α-hydroxylase deficiency.**
As in patients with 11β-hydroxylase deficiency, hypertension is the result of volume expansion mediated by increased levels of DOC. Serum levels of DOC do not correlate entirely with the degree of hypertension, again suggesting that other factors may be involved.

31. **How is CAH diagnosed?**
Patients with various forms of CAH are diagnosed by their clinical features and plasma and urine steroid profiles. In general, the corticotropin stimulation test results in marked elevation of precursor steroids proximal to the deficient enzyme. Neonatal screening for 21-hydroxylase deficiency is available in nearly 20 states in the United States and in many countries worldwide. There is currently no screening program for the hypertensive forms of CAH because of the low incidence of these disorders. Chorionic villus sampling and amniocentesis may be useful in prenatal diagnosis of all forms of CAH in high-risk families.

32. **In which patients with hypertension should CAH be considered in the differential diagnosis?**
All patients with hypertension with the following:
   - Hypokalemic metabolic alkalosis
   - Abnormal external genitalia (virilized female, incompletely virilized male, or infantile female)
   - History of infertility.

33. **Discuss the treatment for CAH.**
In general, CAH is treated with long-term administration of hydrocortisone at a dose of 10 to 15 mg/m^2/day. This provides negative feedback to the pituitary, which decreases corticotropin release, and corrects excessive mineralocorticoid and sex-steroid synthesis. In salt-wasting forms of CAH, such as 21-hydroxylase deficiency, administration of fludrocortisone and sodium chloride is usually necessary. Virilized females with 11β-hydroxylase deficiency require surgical correction of the external genitalia. Sex steroids are necessary in patients with hypogonadotropic hypogonadism, such as in 17α-hydroxylase deficiency. Maternal treatment with dexamethasone during pregnancy has been successful in preventing abnormal fetal genital development. On the horizon is gene therapy, which works in adrenocortical cell lines and animal models.

34. **Which antihypertensive agents are most often used for patients with hypertension and CAH?**
Potassium-sparing diuretics (spironolactone, possibly eplerenone, or amiloride) and calcium antagonists are used most often.

35. **Which antihypertensive agents should be avoided?**
Because renin is suppressed, angiotensin-converting enzyme inhibitors, direct renin inhibitors, and angiotensin receptor blockers are unlikely to be effective. Thiazide diuretics should be avoided because of the increased risk of hypokalemia.

PHEOCHROMOCYTOMA

36. **What is pheochromocytoma?**
Pheochromocytoma is a catecholamine-producing tumor arising from the chromaffin cells of the sympathetic nervous system derived embryonically from the primitive neural crest cells; they are so named because they stain brown with chromium salts. Most pheochromocytomas are found in the adrenal gland; the second most common site is the organ of Zuckerkandl (ganglia at the bifurcation of the aorta), although paraganglionomas (which have very similar presenting features, evaluation, and treatment) can arise anywhere along the parasympathetic chain.

37. **What is the incidence of pheochromocytoma?**
In population-based studies in Denmark, Sweden, Spain, Australia, and Rochester, Minnesota, the annual incidence is about 1.5 to 2.1 cases per million population.

38. **What catecholamines are produced by pheochromocytoma?**
Most pheochromocytomas secrete primarily norepinephrine. Epinephrine-secreting tumors are more commonly malignant or extra-adrenal in location. Very rarely, a tumor is deficient in dopamine beta-hydroxylase; this causes secretion of large amounts of dopamine. Pheochromocytomas also store and secrete many peptides: endogenous opioids, endothelin, erythropoietin, parathyroid hormone–related protein, neuropeptide-Y, and chromogranin-A; the latter has been used as a diagnostic marker.

39. **What are the clinical manifestations of pheochromocytoma?**
The most common finding is hypertension, which occurs in more than 90% of patients and which is paroxysmal in 25% to 33% of cases. This is often accompanied (especially in paroxysmal hypertension) by other signs and symptoms of catecholamine excess: tachycardia, headache, tremor, sweating, and pupillary dilatation. Orthostatic hypotension may occur from decreased sympathetic reflexes, after downregulation of adrenergic receptors. Weight loss may result from chronic hypermetabolism. Hyperglycemia may occur as a consequence of the inhibitory effects of catecholamines on pancreatic beta cells.

40. **What are the five H's associated with pheochromocytoma?**
This mnemonic derives from five of the following clinical manifestations:

- **H**ypertension
- **H**eadache
- **H**yperhidrosis
- **H**yperglycemia
- **H**ypermetabolism

A large French series suggested that the three on the left are present in 95% of cases diagnosed in that country.

41. **What is the "rule of ten (percent)"?**
Classically, each of the following accounts for about 10% of all pheochromocytomas:

- Bilateral (in **both** adrenal glands)
- Extra-adrenal
- Malignant
- Familial (associated with multiple endocrine neoplasia [MEN] syndromes)
- Pediatric

In reality, few large series show the expected 10% incidence; recent data suggest that about 20% of pheochromocytomas are heredofamilial (see next question).

42. **What conditions are associated with pheochromocytoma?**
    - von Recklinghausen's disease (neurofibromatosis)
    - Tuberous sclerosis (de Bourneville's or Pringle's disease)
    - Sturge-Weber syndrome
    - von Hippel-Lindau disease
    - Ataxia telangiectasia
    - MEN syndromes:
      - MEN type 2 (or 2a): pheochromocytoma (usually bilateral, but seldom synchronous), parathyroid adenoma, medullary thyroid carcinoma (which is typically diagnosed first)
      - MEN type 3 (or 2b): pheochromocytoma, medullary carcinoma of thyroid, mucosal neuromas, abdominal gangliomas, Marfanoid body habitus (the prevalence of this syndrome is only about 5% of that of MEN 2 or 2a)
    - Familial paraganglionoma (typically associated with mutations in the succinate dehydrogenase gene)

43. **What are some clinical clues to the diagnosis of pheochromocytoma?**
    - Sustained or paroxysmal hypertension associated with triad of headache, palpitations, and diaphoresis
    - Hypertension and family history of pheochromocytoma
    - Refractory hypertension especially if associated with weight loss
    - Sinus tachycardia
    - Orthostatic hypotension
    - Recurrent cardiac dysrhythmias
    - Features of MEN type 2 (or 2a) or 3 (or 2b)
    - Hypertensive crises during surgery or anesthesia (typically during induction)
    - Pressor response to a beta-blocker
    - Incidentally discovered adrenal mass

44. **What are the most common causes of death of patients with pheochromocytoma?**
    - Myocardial infarction
    - Malignant cardiac dysrhythmias
    - Cerebrovascular accident
    - Renal failure
    - Dissecting aortic aneurysm

45. **Elaborate on the biochemical screening for pheochromocytoma.**
    Plasma metanephrines have the highest sensitivity (~96%), but a low specificity (~85%), so this test is most appropriate for patients at very high risk (e.g., those with family histories or strong histories and a positive scan). A 24-hour urine collection for fractionated metanephrines can be recommended for patients at low risk; vanillylmandelic acid (false-positive rate in patients at low risk ~15%) and total catecholamines can be added for those at higher risk. Collecting a 24-hour urine after a "spell" can increase the sensitivity of urinary tests. Biochemical assays are now much more sophisticated than in decades past; it is no longer necessary to consume a special diet before and during the collection.

46. **What are the potential sources of error in chemical screening tests?**
    Plasma levels of catecholamines and metabolites may be falsely elevated with any type of stress. In patients with paroxysmal hypertension, urinary concentration of catecholamines and their metabolites may be normal if the 24-hour urine is collected when the patient is normotensive and asymptomatic. Common drugs that affect catecholamine and metabolite levels are listed in Table 65-1.

TABLE 65-1. COMMON DRUGS THAT AFFECT CATECHOLAMINE AND METABOLITE LEVELS

Increase	Decrease
Tricyclic antidepressants	Metyrosine
Amphetamine(s)	Methylglucamine
Beta-blockers (labetalol, sotalol)	Reserpine
Benzodiazepines	
L-dopa, methyldopa	
Ethanol	
Withdrawal from clonidine and other alpha-agonists	

47. **What tests should be performed in equivocal cases?**
    A number of pharmacologic tests can be performed but are usually not necessary (Table 65-2).

48. **What studies are used to localize a pheochromocytoma?**
    Imaging studies are generally indicated only after biochemical screening is positive. Using a scan as a screening test increases the risk of discovering an "incidentaloma" (i.e., a nonfunctioning tumor). CT scan or MRI of the abdomen are about 95% sensitive and 65% specific; the T2-weighted MRI has a higher specificity because chromaffin tumors usually "light up." ^{123}I-metaiodobenzylguanidine (MIBG) scintigraphy is about 80% sensitive and 99% specific for chromaffin tissue; it is usually used for large (>10 cm) tumors or to evaluate extra-adrenal tumors. When imaging studies are equivocal, somatostatin receptor imaging, positron emission scanning, or even selective venous sampling of the vena cava at various levels can sometimes help locate the tumor.

TABLE 65-2. TESTS FOR PHEOCHROMOCYTOMA

Test	Rationale
Regitine® (phentolamine) test	Phentolamine is an alpha-blocker, and a reduction in blood pressure after its intravenous administration suggests a catecholamine excess. The test is neither sensitive nor specific.
Histamine test	This old test is seldom performed today because it is neither sensitive nor specific and can be dangerous.
Glucagon stimulation test	Glucagon stimulates catecholamine release and raises blood pressure and pulse rate in a patient with a pheochromocytoma. The risk of precipitating a hypertensive crisis can be blocked by prior administration of an alpha-adrenoceptor antagonist.
Clonidine suppression test	Clonidine decreases central sympathetic outflow in normal or nervous subjects but does not suppress autonomous catecholamine production by a tumor. Failure to suppress plasma norepinephrine by more than 50%, and into the normal range, within 2–3 hours after administration of an appropriate dose (0.2–0.3 mg) of clonidine is highly suggestive of a pheochromocytoma.

49. **What is the treatment of choice for pheochromocytoma?**
Surgical removal of the tumor is the treatment of choice and is curative in >90% of cases. Small, single tumors are now most often removed laparoscopically, but large tumors usually require the traditional midline incision, careful inspection of the paravertebral ganglionic chain, and longer recuperation. Medical therapy is used mainly for perioperative management. Chronic medical therapy in the form of α- and (sometimes) β-blockade or inhibition of catecholamine synthesis with α-methyl-paratyrosine can be used for patients with inoperable, recurrent, multicentric, or malignant pheochromocytoma.

50. **Describe perioperative management.**
The goal of preoperative medical therapy is to control blood pressure (for 1 to 4 weeks prior to surgery) and to block the cardiovascular consequences of increased catecholamine levels. Alpha-blockers should be given first; phenoxybenzamine, a long-acting, oral, noncompetitive alpha-blocker, is preferred. The more selective, competitive, postsynaptic alpha$_1$-blockers (prazosin, terazosin, doxazosin) have a shorter duration of action and provide incomplete α-blockade, so failures have been described. When tachycardia or cardiac dysrhythmias persist, a β-adrenergic blocker may be given, but only *after* achieving α-blockade so as to avoid unopposed α-receptor stimulation and further vasoconstriction.

51. **What clinical parameters should be monitored in the postoperative period?**
- Persistent hypertension reflects:
  - Fluid overload
  - Return of autonomic reflexes
  - Inadvertent ligation of renal artery
  - Presence of residual tumor
- Persistent hypotension often reflects:
  - Blood loss
  - Altered vascular compliance
  - Residual effect of preoperative α-blockade
  - Downregulation of adrenoceptors (left over from chronic stimulation preoperatively)
- Hypoglycemia
  - Removal of inhibitory effect of catecholamines on pancreatic beta cells
  - Increased sensitivity of the beta cells to glucose level after tumor removal
  - Cessation of enflurane anesthesia, which leads to reflexive increase in insulin
- Assess risk for familial syndromes and possible genetic testing
  - Serum calcium, calcitonin, and intact parathyroid hormone
  - Ophthalmologist examination for retinal angiomas; consider head CT for cerebellar hemangioblastomas
  - Consider mutation analysis for the *ret* proto-oncogene for familial and other high-risk cases
- Assess risk for residual tumor
  - A screening test that was positive preoperatively should be repeated 1 to 2 weeks after surgery and annually thereafter

52. **What about treatment for malignant pheochromocytoma?**
Malignant pheochromocytoma accounts for less than 10% of all pheochromocytomas. These are usually slow growing and are poorly responsive to radiotherapy or chemotherapy. Surgical debulking is occasionally necessary to decrease catecholamine synthesis. High-dose radioactive MIBG has been used with some success to ablate primary and metastatic sites. Alpha-methyl-tyrosine has been tried in inoperable cases.

KEY POINTS: ENDOCRINE HYPERTENSION

1. Hyperaldosteronism can be either primary (e.g., Conn's adenoma, bilateral adrenal hyperplasia) or secondary (renovascular hypertension, sleep apnea); these are best distinguished by a plasma aldosterone/renin ratio, although the test results in many false positives for primary hyperaldosteronism.

2. Although exogenous administration of corticosteroids is the most common cause of Cushing's syndrome, a basophilic adenoma of the pituitary gland (Cushing's disease) is the most common noniatrogenic cause. It is classically diagnosed by a nonsuppressing low-dose dexamethasone suppression test but by a suppressing high-dose test.

3. Although many treatments for Cushing's syndrome exist, their success largely depends on accurate identification of overproduced hormone and its source; transsphenoidal removal of the pituitary adenoma is still the preferred procedure, as it was in Cushing's time.

4. Congenital adrenal hyperplasia is rarely seen in adults because pediatricians are so efficient at recognizing affected babies and children. For most, low-dose glucocorticoid (and occasional mineralocorticoid) therapy provides effective long-term treatment.

5. Although very rare, patients with pheochromocytoma typically present with hypertension, headaches, and hyperhidrosis. Patients can be diagnosed with either urinary or plasma catecholamine and/or metabolites, pretreated before surgery with alpha-blockers (and occasional beta-blockade), and often cured with surgery. Patients with features of heredofamilial syndromes should have other family members screened for these diseases.

---

53. **What is the prognosis of pheochromocytoma?**
    - 5-year survival:
        - 95% in nonmalignant pheochromocytoma
        - <50% in malignant pheochromocytoma
    - Recurrence rate after surgery is <10% in nonmalignant pheochromocytoma.
    - Successful resection cures hypertension in approximately 75% of affected patients. In the remaining 25%, hypertension persists but is usually much easier to control with standard antihypertensive agents.

BIBLIOGRAPHY

Hyperaldosteronism

1. Calhoun DA, Nishizaka MK, Zaman MA, et al. High prevalence of primary hyperaldosteronism among black and white subjects with resistant hypertension. *Hypertension* 2002;40:892–896.

2. Dluhy RG, Lifton RP. Glucocorticoid-remediable aldosteronism. *J Clin Endo Metab* 1999;84:4341–4344.

3. Funder JW, Carey RM, Fardella C, et al. Case detection, diagnosis, and treatment of patients with primary aldosteronism: An Endocrine Society Clinical Practice Guideline. *J Clin Endo Metab* 2008;93:3266–3281.

4. Lim PO, Young WF, MacDonald TM. A review of the medical treatment of primary hyperaldosteronism. *J Hypertens* 2001;19:353–361.

5. Netzer NC, Stoohs RA, Netzer CM, et al. Using the Berlin questionnaire to identify patients at high risk for the sleep apnea syndrome. *Ann Intern Med* 2009;131:485–491.

6. Rossi GP, Bernini G, Caliumi C, et al. A prospective study of the prevalence of primary hyperaldosteronism in 1125 hypertensive patients. *J Am Coll Cardiol* 2006;48:2293–2300.

7. Rossi GP, Belfiore A, Bernini G, et al. Comparison of the captopril and the saline infusion test for excluding aldosterone-producing adenoma. *Hypertension* 2007;50:424–431.

8. Sawka AM, Young WF, Thompson GB, et al. Primary hyperaldosteronism: Factors associated with normalization of blood pressure after surgery. *Ann Intern Med* 2001;135:258–261.

9. Stewart PM. Mineralocorticoid hypertension. *Lancet* 1999;353:1341–1347.

10. Young WF Jr. Mini review: Primary hyperaldosteronism—Changing concepts in diagnosis and treatment. *Endocrinology* 2003;144:2208–2213.

Cushing's Syndrome and Congenital Adrenal Hyperplasia

1. Arnaldi G, Angeli A, Atkinson AB, et al. Diagnosis and complications of Cushing's syndrome: A consensus statement. *J Clin Endo Metab* 2003;88:5593–5602.

2. Boscaro M, Arnaldi G. Approach to the patient with possible Cushing's syndrome. *J Clin Endo Metab* 2009;94:3121–3131.

3. Boscaro M, Barzon L, Fallo F, et al. Cushing's syndrome. *Lancet* 2001;357:783–791.

4. Findling JW, Raff H. Cushing's syndrome: Important issues in diagnosis and management. *J Clin Endo Metab* 2006;91:3746–3753.

5. Merke DP, Bornstein SR, Avila NA, et al. NIH conference: Future directions in the study and management of congenital adrenal hyperplasia due to 21-hydroxylase deficiency. *Ann Intern Med* 2002;136:320–334.

6. Newell-Price J, Bertagna X, Grossman AR, et al. Cushing's syndrome. *Lancet* 2006;367:1605–1617.

7. Speiser PW, White PC. Congenital adrenal hyperplasia. *N Engl J Med* 2003;349:776–788.

Pheochromocytoma

1. Lenders JW, Eisenhofer G, Mannelli M, et al. Phaeochromocytoma. *Lancet* 2005;366:665–675.

2. Manger WM. The protean manifestations of pheochromocytoma. *Horm Metab Res* 2009;41:658–663.

3. Pacak K, Eisenhofer G, Ahlman H, et al. Pheochromocytoma: Recommendations for clinical practice from the First International Symposium, October 2005. *Nat Clin Pract Endocrinol Metab* 2007;3:92–102.

4. Petri BJ, van Eijck CH, de Herder WW, et al. Phaeochromocytomas and sympathetic paragangliomas. *Br J Surg* 2009;96:1381–1392.

5. Qin Y, Buddavarapu K, Dahia PL. Pheochromocytoma: From genetic diversity to new paradigms. *Horm Metab Res* 2009;41:665–671.

6. Reisch N, Peczkowska M, Januszewicz A, et al. Pheochromocytoma: presentation, diagnosis and treatment. *J Hypertens* 2006;24:2331–2339.

7. Young WF Jr. Adrenal causes of hypertension: pheochromocytoma and primary aldosteronism. *Rev Endocr Metab Disord* 2007;8:309–320.

8. Young WF Jr. The incidentally discovered adrenal mass. *N Engl J Med* 2007;356:601–610.

CHAPTER 66

OTHER FORMS OF SECONDARY HYPERTENSION

William J. Elliott, MD, PhD

1. **Besides renovascular and the traditional endocrine causes of hypertension, what are eight uncommon, but important, causes of secondary hypertension?**
   - Obstructive sleep apnea (typically causing hyperaldosteronism)
   - Drug-induced hypertension (especially nonsteroidal anti-inflammatory drugs, steroids, and/ or other immunosuppressants)
   - Thyroid disorders (hypothyroidism more commonly than hyperthyroidism)
   - Coarctation of the aorta (typically manifested as different blood pressures in the arms or a lower blood pressure in the legs)
   - Hyperparathyroidism (only 10% to 60% of patients with primary hyperparathyroidism have hypertension at diagnosis, and removal of the parathyroid adenoma does not always lower blood pressure)
   - Acromegaly (18% to 60% of patients with acromegaly have hypertension, many have left ventricular hypertrophy, most respond well to antihypertensive drugs, and some have blood pressures that revert to normal when the acromegaly is cured)
   - "Neurogenic" hypertension
   - Liddle's syndrome (a rare genetic disorder that is also called pseudohyperaldosteronism)

2. **What is the usual sequence of diagnostic and therapeutic steps for patients with sleep apnea?**
   Most such patients are overweight or obese, and many have bed partners who note snoring and/or witness apneic episodes during sleep. The Berlin questionnaire is a useful screening tool, but a polysomnographic sleep study is typically required for diagnosis. Cohort studies have shown a significant improvement in survival if continuous positive airway pressure (CPAP) is used during sleep. Blood pressure can typically be reduced impressively with spironolactone or eplerenone; some authorities recommend a serum aldosterone/renin ratio before starting such treatment

3. **What are the most common drug-induced causes of hypertension?**
   On a population basis, the nonsteroidal anti-inflammatory drugs (including agents that are more selective for the second isoform of cyclooxygenase, e.g., celecoxib) are probably the most common just because their use is so widespread. The mechanism of the process is not well worked out, although some alteration in intrarenal prostaglandin metabolism, sodium retention, and edema formation is very likely.

   Anabolic steroids, glucocorticoids, and mineralocorticoids all raise blood pressure, and the usual recommendation is to use the lowest possible dose for the shortest possible time to decrease the risk of long-term consequences (including hypertension and its sequelae).

   Patients with chronic kidney disease or transplant recipients often take other drugs that raise blood pressure; the most common are cyclosporine, erythropoietin, and tacrolimus. Unlike the situation with most drug-induced hypertension, the antihypertensive drug regimen is usually intensified when these drugs raise blood pressure.

   Many "street" drugs can raise blood pressure acutely, as does acute withdrawal from nicotine, heroin, or other opioids. The drugs most often causing hypertension in an

Emergency Department setting are cocaine, methylphenidate (and its congeners, including ephedra, Ma Hwang, and other stimulants), gamma-hydroxybutyrate, and even ketamine and ergotamine. Chronic ingestion of large quantities of alcohol is associated epidemiologically with an increased risk of hypertension; the clinical trial that was designed to show that moderation of alcohol intake reduced blood pressure did not show a significant difference, probably because those assigned to the "control" group also moderated their intake of alcohol when they realized how much they were ingesting.

A large variety of other prescription drugs (e.g., phenylpropanolamines, oral contraceptive pills, venlafaxine) can raise blood pressure. A wide variety of other drugs can interfere with antihypertensive medications either directly or via inhibition of metabolic pathways (typically hepatic cytochrome P_{450} or CYP oxidoreductases).

4. **What are the "usual and customary" antihypertensive treatment strategies for patients who have drug-induced hypertension?**
   See Table 66-1.

5. **What are three primary diseases of the thyroid that can affect blood pressure?**
   - **Hypothyroidism** is the most common thyroid disease that is associated with hypertension (3% of newly diagnosed hypertensives in a classic series from upstate New York), although the mechanism is unclear. After appropriate thyroid replacement, blood pressure typically falls without specific antihypertensive therapy. Because hypothyroidism is a rare cause of secondary hypertension, a serum ultrasensitive thyroid-stimulating hormone is not generally recommended as an initial test for all patients newly diagnosed with hypertension (although other historical and physical findings might justify it).
   - **Hyperthyroidism** typically presents in younger patients with tachycardia, hypertension, a wide pulse pressure, and other traditional signs, but older people sometimes lack one or more of these typical features. The now-standard initial test is a serum ultrasensitive thyroid-stimulating hormone level. Therapy is usually propranolol, which treats the hypertension, tachycardia, and (at least according to traditional pharmacologic teachings, now under assault) inhibits the peripheral conversion of thyroxine (T_4) to triiodothyronine (T_3).
   - **Medullary carcinoma** of the thyroid is not itself a cause of hypertension, but it is often associated with pheochromocytoma in patients with multiple endocrine neoplasias (MEN) of either type 2a (Sipple's syndrome, which includes parathyroid tumors or adenomas in

TABLE 66-1. ANTIHYPERTENSIVE TREATMENTS FOR DRUG-INDUCED HYPERTENSION	
Drug Inducing Hypertension	**Antihypertensive Drug Treatment(s)**
Corticosteroids, mineralocorticoids	Diuretic, angiotensin-converting enzyme inhibitor
Nonsteroidal anti-inflammatory drug	Diuretic, calcium antagonist, maybe alpha-1-blocker
Phenylpropanolamine(s)	Beta-blocker
Nasal decongestant(s)	Alpha-1-blocker or alpha-beta-blocker
Cocaine	Alpha-blocker (typically phentolamine)
Antidepressants (monoamine oxidase inhibitors, serotonin reuptake inhibitors, etc.)	Alpha-blocker, calcium antagonist (?)
Oral contraceptive pills	None; stop oral contraceptive pills instead

about 50% of afflicted patients) or type 2b (which includes submucosal neuromas, hyperplastic nerves, and Marfanoid habitus with a high, arched palate and adrenomedullary disease in about 33%). About 95% of patients with MEN 2b have a single point ("gain of function") mutation (methionine to threonine) in the "rearranged during transfection" (now commonly abbreviated as RET) proto-oncogene allele in the tyrosine kinase domain within chromosome 10q11.2; about half are spontaneous mutations, but older fathers are more commonly implicated as the source.

6. **What is the usual anatomy of coarctation of the aorta, its typical signs, and diagnostic evaluation scheme?**
   Although the congenital localized narrowing of the aorta may occur anywhere between the aortic valve and the abdominal aorta, most occur in adults near or at the location of the former ductus arteriosus (ligamentum arteriosum after regression). It is the fourth leading cause of congenital heart disease, but it is an uncommon cause of hypertension in children and even less common in adults. Physical examination nearly always shows a lower blood pressure in the leg (measured supine, with a cuff over the thigh and auscultating in the popliteal fossa), radial-femoral delay, and diminished pulses in the lower extremities. Continuous cardiac murmurs are common in chronic untreated coarctation as a result of development of collateral blood flow around the narrowing. The classic chest x-ray findings include rib notching (from dilated intercostal arteries on the inferior surfaces of ribs), and the "3 sign" (consisting of a dilated proximal aorta, the coarctation, and the poststenotic dilatation). An esophagram (obtained after swallowing barium) often shows the "reverse 3" sign. The most useful diagnostic test for patients suspected of having a coarctation is an echocardiogram; some centers prefer magnetic resonance angiograms, although some surgeons still require traditional aortography and a full cardiac catheterization in adults to prove the absence of major coronary heart disease and/or other associated congenital anomalies.

7. **What are the recommended treatment options for patients with coarctation of the aorta and their effects on hypertension and mortality?**
   Multiple surgical procedures have been used, including resection of the involved aortic segment with end-to-end reanastomosis, grafting of an overlying aortic flap, and/or placement of a synthetic graft. More recently, balloon angioplasty has been successful in many infants and children, but the procedure can be technically challenging in adolescents and adults. If left untreated, about 50% of patients with coarctation die by age 30; the 30-year survival improves to 93% if successfully repaired before age 5 years. Hypertension is "cured" in about 50% of children who have successful repairs of coarctation. When the coarctation is discovered in an adult, the life expectancy is reduced, primarily because the hypertension is more difficult to control (and often does not disappear after repair), and more target organ damage has already occurred.

8. **What is the relationship between hypertension and hyperparathyroidism?**
   Hypertension occurs in about 10% to 60% of patients with primary hyperparathyroidism; "cure" of hypertension is unpredictable after resection of the usual parathyroid adenoma that caused the hypercalcemia. Oddly enough, other chronic conditions that produce similar levels of hypercalcemia (e.g., sarcoidosis, myeloma, or other malignancies) are not associated with an increased risk of hypertension. This has led to increased attention to serum parathyroid hypertensive factor, which can now be detected in laboratory assays but is not routinely measured in most clinical laboratories.

9. **What is the relationship between hypertension and acromegaly?**
   Although human growth hormone and insulin-like growth factor-1 (somatomedin C) may increase blood pressure a little, most authorities attribute the higher-than-expected prevalence of hypertension in patients with acromegaly to their hypertrophied hearts and

vascular systems. Octreotide and other antagonists of growth hormone have little antihypertensive effect, but long-term antihypertensive treatment for people with acromegaly probably improves their prognosis because most of them die of premature cardiovascular disease.

10. **What is neurogenic hypertension? What are the most common forms?**
Any pathologic process that acutely increases intracranial pressure can cause hypertension and bradycardia (so-called Cushing's reflex). Thus, acute stroke, intracranial tumors, or severe head injury (and occasional patients with quadriplegia and other spinal cord pathology) is often associated with hypertension and worsened blood pressures in those with a prior history of the condition. In most cases, addressing the primary neurologic problem lowers blood pressure, often in as little as 24 hours. The question of whether neurovascular compression of the left ventrolateral medulla can raise blood pressure (presumably by excessive sympathetic nervous system stimulation) has been debated for 25 years.

11. **What is the genetic defect in Liddle's syndrome, and how are such patients treated?**
This autosomal-dominant disorder is caused by hyperactivity of the epithelial sodium channel (ENaC) of the principal cell of the cortical collecting tubule. Most afflicted patients have mutations in genes coding the beta or gamma subunits of the ENaC on chromosome 16p, which result in deletions of proline-rich regions that bind Nedd4 (a regulatory reprocessor that promotes channel degradation). The kidney thus increases its rate of sodium reabsorption, volume expansion, and blood pressure. The clinical presentation is distinguished from hyperaldosteronism by the low serum aldosterone, but hypokalemia, metabolic acidosis, and hypertension are present in both. Treatment with amiloride or triamterene blocks the constituently active ENaC in the collecting tubule, corrects the hypokalemia, and lowers blood pressure. Spironolactone or eplerenone is ineffective because aldosterone is not primarily involved in the pathogenesis of Liddle's syndrome.

KEY POINTS: OTHER SECONDARY CAUSES OF HYPERTENSION

1. Obstructive sleep apnea is becoming a more widely recognized cause of hypertension because we now have methods for efficient screening (with the Berlin questionnaire), diagnosis (with overnight polysomnographic testing, often in the home), and treatment (typically involving aldosterone antagonists), in addition to continuous positive airway pressure during sleep.

2. The most common cause of drug-induced hypertension is the (often self-) administration of nonsteroidal anti-inflammatory drugs; steroids, cyclosporine, erythropoietin, and tacrolimus are taken by fewer patients, but more antihypertensive drugs are usually prescribed when the patient taking these drugs experiences elevated blood pressures.

3. Hypothyroidism is a more common cause of hypertension than hyperthyroidism, but routine testing of serum thyroid stimulating hormone is not warranted at diagnosis for all patients with hypertension.

4. Coarctation of the aorta should be suspected if there is a lower blood pressure in an arm or a leg compared to the other arm; an echocardiogram can confirm the diagnosis in most cases, and endoluminal therapies are available (and are especially useful in younger children).

5. The many single-gene mutations associated with hypertension have taught us a great deal but account for a very tiny fraction of the prevalence of hypertension.

BIBLIOGRAPHY

1. Bondanelli M, Ambrosio MR, degli Uberti EC. Pathogenesis and prevalence of hypertension in acromegaly. *Pituitary* 2001;4:239–249.

2. Calhoun DA, Jones D, Textor S, et al. Resistant hypertension: Diagnosis, evaluation, and treatment: a scientific statement from the American Heart Association Professional Education Committee of the Council for High Blood Pressure Research. *Hypertension* 2008;51:1403–1419.

3. Chan CC, Reid CM, Aw TJ, et al. Do COX-2 inhibitors raise blood pressure more than nonselective NSAIDs and placebo? An updated meta-analysis. *J Hypertens* 2009;27:2332–2341.

4. Danzi S, Klein I. Thyroid hormone and blood pressure regulation. *Curr Hypertens Rep* 2003;5:513–520.

5. Elliott WJ. Drug interactions and drugs affecting blood pressure. *J Clin Hypertens* (Greenwich) 2006;8:731–736.

6. Gus M, Goncalves SC, Martinez D. Risk for obstructive sleep apnea by Berlin questionnaire, but not daytime sleepiness, is associated with resistant hypertension: A case-control study. *Am J Hypertens* 2008;21:832–835.

7. Landau D. Potassium-related inherited tubulopathies. *Cell Mol Life Sci* 2006;63:1962–1968.

8. Marin JM, Carrizo SJ, Vicente E, et al. Long-term cardiovascular outcomes in men with obstructive sleep apnea-hypopnea with or without treatment with continuous positive airway pressure: An observational study. *Lancet* 2005;365:1046–1053.

9. Schlaich MP, Lambert E, Kaye DM, et al. Sympathetic augmentation in hypertension: Role of nerve firing, norepinephrine reuptake, and angiotensin neuromodulation. *Hypertension* 2004;43:169–175.

10. Tanous D, Benson LN, Horlick EM. Coarctation of the aorta: Evaluation and management. *Curr Opin Cardiol* 2009;24:509–515.

WHITE-COAT HYPERTENSION

Madhav V. Rao, MD, and Vijaykumar M. Rao, MD

CHAPTER 67

1. **What is the definition of white-coat hypertension? masked hypertension?**
   By definition, white-coat hypertension (WCH) is defined as continued elevation in blood pressure measurements in a medical setting. It is thought to be a conditioned response resulting from a pressor response incited by the clinical setting. Specifically, office blood pressure readings higher than 140/90 and blood pressure measurements out of office less than 135/85 are consistent with WCH.

   Masked hypertension (MH) is defined as a clinical condition in which a patient's office blood pressure level is < 140/90 but ambulatory or home BP readings are in the hypertensive range.

2. **What is the estimated prevalence of WCH?**
   Whereas the white coat phenomenon has been extensively investigated in patients with essential hypertension and the general population, only a few studies have involved those with chronic kidney disease. In this population, the estimated prevalence of WCH is around 25%.

   In children, there is an estimated prevalence of 10% to 60%, but that depends on the method of diagnosis. As in adults, WCH is more common in children with mild elevation of office blood pressure measurements.

3. **What are the approaches to diagnosing WCH versus sustained hypertension?**
   Utilization of ambulatory blood pressure monitoring is considered the gold standard to distinguish WCH from persistent hypertension. However, using ambulatory blood pressure monitoring for all suspected cases of WCH is cost prohibitive. Alternatively, frequent home blood pressure recordings can be a viable option to ambulatory monitoring.

   Elevated home and ambulatory blood pressure measurements are considered to be better predictors of target-organ damage such as left ventricular hypertrophy or the onset of chronic kidney disease.

4. **When using ambulatory blood pressure monitoring, what is the definition of hypertension?**
   Depending how long the blood pressure measurements are recorded, the definition of hypertension is 135/85 mm Hg over 24 hours, 140/90 mm Hg if only taken during the daytime, or higher than 125/75 mm Hg if only measured while asleep.

   Blood pressure measurements are usually done over 24 to 48 hours. During the daytime the device usually takes a measurement every 15 to 20 minutes and, while asleep, every 30 to 60 minutes.

5. **What is the chance of WCH progressing to sustained hypertension?**
   Investigators in Europe found that patients with early signs of hypertension with no other medical history who would otherwise not be treated showed that carotid intimal medial thickness is greater and grows faster than in normotensive subjects. This pattern does indicate an increased risk of cardiovascular disease and as a result supports tight control

of blood pressure. The European Society of Cardiology/European Society of Hypertension also supports this premise.

Interestingly, when compared to normotensives, plasma homocysteine levels were significantly higher and left ventricular mass index was significantly greater in those with WCH.

6. **Do patients with WCH develop target organ damage?**
Studies investigating whether WCH patients develop cardiovascular target organ damage have been contradictory to say the very least. Ihm et al. demonstrated a significant association between the biochemical markers of myocardial fibrosis (TGF-B1 and procollagen type I propeptide, PIP) and indices of LV dysfunction (LVH, diastolic dysfunction).

The postulated possible mechanisms for the increase risk of cardiovascular complications in WCH include: elevated sympathetic nervous system activity, insulin resistance, and oxidative stress or enodothelial dysfunction.

Even in children with WCH, the left ventricular mass index was demonstrated to be intermediate between that of normotensives and sustained hypertensives.

7. **Once diagnosed, should WCH be treated?**
In a recent 10-year study of 3200 Italian subjects, patients who initially were diagnosed with WCH had a 2.51 odds ratio (1.79–3.54, $p < 0.0001$) of developing sustained hypertension. This implied that WCH could pose a greater risk for the development of sustained hypertension, independent of blood pressure readings at baseline.

Although several studies have reported a possible increase in the risk of future cardiovascular events, e.g., strokes, in subjects with WCH, there remains a current lack of consensus as to how to prevent such events.

At present, treatment of WCH in general remains controversial, and some authors suggest that it may produce excessive lowering of ABP. In the INVEST Study (International Verapamil SR-trandolapril Study), it was demonstrated that lowering DBP < 83 mmHg was associated with excess mortality and coronary events. Whereas it is counterintuitive to withhold therapy that markedly reduces the risk of cardiovascular morbidity and mortality, one has to recognize that "to completely withhold therapy in patients with WCH" is still highly debatable. A randomized controlled trial is needed whereby patients with WCH are randomly assigned to have their blood pressure treated on the basis of office versus ambulatory blood pressure readings. In the opinion of the authors, the prudent course is to approach the patient individually on a case by case basis.

8. **What is the significance of masked hypertension?**
Compared to WCH, masked hypertension is associated with greater chance of sustained hypertension and cardiovascular disease. Similarly, both WCH and masked hypertension should not be regarded as innocent phenomena but as clinical states that require accurate diagnosis and follow up.

9. **What is the formal definition and risks associated with "nondipping" blood pressure?**
Nondipping of the blood pressure is a blunting of the normal drop in blood pressure at night-time. Usually systolic and diastolic blood pressure decrease by 10%. The development of nondipping of blood pressure is associated with an increased risk of left ventricular hypertrophy, progression of chronic kidney disease, cerebrovascular disease, decrease in cognitive function and increase in fatal and nonfatal vascular events. In addition, in patients with diabetes with and without concomitant hypertension, nocturnal nondipping was associated with increased risk of urinary albumin. In a recent study of 100 people with type 2 diabetes who underwent ambulatory blood pressure monitoring, the prevalence of albuminuria was two times higher in the nondipping group.

10. **What is pseudohypertension?**

Pseudohypertension is a sporadic elevation in blood pressure as a result of excessive sclerosis of large blood vessels. It is more common in the elderly because the compliance of the arteries decreases. A method to distinguish between pseudohypertension and true hypertension is to use a diagnostic tool called Osler's maneuver. Osler's maneuver calls for inflating the blood pressure cuff while palpating the radial or brachial artery. When either vessels becomes palpable, then the patient is deemed "Osler's positive," but if either collapses that is "Osler's negative" and not in line with pseudohypertension.

KEY POINTS: WHITE-COAT HYPERTENSION

1. White-coat hypertension (WCH) is defined as continued elevation in blood pressure measurements believed to be a conditioned response resulting from a pressor response incited by the clinical setting.

2. In patients with chronic kidney disease, the estimated prevalence of WCH is around 25%.

3. Utilization of ambulatory blood pressure monitoring is considered the gold standard to distinguish WCH from persistent hypertension.

4. The development of nondipping of blood pressure is associated with an increased risk of left ventricular hypertrophy, progression of chronic kidney disease, cerebrovascular disease, decrease in cognitive function and increase in fatal and nonfatal vascular events.

BIBLIOGRAPHY

Agarwal R. Home and ambulatory blood pressure monitoring in chronic kidney disease. *Curr Opin Nephrol Hypertens* 2009;18:507–512.

Andersen MJ, Khawandi W, Agarwal R. Home blood pressure monitoring in chronic kidney disease. Am J Kidney Dis 2005;45:994–1001.

Ihm S-H, Youn H-J, Park C-S, et al. Target organ status in white coat hypertensives—usefulness of serum procollagen type I propeptide in the respect of left ventricular dysfunction. *Circulation* 2009;73:100–105.

Kaplan NM. Ambulatory blood pressure monitoring and white coat hypertension in adults. Uptodate 2009.

Mancia G, De Backer G, Dominiczak G, et al. 2007 ESH-ESC Task Force On the Management of Arterial Hypertension. *J Hypertens* 2007;25:1751–1762.

Mancia G, Bombelli M, Facchettia R, et al. Long-term risk of sustained hypertension in white-coat or masked hypertension. *Hypertension* 2009;54:226–232.

Messerli FH, Ventura HO, Amodeo C. Osler's maneuver and pseudohypertension. *New Engl J Med* 1985;312: 1548–1551.

Papadopoulous DP, Makris TK. Masked hypertension definition, impact outcomes: a critical review. *J Clin Hypertens* 2007;9:956–963.

Pickering TG, Coats A, Mallion JM, et al. Task Force V: White coat hypertension. *Blood Pressure Monit* 1999;4(6):333–341.

Puato M, Palatini P, Zanardo M, et al. Increase in carotid intima-media thickness in grade I hypertensive subjects: White-coat hypertension versus sustained hypertension. *Hypertension* 2008;51(5):1300–1305.

Sommerfield AJ, Robinson L, Padfield PL, et al. Clinical variables associated with non-dipping of nocturnal blood pressure in type 2 diabetes. *Br J Diabetes Vasc Dis* 2008;8:236–240.

Stergiou GS, Yiannes NJ, Rarra VC, et al. White-coat hypertension and masked hypertension in children. *Blood Pressure Monit* 2005;10:297–300.

CHAPTER 68

ISOLATED SYSTOLIC HYPERTENSION

Anna Oliveras, MD, PhD, and Daniel Batlle, MD

1. **Define isolated systolic hypertension.**
   Isolated systolic hypertension (ISH) is defined in international guidelines (both the Joint National Committee seventh report [JNC 7] and the current European Cardiology/Hypertension Societies [EHS and EHC] guidelines) as systolic blood pressure (SBP) ≥140 mm Hg and diastolic blood pressure (DBP) <90 mm Hg.

2. **In which age(s) group(s) is ISH prevalent?**
   ISH has historically been recognized as more prevalent in the elderly. However, there is now firm evidence that ISH is also the predominant form of hypertension in adolescents and young adults. In fact, ISH in young adults in the United States has a higher prevalence than systolic/diastolic hypertension. Moreover, ISH is the most common abnormality in patients with hypertension and comorbid conditions (coronary artery disease, stroke, diabetes mellitus, chronic kidney disease, and peripheral artery disease). ISH may also occur in conditions associated with elevated cardiac output, such as anemia, hyperthyroidism, aortic insufficiency, arteriovenous fistula, and Paget's disease of bone.

3. **How common is ISH? What is the epidemiology of ISH?**
   ISH is present in about two thirds of patients with hypertension 60 years and older and in about three quarters of persons 75 years and older. If we exclusively focus on hypertensive subjects, ISH accounts for more than 75% of those aged 50 to 59, approximately 80% of hypertension in those aged 60 to 69, and approximately 90% of those with hypertension aged 70 years and older. Furthermore, ISH is the most common type of uncontrolled hypertension, with a rate of 87% of patients aged ≥60 years with poor blood pressure (BP) control.

   It has been shown that normotensive persons reaching age 65 have a 90% lifetime risk of developing hypertension—almost exclusively of the ISH subtype—if they live another 20 to 25 years.

4. **What are some misconceptions about high BP and age?**
   The concept that SBP increases with age should be considered a pathophysiologic concept. Once considered a benign consequence of aging, ISH has been associated with coronary and cerebrovascular morbidity and mortality.

5. **Describe the relationship between BP and age.**
   DBP increases with age up to about 50 to 60 years, after which it begins to decrease. SBP, however, continues to rise with increasing age, mainly as a result of the functional and structural changes in the arterial vasculature.

6. **Explain the pathophysiology for age-related changes in BP.**
   In patients younger than 50 years, in whom diastolic hypertension predominates, increased peripheral resistance is the major mechanism for elevated BP. In older persons, arterial compliance, especially large artery compliance, is decreased. This increased arterial stiffness mediates elevations in SBP and is also associated with decreases in DBP. Aging of the

cardiovascular system is accompanied by activation of the renin-angiotensin system, endothelial dysfunction, progressive deposition of calcium salts, fraying and fragmentation of elastin, and an increase in the number and cross-linking of collagen fibers that increase the rigidity of the vessel wall and, consequently, vascular remodeling. This process leads to an increase in large artery stiffness and an increase in arterial wave reflections from the vascular resistance bed to the heart. These processes in daily clinical practice translate to an increase in SBP and cause the age-related increase in pulse pressure (PP) (i.e., the difference between SBP and DBP). Furthermore, the BP elevation itself can promote further arterial stiffening and impair endothelium-dependent vasodilatation.

7. **Which are the most important clinical implications of ISH in the elderly?**
ISH could be regarded as the hallmark or clinical sign of an underlying silent atherosclerotic cardiovascular disease. After the sixth decade of life (a) increased PP is a surrogate marker for large artery stiffness and for vascular aging (arteriosclerosis); (b) prehypertension and hypertension, left untreated, accelerate the rate of vascular aging by more than 15 years; and (c) large artery stiffness rather than vascular resistance becomes the dominant hemodynamic factor in both normotensive and hypertensive subjects from age 50 onward.

8. **What is the relationship between pulse pressure, age, and ISH?**
Central artery stiffening with aging is the driving force that results in increased PP and, ultimately, the development of ISH. It is possible that PP reflects both central aortic properties and peripheral wave reflections. Demographic differences such as age, but also height, weight, and obesity, may account for the relative contributions of the two mechanisms.

9. **Are essential hypertension and ISH two distinct disorders?**
Hardening of large arteries and increased PP are the main traits that differentiate ISH from diastolic or systolic–diastolic hypertension, which is commonly referred to as essential hypertension. Other differences between both forms of hypertension is that patients with ISH appear to be more salt sensitive and have lower levels of plasma renin and angiotensin II.

10. **Is the PP an independent predictor of morbidity?**
Yes. The widening of PP is thought to be associated with organ damage, cardiac and vascular disease, and an increased risk of mortality. ISH with increased PP has been associated with several cardiovascular events:
- **Cardiac complications:** left ventricular hypertrophy, atrial fibrillation, systolic and diastolic dysfunction, and heart failure
- **Large artery complications:** myocardial infarction, both hemorrhagic and thrombotic stroke
- **Microvascular complications:** white matter lesions, leading to cognitive impairment, and progressive chronic renal disease

Moreover, increased PP predicts coronary heart disease risk better than either SBP or DBP in normotensive and untreated hypertensive subjects aged 50 to 79 years in the original Framingham cohort. The importance of SBP elevation as a powerful predictor of cardiovascular outcome was emphasized in three major randomized, placebo-controlled trials published in the 1990s: Systolic Hypertension in the Elderly Program (SHEP), Systolic Hypertension in China (Syst-China), and Systolic Hypertension in Europe (Syst-Eur).

11. **Which predicts cardiovascular risk more precisely: systolic or diastolic BP?**
SBP is recognized as a stronger predictor of risk (mortality and cardiovascular complications and also renal disease) than DBP in persons older than 50 years. This is supported by accumulated evidence documenting the vascular risks associated with elevated SBP levels, the greater difficulty in controlling elevated SBP compared with elevated DBP, and the high prevalence of ISH in older persons. This condition, once considered a benign consequence of aging, was strongly associated in the Multiple Risk Factor Intervention Trial (MRFIT) with

a relative risk of stroke of 8.21 for men in the 10th decile of SBP compared with 4.39 for men in the 10th decile of DBP.

12. **Does antihypertensive therapy ameliorate this risk?**
Yes. A 2 mm Hg mean lower SBP has been shown to be equivalent to a 7% lower risk of death from ischemic heart disease and a 10% lower risk of stroke. The landmark clinical trials SHEP, SYST-Eur, and Syst-China support the treatment of ISH. A meta-analysis that examined a subset of patients with ISH from these three trials showed that there was a 23% reduction in cardiovascular events associated with treatment of systolic hypertension compared with no treatment in elderly patients. New trials, LIFE, SCOPE (with a high number of subjects with ISH), SHELL and INSIGHT, confirm these results. Moreover, another meta-analysis showed that the benefits of active treatment, in terms of risk reduction for all cardiovascular events, stroke and myocardial infarction, was mainly the result of lowering of SBP and independent of lowering DBP to <70 mm Hg.

13. **Does antihypertensive treatment benefit all patients with ISH equally?**
Evidence for drug treatment benefit is stronger in patients with ISH with SBP ≥160 mm Hg and weaker for patients with SBP 140 to 159 mm Hg at low global cardiovascular risk (absence of diabetes, target organ damage, associated cardiovascular or renal disease, and other risk factors).

14. **When treating ISH, what is the target BP?**
Systolic hypertension in the elderly should be aggressively treated to target blood pressure. The therapeutic approach goals for ISH are similar to those recommended for most other types of hypertension. The recommended target level of blood pressure is below 140/90 mm Hg. However, treatment of systolic hypertension in older adults remains disappointing given that therapeutic goals often are not reached.

15. **What about the so-called J-curve phenomenon for treating ISH?**
A meta-analysis of clinical trials indicated that the increased risk of coronary events at low DBP was not related to the treatment or the pressure levels and was probably explained by serious illnesses that were causing the low BP. Although reducing DBP to very low levels might be harmful in some cases, the overall benefits of antihypertensive therapy in patients with ISH, including the reduction in coronary heart disease, are well documented. PP is a stronger risk factor than SBP in patients with ISH when DBP is <70 mm Hg. The J-curve of increase in cardiovascular events has occurred both with and without antihypertensive therapy. Several mechanisms may explain why a low DBP in combination with an elevated SBP is associated with increased cardiovascular risk at the lower range of DBP. In fact, the suggestion that very low DBP could be considered a marker more than a cause of cardiovascular events is reinforced by a retrospective analysis of SHEP (no excess of mortality when DBP was lowered to <60 mm Hg).

16. **Should ISH be treated in the elderly and in the very old (aged 85 or more)?**
Yes. Most benefits of SBP reduction extend to all age strata of the elderly population including subjects aged ≥80 years. In octogenarians, SBP lowering is associated with a significant reduction in all cardiovascular endpoints other than coronary events. The recent results from the HYpertension in the Very Elderly Trial (HYVET) study of patients aged ≥80 with sustained SBP of 160 mm Hg or more showed that lowering blood pressure to a target of 150/80 mm Hg resulted in a 30% reduction in the rate of stroke; 39% reduction in the rate of death from stroke; and 21%, 23%, and 64% reduction in the rates of death from any cause, death from cardiovascular causes, and in the rate of heart failure, respectively.

17. **Should the treatment of ISH be addressed to lower PP?**
Treating patients with the aim of reducing PP, even if theoretically correct, cannot be recommended because drug-induced changes of this parameter have not been studied in any intervention trial.

18. **What about adjunctive therapy?**

Elderly patients who have been diagnosed with uncomplicated ISH (moderate or low risk) should be prescribed lifestyle modifications. Weight loss of at least 5 kg (even in those of normal body weight) and sodium restriction to a daily intake of 100 mmol (6 g of sodium chloride) have been shown to be effective in elderly patients with hypertension. Apart from lowering BP, lifestyle modifications have shown other benefits, such as improvement of brachial artery compliance and distensibility, insulin sensitivity, and lipid profile with weight loss over 6 months and rapid improvement of large elastic artery compliance with sodium restriction.

19. **What is the optimal drug treatment of ISH?**

Drugs should be started at the lowest effective dose and titrated slowly to reach optimal control of SBP. This cautious approach is even more advisable in elderly patients because of the increased risk of orthostatic hypotension and other drug-related adverse effects. Compelling indications may favor some drug classes. The JNC 7 guidelines recommend thiazide-type diuretics as initial drug therapy for most patients with ISH unless there are specific contraindications for their use. The joint guidelines of ESH and ESC do not give preference to diuretics and recommend any of the five major classes of antihypertensive drugs for first-line therapy. Recent guidelines from Great Britain argue against the use of both diuretics and β-blockers for initial therapy and favor angiotensin-converting enzyme inhibitors, angiotensin receptor blockers, or calcium channel blockers. Despite some differences in recommendations, all of these guidelines emphasize that the major benefits of therapy are related to lowering blood pressure and controlling hypertension.

Most of these patients will require multiple drug therapies to achieve the substantial reductions in SBP needed to reach target levels. Multiple drug regimens are well tolerated in older patients, and several combinations have shown to achieve greater BP reductions than monotherapy. Moreover, preference should be given to long-acting molecules, which are safer and ensure better compliance with treatment.

KEY POINTS: ISOLATED SYSTOLIC HYPERTENSION

- Isolated systolic hypertension (ISH) is mostly prevalent in the elderly. However, there is now firm evidence that ISH is also the predominant form of hypertension in adolescents and young adults.
- Hardening of large arteries and increased pulse pressure are the main traits that differentiate ISH from diastolic or systolic-diastolic hypertension in the elderly.
- SBP is recognized as a stronger predictor of risk (mortality and cardiovascular complications, and also renal disease) than diastolic blood pressure in persons older than 50 years.
- ISH should also be treated in the elderly and in the very old (aged 85 or more). Most benefits of SBP reduction extend to all age strata of the elderly population including subjects aged 80 years.
- Weight loss of about 5 Kg (even in those of normal bodyweight) and sodium restriction to a daily intake of 100 mmol (6g of sodium chloride) have been shown to be effective in elderly patients with hypertension. As for drugs, there is a good scientific rationale for using agents that act on the renin-angiotensin system in the treatment of ISH.

20. **What about blocking the renin-angiotensin system (RAS) in the elderly with ISH?**

The RAS plays a significant role in the pathogenesis and progression of systolic hypertension. Currently, there is a good scientific rationale for using agents that act on the RAS in the treatment of ISH. Clearly, in ISH complicated by left ventricular hypertrophy or with associated diabetic or nondiabetic kidney disease, drugs that block the RAS should be used in the higher doses that have been demonstrated to be organ protective.

BIBLIOGRAPHY

1. Beckett NS, Peters R, Fletcher AE, et al. HYVET Study Group. Treatment of hypertension in patients 80 years of age or older. *N Engl J Med* 2008;358:1887–1898.

2. Boutitie F, Gueyffier F, Pocock S, et al. J-shaped relationship between blood pressure and mortality in hypertensive patients: New insights from a meta-analysis of individual-patient data. *Ann Intern Med* 2002;136:438–448.

3. Chobanian AV. Isolated systolic hypertension in the elderly. *N Engl J Med* 2007;357:789–796.

4. Chobanian AV, Bakris GL, Black HR, et al. Joint National Committee on Prevention, Detection, Evaluation, and Treatment of High Blood Pressure. National Heart, Lung, and Blood Institute; National High Blood Pressure Education Program Coordinating Committee. Seventh report of the Joint National Committee on Prevention, Detection, Evaluation, and Treatment of High Blood Pressure. *Hypertension* 2003;42:1206–1252.

5. Duprez DA. Systolic hypertension in the elderly: Addressing an unmet need. *Am J Med* 2008;121:179–184.

6. Franklin SS. The pathobiology of isolated systolic hypertension. *Hipertens Riesgo Vasc* 2010;27:23–26.

7. Grebla RC, Rodríguez CJ, Borrell LN, et al. Prevalence and determinants of isolated systolic hypertension among young adults: The 1999–2004 US National Health and Nutrition Examination Survey. *J Hypertens* 2010;28:15–23.

8. Izzo JL, Levy D, Black HR. Importance of systolic blood pressure in older Americans. *Hypertension* 2010;35:1021–1024.

9. Lee HW, Karam J, Hussain B, et al. Vascular compliance in hypertension: Therapeutic implications. *Curr Diabetes Rep* 2008;8:208–213.

10. Lewington S, Clarke R, Qizilbash N, et al; Prospective Studies Collaboration. Age-specific relevance of usual blood pressure to vascular mortality: a meta-analysis of individual data for one million adults in 61 prospective studies. *Lancet* 2002;360:1903–1913.

11. Mancia G, De Backer G, Dominiczak A, et al. 2007. Guidelines for the Management of Arterial Hypertension: The Task Force for the Management of Arterial Hypertension of the European Society of Hypertension (ESH) and of the European Society of Cardiology (ESC). *J Hypertens* 2007;25:1105–1187.

12. Mancia G, Laurent S, Agabiti-Rosei E, et al. Reappraisal of European guidelines on hypertension management: A European Society of Hypertension Task Force document. *J Hypertens* 2009;27:2121–2158.

13. McEniery CM, Yasmin WS, Maki-Petaja K, et al. *Hypertension* 2005;46:221–226.

14. Neutel JM, Gilderman LI. Hypertension control in the elderly. *J Clin Hypertens* (Greenwich) 2008;10:33–39.

15. O'Rourke MF, Nichols WW. Aortic diameter, aortic stiffness, and wave reflection increase with age and isolated systolic hypertension. *Hypertension* 2005;45:652–658.

16. Pannarale G. Optimal drug treatment of systolic hypertension in the elderly. *Drugs Aging* 2008;25:1–8.

17. Sorof JM. Prevalence and consequence of systolic hypertension in children. *Am J Hypertens* 2002;15:57S–60S.

18. Staessen JA, Gasowski J, Wang JG, et al. Risks of untreated and treated isolated systolic hypertension in the elderly: Meta-analysis of outcome trials. *Lancet* 2000;355:865–872.

19. Stamler J, Stamler R, Neaton JD. Blood pressure, systolic and diastolic, and cardiovascular risks: US population data. *Arch Intern Med* 1993;153:598–615.

20. Vasan RS, Beiser A, Seshadri S, et al. Residual lifetime risk for developing hypertension in middle-aged women and men: The Framingham Heart Study. *J Am Med Assoc* 2002;287:1003–1010.

21. Wang J, Staessen JA, Franklin SS, et al. Systolic and diastolic blood pressure lowering as determinants of cardiovascular outcome. *Hypertension* 2005;45:907–913.

22. Wong ND, López VA, L'Italien G, et al. Inadequate control of hypertension in US adults with cardiovascular disease comorbidities in 2003–2004. *Arch Intern Med* 2007;167:2431–2436.

CHAPTER 69

HYPERTENSION IN AFRICAN AMERICANS

David Martins, MD, and Keith C. Norris, MD

1. **What are some of the key lifestyle changes to optimize blood pressure and blood sugar control and preserve renal function in African American patients?**
   - **Healthy diet:** low fat, low sodium, high potassium, and adequate calcium intake
   - **Regular physical activity:** Increase physical activity as part of the daily routine by undertaking an enjoyable physical activity for 30 to 45 minutes per day for 3 to 5 days per week
   - **Weight maintenance:** monitor body weight, maintain a healthy body mass index, and maintain weight by making permanent changes in the daily diet
   - **Stress reduction:** Develop coping skills for specific stressors in work and/or home environment with meditation, relaxation, yoga, biofeedback, etc.
   - **Smoking cessation:** Ensure smoke-free environment

2. **What are some of the key approaches to achieve healthy dietary changes in African American patients?**
   - Consider culturally appropriate nutritional substitutions.
   - Eat more broiled (grilled) and steamed foods.
   - Eat more grains, fresh fruits, and vegetables.
   - Eat fewer fats and use healthier fats, such as olive oil.
   - Eat fewer processed foods, fast foods, and fried foods.
   - Read labels and pay attention to the sodium, potassium, and fat content of foods.
   - Do not season foods with smoked meats, such as bacon and ham hocks.
   - If lactose intolerant, try lactose-free milk or yogurt or drink calcium-fortified juices or soy milk.
   - Limit alcohol consumption to <2 beers, 1 glass of wine, or 1 shot of hard liquor per day.
   - Limit the intake of sugar-sweetened beverages and juices.

3. **When should antihypertensive drug therapy be initiated in African American patients with renal disease?**
   Pharmacotherapy should be initiated promptly for persistent elevation in blood pressure despite the therapeutic lifestyle changes. The duration of therapeutic lifestyle changes prior to the initiation of pharmacotherapy depends on the level of blood pressure and the comorbidities.

   Antihypertensive drug therapy is recommended for persistent blood pressure elevation higher than 130/80 mm Hg in patients with renal disease.

4. **What is the relationship between blood pressure level and renal disease among African American patients?**
   African Americans exhibit some of the highest incidence and prevalence of high blood pressure in the world. High blood pressure predisposes to renal disease, and renal disease predisposes to high blood pressure. The vicious cycle of high blood pressure and renal disease among African Americans accounts in part for the six-fold increase in the incidence of hypertension-related ESRD in this population compared to the Caucasian population. Aggressive and appropriate screening for elevated blood pressure and renal disease among African Americans will minimize the role of this vicious cycle in the rapid progression of renal disease

5. **What is the role of diabetes in renal disease among African American patients?**
High blood pressure and diabetes account for about of two thirds of the new cases of ESRD. Diabetes alone accounts for nearly half of new ESRD cases. Increased rates of poor diabetes control among African Americans accelerate diabetes-related renal injury. Increased rates of hypertension and poorer blood pressure control further contribute to the rapid progression of renal disease among African American patients with diabetes.

6. **What are some of the effective antihypertensive drugs for controlling blood pressure in African American patients with renal disease?**
   - Diuretics (loop diuretics if glomerular filtration rate [GFR] <30 mL/min)
   - Renin-angiotensin system inhibitors
   - Calcium channel blockers
   - Centrally acting sympatholytic agents
   - Direct vasodilators

7. **What should the goal of blood pressure treatment be among African American patients with renal disease?**
The optimum blood pressure level is 120/80 mm Hg. The recommended blood pressure treatment goal in patients with hypertension and renal disease is <130/80 mm Hg. Many patients will require three to four medications to achieve this treatment goal. Blood pressure control should be optimized in African Americans with renal disease for the best renal outcome.

8. **What is the role of the low renin status in renal disease among African Americans?**
Low renin status is more prevalent among African Americans and the elderly. The salt sensitivity associated with low renin status may predispose African Americans to a greater rise in blood pressure on a high-salt diet. A suboptimal blood pressure response to weight loss has also been associated with low renin status. Low systemic renin status may be a result of a paradoxical hyperactivation of the autocrine renin-angiotensin system (e.g., intrarenal, vascular) and the upregulation of the angiotensin II type 1 (AT1) receptors and downregulation of systemic renin. This paradoxical finding, which appears to be more prevalent among African Americans, creates a profile of low systemic renin as result of increased local renin-angiotensin activation leading to an accelerated progression of renal and vascular disease.

KEY POINTS: RENAL DISEASES IN AFRICAN AMERICANS

1. The incidence and prevalence of renal disease are highest among African Americans.
2. Renal disease among African Americans is characterized by an earlier onset and a more rapid progression to end-stage renal disease.
3. High blood pressure and diabetes account for more than two thirds of the new cases of end-stage renal disease.
4. Renal disease progression can be effectively prevented and/or attenuated by appropriate blood pressure and blood sugar control among African Americans.

9. **What is the incidence of end-stage renal disease in African Americans?**
African Americans represent about 10% of the U.S. population but account for more than a third of the end-stage renal disease (ESRD) population. In general African Americans are almost four times more likely than Caucasians to develop ESRD. Among men aged 20 to 39 years, African Americans are ~15 times more likely to develop ESRD secondary to hypertension than age-matched Caucasian men.

10. **What are the risk factors for ESRD among African Americans?**
Many biologic and socioeconomic variables might influence the onset and progression of renal disease among African Americans. The *MHY9* gene is associated with non diabetic kidney disease, and 60% of African Americans carry the variations of the *MHY9* gene associated with increased risk of chronic kidney disease (CKD) compared to only 4% of Caucasians. The high rates of low socioeconomic status and lack of health insurance among ethnic minorities contribute to poor blood pressure and blood sugar control that accelerate the onset and progression of kidney disease. High blood pressure accounts for nearly a third and diabetes accounts for nearly half of the new cases of ESRD among African Americans. Despite these apparent associations, only about 10% of African Americans with high blood pressure recognize renal disease as a consequence of poor blood pressure control. High rates of low health literacy and lack of awareness of CKD risk factors among ethnic minority populations lead to suboptimum self-management attempts to reduce risk and preserve kidney function.

11. **Do African American patients with ESRD have a higher mortality rate?**
Although African Americans in the general population have higher rates of overall premature morbidity and mortality, including cardiovascular diseases, African American patients with ESRD actually have a lower mortality rate than age-adjusted white counterparts. The reasons are not clear but may be linked to a reverse epidemiology of cardiovascular disease seen in patients with chronic diseases.

12. **Does the use of recombinant human erythropoietin predispose African American patients with ESRD to cardiovascular disease?**
Cardiovascular disease is the leading cause of death among patients with ESRD, and high blood pressure is a major risk factor for cardiovascular disease. Higher doses of recombinant human erythropoietin in the management of anemia in African American patients with ESRD may worsen high blood pressure and increase vascular thrombosis. However, African American patients with ESRD do not have an increased risk for cardiovascular death.

13. **What is the mechanism for the pressor effect of recombinant human erythropoietin?**
The mechanisms underlying the pressor effect of recombinant human erythropoietin are not completely understood, but the increased blood viscosity, reversal of hypoxic vasodilation, and increase in red cell mass associated with the use of recombinant human erythropoietin have been postulated as potential mechanisms in addition to a direct effect of recombinant human erythropoietin on the vasculature.

14. **What is a practical approach for treating high blood pressure in African American patients with renal disease?**
Target blood pressure should be <130/80 mm Hg, and expect to use two or more agents to achieve this goal. Therapy should include an angiotensin-converting enzyme inhibitor or an angiotensin receptor blocker along with a diuretic. If hypertension is refractory to therapy, monitor adverse effects, evaluate sociocultural factors (e.g., insurance status and medication plan), consider secondary causes of hypertension, and assess adherence to medication and sodium restriction (perhaps by use of 24-hour urine sodium collection). The diuretic should be thiazide-type if the estimated GFR (eGFR) is >30 mL/min and a loop diuretic (usually administered two to three times day) if eGFR <30 mL/min.

15. **What is the role of sickle cell trait in the rapid progression of renal disease among African Americans?**
Sickle cell trait (HbAS) has a prevalence of about 8% among African Americans compared to 0.046% in non-African Americans. The presence of sickle cell trait has been associated with certain asymptomatic progressive renal structural changes and significant functional impairment. Indeed, prevalence of HbAS among African Americans with ESRD is twice that in the general African American population (15% versus 7%), raising the possibility that sickle

cell trait may contribute to a decline in kidney function, either alone or in conjunction with other known risk factors for renal disease, although the exact mechanism(s) is unclear.

CONTROVERSY

16. **Is blood pressure response to antihypertensive therapy different in African Americans?**
    African Americans have been shown to exhibit lesser blood pressure reductions on monotherapy with renin-angiotensin system inhibition compared to Caucasians, but there are no differences in the cardiorenal benefits of renin-angiotensin system inhibition across racial/ethnic categories. Controlling blood pressure to target levels with a regimen that includes renin-angiotensin system inhibition in both African Americans and Caucasians with CKD is associated with comparable improvements in cardiorenal outcomes, including a similar decrease in renal protein excretion.

17. **Is there evidence of ethnic differences in clinical outcomes based on hypertensive treatment regimens in persons with renal disease?**
    No clinically relevant ethnic differences in outcomes have been noted in patients with hypertension and CKD following most randomized, controlled, evidence-based, pharmacologic interventions for blood pressure control. However, the paucity of data with adequate numbers of African American study participants reinforces the need to achieve greater ethnic diversity in clinical trials. In addition to considering the clinical evidence when treating hypertensive renal disease, clinicians should pay detailed attention to potential cultural and socioeconomic influences that disproportionately affect adherence among ethnic minority patients.

BIBLIOGRAPHY

1. Derebail VK, Nachman PH, Key NS, et al. High prevalence of sickle cell trait in African Americans with ESRD. *J Am Soc Nephrol* 2010;21(3):413–417.

2. Douglas JG, Bakris GL, Epstein M, et al., for the Hypertension in African Americans Working Group of the International Society on Hypertension in Blacks. Management of high blood pressure in African Americans: Consensus statement of the Hypertension in African Americans Working Group of the International Society on Hypertension in Blacks. *Arch Intern Med* 2003;163(5):525–541.

3. Joint National Committee on Prevention, Detection, Evaluation, and Treatment of High Blood Pressure. 3. The seventh report of the joint National Committee on Prevention, Detection, Evaluation and Treatment of High Blood Pressure. *JAMA* 2003;289:2560–2572.

4. K/DOQI clinical practice guidelines for chronic kidney disease: Evaluation, classification, and stratification. *Kidney Int* 2005;67(6):2089–2100.

5. National Kidney Disease Education Program. NKDEP Survey of African-American Adults' Knowledge, Attitudes and Behaviors Related to Kidney Disease. Bethesda, MD: National Institutes of Health, U.S. Department of Health and Human Services, 2003.

6. Norris K, Nissenson AR. Race, gender, and socioeconomic disparities in CKD in the United States. *J Am Soc Nephrol* 2008;19:1261–1270.

7. Norris KC, Tareen N, Martins D, et al. Implications of ethnicity for the treatment of hypertensive kidney disease, with an emphasis on African Americans. *Nat Clin Pract Nephrol* 2008;4(10):538–549.

8. US Renal Data System. Bethesda, MD: National Institutes of Health, National Institute of Diabetes and Digestive and Kidney Diseases, 2005.

REFRACTORY HYPERTENSION

C. Venkata S. Ram, MD, and Edgar V. Lerma, MD

CHAPTER 70

1. **Define refractory or resistant hypertension.**

   True refractory or resistant hypertension is somewhat uncommon in the modern management of hypertension. A majority of patients with primary hypertension respond favorably to multiple antihypertensive drugs. Definitions vary, but hypertension is considered refractory if the blood pressure (BP) cannot be reduced below target levels (Table 70-1) in patients who are compliant with an optimal triple-drug regimen that includes a diuretic. In literature the terms "refractory" and "resistant" are used interchangeably. In patients with isolated systolic hypertension (ISH), refractoriness has been traditionally defined as a failure of multiple antihypertensive drugs to reduce systolic blood pressure below 160 mm Hg, but recent observations strongly indicate that the target level for systolic blood pressure should be ≤140 mm Hg. Whereas refractory hypertension may be still encountered in specialized hypertension centers, its prevalence in the general population of patients with hypertension is probably quite low; most patients with chronic uncomplicated hypertension respond to appropriate (combination) therapy.

   If a patient's BP is not controlled on multiple antihypertensive drugs but one of them is not a diuretic, it should not be diagnosed as "refractory" hypertension.

   It is worthwhile remembering that an "optimal" dose may not necessarily equate to a "full" dose. An optimal dose is the highest dose tolerated by the patient or a dose governed by concomitant conditions such as chronic kidney disease, congestive heart failure, diabetes, and the like.

2. **Discuss the epidemiology of refractory hypertension.**

   Although not representing typical office practices, the data from the Anti-hypertensive and Lipid-Lowering Treatment to Prevent Heart Attack Trial (ALLHAT) provides a valuable estimate of the prevalence of refractory hypertension in the community setting. In ALLHAT, 34% of the study participants had BP >140/90 mostly on two medications, with 27% requiring three or

TABLE 70-1. JNC 7 CLASSIFICATIONS

BP Classification	SBP mm Hg		DBP mm Hg
Normal	<120	and	<80
Prehypertension	120–139	or	80–89
Stage I hypertension	140–159	or	90–99
Stage II hypertension	≥160	or	≥100

JNC 7 = seventh report of the Joint National Committee on Prevention, Detection. Evaluation and Treatment of High Blood Pressure; BP = blood pressure; DBP = diastolic blood pressure; SBP = systolic blood pressure.

more medications. Based on the 5-year observations in ALLHAT, we estimate that the incidence of refractory hypertension was approximately 15%. In the Controlled ONset Verapamil INvestigation of Cardiovascular End Points (CONVINCE), 18% of the patients had a BP level >140/90 mm Hg on three or more medications.

Patients with diabetes are more resistant to antihypertensive drugs than nondiabetic subjects, thus requiring more antihypertensive drugs to achieve goal BP.

3. **What are the most common causes of refractory hypertension?**
When a patient with hypertension demonstrates refractoriness to standard antihypertensive drug therapy, proper management requires identification of possible etiologies (Table 70-2). Before making drastic therapeutic changes, certain questions should come to the physician's mind:
- Does the patient truly have "refractory" hypertension?
- Are there any patient/environmental factors?
- Does the patient have pseudoresistance?
- Are there adverse drug reactions or drug/food interactions?

TABLE 70-2.   CAUSES OF REFRACTORY HYPERTENSION

Pseudoresistance
- White-coat hypertension
- Pseudohypertension in older patients
- Use of small cuff in patients who are obese

Nonadherence to prescribed therapy

Volume overload

Drug-related causes
- Doses too low
- Wrong type of diuretic
- Inappropriate combinations
- Drug actions and interactions
  - Sympathomimetics
  - Nasal decongestants
  - Appetite suppressants
  - Cocaine
  - ? Caffeine
  - Oral contraceptives
  - Adrenal steroids
  - Licorice (as may be found in chewing tobacco)
  - Cyclosporine, tacrolimus
  - Erythropoietin
  - Antidepressants
  - Nonsteroidal anti-inflammatory drugs

Concomitant conditions
- Obesity
- Sleep apnea
- Ethanol intake of more than 1 oz (30 mL) per day
- Anxiety, hyperventilation

Secondary causes of hypertension (e.g., renovascular hypertension, adrenal causes, and renal disease, etc.)

- Does the patient have a secondary form of hypertension such as adrenal or renovascular hypertension?
- Are there any identifiable mechanisms (pressors) that are responsible for elevating the arterial blood pressure despite antihypertensive drug therapy?

4. **What is pseudoresistant hypertension?**
It is not uncommon to see patients whose clinic/office blood pressure levels may be higher than the levels obtained outside the office setting, so-called white-coat hypertension. Although white-coat hypertension is usually considered in the context of mild hypertension (stage I), in some cases, refractory hypertension may be indicative of white-coat hypertension. Patients who may have refractory white-coat hypertension do not demonstrate target organ damage despite seemingly very high blood pressure readings in the office/clinic. The disparity between the degree of hypertension and the lack of target organ damage can be supported by the measurement of serial home blood pressure levels and or by obtaining ambulatory blood pressure recordings.

Another possible source of erroneous blood pressure measurement is a condition termed pseudohypertension, seen sometimes in the elderly individuals. Persistently high readings in the absence of target organ damage or dysfunction may indicate pseudohypertension. This condition is a result of the fact that the hardened and sclerotic artery is not compressible, hence falsely elevated pressures are recorded (the Osler phenomenon). Because of thickened calcified arteries, a greater pressure is required to compress the sclerotic vessels. There is little doubt that pseudohypertension does occur in older individuals, but its exact prevalence is not known. Although some have advocated the use of intra-arterial blood pressure determination as a means of accurately making the diagnosis of this aberration, we do not recommend this procedure to document pseudohypertension; it is simply not practical. A more common example of pseudoresistance is measurement artifact, which occurs when the blood pressure is taken with a small cuff in people with large arm diameters. With the patient in the seated position and the arm supported at heart level, the blood pressure should be taken with an appropriate cuff size to ensure accurate determination. The bladder within the cuff should encircle at least 80% of the arm diameter. One has to be cautious before dismissing an elevated reading as a measurement artifact, however, because patients with truly refractory hypertension experience a high rate of cardiovascular and other complications.

Mejia AD, Egan BM, Schork NJ, et al. Artefacts in measurement of blood pressure and lack of target organ involvement in the assessment of patients with treatment-resistant hypertension. *Ann Intern Med* 1990;112:270–277.

Messerli FH, Ventura HO, Amodeo C. Osler's maneuver and pseudohypertension. *N Engl J Med* 1985;312:1548–1551.

Thibonnier M. Ambulatory blood pressure monitoring: When is it warranted? *Postgrad Med* 1992;91:263–274.

Veglio F, Rabbia F, Riva P, et al. Ambulatory blood pressure monitoring and clinical characteristics of the true and white-coat resistant hypertension. *Clin Exp Hypertens* 2001;23(3):203–211.

Verdecchia P. Using out of office blood pressure monitoring in the management of hypertension. *Curr Hypertens Rep* 2001;3(5):400–405.

5. **How can one define "noncompliance" as a cause of refractory hypertension?**
Failure to follow a prescribed regimen is perhaps the most common reason to achieve goal BP levels. There may be valid reasons for patients' noncompliance, such as side effects, costs, complexity of the drug regimen, and lack of understanding. Social, economic, and personal factors may also play a role in noncompliance. Noncompliance is a complex phenomenon that is not easily discerned in clinical practice.

6. **How does volume overload contribute to refractory hypertension?**
Volume overload from any underlying mechanism may not only increase the blood pressure, but also may offset the effectiveness of antihypertensive drugs. Excessive salt intake retention increases the plasma volume and causes resistance to antihypertensive drugs and can actually raise the blood pressure in some patients. Elderly and African American patients are particularly sensitive to fluid overload, as are patients with renal insufficiency and congestive

heart failure. Some antihypertensive drugs, such as direct vasodilators, antiadrenergic agents, and most of the nondiuretic antihypertensive drugs, cause plasma and extracellular fluid expansion, thus interfering with blood pressure control. Of all the nondiuretic antihypertensive drugs, angiotensin-converting enzyme (ACE) inhibitors, angiotensin receptor blockers, and calcium antagonists are least likely to cause fluid retention. Antihypertensive responsiveness can be regained by restricting the sodium intake; adding or increasing the dose of diuretic; and, in some instances, switching to a loop diuretic from thiazides.

Dustan HP, Tarazi RM, Bravo EL. Dependence of arterial pressure on intravascular volume in treated hypertensive patients. *N Engl J Med* 1972;286:861–866.

7. **What are the common drug-related causes of refractory hypertension?**
Hypertension may be seemingly refractory if the antihypertensive drugs are used in suboptimal doses or when an inappropriate diuretic is used (e.g., using a thiazide-type diuretic as opposed to a loop diuretic in patients with renal insufficiency, congestive heart failure, and in those who are taking potent vasodilators such as minoxidil or hydralazine). Inappropriate combinations can also limit their therapeutic potential. Adverse drug–drug interactions can raise the blood pressure in patients with and without hypertension. Such adverse interactions (Table 70-3) can occur as a result of alterations in drug pharmacokinetics or in pharmacodynamics of concomitant drugs administered for different indications. One typical example of an adverse drug interaction is between indomethacin and beta blockers, diuretics, and ACE inhibitors. Tricyclic antidepressants (no longer widely used) have a significant interaction with sympathetic blocking agents. Hypertension associated with renal insufficiency is often difficult to treat; patients with hypertension and reduced renal function generally require concomitant therapy with a loop diuretic such as furosemide because the thiazide diuretics do not work that well in such patients.

Of all the drugs listed in Table 70-3, the nonsteroidal anti-inflammatory drugs are important because of the frequency with which they are used in clinical practice; these drugs attenuate the vasodilatory actions of (intrarenal) prostaglandins, thus inhibiting natriuresis and causing volume expansion and therefore resulting in blood pressure elevation. Hence, in patients with refractory or severe hypertension, nonsteroidal anti-inflammatory drugs should be avoided if possible. Estrogen as a component of oral contraceptive preparations may raise the blood pressure, but hormonal replacement therapy has no significant adverse effect on blood pressure.

Fierro-Carrion G, Ram CVS. Nonsteroidal anti-inflammatory drugs (NSAIDs) and blood pressure. *Am J Cardiol* 1980;80:775–776. (This article covers the pathophysiologic adverse interactions between the drugs and the blood pressure.)

TABLE 70-3. DRUG INTERACTIONS THAT MAY LEAD TO RESISTANT HYPERTENSION	
Antihypertensive Agents	**Interacting Drugs**
Hydrochlorothiazide	Cholestyramine
Propranolol	Rifampin
Guanethidine	Tricyclics
Angiotensin-converting enzyme inhibitors	Indomethacin
Diuretics	Indomethacin
All drugs	Cocaine
	Tricyclics
	Phenylpropanolamine

8. **What other comorbid conditions contribute to refractory hypertension?**
It has been reported that cigarette smoking can interfere with BP control mechanisms. Obesity often is a major factor in the genesis of refractory hypertension. Obstructive sleep apnea (OSA) is being increasingly recognized as a possible factor in the development of resistant hypertension. Excessive alcohol consumption (more than 1 oz or 30 mL daily) clearly raises the systemic blood pressure, sometimes to dangerously high levels. We have sometimes witnessed panic attacks and hyperventilation as possible causative factors for refractory hypertension. Similarly, chronic pain may aggravate with BP levels.

Bloxham CA, Beevers DG, Walker JM. Malignant hypertension and cigarette smoking. *Br Med J* 1997;1:581–583.

Lavie P, Hoffstein V. Sleep apnea syndrome: A possible contributing factor to resistant hypertension. *Sleep* 2001;24(6):721–725. (This article covers the possible implications of sleep disorders in increasing the blood pressure.)

Tuomilehto J, Enlund H, Salonen JG, et al. Alcohol, patient compliance and blood pressure control in hypertensive patients. *Scand J Soc Med* 1984;12:177–181.

9. **What are the secondary causes of hypertension?**
In a small percentage of patients with refractory hypertension, the underlying cause may be a secondary form of hypertension such as renovascular hypertension or other possible etiologies (Table 70-4). Patients with a secondary form of hypertension may present with drug-resistant hypertension. The sudden loss of effectiveness of previously effective antihypertensive regimen should raise the suspicion of renovascular disease or other secondary forms of hypertension. (A more detailed discussion on this subject matter is presented in Chapters 65 to 67.)

van Jaarsveld BC, Krijnen P, Derkx FH, et al. Resistance to antihypertensive medication as predictor of renal artery stenosis: Comparison of two drug regimens. *J Hum Hypertens* 2001;15(10):669–676. (This paper reveals that a secondary cause such as renal artery stenosis may be responsible for resistant hypertension.)

10. **What are the treatment options for refractory hypertension?**
Rational management of refractory hypertension requires a systematic approach based on the causative considerations described in the foregoing discussion. It should be re-emphasized that because uncontrolled hypertension can cause significant morbidity and mortality, aggressive therapeutic management should be implemented. An overall management approach should be based on careful evaluation and rational medical therapy, which may be complex.

11. **How should refractory hypertension be evaluated?**
When the patient's BP does not respond satisfactorily to appropriate therapy, one has to consider whether the patient has pseudoresistance as a result of white-coat hypertension, pseudohypertension in the elderly, or a measurement artifact. In some individuals, therefore, it is appropriate to obtain home BP readings and/or 24-hour ambulatory BP recordings to document the degree of hypertension outside the office/clinic setting. In individuals who are obese, BP should always be measured with a large cuff. Once the validity of the BP measurement is confirmed, it is critical to ascertain the patient's adherence to a prescribed regimen; nonadherence to treatment must be considered before extensive and unnecessary evaluation is undertaken. Factor(s) responsible for noncompliance should be identified and

TABLE 70-4. SOME EXAMPLES OF SECONDARY FORMS OF HYPERTENSION THAT MAY BE RESISTANT TO CONVENTIONAL ANTIHYPERTENSIVE THERAPY

Renovascular hypertension	Hyperthyroidism
Primary aldosteronism	Hyperparathyroidism
Pheochromocytoma	Aortic coarctation
Hypothyroidism	Renal disease

corrected, if possible. The treatment should be simplified to encourage patient participation. Often a firm dialogue with the patient and the family can reveal whether compliance is the cause.

Correction of volume overload is one of the key strategies in managing resistant hypertension. Excessive salt intake must be curtailed. Adequate diuretic therapy should be implemented based on clinical circumstances. The dosage and the choice of the diuretic should be appropriately modified. Patients with concomitant congestive heart failure or renal insufficiency require optimal volume control to achieve adequate BP control. The doses of antihypertensive drugs should be titrated systematically to determine whether the patient is responding to the treatment. Drug interactions should be considered and eliminated in the treatment of hypertension. A complete list should be made of drugs that could increase the blood pressure such as steroids, oral contraceptives, sympathomimetics, nasal decongestants, cocaine, appetite suppressants, and so on. Patients should be counseled about alcohol consumption, weight control, salt intake, and regular physical activity. Conditions such as obstructive sleep apnea or chronic pain should be vigorously addressed.

Secondary causes of hypertension such as those listed in Table 70-4 should be considered in the overall evaluation of patients with resistant hypertension. Based on the clinical characteristics, renovascular hypertension should be pursued in patients with truly refractory hypertension. Other causes such as primary hyperaldosteronism, pheochromocytoma, Cushing's syndrome, coarctation of aorta, and renal disease should be considered based on the clinical course, follow-up, and laboratory findings. If an underlying cause is found, it should be corrected, if possible, to permit better BP control. Patients with refractory hypertension experience and suffer from a high degree of target organ damage.

Addison C, Varney S, Coats A. The use of ambulatory blood pressure monitoring in managing hypertension according to different treatment guidelines. *J Hum Hypertens* 2001;15(8):535–558.

Chobanian AV, Bakris GL, Black HR, et al.; Joint National Committee on Prevention, Detection, Evaluation, and Treatment of High Blood Pressure, National Heart, Lung, and Blood Institute; National High Blood Pressure Education Program Coordinating Committee. The seventh report of the Joint National Committee on Prevention, Detection. Evaluation and Treatment of High Blood Pressure. *Hypertension* 2003;41:1206–1252. (This is the latest report from the Joint National Committee, which includes a description of refractory hypertension.)

Cuspidi C, Macca G, Sampieri L, et al. High prevalence of cardiac and extracardiac target organ damage in refractory hypertension. *J Hypertens* 2001;19(11):2063–2070.

Eraker S, Kirscht J, Becker M. Understanding and improving patient compliance. *Ann Intern Med* 1984;100:258–268.

Felmeden DC, Lip GY. Resistant hypertension and the Birmingham Hypertension Square. *Curr Hypertens Rep* 2001;3(3):203–208.

Graves J. Management of difficult-to-control hypertension. *Mayo Clin Proc* 2000;75:278–284.

Nuesch R, Schroeder K, Dieterle T, et al. Relation between insufficient response to antihypertensive treatment and poor compliance with treatment: A prospective case-control study. *Br Med J* 2001 Jul 21; 323(7305):142–146.

Setaro J, Black H. Refractory hypertension. *N Engl J Med* 1992;327:534–547. (This paper addresses the low incidence of truly refractory hypertension in a referral center.)

12. **Describe the drug treatment of refractory hypertension.**
When a correctable cause is not found, patients with refractory hypertension require aggressive and diligently considered drug therapy to control the BP. The first step is to optimize the existing therapy either by increasing the dosages or by changing to different combinations and observing the patient for a few weeks. In the event the BP still remains uncontrolled, effective diuretic therapy should be implemented. Assuming that the hypertension has failed to respond to conventional therapies, consideration should be given to the use of hydralazine or minoxidil (in conjunction with a β-blocker and a diuretic). Because direct vasodilators cause significant reflex activation of sympathetic nervous system and fluid retention, their use should be accompanied by coadministration of a β-blocker and a diuretic (usually a loop diuretic). We generally give a trial of hydralazine therapy before choosing minoxidil therapy. Occasionally, further reductions in the BP can be secured by adding a fourth

agent such as oral or transdermal clonidine. In patients with advanced renal impairment, dialysis might be required for adequate control of BP. Recent observations suggest that in some patients with resistant hypertension, aldosterone levels may be inappropriately high; this may worsen BP control not only in patients with classical primary hyperaldosteronism, but also those without the syndrome with relatively high aldosterone levels. Thus, it seems reasonable to offer a trial of aldosterone antagonist therapy (as an add-on) for patients with resistant hypertension. Carefully performed clinical studies have confirmed the usefulness of adding an aldosterone antagonist in the management of refractory hypertension. Recent research findings suggest that aldosterone may play a possible contributory role in the pathogenesis of refractory hypertension. Whether this is a direct effect of aldosterone itself on the peripheral vascular resistance or is a result of its humorally mediated volume expansion is not clear. Aldosterone promotes vascular inflammation and vessel stiffness, which may contribute, in part, to its effects on systemic blood. Although, in a small number of selected patients, workup for primary hyperaldosteronism is indicated, therapeutic response to aldosterone antagonists in refractory hypertension occurs irrespective of aldosterone levels. It also has been proposed that the pathogenesis of obstructed sleep apnea may be explained by inappropriate vascular actions of aldosterone. Therefore, aldosterone antagonism may be an option in the management of OSA in addition to the correction of underlying respiratory disturbance. OSA may be associated with refractory hypertension; whether uncontrolled hypertension results from obesity or OSA is hard to distinguish clinically. Nevertheless, correction of breathing disorders may be a necessary tool in the therapeutic management of refractory hypertension associated with OSA.

Calhoun DA. Use of aldosterone antagonists in resistant hypertension. *Prog Cardiovasc Dis* 2006;48:387–396. (Rationale for the application of aldosterone antagonists is discussed in this publication.)

Drager LF, Pereira AC, Barreto-Filho JA, et al. Phenotypic characteristics associated with hypertension in patients with obstructive sleep apnea. *J Hum Hypertens* 2006;20(7):523–528. (This article provides a description of patients with resistant hypertension who have sleep apnea syndrome.)

Gaddam KK, Pratt-Ubunama MN, Calhoun DA. Aldosterone antagonists: Effective add-on therapy for the treatment of resistant hypertension. *Expert Rev Cardiovasc Ther* 2006;4:353–359.

Norman D, Loredo JS, Nelesen RA, et al. Effects of continuous positive airway pressure versus supplemental oxygen on 24 hour ambulatory blood pressure. *Hypertension* 2006;47:840–845.

Sartori M, Calo LA, Mascagna V, et al. Aldosterone and refractory hypertension: A prospective cohort study. *Am J Hypertens* 2006;19:373–379.

Wolk R, Somers VK. Obesity-related cardiovascular disease: Implications of obstructive sleep apnea. *Diabetes Obes Metab* 2006;8:250–260.

KEY POINTS: REFRACTORY HYPERTENSION

1. In most patients with chronic primary hypertension, blood pressure (BP) can be controlled with changes in lifestyle and with one or two drugs; in some, however, the BP remains uncontrolled even on a three-drug regimen. These patients have refractory or resistant hypertension.

2. If a patient's BP is not controlled with multiple antihypertensive drugs but one of them is not a diuretic, it should not be diagnosed as "refractory" hypertension.

3. In the management of refractory hypertension, it is essential to determine the potential cause(s) for the failure of the patient to respond to an appropriate regimen. If an identifiable cause is not found or cannot be corrected, suitable changes should be made in the treatment plan including effective diuretic therapy and proper utilization of potent classes of antihypertensive drugs such as direct vasodilators.

4. The problem of refractory hypertension can be treated successfully in a systematic fashion and on a rational basis.

CHAPTER 71

HYPERTENSIVE EMERGENCIES

William J. Elliott, MD, PhD

1. **How does a "hypertensive emergency" differ from "hypertensive urgency"?**
   A "hypertensive emergency" is a clinical situation in which severely elevated blood pressure is associated with acute, progressive target organ damage that needs to be treated immediately with the safe and controlled reduction of blood pressure. "Hypertensive urgencies" (if they truly exist) are characterized by elevated blood pressures but in a patient who has no acute, progressive target organ damage; these are typically treated with oral antihypertensive medications and close follow-up thereafter. Typical scenarios that are hypertensive emergencies include the following:
   - Hypertensive encephalopathy (typically a diagnosis of exclusion; see later)
   - Acute left ventricular failure and/or pulmonary edema (see later)
   - Subarachnoid or intracerebral hemorrhage
   - Acute aortic dissection (for which the target blood pressure is <120/70 mm Hg, within 20 minutes; see later)
   - Acute myocardial infarction or acute coronary syndrome
   - Adrenergic crisis (e.g., pheochromocytoma, phencyclidine, or cocaine overdose; see later)
   - Glomerulonephritis or acute renal failure
   - Epistaxis, gross hematuria, or threatened suture lines after vascular surgery
   - Eclampsia

   The absolute level of blood pressure does not distinguish between emergencies and urgencies. Patients who were previously normotensive can develop a hypertensive emergency with a blood pressure that is only 30 to 50 mm Hg higher than their usual and customary blood pressure (e.g., 160/100 in a woman with pre-eclampsia). Conversely, some patients with chronic hypertension remain asymptomatic and might qualify as only hypertensive urgencies, even with a blood pressure of 250/150 mm Hg. Seldom, if ever, does such a high blood pressure require hospitalization if there is no acute target organ damage.

2. **What is "malignant hypertension," and how does it differ from "accelerated hypertension"?**
   Malignant hypertension is the term historically given when severely elevated blood pressure was accompanied by retinal hemorrhages, exudates, and, originally, papilledema. The term arose in the 1920s when no effective treatment was available because the prognosis of patients with this condition was similar to that of those with cancer. Now that treatment is possible and effective, the term is used predominantly by hospital-based DRG coders. In the last millennium, "accelerated hypertension" was severely elevated blood pressure without papilledema; this term is now only rarely used outside its historical context.

3. **What are the epidemiologic characteristics of patients who present with a hypertensive emergency?**
   Most such patients have a history of stage 2 hypertension that has not been adequately treated, most commonly as a result of nonadherence to prescribed medication. In the last millennium, patients presenting with "malignant hypertension" typically had very high blood pressures (before treatment) and were often cigarette smokers. Secondary hypertension, especially renovascular hypertension, was often found in patients with Keith-Wagener-Barker

Grade III (hemorrhages/exudates) or IV (frank papilledema) retinopathy; chronic kidney disease was also very common in such patients in the 1970s.

4. **What is the pathophysiology of "malignant hypertension"?**
A rapid and sustained rise in blood pressure causes endothelial dysfunction and then frank arteritis, leading to platelet and fibrin deposition within the vessel and eventually fibrinoid necrosis. The juxtaglomerular apparatus of the kidney releases renin when it senses relative ischemia, which increases circulating angiotensin II levels, and causes severe vasoconstriction. The kidney responds to the elevated blood pressure with natriuresis, causing relative volume depletion and further activating the renin-angiotensin-aldosterone system. These events typically reinforce each other and lead to the "vicious cycle" of increasing blood pressure and worsening vascular function.

5. **What were the typical pathologic findings in "malignant hypertension?"**
The patient's blood vessels undergo myointimal proliferation (and medial thickening, leading to the "onion-skin" appearance) and fibrinoid necrosis. If the process is chronic, vascular smooth muscle hypertrophy occurs and collagen deposits in the small vessels and arterioles; this process usually takes too long to occur in larger arteries.

6. **Historically, what were the common clinical features of "malignant hypertension?"**
Typically the blood pressure was very high (often diastolic >140 mm Hg). The optic fundi showed bilateral papilledema, often with hemorrhages and exudates in the periphery. Hypertensive encephalopathy was common, usually preceded by headache, somnolence, visual changes, and confusion. Microangiopathic hemolytic anemia, with schistocytes and helmet cells on peripheral smear, and increased serum lactate dehydrogenase often were associated with fibrinoid necrosis of arterioles. Normal renal function was distinctly unusual; most patients had oliguria, azotemia, proteinuria, and (usually microscopic) hematuria. The major reason malignant hypertension is not so common today is that, in early studies, even a single antihypertensive drug reduced the risk of this problem by more than 90%.

7. **How does one diagnose hypertensive encephalopathy?**
Such patients typically present with very high blood pressures and an altered mental status. The optic fundi can provide a strong clue if Grade III or IV retinopathy is seen. Usually other evidence of hypertensive target-organ damage is present (e.g., hematuria, elevated serum creatinine, electrocardiographic evidence of left ventricular hypertrophy). Although the differential diagnosis in such a patient is long and complex, consideration can be given to starting a short-acting, easily titratable, intravenous antihypertensive agent while transporting the patient to the computed tomography scanner. It is often rewarding to see an improvement in central nervous system function after the blood pressure is reduced even by 10%. However, other causes of stupor and coma have to be considered and appropriately evaluated and eliminated before one can be certain of the diagnosis of hypertensive encephalopathy.

8. **What are the major principles of treating a patient with a hypertensive emergency?**
The most important thing to remember is that the patient has had the autoregulatory capacity of vascular beds "reset," with the pressure-flow curve shifted up and to the right, compared to normal, during the days to weeks before the medical encounter. This allowed them, over time, to constrict and continue to deliver an appropriate (if not quite normal) flow of blood and oxygen, despite the very high blood pressures. The major idea of treatment is to gradually reduce the blood pressure for a sufficient time period to allow these vascular beds to adjust to the "new, lower" pressure, without causing a precipitous decline in blood flow.

Most authorities recommend admission to an intensive care unit, although a method to monitor blood pressure (intra-arterial line versus automated oscillometric device), an intravenous line to deliver the antihypertensive agent, and an attentive physician can begin the process in the Emergency Department.

No trials have been done to establish a blood pressure target (Table 71-1), but most authorities recommend a decrease in mean arterial pressure by about 10% in the first hour and no more than 25% during the first 2 hours. Most patients tolerate a blood pressure of about 160 to 180/100 mm Hg well after the first 2 hours or so, but the antihypertensive medication dose should be individualized and should be reduced if deterioration occurs when the blood pressure is decreased "too fast" or "too far." After the blood pressure has been stabilized (usually for 6–24 hours) and after oral treatment is administered, intravenous antihypertensive therapy can be withdrawn.

9. **What drugs are used for treatment of hypertensive emergencies?**
   Fortunately, many drugs are available (Table 71-2), each with their own advantages and disadvantages. Nitroprusside is the most widely available, has the shortest time to effect, and can be easily titrated up or down as needed. It breaks down to cyanide and thiocyanate, which can cause metabolic acidosis, an anion gap, blurred vision, tinnitus, and/or confusion; the risk of these adverse effects increases with the dose and duration of infusion. The newer agents— esmolol, fenoldopam, and clevidipine—are reasonably short-acting agents that are a beta blocker, dopamine-1 agonist, and calcium antagonist, respectively; these attributes can be helpful in certain clinical scenarios (see Table 71-1).

10. **What is the long-term prognosis of patients with a hypertensive emergency?**
    With prompt and effective therapy, it depends more on renal function at presentation (the higher the serum creatinine, the greater the risk of dialysis) and the ability of the patient to take prescription antihypertensive drugs. Although the prognosis was dismal (10% 1-year survival) before antihypertensive drug therapy was available, most recent series show higher than 95% 1-year survival rates. Although renal function sometimes deteriorates acutely during and after blood pressure lowering (except, perhaps, with fenoldopam), some patients have recovered enough renal function to discontinue dialysis if the blood pressure can be well controlled on an outpatient basis.

11. **How does a hypertensive emergency with aortic dissection differ from others?**
    Such patients typically present with a characteristic history of chest or back pain, often described as "tearing" or "ripping," with radiation to the arms or upper abdomen. Typically blood pressures are lower in the legs than in the arms, and a murmur of acute aortic regurgitation may be present. A chest x-ray may show nothing, a widened aortic shadow, or a widened mediastinum; in appropriate patients, consideration should be given to initiating therapy before the imaging study (transesophageal echocardiogram, computed tomogram of the chest) is completed.
    Therapy for aortic dissection differs in three important ways from other hypertensive emergencies. Therapy should include a beta blocker (unless otherwise contraindicated) to decrease the shear forces driving the dissection. The blood pressure target is <120 mm Hg systolic, and it should be achieved within 20 minutes of starting therapy to minimize progression. A cardiothoracic surgeon should be consulted quickly; type A dissections (proximal to the aortic arch) nearly always require emergent surgery, sometimes including valve replacement.

12. **How does a hypertensive emergency with acute left ventricular failure differ from other hypertensive emergencies?**
    These patients typically present with dyspnea; cough; frothy, pink-tinged sputum; and hypoxia. Physical examination nearly always shows distended neck veins, râles in most of the lung fields, and an S_3. Chest x-ray typically shows pulmonary vascular redistribution, hilar congestion, and diffuse infiltrates in most of the lung fields. Prompt therapy with oxygen, intravenous loop diuretics, morphine, and nitroglycerin are usually effective acutely, although nitroprusside may be added to help lower both preload and afterload if nitroglycerin is an insufficient hypotensive agent. Appropriate evaluation of the reason for the acute decompensated heart failure is appropriate during the intensive care unit stay. Intravenous enalaprilat has been shown in a small study to improve prognosis in these patients, but its hypotensive effect is variable and may lead to acute hypotension that is difficult to reverse.

TABLE 71-1. TYPES OF HYPERTENSIVE EMERGENCIES, WITH SUGGESTED DRUG THERAPY AND BLOOD PRESSURE TARGETS

Type of Emergency	Drug of Choice	Blood Pressure Target
Aortic dissection	Beta blocker + nitroprusside*	120 mm Hg systolic in 20 minutes (if possible)
CARDIAC		
Ischemia/infarction	Nitroglycerin, nitroprusside, nicardipine, or clevidipine	Cessation of ischemia
Heart failure (or pulmonary edema)	Nitroprusside* and/or nitroglycerin	Improvement in failure (typically only a 10% to 15% decrease is required)
HEMORRHAGIC		
Epistaxis, gross hematuria, or threatened suture lines	Any (perhaps with anxiolytic agent)	To decrease bleeding rate (typically only 10% to 15% reduction over 1–2 hours is required)
OBSTETRIC		
Eclampsia or pre-eclampsia	MgSO₄, hydralazine, methyldopa	Typically <90 mm Hg diastolic but often lower
CATECHOLAMINE EXCESS STATES		
Pheochromocytoma	Phentolamine	To control paroxysms
Drug withdrawal	Drug withdrawn	Typically only one dose necessary
Cocaine (and similar drugs)	Phentolamine	Typically only 10% to 15% reduction over 1–2 hours
RENAL		
Major hematuria or acute renal impairment	Fenoldopam	0% to 25% reduction in mean arterial pressure over 1–12 hours
NEUROLOGIC		
Hypertensive encephalopathy	Nitroprusside*	25% reduction over 2–3 hours.
Acute head injury/ trauma	Nitroprusside*	0% to 25% reduction over 2–3 hours (controversial)

*Some physicians prefer an intravenous infusion of clevidipine, fenoldopam, or nicardipine, none of which has potentially toxic metabolites, over nitroprusside. Acute improvements in renal function occur during therapy with fenoldopam but not with nitroprusside.
Adapted from Elliott WJ. Management of hypertensive emergencies. *Curr Hypertens Rep* 2003;5: 486–492.

TABLE 71-2. USEFUL DRUGS FOR HYPERTENSIVE EMERGENCIES

Drug	Onset of Action	Elimination Half-Life	Usual Dose (IV)	Positive Attributes	Risks
Sodium nitroprusside	Seconds	~2 minutes	0.25–8.0 µg/kg/min	Very effective; fast-acting, easily titrated or stopped	Photosensitive; metabolized to cyanide and thiocyanate
Nitroglycerin	2–5 minutes	1–4 minutes	5–100 µg/min	Useful for coronary ischemia	Methemoglobinemia; special tubing needed
Labetalol	5–10 minutes	5–6 hours	20–80 mg bolus every 10–15 minutes, or 0.5–2.0 mg/min infusion	Useful for coronary ischemia; oral formulation available	Asthma, acute left ventricular dysfunction
Enalaprilat	15–30 minutes	11 hours	1.25–5.0 mg every 6 hours	Useful in left ventricular dysfunction	Avoid in acute myocardial infarction
Nicardipine	2–5 minutes	45 minutes, 14 hours	5 mg/hour, increased to 15 mg/hour	Useful for cardiac ischemia	Interacts with cimetidine, cyclosporine; oral formulation available
Esmolol	5–10 minutes	9 minutes	250–500 µg/kg/min for 1 minute, then 50–100 µg/kg/min	Useful for aortic dissection and perioperative state	Asthma, left ventricular dysfunction
Fenoldopam	2–5 minutes	5 minutes	0.1–0.3 µg/kg/min initially, increase 0.1–0.2 every 15 minutes	Improves several parameters of renal function	Raises intraocular pressure; may cause hypokalemia
Clevidipine	2–4 minutes	~1 minute	1–2 mg/hour, increased every 90 seconds	Useful for cardiac ischemia, perioperative state	Photosensitive; comes in lipid emulsion

KEY POINTS: HYPERTENSIVE EMERGENCIES

1. Hypertensive emergencies are clinical scenarios in which acute target organ damage is progressive and which require the blood pressure to be reduced gradually and safely within minutes to hours.

2. The most common clinical scenarios involving hypertensive emergencies include acute myocardial infarction, pulmonary edema, intracranial hemorrhage, glomerulonephritis, eclampsia, adrenergic crisis, uncontrolled bleeding, or hypertensive encephalopathy.

3. The standard recommendation for lowering blood pressure in the setting of a hypertensive emergency is to lower mean arterial pressure by about 10% in the first hour and a further 10% to 15% in the next hour—**NOT** <140/90 mm Hg.

4. Although many intravenous antihypertensive drugs can be used for hypertensive emergencies, the pharmacokinetic advantages of sodium nitroprusside (very short onset of action, very short elimination half-life) usually outweigh the risk of cyanide or thiocyanate poisoning, which are more common with high doses or long durations of therapy.

5. Acute aortic dissection differs from all other hypertensive emergencies because the blood pressure target is <120/80 mm Hg within 20 minutes of diagnosis and an intravenous beta blocker is used to decrease the shear stress on the ruptured intimal flap.

13. **How does an adrenergic crisis differ from other hypertensive emergencies?**
These patients present with an acutely increased alpha-adrenergic tone, typically because of excess catecholamines or their congeners. Abrupt withdrawal of oral alpha-2 adrenergic agonists (e.g., clonidine, guanabenz, guanfacine), cocaine and/or amphetamine ingestion, or the ingestion of tyramine-containing foodstuffs during monoamine oxidase inhibitor therapy are all good examples. These patients are usually treated successfully with phentolamine (or the alpha-2 agonist that they stopped abruptly), although some physicians prefer labetalol, which also has beta-adrenergic inhibitory effects.

14. **Are there some drugs that should not be used to treat hypertensive emergencies?**
Generally, drugs that can cause precipitous hypotension and cannot be recalled or stopped should be avoided. Nifedipine capsules once were widely used for hypertensive urgencies and even emergencies, but the U.S. Food and Drug Administration did not grant this indication because the blood pressure lowering was unpredictable and sometimes caused serious hypotension, shock, and death. Most physicians prefer to use drugs that have a short "time to effect," can be easily titrated, and have a short "off time" just in case the blood pressure drops and the medication has to be reduced in dosage or stopped altogether. Drugs with a long elimination half-life, even when given intravenously, are more likely to cause a problem in these conditions.

BIBLIOGRAPHY

1. Agabiti-Rosei E, Salvetti M, Farsang C. European Society of Hypertension Scientific Newsletter: Treatment of hypertensive urgencies and emergencies. *J Hypertens* 2006;24:2482–2485.
2. Deeks ED, Keating GM, Kearn SJ. Clevidipine: A review of its use in the management of acute hypertension. *Am J Cardiovasc Drugs* 2009;9:117–134.
3. Elliott WJ. Clinical features in the management of selected hypertensive emergencies. *Prog Cardiovasc Dis* 2006;48:316–325.
4. Feldstein C. Management of hypertensive crises. *Am J Ther* 2007;14:135–139.

5. Flanigan JS, Vitberg D. Hypertensive emergency and severe hypertension: What to treat, who to treat, and how to treat. *Med Clin North Am* 2006;90:439–451.
6. Grassi D, O'Flaherty M, Pellizzari M, et al.; for the REHASE Program Investigators. Hypertensive urgencies in the emergency department: Evaluating blood pressure response to rest and to antihypertensive drugs with different profiles. *J Clin Hypertens (Greenwich)* 2008;10:662–667.
7. Moser M, Izzo JL Jr, Bisognano J. Hypertensive emergencies. *J Clin Hypertens (Greenwich)* 2006;8:275–281.
8. Perez MI, Musini VM. Pharmacologic interventions for hypertensive emergencies: A Cochrane systematic review. *J Hum Hypertens* 2008;22:596–607.
9. Ram CV, Silverstein RL. Treatment of hypertensive urgencies and emergencies. *Curr Hypertens Rep* 2009;11:307–314.
10. Varon J. The diagnosis and treatment of hypertensive crises. *Postgrad Med* 2009;121:5–13.

PHARMACOLOGIC TREATMENT OF HYPERTENSION

C. Venkata S. Ram, MD, and Edgar V. Lerma, MD

CHAPTER 72

1. **When is pharmacologic treatment of hypertension indicated?**

   When an individual's blood pressure (BP) does not fall below goal after a suitable period of intensive lifestyle modifications, antihypertensive drug therapy is universally recommended. Various guideline committees recommend different initial therapies, but there is general agreement that antihypertensive drug therapy is one of the major reasons for the decline in stroke and coronary heart disease mortality over the past 50 years. Compared to placebo or no treatment, active drug treatment in clinical trials significantly reduced fatal or nonfatal stroke by ~33%, myocardial infarction by ~15%, heart failure by ~36%, and all-cause mortality by ~12%. Most recent meta-analyses suggest that the cardiovascular protective effects of all antihypertensive drugs can be most easily attributed to their BP-lowering properties, despite the fact that they do so by different molecular mechanisms.

   Canadian Hypertension Education Program. Recommendations—2010. Available at: http://hypertension.ca/chep/recommendations-2010/. Accessed March 21, 2010.

   Chobanian AV, Bakris GL, Black HR, et al. Seventh Report of the Joint National Committee on Prevention, Detection, Evaluation and Treatment of High Blood Pressure. National High Blood Pressure Education Program Coordinating Committee. *Hypertension* 2003;42:1206–1252.

   Littlejohns P, Ranson P, Sealey C, et al.; for the National Collaborating Centre for Chronic Conditions. Hypertension: Management of hypertension in adults in primary care (partial update of NICE Clinical Guideline 18). National Institute for Health and Clinical Excellence. Available at www.nice.org.uk/page.aspx?o=278167. Accessed June 25, 2006.

   Mancia G, De Backer G, Dominiczak A, et al. 2007 Guidelines for the management of arterial hypertension. Task Force for the Management of Arterial Hypertension of the European Society of Hypertension and the European Society of Cardiology. *J Hypertens* 2007;25:1105–1187.

   Turnbull F; for the Blood Pressure Lowering Treatment Trialists' Collaboration. Effects of different blood-pressure-lowering regimens on major cardiovascular events: Results of prospectively-designed overviews of randomised trials. *Lancet* 2003;362:1527–1535.

   Turnbull F; for the Blood Pressure Lowering Treatment Trialists' Collaboration. Blood pressure-dependent and independent effects of agents that inhibit the renin-angiotensin system. *J Hypertens* 2007;25:951–958.

   Turnbull F, Neal B, Ninomiya T, et al.; for the Blood Pressure Lowering Treatment Trialists' Collaboration. Effects of different regimens to lower blood pressure on major cardiovascular events in older and younger adults: Meta-analysis of randomised trials. *BMJ* 2008;336:1121–1123.

2. **What are the current recommended goals for treatment of hypertension?**

   Although epidemiologic data indicate that a BP <115/75 mm Hg is associated with the lowest risk of cardiovascular morbidity and mortality, several recent studies have concluded that "lower BP" is not necessarily better to prevent cardiovascular events. Traditionally, the BP target has been <140/90 mm Hg for all patients with hypertension; more recently, a target of <130/80 mm Hg has been recommended for patients with diabetes, people with chronic kidney disease (CKD), or those with established heart disease. These targets are controversial because the evidence base for each consists of subgroup analyses of clinical trials and/or extrapolations from other therapeutic areas (e.g., lipid-lowering therapy, for which a progressively lower target is beneficial for patients at higher risk). Relatively few outcome-based clinical trials have been done that randomized subjects with hypertension to different BP targets. A recent exception is the Action to Control Cardiovascular Risk in Diabetes blood pressure (ACCORD-BP) trial, which showed no significant benefit in patients with hypertension and diabetes randomly assigned to a systolic BP target of <120 mm Hg. Because of the lack of direct clinical trial evidence, various guidelines offer different BP targets for different hypertensive subgroups, although most agree that higher-risk subjects ought to be treated to a lower-than-usual BP.

ACCORD Study Group, Cushman WC, Evans GW, et al. Effects of intensive blood-pressure control in type 2 diabetes mellitus. *N Engl J Med* 2010;29;362(17):1575–1585.

Age-specific relevance of usual blood pressure to vascular mortality: A meta-analysis of individual data for one million adults in 61 prospective studies. Prospective Studies Collaborative. *Lancet* 2002;360:1903–1913.

American Diabetes Association. Executive summary: Standards of medical care in diabetes—2010. *Diabetes Care* 2010;33:S4–S10.

Arguedas JA, Perez MI, Wright JM. Treatment blood pressure targets for hypertension. *Cochrane Database Syst Rev* 2009;3:CD004349.

Levey AS, Rocco MV, Anderson S, et al. K/DOQI clinical practice guidelines on hypertension and antihypertensive agents in chronic kidney disease. *Am J Kidney Dis* 2004;43 (Suppl 1):S1–S290.

Rosendorff C, Black HR, Cannon CP, et al. Treatment of hypertension in the prevention and management of ischemic heart disease. A Scientific Statement from the American Heart Association Council for High Blood Pressure Research and the Councils on Clinical Cardiology and Epidemiology and Prevention. *Circulation* 2007;115:2761–2788.

3. **What have we learned about monotherapy for hypertension?**
   There is growing awareness that a small minority of patients with hypertension reach their BP targets using only a single drug. In reality, therefore, guidelines that offer different recommendations for initial therapy of hypertension tend to converge once the initial drug's effect on BP is found to be insufficient. The most widely used classes of initial antihypertensive therapy include (in historical order) diuretics, calcium antagonists, angiotensin-converting enzyme (ACE) inhibitors, and angiotensin receptor blockers (ARBs). Some would place β-blockers second in this list, but recent meta-analyses (based in large part on clinical trials that used atenolol) suggest that an initial β-blocker is significantly inferior to other antihypertensive drugs in preventing cardiovascular events in patients with hypertension (Table 72-1).

   Most guideline committees agree that if a patient has a condition for which a specific type of antihypertensive drug improves prognosis, that medication can be used as initial therapy to lower BP. A hypertensive survivor of a recent myocardial infarction, for example, would benefit from a β-blocker to reduce the risk of death or recurrent infarction, so a β-blocker would be appropriate initial antihypertensive therapy in such a case. All guideline committees recognize the existence and importance of contraindications (including allergies), even for drugs that might otherwise be first-line choices. For patients with uncomplicated hypertension, different guideline committees disagree about the most appropriate initial therapy. In the United States, the Antihypertensive and Lipid-Lowering Treatment to Prevent Heart Attack Trial (ALLHAT) influenced the authors of the Seventh Report of the Joint National Committee on Prevention, Detection, Evaluation, and Treatment of High Blood Pressure (JNC 7) to recommend a low dose of a thiazide or thiazide-like diuretic for "most" uncomplicated Stage 1 (BP 140–159/90–99 mm Hg) hypertensives. In the United Kingdom, the Anglo-Scandinavian Cardiac Outcomes Trial (ASCOT) favored the calcium antagonist ± ACE inhibitor arm over the β-blocker ± diuretic arm, so their guidelines recommend a calcium channel blocker (CCB) or diuretic for older or African American patients with hypertension or an ACE inhibitor for younger, white patients. The European guidelines recognize that few will attain their individual BP target with monotherapy and therefore emphasize appropriate combinations more than initial treatment recommendations.

Dahlöf B, Sever PS, Poulter NR, et al. Prevention of cardiovascular events with an antihypertensive regimen of amlodipine adding perindopril as required versus atenolol adding bendroflumethiazide as required, in the Anglo-Scandinavian Cardiac Outcomes Trial-Blood Pressure Lowering Arm (ASCOT-BPLA): A multicentre randomised controlled trial. *Lancet* 2005;366:895–906.

TABLE 72-1. EFFECTS OF DIFFERENT CLASSES OF ANTIHYPERTENSIVE AGENTS ON SURROGATE MARKERS OF CARDIOVASCULAR DISEASE

	Central α-Agonists	α-Blockers	α-, β-Blocker	Vasodilator	β-Blockers	ACE Inhibitors	ATRAs	CCBs	Diuretics
METABOLIC									
LDL cholesterol	↑	↑	↑	↑	↑*↑	↑	↑	↑	↑
HDL cholesterol	↑	↓	↑	↑	↑↓	↑	↑	↑	↑
Insulin resistance	↑	↓	↑↓	↑↓	↑↓	↓	→	↑	↑↓
Glucose control	↑	↑	↑	↑	↑↓	↑↓	↑	=↓↑	↑↓
CARDIOVASCULAR									
Left ventricular hypertrophy	→	→	→	↑↓	→	→	→	→	↑↓
RENAL									
Microalbuminuria	↑	↑	↑↓	↑↓	↑↓	↓↓	↓↓	†↓↑↓	↑↓

* Only β-blockers with intrinsic sympathomimetic activity; only when used in high doses (e.g., 480 mg/day diltiazem, 480 mg/day verapamil, 90 mg/day nifedipine).

† Only nonhydropyridine calcium channel blockers (verapamil, diltiazem).

ACE = angiotensin-converting enzyme; ATRAs = angiotensin II receptor antagonists; CCBs = calcium channel blockers; LDL = low-density lipoprotein; HDL = high-density lipoprotein; → = no effect; ↑ = increase; ↓ = decrease.

From Johnson RJ, Feehally J. *Comprehensive Clinical Nephrology*, 2nd ed. Philadelphia: Mosby, 2003.

Lindholm LH, Carlberg B, Samuelsson O. Should β-blockers remain first choice in the treatment of primary hypertension? A meta-analysis. *Lancet* 2005;366:1545–1553.

Major outcomes in high-risk hypertensive patients randomized to angiotensin-converting enzyme inhibitor or calcium channel blocker vs. diuretic: The Antihypertensive and Lipid Lowering Treatment to Prevent Heart Attack Trial (ALLHAT). The ALLHAT Officers and Coordinators for the ALLHAT Collaborative Research Group. *JAMA* 2002;288:2981–2997.

Wiysong CS, Bradley H, Mayosi B, et al. Beta-blockers for hypertension. *Cochrane Database Syst Rev* 2007;1:CD002003.

4. **Is combination therapy better than monotherapy?**
   Recent meta-analyses have suggested that, for most antihypertensive drug classes, combining two different classes of drugs at moderate doses is more likely to lower BP than pushing to any one drug to its maximum dose. This may also be advantageous to avoid common adverse effects. The combination of a low-dose diuretic and an ACE inhibitor, ARB, or a (direct) renin inhibitor (DRI) is likely to maintain eukalemia and perhaps euglycemia. Combining a CCB with an ACE inhibitor, or probably an ARB, tends to reduce incidence and severity of pedal edema seen with higher-dose CCBs. Many single-pill combinations are marketed that contain such agents; this has the potential to improve long-term adherence to antihypertensive drug therapy, which is necessary for optimal cardiovascular risk reduction. Although JNC 7 recommended that combination therapy usually include a diuretic, the results of the recent Avoiding Cardiovascular events through COMbination therapy in Patients LIving with Systolic Hypertension (ACCOMPLISH) trial are likely to broaden the choices for combination therapy in the next set of U.S. guidelines. The U.S. Food and Drug Administration has recently approved several single-pill combination products for first-line therapy, typically when the probability of achieving goal BP with a single agent is small.

Jamerson K, Weber MA, Bakris GL, et al.; for the ACCOMPLISH Trial Investigators. Benazepril plus amlodipine or hydrochlorothiazide for hypertension in high-risk patients. *N Engl J Med* 2008;359:2417–2428.

Law MR, Morris JK, Wald NJ. Use of blood pressure lowering drugs in the prevention of cardiovascular disease: Meta-analysis of 147 randomised trials in the context of expectations from prospective epidemiological studies. *BMJ* 2009;338:b1665 doi:101136/bmj.b1665.

Wald DS, Law M, Morris JK, et al. Combination therapy versus monotherapy in reducing blood pressure: Meta-analysis on 11,000 participants from 42 trials. *Am J Med* 2009;122:290–300.

5. **What different classes of antihypertensive agents are currently available?**
   Diuretics, calcium channel blockers, ACE inhibitors, ARBs, DRIs, β-blockers, and α-blockers are available.

6. **Discuss the use of diuretics.**
   Diuretics were the first drug class to show benefits in patients with hypertension, although they were usually used in combination with other agents, even in the early trials. They primarily work by reducing extracellular sodium and volume, although some also have vasodilatory properties, perhaps at the calcium channel. Thiazide and thiazide-like diuretics, which act primarily in the distal convoluted tubule, are the most widely used, particularly in patients with normal renal function, although the doses in current use are much lower than those used in early clinical trials. The lower doses reduce the incidence and severity of adverse effects, particularly hypokalemia, which is blamed for some of the long-term metabolic effects of thiazides. The BP-lowering effects of diuretics can be overcome with dietary or other sources of sodium and with the use of nonsteroidal anti-inflammatory drugs (NSAIDs). Most authorities agree that chlorthalidone is both more potent in lowering BP and has a longer duration of action than hydrochlorothiazide (HCTZ); these properties may account for the seemingly disparate results of ALLHAT (in which chlorthalidone was "superior in preventing one or more major forms of cardiovascular disease") compared to ACCOMPLISH (in which the benazepril + HCTZ arm fared worse than the benazepril + amlodipine arm).

   Diuretics that act primarily in the thick ascending limb of the loop of Henle (so-called "loop diuretics") are usually required for patients with Stage 3 and higher CKD. They are also often used for patients with heart failure but are typically given twice daily. If short-acting furosemide or bumetanide is given once daily, fluid accumulation can occur during the 12 to 18 hours before the morning dose, particularly if the evening meal contains most of the day's dietary sodium. Both loop and thiazide diuretics are sulfonamides, so they are usually contraindicated for people with true sulfa allergies. For these people, oral ethacrynic acid has again become available for twice-daily use.

Although several potassium-sparing diuretics are available, they are used mostly in combination with thiazides. The two aldosterone inhibitors, spironolactone and eplerenone, are used largely in patients with heart failure or hyperaldosteronism (either idiopathic or as a result of sleep apnea).

Elliott WJ, Grimm RH Jr. How to use diuretics in clinical practice—One opinion. *J Clin Hypertens* (Greenwich) 2008;10:856–862.

Wall GC, Gibner D, Craig S. Ethacrynic acid and the sulfa-sensitive patient. *Arch Intern Med* 2003;163: 116–117.

7. Discuss the use of calcium channel blockers.

The many available CCBs can be divided pharmacologically into two subgroups: dihydropyridines (nifedipine) and the nondihydropyridines (verapamil and diltiazem and related compounds). The latter typically have negative inotropic and chronotropic properties, whereas the former are more vasoselective and can increase heart rate, especially acutely if immediate-release preparations are given. All CCBs inhibit the flux of calcium into smooth muscle cells, resulting in vasodilation. Many CCBs are approved for patients with angina pectoris. Verapamil can cause dose-related constipation, and immediate-release dihydropyridine compounds can cause flushing, tachycardia, and dose-dependent pedal edema; only the latter is seen with long-acting preparations. The BP-lowering of CCBs is generally little affected by dietary sodium or NSAIDs. Although studies in the last millennium suggested that CCBs were associated with a significantly higher risk of cardiovascular events than other antihypertensive drug classes, recent meta-analyses of comparative clinical trials indicate that they are as effective in preventing both stroke and coronary heart disease as diuretics, although the risk of heart failure is significantly increased (by about 44%), whether dihydropyridine or not. This may be a result, in part, of the propensity (especially for dihydropyridine compounds) to cause dose-dependent pedal edema and for verapamil and diltiazem to reduce left ventricular ejection fraction.

Elliott WJ, Basu S, Meyer PM. Initial drugs for stroke prevention in hypertensive patients: Network and Bayesian meta-analyses of clinical trial data (abstract). *J Clin Hypertens* (Greenwich) 2009;11(Suppl A):A7.

Elliott WJ, Basu S, Meyer PM. Initial drugs for coronary heart disease prevention in hypertensive patients: Network and Bayesian meta-analyses of clinical trial data (abstract). *J Clin Hypertens* (Greenwich) 2009;11(Suppl A):A7.

Elliott WJ, Basu S, Meyer PM. Initial drugs for heart failure prevention in hypertensive patients: Network and Bayesian meta-analyses of clinical trial data (abstract). *Circulation* 2008;118 (Suppl 2):S886.

Pahor M, Psaty BM, Alderman MH, et al. Health outcomes associated with calcium antagonists compared with other first-line antihypertensive therapies: A meta-analysis of randomised controlled trials. *Lancet* 2000;356:1949–1951.

Psaty BM, Heckbert SR, Koepsell TD, et al. The risk of myocardial infarction associated with antihypertensive drug therapies. *JAMA* 1995;274:620–625.

8. Discuss the use of ACE inhibitors.

ACE inhibitors inhibit the conversion of angiotensin I to angiotensin II, thereby producing vasodilation and lowering BP. Because the hydrolysis of bradykinin is also inhibited by these drugs, cough (7% to 12%) and angioedema (0.7%) can occur. Like any drug that inhibits the renin-angiotensin system, ACE inhibitors can cause acute renal failure in patients with renal artery stenosis, and they are teratogenic. These drugs cause birth defects, even if given during the first trimester of pregnancy.

ACE inhibitors are usually effective in lowering BP, but their efficacy is reduced by dietary or other sources of sodium, and renal function may be further threatened if given with NSAIDs. In clinical trials, they are among the most effective drugs in preventing coronary heart disease, which some believe is a "benefit beyond BP control." ACE inhibitors are also very useful for patients with heart failure or CKD (particularly type 1 diabetics and nondiabetic CKD). All ACE inhibitors are generically available, so they are often favored by formulary committees over other inhibitors of the renin-angiotensin system for financial reasons.

Cooper WO, Hernandez-Diaz S, Arbogast PG, et al. Major congenital malformations after first-trimester exposure to ACE inhibitors. *N Engl J Med* 2006;354:2443–2451.

Verdecchia P, Reboldi G, Angeli F, et al. Angiotensin-converting enzyme inhibitors and calcium channel blockers for coronary heart disease and stroke prevention. *Hypertension* 2005;46:386–392.

9. **Discuss the use of angiotensin receptor blockers.**

   ARBs inhibit the binding of angiotensin II to its subtype 1 receptor, which also results in vasodilation and BP lowering. They do not cause as much cough or angioedema as ACE inhibitors, although the risks of teratogenicity or acute renal failure in the setting of renal artery stenosis seen with ACE inhibitors are not diminished. Some ARBs have been approved for type 2 diabetic nephropathy and heart failure with diminished left ventricular function, either alone or in combination with ACE inhibitors. Several recent clinical trials of ARBs have provided disappointing results, either compared to CCBs (VALUE) or placebo (TRANSCEND, PRoFESS). The design of these trials has been criticized because either the dose was too low to cause equivalent BP lowering (e.g., VALUE), or the randomized agents were given in addition to other antihypertensive and other preventive therapies rather than as initial treatments (TRANSCEND, PRoFESS). There are no direct comparisons of diuretics with ARBs because nearly all the ARB trials used a diuretic as second-line therapy. The major advantage of ARBs seems to be their relatively benign adverse effect profile; this probably accounts for why they have the highest persistence rates of all antihypertensive agents in general clinical practice. The combination of an ARB plus an ACE inhibitor was found to lower BP only a little more than either drug alone, not significantly improve clinical outcomes, and be associated with a much higher rate of adverse effects (especially renal) in the ONTARGET trial.

Brenner BM, Cooper ME, de Zeeuw D, et al. Effects of losartan on renal and cardiovascular outcomes in patients with Type 2 diabetes and nephropathy. Reduction of Endpoints in Non-Insulin Dependent Diabetes Mellitus with the Angiotensin II Antagonist Losartan (RENAAL) Study Group. *N Engl J Med* 2001;345: 861–869.

Julius S, Kjeldsen S, Weber M, et al. Outcomes in hypertensive patients at high cardiovascular risk treated with regimens based on valsartan or amlodipine: The VALUE randomised trial. *Lancet* 2004;363:2022–2031.

Lewis EJ, Hunsicker LG, Clarke WR, et al. Renoprotective effect of the angiotensin-receptor antagonist irbesartan in patients with nephropathy due to Type 2 diabetes. Collaborative Study Group. *N Engl J Med* 2001;345:851–860.

Maggioni AP, Anand I, Gottlieb SO, et al. Val-HeFT Investigators (Valsartan Heart Failure Trial). Effects of valsartan on morbidity and mortality in patients with heart failure not receiving angiotensin-converting enzyme inhibitors. *J Am Coll Cardiol* 2002;40:1414–1421.

McMurray JJV, Östergren J, Swedberg K, et al. Effects of candesartan in patients with chronic heart failure and reduced left-ventricular systolic function taking angiotensin-converting-enzyme inhibitors: The CHARM-Added trial. CHARM Investigators and Committees. *Lancet* 2003;362:767–771.

Telmisartan, ramipril or both in patients at high risk for vascular events. ONTARGET Investigators. *N Engl J Med* 2008;358:1547–1549.

Yusuf S; for the Telmisartan Randomised AssessmeNt Study in ACE iNtolerant subjects with cardiovascular Disease (TRANSCEND) Investigators. Effects of the angiotensin-receptor blocker telmisartan on cardiovascular events in high-risk patients intolerant to angiotensin-converting enzyme inhibitors: A randomised controlled trial. *Lancet* 2008;371:1174–1183.

Yusuf S, Diener H-C, Sacco R, et al.; for the PRoFESS Study Group. Telmisartan to Prevent Recurrent Stroke and Cardiovascular Events. *N Engl J Med* 2008;359:1225–1237.

10. **Discuss the use of (direct) renin inhibitors.**

    In the past few years, compounds that inhibit the binding of renin to angiotensinogen and block the production of angiotensin I have been developed. These compounds block the renin-angiotensin system at its rate-limiting step and lower BP in a slightly dose-dependent fashion. The first compound of this class (aliskiren) to market has an excellent tolerability profile and combines well with a low-dose diuretic, a CCB, and even with an ARB, although hyperkalemia and impaired renal function have been seen. Because this is a new class of drugs, no long-term outcomes studies are available, but the compound has benefit in short-term trials using surrogate outcomes in heart failure, albuminuria, and left ventricular hypertrophy.

McMurray JJV, Pitt B, Latini R, et al.; for the ALOFT Investigators. Effects of the oral direct renin inhibitor aliskiren in patients with symptomatic heart failure. *Circ Heart Fail* 2008;1:17–24.

Oparil S, Yarows SA, Patel S, et al. Efficacy and safety of combined use of aliskiren and valsartan in patients with hypertension: A randomised, double-blind trial. *Lancet* 2007;370:221–229.

Parving H-H, Persson F, Lewis JB, et al.; for the AVOID Study Investigators. Aliskiren combined with losartan in type 2 diabetes and nephropathy. *N Engl J Med* 2008;358:2433–2446.

Solomon SD, Appelbaum E, Manning WJ, et al.; for the ALLAY Trial Investigators. Effect of the direct renin inhibitor, aliskiren, the angiotensin receptor blocker, losartan, or both, on left ventricular mass in patients with hypertension and left ventricular hypertrophy. *Circulation* 2009;119:530–537.

11. **Discuss the use of β-blockers.**
Although traditionally an acceptable first-line therapy for hypertension, β-blockers (particularly atenolol, which has 72% of the clinical trial data) are not currently recommended by either U.S. or U.K. guidelines as initial therapy for patients with uncomplicated hypertension. Four possible mechanisms have been invoked for how β-blockers reduce BP: they inhibit renin release from the juxtaglomerular apparatus of the kidney, diminish tonic sympathetic outflow from the central nervous system, they reduce myocardial contractility, they reduce cardiac output, and they vasodilate (some more than others). Some β-blockers have ancillary properties, including greater selectivity for the β_1-adrenoreceptor, water solubility, intrinsic sympathomimetic activity, membrane-stabilizing activity, or other properties (e.g., α_1-blocking activity, enhancement of nitric oxide bioavailability). Several β-blockers are effective second-line therapy (after ACE inhibitors) for heart failure. Adverse effects include bradycardia, fatigue, bronchoconstriction, dyspnea on exertion, and impairment of recognition of hypoglycemia in brittle diabetics. Many β-blockers decrease high-density lipoprotein cholesterol levels, raise triglycerides, and may impair glucose tolerance. They are nonetheless very useful for reducing pulse rate and BP and are often used in patients with aortic dissection and eight other U.S. Food and Drug Administration–approved indications.

KEY POINTS: PHARMACOLOGIC TREATMENT OF HYPERTENSION

1. Compared to placebo or no treatment, active drug treatment in clinical trials significantly reduced fatal or nonfatal stroke by ~33%, myocardial infarction by ~15%, heart failure by ~36%, and all-cause mortality by ~12%.

2. For most antihypertensive drug classes, combining two different classes of drugs at moderate doses is more likely to lower blood pressure than pushing the dose of any one drug to its maximum.

3. Although traditionally an acceptable first-line therapy for hypertension, β-blockers (particularly atenolol, which has ~72% of the clinical trial data) are not currently recommended by either U.S. or U.K. guidelines as initial therapy for patients with uncomplicated hypertension.

12. **Discuss the use of.**
α-blockers block neuromuscular transmission by occupying the post-synaptic α_1-adrenoceptor on the smooth muscle cell, causing vasodilation. Their major adverse effects are dizziness, headache, orthostatic hypotension (particularly first-dose hypotension), and an increased risk of falls and hip fractures). Since the early termination of the doxazosin arm of ALLHAT, resulting from a significantly increased risk of combined cardiovascular events (especially heart failure), α-blockers have been relegated to, at best, second-line therapy for uncomplicated

hypertension; doxazosin was used successfully as the third therapy in ASCOT. α-blockers are beneficial (in combination with other antihypertensive drugs) for men with symptoms of benign prostatic hyperplasia and have "favorable" effects on lipids and glucose metabolism.

ALLHAT Officers and Coordinators for the ALLHAT Collaborative Research Group. Diuretic versus alpha-blocker as first-step antihypertensive therapy: Final results from the Antihypertensive and Lipid-Lowering Treatment to Prevent Heart Attack Trial (ALLHAT). *Hypertension* 2003;42:239–246.

13. **Discuss the use of other antihypertensive drugs.**
Clonidine and other centrally acting α_2-agonists (e.g., methyldopa, guanfacine) work by decreasing sympathetic outflow from the central nervous system; in small doses, this causes vasodilation and BP lowering. In larger doses, sedation, dry mouth, drowsiness, and other symptomatic adverse effects occur, which are presumably the reason clonidine was the least well-tolerated drug in the Department of Veterans Affairs monotherapy trial. Sudden discontinuation of short-acting α_2-agonists causes major rebound hypertension, which is best treated by reinstituting therapy. Clonidine is the only transdermal antihypertensive available in the United States.

Direct vasodilators (hydralazine, minoxidil) are typically used with a diuretic and β-blocker to counteract their tendency to cause sodium and fluid retention and reflex tachycardia. Accordingly, these drugs are typically used third-line or higher, as was hydralazine in ALLHAT. Hydralazine is typically limited to ≤300 mg/day because of the risk of lupus; minoxidil causes hair growth that is not well tolerated by most women.

Materson BJ, Reda DJ, Cushman WC. Department of Veterans Affairs Single-Drug Therapy of Hypertension Study. Revised figures and new data. Department of Veterans Affairs Cooperative Study Group on Antihypertensive Agents. *Am J Hypertens* 1995;8:189–192.

CHAPTER 73

NONPHARMACOLOGIC TREATMENT OF HYPERTENSION

Martin J. Andersen, DO, and Rajiv Agarwal, MD

1. **What nonpharmacologic strategies can be used to treat hypertension?**
   Several nonpharmacologic strategies are recommended for improving blood pressure (BP) control among patients with essential hypertension. By extension, similar strategies may be effective among patients with chronic kidney disease (CKD). These strategies include salt restriction, weight loss, exercise, moderation of alcohol intake, and smoking cessation. Obstructive sleep apnea is recognized as an important problem among patients with CKD and its treatment may improve BP control.

   Agrawal V, Vanhecke TE, Rai B, et al. Albuminuria and renal function in obese adults evaluated for obstructive sleep apnea. *Nephron Clin Pract* 2009;113(3):c140–147.

2. **How effective is salt restriction?**
   Dietary sodium (Na) restriction is the single most important dietary advice to patients with CKD. The Institute of Medicine recommends no more than 1.5 g of dietary Na intake per day. However, Americans consume too much sodium—men consume more than 4 g of Na daily, whereas women consume more than 2.5 g. Excess Na intake has been causally linked to hypertension.

   Limiting Na intake may reduce target organ damage, end-stage renal disease, and cardiovascular morbidity and mortality. Limiting dietary Na from 3 g daily to 1.5 g daily reduces blood pressure both in hypertensive and nonhypertensive populations ($-6.7/-3.5$ mm Hg) (limiting Na intake may reduce BP to a greater degree among African Americans compared to other groups). Dietary sodium restriction may also markedly reduce urinary albumin excretion and arterial stiffness. Patients with type II diabetes who restrict dietary Na have lower microalbuminuria and ambulatory blood pressures. Dietary Na restriction to <1.6 g daily can regress left ventricular hypertrophy.

   Although dietary Na restriction is difficult, patients on Na-restricted diets acclimate to their diets after several weeks and begin to prefer low-Na foods. Population-wide reduction in Na intake to 1200 mg daily may translate into significant reductions in cardiovascular mortality and save approximately $10 to 24 billion dollars annually in health care costs. Because three fourths of Na is consumed from processed foods, the food industry and the government will need to work together to meet this goal.

   Bibbins-Domingo K, Chertow GM, Coxson PG, et al. Projected effect of dietary salt reductions on future cardiovascular disease. *N Engl J Med* 2010;362(7):590–599.

   Blais CA, Pangborn RM, Borhani NO, Ferrell MF, Prineas RJ, Laing B. Effect of dietary sodium restriction on taste responses to sodium chloride: a longitudinal study. *Am J Clin Nutr* 1986;44(2):232–243.

   Jula AM, Karanko HM. Effects on left ventricular hypertrophy of long-term nonpharmacological treatment with sodium restriction in mild-to-moderate essential hypertension. *Circulation* 1994;89(3):1023–1031.

   Krikken JA, Laverman GD, Navis G. Benefits of dietary sodium restriction in the management of chronic kidney disease. *Curr Opin Nephrol Hypertens* 2009;18(6):531–538.

   National Academy of Sciences. FDA should set standards for salt added to processed foods, prepared meals. April 20, 2010. http://www8.nationalacademies.org/onpinews/newsitem.aspx?RecordID=12818

   Sacks FM, Svetkey LP, Vollmer WM, et al. Effects on blood pressure of reduced dietary sodium and the Dietary Approaches to Stop Hypertension (DASH) diet. DASH-Sodium Collaborative Research Group. *N Engl J Med* 2001;344(1):3–10.

USDA Center for Nutrition Policy and Promotion. Dietary guidance on sodium: should we take it with a grain of salt? *Nutrition Insights* May 1997.

Vedovato M, Lepore G, Coracina A, et al Effect of sodium intake on blood pressure and albuminuria in Type 2 diabetic patients: the role of insulin resistance. *Diabetologia* 2004;47(2):300–303.

3. **How effective is the Dietary Approaches to Stop Hypertension (DASH) diet?**
   Americans, besides consuming excess salt, eat foods high in saturated fats and low in fiber and potassium (K). Low dietary K predisposes to Na retention, volume expansion, and hypertension. K supplementation can decrease BP in patients with hypertension. The mechanism by which fiber may prevent hypertension is not well delineated, although a recent meta-analysis showed that diets supplemented with fiber lower BP ($-1.13/-1.26$ mm Hg). The DASH diet emphasizes fruits and vegetables and low-fat foods. During an 8-week trial, the DASH diet, in patients with and without hypertension, lowered BPs by $-5.5/-3$ mm Hg. If the DASH diet is coupled with low Na intake (1.5 g daily), BPs will decrease by $-8.9/-4.5$ mm Hg compared to an average American diet. Unfortunately, National Health and Nutrition Examination Survey (NHANES) data show that compliance with the DASH diet is suboptimal. DASH dietary instructions have been published for easy reference. The safety and benefits of the DASH diet in patients with CKD, especially those with advanced CKD and hyperkalemia, remain to be demonstrated.

Appel LJ, Moore TJ, Obarzanek E, et al. A clinical trial of the effects of dietary patterns on blood pressure. DASH Collaborative Research Group. *N Engl J Med* 1997;336(16):1117–1124.

Gallen IW, Rosa RM, Esparaz DY, et al. On the mechanism of the effects of potassium restriction on blood pressure and renal sodium retention. *Am J Kidney Dis* 1998;31(1):19–27.

Krishna GG. Effect of potassium intake on blood pressure. *J Am Soc Nephrol* 1990;1(1):43–52.

Mellen PB, Gao SK, Vitolins MZ, Goff DC Jr. Deteriorating dietary habits among adults with hypertension: DASH dietary accordance, NHANES 1988-1994 and 1999-2004. *Arch Intern Med* 2008;168(3):308–314.

Sacks FM, Svetkey LP, Vollmer WM, et al. Effects on blood pressure of reduced dietary sodium and the Dietary Approaches to Stop Hypertension (DASH) diet. DASH-Sodium Collaborative Research Group. *N Engl J Med* 2001;344(1):3–10.

Streppel MT, Arends LR, van 't Veer P, Grobbee DE, Geleijnse JM. Dietary fiber and blood pressure: a meta-analysis of randomized placebo-controlled trials. *Arch Intern Med* 2005;165(2):150–156.

WebMD. High blood pressure and the DASH diet. http://www.webmd.com/hypertension-high-blood-pressure/dash-diet

4. **How effective is the treatment of obstructive sleep apnea?**
   Patients with obstructive sleep apnea (OSA) experience oxygen desaturation and sympathetic activation. Persistent, untreated OSA leads to hypertension. In the Wisconsin Sleep Cohort Study, 709 patients were followed for 4 years, and those patients with an apnea-hypopnea index of ≥5 had a more than twofold higher risk for hypertension compared to patients with no apnea-hypopnea events. In a retrospective study of 98 patients with OSA, those with resistant hypertension (defined as a BP ≥140/90 and taking three or more antihypertensive medications) saw improvement in mean arterial pressure (MAP) by 5.6 mm Hg after 1 year of continuous positive airway (CPAP) therapy. Of the patients with resistant hypertension, 71% simplified their medication regimen. A trial of 118 males with OSA showed that CPAP reduced ambulatory MAP by 2.5 mm Hg, with the benefits most pronounced in those with severe OSA. It is possible that the treatment of OSA will translate to similar benefits among patients with CKD.

Dernaika TA, Kinasewitz GT, Tawk MM. Effects of nocturnal continuous positive airway pressure therapy in patients with resistant hypertension and obstructive sleep apnea. *J Clin Sleep Med* 2009;5(2):103–107.

Peppard PE, Young T, Palta M, Skatrud J. Prospective study of the association between sleep-disordered breathing and hypertension. *N Engl J Med* 2000;342(19):1378–1384.

Pepperell JC, Ramdassingh-Dow S, Crosthwaite N, et al. Ambulatory blood pressure after therapeutic and subtherapeutic nasal continuous positive airway pressure for obstructive sleep apnoea: a randomised parallel trial. *Lancet* 2002;359(9302):204–210.

5. **What is the role of alcohol in hypertension?**

A morning BP surge is a risk factor for cardiovascular mortality, and studies show that alcohol is a risk factor for stroke—primarily hemorrhagic stroke. A possible mechanism is related to alcohol's circadian effect on BP. Acutely, alcohol ingestion will lower BP resulting from vasodilation. However, hours later, BP rises, possibly as a result of sympathetic activation. A recent Japanese trial demonstrated that ambulatory BPs surged in drinkers shortly after awakening.

The popular press has championed moderate alcohol intake as a treatment to reduce cardiovascular disease risk. Red wine, because of its antioxidant content, has been particularly noted. However, studies show that red wine's purported benefits result from the different drinking habits. Furthermore, the diet of red wine drinkers and those who imbibe primarily beer or spirits differs. Moderate alcohol intake (one to two drinks daily for males and one drink for females) may be beneficial by increasing high-density lipoprotein levels and lowering platelet aggregation. These benefits are seen mostly among older patients. These benefits disappear with higher amounts of alcohol intake or binge drinking. The World Health Organization estimates that worldwide alcohol contributes 16% to the risk of becoming hypertensive.

Klatsky AL. Alcohol and cardiovascular disease--more than one paradox to consider. Alcohol and hypertension: does it matter? Yes. *J Cardiovasc Risk* 2003;10(1):21–24.

Nakashita M, Ohkubo T, Hara A, et al. Influence of alcohol intake on circadian blood pressure variation in Japanese men: the Ohasama study. *Am J Hypertens* 2009;22(11):1171–1176.

Puddey IB, Beilin LJ. Alcohol is bad for blood pressure. *Clin Exp Pharmacol Physiol* 2006;33(9):847–852.

6. **How effective are weight loss and exercise?**

Weight loss and exercise are integral for hypertension control. Americans are increasingly becoming more sedentary and overweight. According to the latest NHANES data, 33% of adult males and 35% of adult females are obese (body mass index >30), and minority women are at highest risk for being obese. Obesity predisposes patients to become hypertensive. Weight loss through exercise improves hypertension because exercise improves antioxidant effects and reduces systemic vascular resistance. The PREMIER trial showed that intensive lifestyle modification, entailing a low-Na DASH diet, weight loss, and exercise, is successful in lowering BP in patients with pressures of 120 to 159/80 to 95 mm Hg. The average improvement, from baseline, was −4.3/2.6 mm Hg. Two recent meta-analyses showed that ~1 kg weight loss translates to an improvement in systolic BP ~1 mm Hg.

As the American population ages and more patients face chronic disease, expert opinion recognizes the importance of exercise to reduce cardiovascular events. Patients with CKD are at high risk because CKD is an independent cardiovascular risk factor. Recent guidelines advocate older patients perform moderate intensity exercise (e.g., walking) for a minimum of 30 minutes 5 days a week or vigorous activity (e.g., jogging) for a minimum of 20 minutes 3 days a week. In a small study of patients with CKD, regular exercise significantly reduced BP. However, once these patients stopped their exercise training, their pressures promptly increased. A recent study of patients with CKD undergoing cardiac rehabilitation showed improvements in weight, physical well-being, and lipid profiles. Finally, a study in which patients with CKD who were obese underwent exercise training, dietary education, and orlistat therapy (a drug that causes fat malabsorption) demonstrated these patients can effectively lose weight. This is important because obesity is a barrier to renal transplantation, and transplantation provides a survival benefit to patients with CKD, as compared to dialysis, through reduction in cardiovascular risk.

Appel LJ, Champagne CM, Harsha DW, et al. Effects of comprehensive lifestyle modification on blood pressure control: main results of the PREMIER clinical trial. *JAMA* 2003;289(16):2083–2093.

Aucott L, Rothnie H, McIntyre L, Thapa M, Waweru C, Gray D. Long-term weight loss from lifestyle intervention benefits blood pressure?: a systematic review. *Hypertension* 2009;54(4):756–762.

Boyce ML, Robergs RA, Avasthi PS, et al. Exercise training by individuals with predialysis renal failure: cardiorespiratory endurance, hypertension, and renal function. *Am J Kidney Dis* 1997;30(2):180–192.

Briones AM, Touyz RM. Moderate exercise decreases inflammation and oxidative stress in hypertension: but what are the mechanisms? *Hypertension* 2009;54(6):1206–1208.

Chobanian AV, Bakris GL, Black HR, et al. The Seventh Report of the Joint National Committee on Prevention, Detection, Evaluation, and Treatment of High Blood Pressure: the JNC 7 report. *JAMA* 2003;289(19): 2560–2572.

MacLaughlin HL, Cook SA, Kariyawasam D, et al. Nonrandomized trial of weight loss with orlistat, nutrition education, diet, and exercise in obese patients with CKD: 2-year follow-up. *Am J Kidney Dis* 2010;55(1):69–76.

McDermott AY, Mernitz H. Exercise and older patients: prescribing guidelines. *Am Fam Physician* 2006;74(3):437–444.

Neter JE, Stam BE, Kok FJ, Grobbee DE, Geleijnse JM. Influence of weight reduction on blood pressure: a meta-analysis of randomized controlled trials. *Hypertension* 2003;42(5):878–884.

Ogden CL, Carroll MD, McDowell MA, Felgal KM. Obesity among adults in the United States—no statistically significant change since 2003-2004. National Center for Health Statistics. http://www.cdc.gov/nchs/data/databriefs/db01.pdf

Petersen AM, Pedersen BK. The anti-inflammatory effect of exercise. *J Appl Physiol* 2005;98(4):1154–1162.

Venkataraman R, Sanderson B, Bittner V. Outcomes in patients with chronic kidney disease undergoing cardiac rehabilitation. *Am Heart J* 2005;150(6):1140–1146.

Weiner DE, Tighiouart H, Amin MG, et al. Chronic kidney disease as a risk factor for cardiovascular disease and all-cause mortality: a pooled analysis of community-based studies. *J Am Soc Nephrol* 2004;15(5): 1307–1315.

KEY POINTS: NONPHARMACOLOGIC TREATMENT OF HYPERTENSION

1. Limiting dietary sodium (Na) from 3 g daily to 1.5 g daily reduces blood pressure (BP) both in hypertensive and nonhypertensive populations and can protect from cardiovascular disease.

2. Patients with obstructive sleep apnea (OSA) have a more than twofold higher risk for hypertension. Continuous positive airway therapy may improve BP, particularly in those patients with severe OSA.

3. Both weight loss and exercise can improve BP control. Moderate intensity exercise (e.g., walking) for minimum of 30 minutes 5 days a week or vigorous activity (e.g., jogging) for a minimum of 20 minutes 3 days a week can improve BP even among older people.

XII. ACID–BASE AND ELECTROLYTE DISORDERS

VOLUME DISORDERS

John B. Stokes, MD, and Mony Fraer, MD

CHAPTER 74

HYPERVOLEMIA

1. **What is hypervolemia?**
    Hypervolemia results from a state of positive balance of sodium and water that produces expansion of the extracellular fluid (ECF) compartments. Most often, hypervolemia is caused by renal retention of sodium (Na) and water. This retention can be primary or secondary. Primary renal sodium retention is caused by renal diseases and conditions characterized by primary excess mineralocorticoid activity. Secondary hypervolemia is associated with a reduction in the effective arterial volume (EAV); the three most common conditions are congestive heart failure, nephrotic syndrome, and cirrhosis. In each of these disorders the body perceives the reduced EAV and the homeostatic mechanisms respond as if there is hypovolemia, causing the kidney to retain Na and water thereby producing ECF volume expansion.

2. **What are the manifestations of hypervolemia?**
    Edema is the most common clinical manifestation of hypervolemia; in fact, the terms are generally synonymous. Specific causes can also produce other manifestations: heart failure produces jugular venous distension and pulmonary crackles, cirrhosis produces ascites, and nephrotic syndrome produces widespread edema. Any severe cause of hypervolemia can produce pleural effusion.

3. **Why does edema develop?**
    The underlying cause of edema is a disturbance in the forces (Starling forces) that maintain a normal balance between the blood volume and the ECF volume. These forces are hydrostatic pressure and oncotic pressure. Heart failure and cirrhosis produce high venous pressure forcing fluid out of the capillaries. Nephrotic syndrome produces a loss of protein (albumin) and thus a loss of oncotic pressure (to keep fluid in the vessels).

4. **How is hypervolemia treated?**
    There is one key strategy to treat hypervolemia: inducing a negative sodium (and water) balance. The three methods to accomplish this goal are dietary sodium restriction, diuretics, and (in the event the kidneys are unable to respond to diuretics) ECF removal by ultrafiltration. One can also remove fluid from the abdominal or thoracic space directly (paracentesis or thoracentesis). To maintain the induced reduction in ECF volume, there has to be a restriction of sodium intake because high dietary salt intake can negate even the best strategy of diuretic therapy or extracorporeal fluid removal.

5. **Is there a limit for volume removal?**
    Diuretics produce fluid loss initially from the intravascular space. This change leads to a reduction in the capillary hydraulic pressure, followed by the mobilization of edema fluid into the vascular space. The rate at which this mobilization occurs is variable. In patients with generalized edema as a result of heart failure or nephrotic syndrome, the edema fluid can be mobilized at the rate of 2 to 3 L/24 hours. However, patients with cirrhosis and ascites without edema are more difficult to manage and the diuresis must be more cautious (daily maximum

of 500 mL) because the mobilization of the fluid occurs via the peritoneal capillaries. More aggressive diuresis may result in low blood pressure, lowered glomerular filtration rate and possible precipitation of the hepatorenal syndrome. However, for people who are symptomatic, removing large volumes of ascites is possible, but one must use counter measures to prevent renal insufficiency.

6. **What are the consequences of excessive volume removal?**
The most serious consequence of too rapid fluid removal is hypotension. The sequence of events starts with a decrease in the return of blood to the heart. As a consequence of the decrease in cardiac filling pressures, cardiac output will fall. A decrease in the EAV leads to impaired tissue perfusion and an activation of neurohormonal systems (renin, norepinephrine, sympathetic nervous system, and vasopressin). The glomerular filtration rate (GFR) could decrease (10% to 20% or more) and azotemia, elevated uric acid levels, or orthostatic symptoms may develop.

7. **How do diuretics work?**
Diuretics are classified based on mechanism and site of action; all diuretics block sodium absorption at one site along the nephron. Each nephron segment possesses specific transport pathways that permit sodium to move across the luminal membrane. There are four main classes of diuretics: thiazides (hydrochlorothiazide, chlorthalidone, and metolazone), loop diuretics (furosemide, bumetanide, torsemide, and ethacrynic acid), potassium-sparing diuretics (amiloride, triamterene, spironolactone, and eplerenone), and carbonic anhydrase inhibitors (Fig. 74-1). Thiazides block the sodium chloride cotransport mechanism across apical plasma membranes of the distal convoluted tubule; they are secreted in the proximal tubule and have a bioavailability of 60% to 70% and a half-life of 12 hours (hydrochlorothiazide) to 30 hours (chlorthalidone). Loop diuretics work by inhibiting the coupled entry of sodium, chloride, and potassium across apical plasma membranes in the thick ascending limb of the loop of Henle, which is responsible for the reabsorption of approximately 25% of filtered sodium; they also act from the tubular lumen and require both filtration and secretion to be effective. The duration of action is about 4 to 8 hours. Potassium-sparing diuretics inhibit sodium absorption in the collecting duct and concomitantly indirectly suppress potassium and proton secretion; they are usually weak diuretics when used alone, but they can be powerful adjuncts to therapy when used in combination with other classes of diuretics. Carbonic anhydrase inhibitors act largely on the proximal tubule; their use is limited by the development of metabolic acidosis.

8. **What is the response to the administration of a loop diuretic?**
If sodium intake is kept constant (e.g., a no-added-salt diet of 2 g of sodium or 80 mEq per day), administering a loop diuretic will produce a negative sodium balance with a large Na excretion and a net decrease in body weight within 4 hours. After 4 to 6 hours, sodium excretion falls as the diuretic is eliminated. At the end of 24 hours the total body Na is less than it was before the diuretic was taken. If the patient continues to receive the loop diuretic daily, by day 3 he or she will achieve a new state of sodium balance at a lower body weight, lower intravascular volume, and blood pressure. In patients with edema, the new steady state may take weeks to become established. The mechanisms that perpetuate this new steady state include activation of the renin-angiotensin-aldosterone system and the sympathetic nervous system (among others). In this steady state, sodium and water excretion are again equal to intake (over a 24-hour period) and the body weight is reduced by the amount lost during the first few days of therapy (1–2 kg in normal patients). Also, the effects of diuretic therapy on electrolytes) stabilize after 2 to 3 weeks in most patients. When loop diuretics are stopped, the mechanisms that maintain the steady state are left unopposed and the patient will gain weight again. Usually, the weight gain overshoots the original weight and the patients can end up with more edema than they started with. This "rebound" volume expansion is a common consequence of intermittent loop diuretic use.

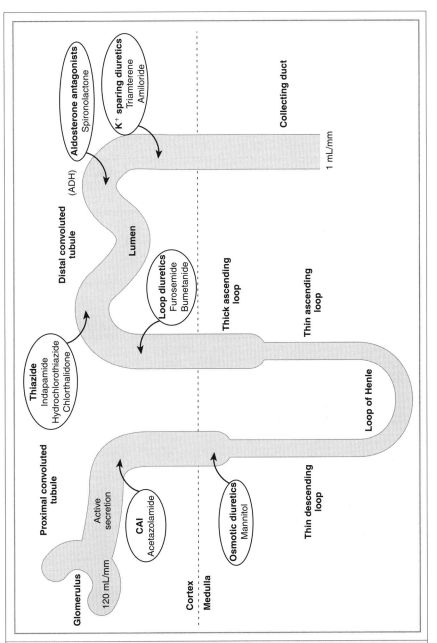

Figure 74-1. Site of diuretic action. (From Kester M, Karpa KD, Quraishi S, et al. *Elsevier's Integrated Pharmacology.* Philadelphia: Mosby, 2007.)

9. **What is an effective diuretic dose?**
   With loop diuretics, there is a dose-response curve. The threshold is the minimum dose required to induce diuresis. Larger doses produce increases in sodium excretion, up to a maximum effective dose (plateau) at which the sodium-chloride-potassium cotransporter is completely inhibited. The maximum effective dose differs based on the underlying condition: heart failure, cirrhosis, nephrotic syndrome, chronic kidney disease, or acute kidney injury. The recommended doses of loop diuretics for these disorders should be adjusted upward if there is concurrent renal insufficiency (Tables 74-1 and 74-2).

10. **What is the response to the administration of a thiazide diuretic?**
    Patients taking thiazide diuretics do not experience variations in urine volume throughout the day like those taking loop diuretics. Thiazides are longer acting and have much less effect on water excretion because of where they act (distal convoluted tubule). They also produce a less pronounced net negative sodium balance. However, there are two consequences of thiazide diuretics that are more common than with loop diuretics. Both types of diuretics produce increases in serum uric acid levels, a consequence of the secondary increase in proximal tubular reabsorption caused by volume contraction. Thiazides are more likely to produce hypokalemia because of their longer duration of action. In addition, thiazides produce increases in proximal tubular calcium reabsorption that result in lower calcium excretion and a positive calcium balance. This secondary effect of thiazides is useful in treating nephrolithiasis, osteopenia, and osteoporosis.

TABLE 74-1.	LOOP DIURETIC DOSE EQUIVALENCIES					
	NORMAL RENAL FUNCTION		RENAL INSUFFICIENCY		INFUSION	
Diuretic Dose (mg)	Initial (oral/IV)	Ceiling* (oral/IV)	Moderate (oral/IV)	Severe* (oral/IV)	Loading	Continuous
Furosemide	40–80/ 20–40	80–240/ 80–200	80–160	200–400/ 160–200	40	10–40
Bumetanide	0.5–1.0	4–8/ 2–4	4–8	8–10	1	0.5–2.0
Torsemide	20	100	20–50	50–100	20	5–20

*The high doses listed are sometimes required, on a temporary basis, for patients with nephrotic syndrome, congestive heart failure, and decompensated cirrhosis.

TABLE 74-2.	THIAZIDE DIURETIC DOSE EQUIVALENCIES	
Diuretic Dose (mg)	Initial	Maximum
Hydrochlorothiazide	25–50	50–100
Chlorthalidone	12.5–25	100
Metolazone	2.5	20
Chlorothiazide	250–500	1000

11. **What is the goal of treatment of edema?**
The purpose of using diuretics is to reduce ECF volume and maintain it at a clinically acceptable level (asymptomatic patient and a stable weight). The decision to use diuretics must be made in context (patient, underlying disease) because a modest amount of edema is, by itself, not life-threatening. The decision to use diuretics should be based primarily on one or more of the following: elevated blood pressure, tense ascites or lower extremity edema, and/or uncomfortable edema with functional consequences. Patients with edema and low blood pressure are particularly challenging to treat because diuretics will virtually always lower blood pressure.

12. **What is the reason for using diuretics in hypertension?**
Diuretics are an effective therapy in most patients with hypertension probably because they reduce the EAV. In patients with normal renal function, thiazide diuretics are as effective as loop diuretics. One can expect a 10 to 15/5 to 10 mm Hg drop in blood pressure in some groups of patients with hypertension. Obese, African American, and elderly patients generally have salt-sensitive hypertension and respond well to diuretics and a low-sodium diet. Potassium-sparing agents can be used as additional therapy and can help to avert the hypokalemia seen with thiazide diuretics. Mineralocorticoid receptor antagonists like spironolactone and eplerenone are useful in resistant hypertension or hypertension secondary to mineralocorticoid excess. Diuretics are almost always necessary for blood pressure control in patients with renal insufficiency. Virtually all such patients—even those with only moderately reduced renal function—are volume expanded. If such patients have hypertension—and most do—diuretics are the cornerstone of therapy. In resistant hypertension, volume expansion can be present in the absence of edema, even when the patient is taking a diuretic; the aim in this setting is removal of fluid until blood pressure control has been attained or the patient develops signs or symptoms of extracellular volume depletion.

13. **Are there special considerations when treating patients with nephrotic syndrome?**
In nephrotic syndrome, the low plasma oncotic pressure causes an oncotic pressure gradient that leads to a low plasma volume (and EAV). This situation sends neurohumoral signals to the kidney to retain sodium. Hypervolemia in these patients can be difficult to treat as a result of diuretic resistance. Combination diuretic therapy is often necessary to achieve results and should be coupled with agents designed to reduce the magnitude of proteinuria (angiotensin-converting enzyme inhibitors or angiotensin receptor antagonists). It is common to see the edema persist even in patients treated with high doses of loop diuretics. If it continues to produce symptoms, and the blood pressure is not too low, it is often useful to add another class of diuretic. The class that should be next considered is a potassium-sparing diuretic (because aldosterone secretion will be high and hypokalemia is common). If this combination does not produce the desired effect, one can add a thiazide-type diuretic. If one adds thiazide diuretics to loop diuretics without first administering potassium-sparing diuretics, one risks precipitating potentially severe hypokalemia. Of the thiazide diuretics, hydrochlorothiazide produces the mildest effect and metolazone produces the most potent effect. Albumin infusion is not effective in increasing diuretic efficacy in patients with nephrotic syndrome.

14. **Are there special considerations when treating patients with congestive heart failure?**
In heart failure, the reduction in cardiac output and tissue perfusion leads to activation of the sympathetic nervous system, renin-angiotensin-aldosterone, and vasopressin, causing sodium and water retention. This leads to an increased ECF volume, but the EAV is low as a result of the low cardiac output. For patients with heart failure, the goal is to achieve an ECF volume at which they do not have symptoms of dyspnea, and they have a normal (or low) blood pressure, minimal edema, and normal jugular venous pressure. Volume removal (by diuresis

or by mechanical means) can lead to a significant increase in cardiac output and patients may notice a relief of fatigue and dyspnea. Home blood pressure, pulse, and weight monitoring are often necessary to maintain optimal blood pressure and cardiac function. Sometimes patients with tenuous heart failure can be taught to adjust the diuretic dose by making prespecified changes based on the weight change beyond a specified range. Any effective therapy involves maintaining a constant low-sodium diet.

KEY POINTS: HYPERVOLEMIA

1. The treatment goal for hypervolemia is to induce a negative sodium (and water) balance.

2. The purpose of using diuretics to treat edema is to reduce extracellular fluid volume and maintain it at a clinically acceptable level.

3. A high salt intake can negate the beneficial effects of diuretics.

4. In congestive heart failure, volume removal can lead to an increase in cardiac output and patients may notice a relief of fatigue and dyspnea.

15. **Are there special considerations when treating patients with decompensated cirrhosis?**

With cirrhosis, there is a nitric-oxide–mediated reduction in systemic vascular resistance in conjunction with blood shunting through varices. The consequence of this state of affairs is a low arterial pressure. Usually, cardiac output and central venous pressure are normal. As a consequence of the hypotension, there is renal vasoconstriction and a compensatory activation of neurohormonal systems as described previously, resulting in water and sodium retention. The ECF volume will increase, and the plasma volume is increased (caused by a dilated splanchnic circulation). However, patients behave as if they are volume depleted because the excess fluid is sequestered in the venous system, the peritoneal cavity, and the extracellular space. Spironolactone is the most effective diuretic because of the high circulating levels of aldosterone. As with many states where edema and ECF volume is high, it may take weeks of therapy to achieve a new steady state. A commonly used regimen is the combination of single morning (minimizes nocturia) oral doses of spironolactone and furosemide; this combination also helps maintain the patient with normokalemia. Thiazide diuretics can be added if the response is inadequate. The therapeutic objective in patients with cirrhosis is to keep the patient comfortable. The large ascites can impair respiration and tense edema can cause skin breakdown. It is important to avoid hypokalemia in patients with cirrhosis because potassium depletion will enhance renal ammonia production, initiate and maintain metabolic alkalosis, and cause/exacerbate hepatic encephalopathy.

HYPOVOLEMIA

16. **What is hypovolemia and is it different from dehydration?**

Hypovolemia is a reduction in the volume of the ECF compartment in relation to its capacity. It can result from sodium and water loss or from water loss alone. With the first scenario, the ECF volume is reduced, leading to decreased tissue perfusion. In the case of water loss only (dehydration), the intracellular body water and the extracellular body water are decreased. As a consequence, with dehydration, it takes more volume to cause the same degree of extracellular volume depletion as sodium and water loss. Hypovolemic shock is a more severe hypovolemic state and occurs most commonly from trauma, hemorrhage, vomiting, diarrhea, burns, pancreatitis, or Addisonian crisis.

17. **What are the extrarenal causes of hypovolemia?**

The most direct cause of extrarenal volume loss is from the intravascular space, as in bleeding. The compensatory responses involve a shift of fluid from the interstitial to the intravascular compartment secondary to altered transcapillary Starling hydraulic forces; in the absence of this shift, the patients will not have a low hemoglobin. As a consequence of this type of loss, the hematocrit and albumin concentrations fall. Extrarenal causes of hypovolemia also occur from fluid losses from the gastrointestinal tract (vomiting, diarrhea) or skin (sweat or severe burns). Although the sodium concentration in sweat is only 20 to 50 mmol/L, a significant sodium deficit and ECF volume contraction can occur in unconditioned people who exercise heavily or who stay in hot environments. ECF may also be sequestered into compartments within the body. These "third-space" losses occur in gastrointestinal obstruction, abdominal surgery, trauma, burns, ascites, pancreatitis, or peritonitis. These extrarenal causes of hypovolemia will invoke neural and hormonal responses that result in renal sodium and water retention, with the aim of restoring intravascular volume and stabilizing the circulation.

18. **What are the renal causes of hypovolemia?**

Excessive renal losses of Na and ECF volume can be caused by overuse of diuretics. Other causes include decreased aldosterone production or cortisol synthesis (Addison's disease). Resistance to the action of aldosterone or intrinsic damage to the kidney can also produce salt wasting. Less common causes of renal salt wasting and hence reduced ECF volume are genetic defects in Na absorption by the kidney. Examples of such defects include Bartter syndrome (thick ascending limb of Henle's loop), Gitelman syndrome (Na/Cl cotransporter in the distal convoluted tubule), and pseudohypoaldosteronism (loss of function of the epithelial Na channel in the collecting duct).

19. **How does one assess a patient's volume status?**

Extravascular volume deficits do not become clinically apparent until they exceed 10% of body weight. The symptoms of mild to moderate volume contraction are nonspecific. Fatigue and lethargy are the most common. More severe volume contraction can produce a low urine output, postural dizziness, excessive thirst, and cramps. Signs of volume contraction include tachycardia, dry axillae, orthostatic hypotension (systolic blood pressure decrease of at least 20 mm Hg or a diastolic blood pressure decrease of at least 10 mm Hg within 3 minutes of standing), and ultimately overt hypotension. Severe volume contraction can produce cool extremities, clammy skin, and cool kneecaps. If the loss of ECF volume is not from hemorrhage, the hematocrit and albumin concentration will be high. In the presence of normal kidney function, volume contraction will cause the kidneys to produce a concentrated urine that is low in sodium (usually less than 10 mEq/L) and chloride. If the volume contraction is prolonged and severe, the GFR can fall with a concomitant rise in serum creatinine. In such cases the blood urea nitrogen can be >20 times the creatinine value, but such a situation may not be present if the person has not been eating. If tissue perfusion is impaired, lactic acidosis may ensue.

20. **What are the difficulties in assessing the volume status?**

Assessing ECF volume and EAV can be challenging; changes in ECF volume of ±5% can be subclinical. The history, physical examination, and routine laboratory tests have limited sensitivity and specificity, and it is better to use a combination of these to diagnose hypovolemia. Both conventional hemodynamic parameters (central venous and pulmonary artery occlusion pressures and mixed venous O_2 saturation) as well as the more sophisticated dynamic indicators (inspiratory decrease in right atrial pressure, expiratory decrease in arterial systolic pressure, respiratory changes in pulse pressure, and respiratory changes in aortic blood velocity) have limitations. Techniques such as left ventricular end-diastolic area by transesophageal echocardiography are also not routinely used. For example, a person in heart failure may have tachycardia, hypotension, cool extremities (and kneecaps), a concentrated urine, and a low urine sodium. Such a person probably has edema. The interpretation of this constellation is that EAV is low (from heart failure) and that ECF is high because of the high hydrostatic pressure in the postcapillary venules. People with sepsis may present with hypotension (from the accompanying vasodilation) but demonstrate warm extremities.

21. **When is the urine sodium concentration not useful in assessing hypovolemia?**
Volume contraction does not always produce a low urine sodium. When metabolic alkalosis is combined with volume contraction, as in vomiting, urine sodium concentration may be high because large amounts of bicarbonate are lost in the urine, obligating the excretion of sodium to maintain electrical neutrality. In this instance the urine will always be alkaline. In these instances, a urine chloride concentration of less than 10 mEq/L more reliably indicates volume depletion. A higher than expected urinary sodium can also occur with renal sodium losses resulting from intrinsic renal disease, use of diuretics, adrenal insufficiency, acute tubular necrosis, or in states of relative hypovolemia with edema.

22. **How is hypovolemia in the elderly different?**
Elderly patients have a lower total body water because of a greater proportion of fat (which contains less water) relative to muscle mass; as a consequence, for any given degree of fluid loss they will have a greater reduction in extracellular fluid volume. Usually, the clinical manifestations of hypovolemia are nonspecific. The degree of weight loss is the most important parameter to be used in assessing their volume status.

23. **What are the acid–base and potassium changes that can be associated with hypovolemia?**
Hypokalemia with metabolic alkalosis frequently accompany vomiting. ECF volume loss from diarrhea is associated with a nonanion gap metabolic acidosis and often with hypokalemia too. Loop and thiazide diuretic–induced hypovolemia is associated with hypokalemia and metabolic alkalosis. Inherited transport defects have presentations that are nearly indistinguishable from chronic use of loop and thiazide diuretics, respectively. The hypokalemia from diuretics is caused by the increase in aldosterone secretion produced by the (intentional) volume contraction together with high Na delivery to the site in the distal nephron (collecting duct) where K secretion occurs. This K deficiency in turn is the major cause of metabolic alkalosis. It is necessary to replace the K deficits before the body (kidney) can correct the metabolic alkalosis.

24. **Give some guidelines for volume replacement therapy in hypovolemia.**
The blood pressure and pulse are the most important parameters to guide the magnitude of fluid replacement, and they must be monitored frequently. The type of fluid given is dependent on the type of fluid that has been lost. Hypotonic solutions (e.g., half normal saline) are preferred in patients with hypernatremia. Patients with hypovolemia and hyponatremia should be administered isotonic saline, and patients with blood loss usually require isotonic fluids, oncotic solutions (albumin or hetastarch), or blood. The body weight lost offers the best estimate of volume losses, but reliable weight values are often not available. Clinical and laboratory parameters must be used to assess the severity of volume depletion (blood pressure, pulse, capillary refill, clinical signs of tissue perfusion, urine output, urine sodium excretion and osmolality, and mental status) and guide the resuscitation. With severe volume depletion or hypovolemic shock, the goal of volume resuscitation is to restore circulating volume to normal and, as a result, improve tissue perfusion and oxygen delivery. A few liters of crystalloids should be given as rapidly as possible. With less severe hypovolemia, the goal is to correct existing abnormalities in plasma electrolytes and volume status. The optimal rate of volume could be 50 to 100 mL per hour in excess of continued losses (equal to the sum of the urine output, estimated insensible losses are 30–50 mL per hour). The selection of the type, amount, and rate of ECF volume replacement is an art; there are no useful formulas to guide such therapy.

25. **Are colloids better than crystalloids for volume replacement?**
No study has demonstrated the superiority of one crystalloid solution over another. Crystalloids are inexpensive, are readily available, are effective, have a long shelf life and incidence of adverse reactions, and come in a variety of formulations. Normal saline (0.9% saline) and lactated Ringer's solution are both commonly used, although the latter may cause hyperkalemia in patients with renal failure. Some patients with severe volume contraction with existing lactic acidosis or hepatic failure cannot metabolize lactate to bicarbonate. Theoretic advantages of colloids (high molecular weight solutions) over crystalloids (electrolyte solutions) when used for volume replacement include lower incidence of pulmonary edema, less reperfusion injury, and a more rapid expansion of the intravascular space (because the large molecules colloid solution remains in the vascular space in contrast to saline, two thirds of which enters the interstitium). However, few studies demonstrate superiority of colloid solutions over crystalloid solutions. Administration of colloid solutions has documented risks: dextrans can cause anaphylactoid reactions and can alter the coagulation system, hetastarch can cause acute kidney injury, and blood can produce many adverse reactions. For most hypovolemic states, albumin infusion has not been clearly shown to be superior to crystalloids. An exception to this general rule is in patients with cirrhosis and tense ascites undergoing large-volume paracentesis; colloids (dextran 70 or albumin) were found to protect against acute kidney injury. In patients with severe hemorrhage, administration of packed red blood cells improves tissue perfusion and oxygen carrying capacity.

26. **What is the effective arterial volume, and why is it important?**
The EAV refers to that part of the ECF that is in the arterial system and is effectively perfusing the tissues (about 700 mL in a 70-kg man). In clinical practice it is an unmeasurable entity and often difficult to assess. Often, it correlates directly with the ECF volume and total body sodium stores. In states of edema secondary to cardiac failure, decompensated cirrhosis, or nephrotic syndrome, the EAV may be independent of the ECF volume, the plasma volume, or even the cardiac output because of redistribution of ECF fluid. In these scenarios, although the ECF compartment is increased, the EAV is low. This leads to hypotension and activation of compensatory mechanism as for a hypovolemic state. Other causes of low EAV are states of vasodilation in response to drugs (e.g., hydralazine, minoxidil), sepsis (peripheral vasodilation and low systemic vascular resistance), or with pregnancy (high nitric-oxide production). The ensuing perception of low intravascular volume can be accompanied by clinical manifestations suggestive of absolute hypovolemia (tachycardia and hypotension) and compensatory responses to it (renal sodium and water retention). The reduction of edema by diuretics causes a decrease in EAV, which in turn is translated into a reduction of ECF volume. Informed management of hypervolemia and hypovolemia requires understanding of these concepts.

KEY POINTS: HYPOVOLEMIA

1. Intravascular volume contraction of less than 5% is usually not symptomatic or detectable.

2. A stable hemoglobin does not rule out bleeding as a source of hypovolemia.

3. The body weight that was lost offers the best estimate of volume losses.

4. There is no proven benefit of usage of colloids over crystalloids for correction of hypovolemia.

5. In states of edema secondary to cardiac failure, decompensated cirrhosis, or nephrotic syndrome, the effective arterial volume may be independent of the extracellular fluid volume.

27. **What is the role of dopamine in oligoanuric acute kidney injury?**
In healthy subjects, low-dose dopamine increases renal blood flow and induces both natriuresis and diuresis. No good studies support the use of renal-dose dopamine as a kidney-protective effect or to improve mortality. A possible reason for this discrepancy may derive from the fact that infused doses do not translate into a reliable plasma level because of the renal failure and altered pharmacokinetics in the critically ill. Also, although dopamine does cause diuresis, other diuretics have fewer adverse effects than dopamine and can be used in the prevention of anuria; despite its renal vasodilatory effect and the increase in cardiac output and blood pressure, dopamine may paradoxically increase the myocardial oxygen consumption. Other adverse effects are that it blunts the hypoxic ventilatory drive, worsens the sick euthyroid, increases the odds ratio of tachyarrhythmias, causes gut ischemia, inhibits lymphocyte proliferation and immunoglobulin synthesis, and decreases serum prolactin and growth hormone secretion.

BIBLIOGRAPHY

HYPERVOLEMIA

1. Andreoli TE. Edematous states: An overview. *Kidney Int* 1997;51(Suppl 59):S2–S10.
2. Bleich M, Greger R. Mechanism of action of diuretics. *Kidney Int* 1997;51:S11–S15.
3. Bock HA, Stein JH. Diuretics and the control of extracellular fluid volume: Role of counterregulation. *Semin Nephrol* 1988;8:264.
4. Brater DC. Diuretic therapy. *N Engl J Med* 1988;339:387.
5. Brater DC. Pharmacology of diuretics. *Am J Med Sci* 2000;319:38–50.
6. Brater DC. Use of diuretics in cirrhosis and nephrotic syndrome. *Semin Nephrol* 1999;19:575–580.
7. Cadnapaphornchai MA, Gurevich AK, Weinberger HD, et al. Pathophysiology of sodium and water retention in heart failure. *Cardiology* 2001;96:122–131.
8. Ellison DH. Diuretic drugs and the treatment of edema: From clinic to bench and back again. *Am J Kidney Dis* 1994;23:623.
9. Humphreys MH. Mechanisms and management of nephrotic edema. *Kidney Int* 1994;45:266.
10. Ernst ME, Moser M. Use of diuretics in patients with hypertension. *N Engl J Med* 2009;361(22):2153–2156.
11. Faris R, Flather M, Purcell H, et al. Current evidence supporting the role of diuretics in heart failure: A meta analysis of randomised controlled trials. *Int J Cardiol* 2002;82:149–158.
12. Gines P, Cardenas A, Arroyo V, et al. Management of cirrhosis and ascites. *N Engl J Med* 2004;350:1646–1654.
13. Ikram H, Chan W, Espiner EA, et al. Hemodynamic and hormone responses to acute and chronic furosemide therapy in congestive heart failure. *Clin Sci* 1980;59:443.
14. Loon NR, Wilcox CS, Unwin RJ. Mechanism of impaired natriuretic response to furosemide during prolonged therapy. *Kidney Int* 1989;36:682–689.
15. Martin PY, Schrier RW. Sodium and water retention in heart failure: Pathogenesis and treatment. Review. *Kidney Int* 1997;51(Suppl 59):S57–S61.
16. Rasool A, Palevsky PM. Treatment of edematous disorders with diuretics. *Am J Med Sci* 2000;319:25–37.
17. Schrier RW, Gurevich AK, Cadnapaphornchai MA. Pathogenesis and management of sodium and water retention in cardiac failure and cirrhosis. *Semin Nephrol* 2001;21:157–172.
18. Schrier RW. Pathogenesis of sodium and water retention in high-output and low-output cardiac failure, nephrotic syndrome, cirrhosis, and pregnancy (1). Review. *N Engl J Med* 1988;319:1065–1072. [Published erratum appears in *N Engl J Med* 1989;320(10):676.]
19. Wilcox CS. New insights into diuretic use in patients with chronic renal disease. *J Am Soc Nephrol* 2002;13:798.

HYPOVOLEMIA

1. Choi PTL, Yip G, Quinonez LG, et al. Crystalloids vs. colloids in fluid resuscitation: A systematic review. *Crit Care Med* 1999;27:200.
2. Erstad BL, Gales BJ, Rappaport WD. The use of albumin in clinical practice. *Arch Intern Med* 1991;151:901.

3. Finfer S, Bellomo R, Boyce N, et al. A comparison of albumin and saline for fluid resuscitation in the intensive care unit. *N Engl J Med* 2004;350:2247–2256.

4. Gould SA, Sehgal LR, Sehgal HL, et al. Hypovolemic shock. *Crit Care Clin* 1993;9:239–259.

5. Imm A, Carlson RW. Fluid resuscitation in circulatory shock. *Crit Care Clin* 1993;9:313–333.

6. McGee S, Abernethy WB, Simel DL. Is this patient hypovolemic? *JAMA* 1999;281:1022.

7. Pinsky MR, Brophy P, Padilla J, et al. Fluid and volume monitoring. *Int J Artif Organs* 2008;31(2):111–126.

8. Schierhout G, Roberts I. Fluid resuscitation with colloid or crystalloid solutions in critically ill patients: A systematic review of randomised trials. *BMJ* 1998;316:961.

9. Schenarts PJ, Sagraves SG, Bard MR, et al. Low-dose dopamine: a physiologically based review. *Curr Surg* 2006;63(3):219–225.

10. Tommasino C, Picozzi V. Volume and electrolyte management. *Best Pract Res Clin Anaesthesiol* 2007;21(4):497–516.

11. Vincent JL, Weil MH. Fluid challenge revisited. *Crit Care Med* 2006;34(5):1333–1337.

12. Waikar SS, Chertow GM. Crystalloids versus colloids for resuscitation in shock. *Curr Opin Nephrol Hypertens* 2000;9:501–504.

CHAPTER 75

GENETIC DISORDERS OF SODIUM TRANSPORT

Supriya Maddirala, MD, and David H. Ellison, MD

1. **What are monogenic or Mendelian forms of hypertension?**

   Essential hypertension, which is the most prevalent form of hypertension, results from multiple gene–gene and gene–environment interactions. The genes that predispose an individual to essential hypertension have not been identified. Secondary hypertension is the result of an identifiable cause; the most common cause is primary hyperaldosteronism, arising from an adrenal adenoma or bilateral adrenal hyperplasia and accounts for 8% to 13% of cases of resistant hypertension. Monogenic forms of hypertension, in contrast, are exceedingly rare. They result from mutations in single genes and are inherited in Mendelian patterns. These genetic mutations nearly all affect electrolyte transport in the distal nephron or synthesis/activity of mineralocorticoids, ultimately leading to increased absorption of sodium and chloride, volume expansion, and hypertension.

2. **Which clinical characteristics support the diagnosis of monogenic hypertension?**

   Monogenic hypertension should be considered in young patients who present with severe or refractory hypertension, in individuals with a family history of early-onset hypertension or cerebrovascular accidents, or in individuals with hypertension and specific biochemical abnormalities (e.g., changes in renin, aldosterone, and potassium (K^+) values.)

3. **How many single-gene mutations have been recognized thus far that result in monogenic hypertension?**

   Seven single-gene mutations have been identified as the cause of hypertensive disorders. Each disorder can be described based on characteristics of age of onset, inheritance pattern, biochemical changes, and response to specific treatment (Table 75-1).

4. **How do changes in renin and aldosterone help in the diagnosis of monogenic forms of hypertension?**

   A low renin value is shared by these disorders. Aldosterone activity may be increased or decreased. A high level of aldosterone expression is seen in familial hyperaldosteronism I and II (FH I & II). Both familial and sporadic forms of primary hyperaldosteronism typically exhibit a serum aldosterone-renin ratio (ARR) > 30 and a serum aldosterone value ≥15 ng/dL. Because this initial approach lacks adequate positive and negative predictive values, a 24-hour urine aldosterone measurement of greater than 14 ng is needed to confirm the diagnosis in the setting of a high salt intake (urine Na^+ should exceed 200 mEq/day).

5. **Describe the first recognized cause of monogenic hypertension resulting from a single-gene mutation.**

   Familial hyperaldosteronism (FH-I) is an autosomal-dominant hypertensive disorder resulting from a hybrid gene located on chromosome 8. The defective gene consists of the regulatory gene of 11β-hydroxylase gene, *CYP11B1,* and the structural region of aldosterone synthase gene, *CYP11B2.* Angiotensin-II (Ang-II) induces the production of aldosterone by stimulating *CYP11B2,*

TABLE 75-1. MONOGENIC LOW RENIN HYPERTENSION

Disorder	Site of Mutation	Inheritance	Plasma Aldosterone	Serum K+	Genetic Test	Treatment
Familial hyperaldosteronism-I (FH-I) or glucocorticoid remediable hyperaldosteronism	Aldosterone synthase	AD	High	Low	Commercial	Glucocorticoids
Familial hyperaldosteronism-II (FH-II)		AD	High	Low/nl	Research	Spironolactone Eplerenone
Syndrome of apparent mineralocorticoid excess (SAME)	HSD 11β2	AR	Low	Low/nl	Commercial	Spironolactone Dexamethasone
Congenital adrenal hyperplasia (CAH)		AR	Low	Low/nl	Research	Glucocorticoids
Hypertension with severe exacerbation in pregnancy (Geller syndrome)	NR3C2 (MCR?)	Unknown	Low	Low/nl	Research	Delivery
Liddle syndrome	β- or γ-ENaC	AD	Low	Low/nl	Commercial	Amiloride Triamterene
Familial hyperkalemic hypertension (pseudohypoaldosteronism-II [PHA-II] or Gordon syndrome)	WNK1, WNK4, locus 3	AD	Variable	High	Research	Thiazide Low-sodium diet

HSD = hydroxysteroid dehydrogenase; MCR = mineralocorticoid receptor; ENaC = epithelial sodium channel; AD = autosomal dominant; AR = autosomal recessive.
Adapted from Mount D, Pollak M. *Molecular and Genetic Basis of Renal Disease: A Companion to Brenner and Rector's The Kidney.* Philadelphia: Elsevier Health Sciences, 2007.

whereas ACTH stimulation of *CYP11B1* leads to cortisol production. The chimeric gene results in adrenocorticotropic hormone (ACTH)–stimulated production of mineralocorticoids in the zona fasciculata instead of the zona glomerulosa; thus, mineralocorticoid production is unresponsive to its traditional regulators, angiotensin II and K^+.

Plasma renin is reduced, whereas aldosterone level is increased. Hypokalemia, although common, is seen in only half of all patients with FH-I. Given the severity of hypertension at presentation, patients suffer hemorrhagic strokes from ruptured aneurysms. Hence, cerebral magnetic resonance angiography is a requisite in these patients at the time of diagnosis; it should be repeated every 5 years. Low doses of glucocorticoids suppress ACTH and aldosterone production and thereby serve an important therapeutic role. Amiloride and spironolactone are also effective.

6. **What is the distinction between familial hyperaldosteronism-II (FH-II) from primary hyperaldosteronism?**
   It is difficult to distinguish FH-II from primary hyperaldosteronism attributable to bilateral adrenal hyperplasia. However, the diagnosis should be considered for patients with hypokalemia, metabolic alkalosis, low renin and high aldosterone activity, *and* a strong family history for hypertension. The defective gene is found on chromosome 7p22. Although glucocorticoid administration ameliorates hypertension in FH-I, it is ineffective in FH-II. Thus the response to dexamethasone, in addition to genetic testing, helps to exclude other familial causes of primary hyperaldosteronism. FH-II responds well to spironolactone.

7. **How can cortisol biosynthesis lead to hypertension and hypokalemia?**
   Both cortisol and aldosterone activate the mineralocorticoid receptor (MCR). Serum cortisol levels are typically 10-fold greater than aldosterone levels; in aldosterone-sensitive cells, however, the enzymatic action of 11β-hydroxysteroid dehydrogenase-2 (11β-HSD-2) converts the cortisol to cortisone, a form without effect on the MCR. If cellular cortisol levels exceed aldosterone levels, the receptor is stimulated and hypertension and hypokalemia ensue.

8. **Which inherited and acquired conditions lead to excess cortisol levels and hypertension?**
   The syndrome of apparent mineralocorticoid excess (SAME) is characterized by hypertension and hypokalemia. It is caused by loss-of-function mutations in the 11β-hydroxysteroid dehydrogenase, which allow concentrations of cortisol to rise in distal cells. An elevated urine cortisol to cortisone ratio establishes the diagnosis. The mainstay of therapy hinges on MCR blockade with spironolactone. Adjunctive therapy includes K^+ supplementation and low Na^+ diet.

   An acquired form of the disease is more common. Black licorice contains glycyrrhetinic acid, which inhibits 11β-HSD-2, with resultant failure to inactivate cortisol in the distal nephron. Patients with excess cortisol production arising from a variety of causes, including ectopic ACTH release, present with hypertension and metabolic alkalosis. They may also have "Cushingoid features," helping to distinguish hypertension resulting from hypercortisolism from other causes of low-renin, low-aldosterone hypertension. A positive dexamethasone suppression test result is also useful in establishing the diagnosis.

9. **What is the only gain of function mutation described for the mineralocorticoid receptor?**
   In Geller syndrome, a single mutation activates and alters the binding properties of the MCR. There are changes in the affinity for 21-hydroxylated ligands, aldosterone, and cortisol, but more important, the receptor also exhibits enhanced affinity for steroids lacking the hydroxyl group, such as progesterone, which circulates at high levels during pregnancy. Hence, affected patients develop hypokalemia and early-onset hypertension, which, in females, is exacerbated by pregnancy, often requiring premature delivery in the absence of pre-eclampsia. Spironolactone has been shown to have a paradoxical increase in receptor function and thus should not be considered for therapy. Amiloride and triamterene, which block epithelial sodium channel (ENaC), may be more effective.

10. **What is Liddle syndrome?**

The phenotype of Liddle syndrome, sometimes referred to as pseudoaldosteronism, includes hypertension, hypokalemia, and metabolic alkalosis. It is a rare autosomal-dominant condition involving a mutation in the gene for the ENaC of the connecting tubule and collecting duct. This amiloride-sensitive sodium channel comprises three subunits and is responsible for Na^+ reabsorption in the apical membrane of the collecting duct. A gain-of-function mutation of ENaC (β or γ subunits) leads to an inability to retrieve the channel from the apical membrane and increases its activation, resulting in a mineralocorticoid excess–like state. As a consequence, K^+ excretion is augmented, Na^+ reabsorption is increased, and volume expansion ensues. Unlike primary aldosteronism, aldosterone levels are reduced—hence the term pseudoaldosteronism (Table 75-2).

11. **A patient with hypertension is found to have hyperkalemia, metabolic acidosis, and low plasma renin and aldosterone levels. Which disorder would be consistent with these findings?**

Familial hyperkalemic hypertension (FHHt) results from autosomal-dominant transmission and is also known as pseudohypoaldosteronism type II (PHA-II) or Gordon syndrome. In addition to high blood pressure and hyperkalemia, patients develop hyperchloremic metabolic acidosis. Aldosterone levels are typically in the low normal range, reflecting the opposing effects of hyperkalemia, which normally stimulates aldosterone release, and extracellular fluid volume expansion, which normally inhibits it.

12. **What is the genetic defects that result in the clinical and biochemical profiles of FHHt (Gordon syndrome)?**

The disorder has been ascribed to molecular defect of protein kinases WNK4 and WNK1. The WNK4 mutation leads to increased expression and activity of the thiazide-sensitive NaCl cotransporter and hyperplasia of the distal convoluted tubule. In addition, mutant WNK4 results in increased removal of ROMK from the cell surface in the collecting duct, which may contribute to decreased K^+ secretion. Increased Cl^- permeability through the paracellular pathway was postulated to play a role, but this was not confirmed in a mouse model.

WNK1 mutations also cause FHHt. WNK1 typically inhibits WNK4 and also phosphorylates another kinase, SPAK. The WNK1 mutations appear to enhance WNK1 effects, leading to the clinical manifestations of FHHt. Both high blood pressure and hyperkalemia respond extremely well to thiazide diuretics.

13. **Do mutations in Na^+ and K^+ transport proteins cause salt wasting and hypotension?**

Although some mutations of distal nephron genes cause monogenic forms of hypertension, other mutations of the same pathways lead to salt wasting and hypotension (Table 75-3).

14. **Is pseudohypoaldosteronism type I (PHA I) also characterized by hypertension and aldosterone deficiency similar to PHA II?**

Both PHA-I and PHA-II exhibit hyperkalemia and metabolic acidosis. However, PHA-I is characterized by salt and volume depletion and high circulating aldosterone, whereas PHA-II is characterized by hypertension; as noted earlier, aldosterone levels are typically low normal. The severity of the clinical findings of PHA I depends on the mode of transmission. The autosomal-recessive form, from mutations of any of the three subunits of ENaC, causes life-threatening consequences as a result of salt wasting despite increased aldosterone levels. Affected patients may also develop extrarenal manifestations including cutaneous lesions from excess salt concentration in sweat and respiratory infections. Salt repletion and K binding resins are requisite lifelong to maintain electrolyte and volume balance. The autosomal-dominant inheritance pattern of PHA I from inactivating mutation of the MCR and clinical features are limited to renal transport abnormalities and typically disappear. In these patients, aldosterone levels are chronically elevated, even after resolution of the salt wasting. Autosomal-recessive PHA-I is a mirror image of Liddle syndrome, and autosomal-dominant PHA-I is opposite that of Geller syndrome. Both sporadic and familial cases have been described for PHA-I.

TABLE 75-2. FEATURES OF LIDDLE SYNDROME, APPARENT MINERALOCORTICOID EXCESS (AME) AND GLUCOCORTICOID REMEDIABLE ALDOSTERONISM (GRA)

| Feature | SYNDROMES WITH HYPOKALEMIA, METABOLIC ALKALOSIS, AND HYPERTENSION | | |
	Liddle Syndrome	AME	GRA
Inheritance	Autosomal dominant	Autosomal recessive	Autosomal dominant
Chief features	Significant hypertension, polyuria, growth retardation	Low birthweight, early-onset hypertension, polyuria, growth restriction	Significant hypertension, hemorrhagic stroke
Plasma aldosterone	Reduced	Reduced	Elevated
Plasma renin activity	Reduced	Reduced	Reduced
Urinary mineralocorticoid metabolites	Normal	Elevated ratios of THF + alloTHF to THE; free cortisol to cortisone	Elevated cortisol C-18 oxidation products
RESPONSE TO			
Glucocorticoids	No	Satisfactory	Satisfactory
Triamterene	Satisfactory	Satisfactory	Satisfactory
Spironolactone	No	Satisfactory	Satisfactory

THF = tetrahydrocortisol; THE = tetrahydrocortisone.
From Johnson RJ, Feehally J. *Comprehensive Clinical Nephrology*, 2nd ed. Philadelphia: Mosby, 2003.

TABLE 75-3.   MUTATIONS OF NA⁺ TRANSPORT ACROSS THE DISTAL NEPHRON RESULTING IN RENAL SALT WASTING

Disorder	Site of Mutation	Inheritance	Serum K⁺	Plasma Aldosterone
Gitelman syndrome	NCC	AR	Low	High
Bartter syndrome	NKCC2, ROMK, CLC-Kb, CLC-Ka, Barttin	AR	Low	High
Pseudohypoaldosteronism-I (PHA I)	NR3C2 (MCR)	AD	High	High
Pseudohypoaldosteronism-I (PHA I)	α-, β-, or γ-ENaC	AR	High	Very High

NCC = NaCl cotransporter; AR= autosomal recessive; MCR = mineralocorticoid receptor; AD = autosomal dominant.
Adapted from Mount D, Pollak M. *Molecular and Genetic Basis of Renal Disease: A Companion to Brenner and Rector's The Kidney.* Philadelphia: Elsevier Health Sciences, 2007.

15. **What are the characteristics of Bartter and Gitelman syndromes?**
Bartter and Gitelman syndrome are inherited disorders of salt reabsorption, leading to ECF volume depletion and normal to low blood pressure. The clinical phenotypes can be classified according to the predominant site of deficient salt transport.

Gitelman syndrome typically presents with hypokalemic alkalosis. The arterial pressure is typically low normal and the serum magnesium is reduced. The urinary calcium excretion is suppressed. The syndrome (DC1-type) results from mutation of the gene (*SLC12A3*) that encodes the thiazide-sensitive NaCl cotransporter (NCC) in the distal convoluted tubule. Some patients presenting with similar characteristics (DC2-type) have mutations in a basolateral chloride channel (*CLC-Kb*) instead.

Bartter syndrome comprises disorders from reduced NaCl reabsorption along the thick ascending limb of Henle (TAL). Patients often present during infancy with salt wasting, depletion of the extracellular fluid volume, and failure to thrive. The defective genes encode the luminal bumetanide-sensitive Na-K-2Cl cotransporter (L1-type, *NKCC2*) or the luminal potassium conductance channel ROMK (L2-type, *KCJN1*). Compound disorders display mixed phenotypic features; these include L-DC1-type (from mutations in CLCNKB gene and CLC-Kb) and the L-DC2-type (from mutations in the β subunit of ClC [*BSND*]). The BSND gene encodes the protein Barttin (β-subunit of CLC-K), an essential subunit for the basolateral Cl⁻ channels; because it is also necessary for hearing, these patients also develop sensorineural deafness.

16. **Which clinical features are shared by patients with Bartter and Gitelman syndromes? How can the two conditions be differentiated?**
Gitelman syndrome is relatively common (estimated disease frequency 1:40,000). It typically presents after puberty with hypokalemic alkalosis. Most individuals have nonspecific symptoms, but severe manifestations, such as tetany or cardiac arrhythmias, can occur if the hypokalemia is severe. Hypocalciuria and hypomagnesemia are characteristic features of Gitelman syndrome. Paralysis and prolonged QT interval with malignant arrhythmias have been observed and ascribed to electrolyte abnormalities.

Bartter syndrome often presents at or near birth with polyuria, dehydration, and failure to thrive. Affected individuals also have findings akin to a nephrogenic diabetes insipidus and hypercalciuria. Depending on whether the individual has L1-type or L2-type disease, the initial presentation may include either hypokalemia or hyperkalemia, but hypokalemia eventually supervenes.

Urinary Ca^{2+} excretion and change in urinary Cl^- excretion after thiazide administration are useful diagnostic tools. Urinary Ca^{2+} excretion is increased in Bartter syndrome, in contrast with the hypocalciuria evident in patients with Gitelman syndrome. A lack of change in urinary Cl^- with thiazide administration allows a distinction to be made between the two conditions (Table 75-4).

Because there are uncommon disorders it is important, especially in adults, to exclude surreptitious vomiting and diuretic use.

KEY POINTS: SODIUM TRANSPORT MUTATIONS IN THE DISTAL NEPHRON ✓

1. Monogenic hypertension results from a mutation in a single gene, typically one that affects electrolyte transport in the distal nephron.

2. Patients with monogenic hypertension present at a young age with severe or refractory hypertension, have a strong family history of hypertension, and have typical changes in serum electrolytes.

3. Excess sodium absorption is characteristic of all genetic mutations that cause hypertension with low renin. Whereas metabolic alkalosis and hypokalemia are most common, a phenotypic variant with hyperkalemia and hyperchloremic acidosis can also be observed.

4. Mutations of Na^+ transport also lead to renal salt wasting. Patients with Bartter or Gitelman syndrome present typically manifest with hypokalemia and metabolic alkalosis. Patients with pseudohypoaldosteronism-I develop salt wasting with hyperkalemia and nongap metabolic acidosis.

TABLE 75-4.   FEATURES DIFFERENTIATING BARTTER AND GITELMAN SYNDROMES

Feature	Neonatal Bartter Syndrome	Classic Bartter Syndrome	Gitelman Syndrome
Age at onset	Neonatal period	Infancy/childhood	Childhood/later
Maternal hydramnios	Common	Rare	Absent
Polyuria, polydipsia	Marked	Present	Rare
Dehydration	Present	Often present	Absent
Tetany	Absent	Rare	Present
Growth retardation	Present	Present	Absent
Urinary calcium	Very high	Normal or high	Low
Nephrocalcinosis	Present	Rare	Absent
Serum magnesium	Normal	Occasionally low	Low
Urine prostaglandins	Very high	High or normal	Normal
Response to indomethacin	Good	Good	Rare

From Johnson RJ, Feehally J. *Comprehensive Clinical Nephrology,* 2nd ed. Philadelphia: Mosby, 2003.

BIBLIOGRAPHY

1. Adachi M, Asakura Y, Sato Y, et al. Novel SLC12A1 (NKCC2) mutations in two families with Bartter syndrome type 1. *Endocr J* 2007;54(6):1003–1007.
2. Akinci B, Celik A, Saygili F, et al. A case of Gitelman's syndrome presenting with extreme hypokalaemia and paralysis. *Exp Clin Endocrinol Diab* 2009;117(2):69–71.
3. Aoi N, Nakayama T, Tahira Y, et al. Two novel genotypes of the thiazide-sensitive Na-Cl cotransporter (SLC12A3) gene in patients with Gitelman's syndrome. *Endocrine* 2007;31(2):149–153.
4. Cheng CJ, Shiang JC, Hsu YJ, et al. Hypocalciuria in patients with Gitelman syndrome: Role of blood volume. *Am J Kidney Dis* 2007;49(5):693–700.
5. Colussi G, Bettinelli A, Tedeschi S, et al. A thiazide test for the diagnosis of renal tubular hypokalemic disorders. *Clin J Am Soc Nephrol* 2007;2(3):454–460
6. Garovic VD, Hilliard AA, Turner ST.. Monogenic forms of low-renin hypertension. *Nat Clin Pract Nephrol* 2006; 11(2):624–630.
7. Geller DS, Farhi A, Pinkerton N, et al. Activating mineralocorticoid receptor mutation in hypertension exacerbated by pregnancy. *Science* 2000;289(5476):119–123.
8. Huyet J, Pinon GM, Fay MR, et al. Structural basis of spirolactone recognition by the mineralocorticoid receptor. *Mol Pharmacol* 2007;72:563–571.
9. Krämer BK, Bergler T, Stoelcker B, et al. Mechanisms of disease: The kidney-specific chloride channels ClCKA and ClCKB, the Barttin subunit, and their clinical relevance. *Nat Clin Pract Nephrol* 2008;4(1):38–46.
10. Mosso L, Carvajal C, González A, et al. Primary aldosteronism and hypertensive disease. *Hypertension* 2003;42:161–165.
11. Mount D, Pollak M. *Molecular and Genetic Basis of Renal Disease: A Companion to Brenner and Rector's The Kidney.* Philadelphia: Elsevier Health Sciences, 2007.
12. Nozu K, Inagaki T, Fu XJ, et al. Molecular analysis of digenic inheritance in Bartter syndrome with sensorineural deafness. *J Med Genet* 2008;45(3):182–186.
13. Pachulski RT, Lopez F, Sharaf R. Gitelman's not-so-benign syndrome. *N Engl J Med* 2005;353(8):850–851.
14. Rafestin-Oblin ME, Souque A, Bocchi B, et al. The severe form of hypertension caused by the activating S810L mutation in the mineralocorticoid receptor is cortisone related. *Endocrinology* 2003;144(2):528–533.
15. Seyberth HW. An improved terminology and classification of Bartter-like syndromes. *Nat Clin Pract Nephrol* 2008;10:560–567.
16. Strautnieks SS, Thompson RJ, Gardiner RM, et al. A novel splice-site mutation in the gamma subunit of the epithelial sodium channel gene in three pseudohypoaldosteronism type 1 families. *Nat Genet* 1996;13(2): 248–250.
17. Xie J, Craig L, Cobb MH, et al. Role of with-no-lysine [K] kinases in the pathogenesis of Gordon's syndrome. *Pediatr Nephrol* 2006;21:1231–1236.
18. Yang S, Morimoto T, Rai T, et al. Molecular pathogenesis of pseudohypoaldosteronism type II: Generation and analysis of a Wnk4D561A/+ knockin mouse model. *Cell Metab* 2007;5:331–344.

CHAPTER 76

HYPONATREMIA AND HYPERNATREMIA

Tomas Berl, MD, and Jeffrey Thomas, MD

1. **Is the serum sodium a reflection of total body sodium?**
   No.

2. **Then what is it a reflection of?**
   It is a reflection of the relative concentration of sodium in water in a liter of plasma. Disorders of total body sodium reflect disturbances in extracellular fluid (ECF) volume because sodium is the predominant cation in ECF, as was discussed in Chapter 74. Increases (hypernatremia) and decreases (hyponatremia) in serum sodium concentration can therefore occur in settings of low, normal, and high total body sodium. The term dehydration, which strictly speaking reflects loss of total body water resulting in hypernatremia, is often misused to describe hypovolemic states. The assessment of total body sodium is an important component of the approach to the diagnosis and treatment of dysnatremic disorders. Dysnatremias are reflected in alterations in plasma osmolality.

3. **How is plasma osmolality determined?**
   Plasma osmolality can be either measured by an osmometer or calculated using the following formula:

   $$\text{Plasma osmolality (mOsm/kg)} = 2[\text{Na}](\text{mEq/L}) + \text{urea (mg/dL)}/2.8 + \text{glucose (mg/dL)}/18$$

   Please note the central role of the sodium concentration as the primary determinate of plasma osmolality based on this equation. Normally, the measured plasma osmolality is no more than 10 mOsm/kg higher than the calculated plasma osmolality. If the measured osmolality greatly exceeds 10 mOsm, an osmolar gap reflecting the presence of an osmotically active substance is not routinely measured in the ECF.

4. **Is there a difference between tonicity and osmolality?**
   Yes. Tonicity is determined by the presence of impermeable solutes such as sodium and chloride in the ECF. Such solutes set up osmotic gradients that cause water movement across cell membranes. In contrast, solutes that are permeable to cell membranes (alcohols, urea) contribute to the measured osmolality of body fluids but do not cause water movement and therefore are not effective solutes and do not contribute to tonicity.

5. **Does hypernatremia always reflect hyperosmolality?**
   Yes. Not only are patients with hypernatremia hyperosmolar, but they are also hypertonic. In contrast, not every patient with hyperosmolality is hypertonic. Such is the case with alcohol ingestion and azotemia.

6. **Does hyponatremia always reflect hypo-osmolality?**
   No. Hyponatremia can also occur with normal or even hyperosmolality.

7. **In what clinical settings does hyponatremia occur with normal or high plasma osmolality?**
   This occurs in three settings:
   - **Pseudohyponatremia.** Sodium determination in plasma reflects its presence in the water component of plasma. When solids such as lipids and proteins circulate in greatly elevated amounts, they occupy a volume that falsely dilutes the measured sodium concentration. Neither the flame photometer nor indirect potentiometry with ion-specific electrodes resolves this discrepancy. Only direct potentiometry with undiluted sample will provide the accurate measurement of serum sodium in the water component. An experimentally derived formula has been proposed to calculate the change in plasma water content brought about by protein and lipids. The protein and lipid concentrations are in kg/L:

     $$\text{Plasma water content} = 0.991 - (0.73 \times [\text{protein}]) - (1.03 \times [\text{lipid}])$$

   - **Translocational hyponatremia.** This reflects the translocation of water from cells into the ECF diluting plasma sodium concentration. This occurs primarily with glucose in the setting of uncontrolled diabetes but can also occur with use of mannitol. The plasma sodium concentration is increased by approximately 1.6 mEq/L of every 100 mg/dL of glucose above normal.
   - **Renal failure.** The presence of azotemia in renal failure contributes to the measured plasma osmolality, albeit not to the effective plasma tonicity. Thus patients with renal failure who are hyponatremic have true hypotonicity.

8. **What is the diagnostic approach to the patient with hypotonic hyponatremia?**
   Once it is established that the hyponatremia is hypotonic, it is helpful to determine whether the patient is or is not diluting the urine. To this end, a urinary osmolality of <100 mOsm/kg reflects intact diluting mechanism. A urinary osmolality of >100 mOsm/kg suggests a diluting defect.

9. **What is the approach to the patient with hyponatremia with urinary osmolality of <100 mOsm/kg?**
   The ability of the kidney to dilute the urine protects against hypotonic states and allows for the very generous intake of water of up to >20 L per day. The kidneys are able to excrete 15% to 18% of daily glomerular ultrafiltrate as free water (daily glomerular filtration rate [GFR] is 180 L × 15% = 27 L). When this limit is exceeded, water is retained and the patient can become hyponatremic. This is known as water intoxication or psychogenic polydipsia.
   This generous flexibility for water intake is dependent on normal solute. The average Western diet contains approximately 800 mOsm of solute. This is derived from the dietary content of sodium (150 mEq/day), potassium (50 mEq/day), and accompanying anions, which accounts for 400 mOsm per day. An approximately equivalent contribution is provided by urea from protein catabolism (50 mmol/day) and dietary intake of protein that generates 50 mmol per 10 g (80 g average dietary intake × 50 mmol = 400 mmol). At an average urinary osmolality of 50 mOsm/kg, these 800 mOsm can be excreted in 16 L of urine. However, if the solute intake is limited and solute excretion decreases, for example, to only 200 mOsm, even in the face of the same urinary dilution, the maximal urine flow is limited to 4 L per day. If more than this volume of fluid is ingested, then hyponatremia will ensue. This is the case with the "tea and toast" diet and beer potomania.

10. **What is the approach to the patient with hyponatremia with urinary osmolality of >100 mOsm/kg?**
    The presence of urine osmolality of >100 mOsm/kg in a patient who is hypotonic and hyponatremic reflects a defect in urinary dilution. These patients can be approached by an assessment of total body sodium (i.e., hypovolemic, euvolemic, or hypervolemic as depicted in Fig. 76-1).

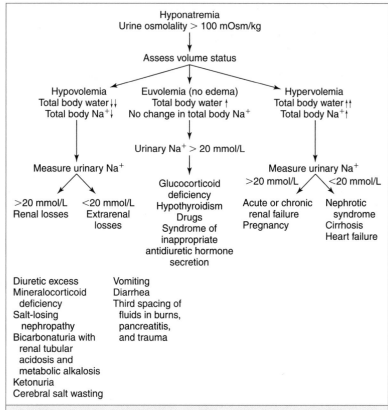

Figure 76-1. Diagnostic approach to the patient with hypotonic hyponatremia. (Modified from Chonchol M, Berl T. Hyponatremia. In: Hamm L, DuBose T (eds.). *Acid-Base and Electrolyte Disorders: A Companion to Brenner & Rector's The Kidney.* Philadelphia: Saunders, 2002, p. 231.)

11. **What is the incidence of hyponatremia?**
    The incidence and prevalence of hyponatremia vary dramatically with the level of serum sodium used to define the disorder and the setting in which the measurement is done (acute care hospital or ambulatory care). A recent report involving almost 100,000 hospitalized patients observed a sodium of <135 mEq/L in 14.5% of patients at initial measurement. These patients had higher in-hospital, 1-year, and 5-year mortalities with multivariate analysis.

12. **What is the syndrome of inappropriate antidiuretic hormone secretion?**
    As shown in Figure 76-1, syndrome of inappropriate antidiuretic hormone secretion (SIADH) is a form of euvolemic hyponatremia that occurs independently of adrenal, thyroid, cardiac, hepatic, and renal diseases and is not caused by the concomitant administration of drugs that stimulate the hormone's release or enhance its action. Likewise, there is an absence of osmotic or volume stimulus. It is therefore a setting of unprovoked vasopressin release. This occurs in a large variety of central nervous system disorders, pulmonary disorders, and tumors. In a patient with new onset of hyponatremia from SIADH, a search for an underlying tumor and especially a small cell carcinoma of the lung with a chest CT is indicated. On rare occasions a tumor becomes evident later in the course, but the frequency with which a tumor workup should be undertaken if the initial one is negative has not been established.

Because of water expansion, the urine sodium concentration is generally >20 mmol/L, but it can be lower in the face of concomitant volume contraction or poor solute intake. In large measure the urinary sodium excretion reflects the sodium intake. In some series, the uric acid has been recognized to be low (<4 mg/dL), probably reflecting a high fractional excretion of urate. Thus the diagnosis of SIADH can be made in a patient with euvolemia whose effective extracellular osmolality is <270 mOsm/kg as the urinary osmolality exceeds 100 mOsm/kg. The urinary sodium is elevated (>40 mEq/L) in the face of normal sodium intake, and adrenal, thyroid, renal, and pituitary disease have to be ruled out. A confirmatory vasopressin level can be obtained but is not necessary as the elevated urinary osmolality is in essence a bioassay for the presence of the hormone in the circulation.

13. **What are the clinical manifestations of hyponatremia?**
Because the underlying pathology of hyponatremia is cell swelling, the size limitations of the brain cause most of the symptoms. The rate at which hyponatremia develops is an important determinant of symptoms. Severe acute hyponatremia of <48 hours duration can be associated with seizures, coma, neurogenic pulmonary edema, and tentorial herniation particularly when adaptive mechanisms fail to operate. After 48 hours, solute losses from the brain attenuate the degree of cerebral swelling and symptoms are less dramatic—anorexia, nausea, vomiting, muscle cramps, and only when very severe also seizures. Many patients with chronic hyponatremia are deemed to be "asymptomatic." Recent observational and case-controlled studies have suggested that such patients may have subtle neuropsychiatric disturbances, gait disturbances, increased risk for falls, and increased risk for fractures. The risk for the latter complication may be aggravated by an effect of hyponatremia on bone mineral content.

14. **How is hyponatremia treated?**
Treatment is based on the etiology of the hyponatremia.
Because the underlying etiology of **hypovolemic hyponatremia** disorders is a deficit of total body sodium and a decrease in blood volume leading to the nonosmotic release of vasopressin, the treatment requires volume repletion with saline.

Hypervolemic hyponatremia disorders are characterized by decreased effective blood volume (heart failure) or peripheral dilatation (cirrhosis). These hemodynamic disorders lead to nonosmotic vasopressin release, which underlies the diluting defect in most of these patients. The treatment revolves around restriction of both sodium and water. Two vasopressin antagonists have been approved for treatment in these settings: conivaptan and tolvaptan. Both drugs cause a prompt aquaresis characterized by an increase in urine volume and decrease in urinary osmolality. Neither alters sodium excretion. Although Tolvaptan is a pure V2 antagonist approved for oral use, conivaptan is both a V1/V2 antagonist and is approved for short-term (4-day) intravenous use only. Both drugs are well tolerated overall. Their main side effects relate to their aquaretic action: thirst polyuria and dry mouth. Tolvaptan has been found to maintain its efficacy both in short-term (30 days) and long-term (up to 2 years) trials. Conivaptan should be used with caution in patients with cirrhosis given its V1 antagonist activity.

Treatment of **euvolemic hyponatremia** should begin with withdrawal of offending drugs and treatment of underlying endocrinopathies (adrenal, thyroid). In SIADH, water restriction has been the cornerstone for the treatment of this syndrome for many decades. This restriction has to be unduly severe in patients with a severe form of this syndrome characterized by a ratio of

$$\frac{UNa + Uk}{PNa} \text{ greater than } 1$$

Compliance with this regimen is poor because many patients also have a defective thirst mechanism. In addition, when the ratio of this formula exceeds 1, the administration of isotonic saline will result in a further decrement in serum sodium because the NaCl will be excreted in a volume lower than the one infused, culminating in net water retention. The correction of the hyponatremia requires that net negative free water balance be achieved. Thus the Na + K of the solution given must be higher than that of the excreted urine.

An increase in solute load and excretion with urea allows for the excretion of a larger volume of urine and is effective but is poorly tolerated. Solute excretion can also be increased with saline tablets accompanied by loop diuretics to prevent positive sodium balance and allow for the excretion of free water. Both lithium and demeclocycline inhibit the renal action of vasopressin and particularly the latter has been used in patients with this syndrome. The aforementioned vasopressin antagonists may be ideal agents for patients with SIADH. In the Tolvaptan trials an increment of approximately 7 to 8 mEq/L was observed.

15. **At what rate should hyponatremia be corrected?**
This is determined by the duration of hyponatremia and the presence or absence of symptoms.

Based on animal studies and clinical observations, hyponatremia has been classified as acute if it is of <48 hours duration. When symptomatic, such patients (particularly premenstrual females and children) are prone to severe cerebral edema and its neurologic consequences and should be treated emergently. The primary treatment for rapid correction of sodium involves the administration of hypertonic saline to minimize brain edema. Recent studies suggest that elevations of serum sodium by 4 to 6 mmol may be sufficient to prevent tentorial herniation and can significantly decrease intracranial pressure. Thus, although full and rapid correction may be safe in these patients, it is not necessary.

When the duration of hyponatremia exceeds 48 hours or is of unknown duration, careful attention to the rate of correction is necessary. The brain has likely undergone an adaptive response to the hypotonic state to minimize cerebral edema. This adaptation involves the loss of sodium chloride, potassium, and osmolytes (glutamate, sorbitol, betaine, and especially inositol). These brains are sensitive to correction rates that exceed 10 to 12 mmol per 24 hours or 18 mmol in 48 hours because the restoration of the aforementioned inert solutes is frequently sluggish or delayed, causing cerebral water losses. The serum sodium in symptomatic patients with chronic hyponatremia can also be treated with hypertonic saline or with normal saline in conjunction with a loop diuretic to generate renal free water losses. By this approach, the solute losses generated by the loop diuretic are returned to the patient in a lower volume of either hypertonic or normal saline, resulting in net electrolyte free water losses. Vasopressin antagonists are alternative options for treatment because they appear to increase serum sodium by 6 to 8 mmol per 24 hours in most reported studies. Whichever approach is used, serum sodium needs to be carefully monitored every 2 to 4 hours along with urine volume to prevent overcorrection. If overcorrection occurs, serum sodium should be relowered by administration of water with or without DDAVP (1-deamino-8-D-arginine vasopressin, or desmopressin acetate).

Patients who present without overt symptoms of hyponatremia almost always have had the disorder for >48 hours. Because of the recent recognition that these patients, despite appearing asymptomatic, are at risk for falls and fractures, it has been suggested that elderly individuals with serum sodium of <125 mEq/L should have these electrolyte disorder corrected. Data to support that such correction would result in decreased falls and fractures are lacking, but gait disturbances have been found to improve with such an approach.

16. **What is the diagnostic approach to the patient with hypernatremia?**
As was the case with hyponatremia, patients with hypernatremia can have a low, normal, or high total body sodium. An assessment of volume status is helpful in these patients (Fig. 76-2).

17. **How does hypernatremia develop?**
Although a defect in urinary dilution underlies the etiology of most hyponatremic disorders, a defect in urinary concentration is responsible at least in part for the development of hypernatremia. The urinary concentrating mechanism is highly dependent on the generation of interstitial hypertonicity. The failure to generate hypertonic medulla, as occurs with acute or

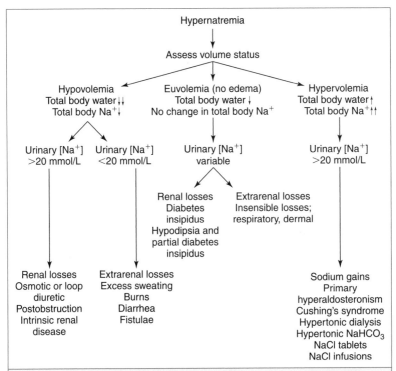

Figure 76-2. Diagnostic approach to the patient with hypernatremia. (Modified from Bichet D, Mallie JP. Hypernatremia and the polyuric disorders. In: Hamm L, DuBose T (eds.). *Acid-Base and Electrolyte Disorders: A Companion to Brenner & Rector's The Kidney.* Philadelphia: Saunders, 2002, p. 242.)

chronic renal failure, the use of loop diuretics, or poor protein intake, places such patients at risk to develop hypernatremia. Likewise, the concentrating mechanism is highly dependent on the ability of collecting ducts to become water permeable under the influence of vasopressin, which is impaired in diabetes insipidus. However, in these disorders hypernatremia would remain mild (sodium up to 145 mEq/L) if the hypertonic response to thirst is intact because increased water intake can compensate for increased urinary water losses (polyuria) and prevent development of severe hypernatremia.

18. **What is polyuria and how should it be approached?**
Polyuria is defined as the excretion of more than 3 L of urine per day. A determination of urinary osmolality can differentiate between hypotonic polyuria caused primarily by the excretion of free water or a polyuria driven by high solute excretion. In the former setting the urinary osmolality is lower than plasma and frequently below 100 mOsm/Kg. This can be a result of diabetes insipidus or primary polydipsia. In contrast, a solute-driven polyuria is characterized by the excretion of a urine more concentrated than plasma. Because the normal solute consumption requires the excretion of no more than 900 mOsm/day, this can be achieved in 3 L of urine excreted at 300 mOsm/L (osmolar excretion rate = urinary osmolality × volume). Thus a patient whose urine output is 5 L with a urinary osmolality 400 mOsm/L is excreting 2000 m osmoles per day— a solute diuresis. This can occur, for example, in uncontrolled diabetes mellitus.

19. **What is diabetes insipidus?**

Diabetes insipidus is a disorder of vasopressin secretion (neurogenic diabetes insipidus), vasopressin action (nephrogenic diabetes insipidus), or accelerated breakdown of the hormone by vasopressinase (gestational diabetes insipidus). The most frequent causes of central and nephrogenic diabetes insipidus are listed in Table 76-1.

Neurogenic and nephrogenic diabetes insipidus can be differentiated by the response to water restriction followed by the administration of vasopressin or an analogue. The patient with neurogenic diabetes insipidus will have a robust response to the exogenous hormone. Some patients with the disorder have a partial defect in vasopressin secretion and can attain a moderately concentrated urine when water restricted, but they also will increase their urinary osmolality by >10% when given vasopressin. In contrast, the patient with nephrogenic diabetes insipidus will display no such response to the exogenously administered hormone and will remain with unchanged urine tonicity.

Of the listed causes of central diabetes insipidus, the idiopathic variety is characterized by an acute onset and the penchant for ice cold water. An autoimmune etiology has been suggested. Most patients with acquired nephrogenic diabetes insipidus can usually concentrate their urine to isotonicity. This is not the case in congenital diabetes insipidus, which comes in two forms related to mutations in the pathway of the cellular action of vasopressin. The most common of these (90%) is the X-linked variety with mutations in the vasopressin-2 receptor. Patients with this mutation are unable to generate cyclic adenosine monophosphate (AMP), the signaling molecule of this receptor. Less frequent (10%) is the autosomal-recessive mutation of the vasopressin-dependent water channel (aquaporin 2). These patients cannot insert the water channel in the luminal membrane, a step that is critical to render the collecting duct permeable to water.

TABLE 76-1.	CAUSES OF DIABETES INSIPIDUS	
	Causes of Neurogenic Diabetes Insipidus	Causes of Nephrogenic Diabetes Insipidus
Hereditary	Autosomal dominant Autosomal recessive	X-linked Autosomal recessive
Acquired	Idiopathic Head trauma Hypophysectomy Brain tumors (primary or metastatic) Infections (encephalitis, meningitis, Guillain-Barré syndrome) Vascular (cerebral aneurysm, cerebral thrombosis or hemorrhage, sickle cell disease, postpartum necrosis [Sheehan syndrome]) Granulomas (sarcoid, Wegener granulomatosis, tuberculosis, syphilis)	Acute or chronic kidney disease Electrolyte disorders (hypokalemia, hypercalcemia) Drugs (lithium, demeclocycline, amphotericin, foscarnet, osmotic diuretics, furosemide and ethacrynic acid) Sickle cell disease Dietary abnormalities (excessive water intake, decreased sodium chloride or protein)

Modified from Berl T, Schrier R. In Schrier R (ed.). *Renal and Electrolyte Disorders,* 7th ed. Philadelphia: Lippincott Williams & Wilkins, 2010, pp. 16 and 21.

20. **How is diabetes insipidus treated?**
    The treatment of neurogenic diabetes insipidus centers on hormone replacement, primarily with DDAVP. Those with a partial defect can be treated with drugs that enhance the peripheral action of the hormone, such as chlorpropamide or carbamazepine. Nephrogenic diabetes insipidus is more challenging to treat. In children a low-sodium diet to induce volume contraction, then maintained with diuretics, has been used. This enhances proximal fluid reabsorption leading to decreased delivery of tubular fluid to the distal nephron and thereby decreased urine flow. Some patients respond to nonsteroidal anti-inflammatory agents. In the particular setting of Li-induced nephrogenic diabetes insipidus, amiloride ameliorates the condition as Li also enters the cell by the amiloride sensitive sodium channel.

21. **Who is prone to develop hypernatremia?**
    As mentioned earlier, it is not surprising that those individuals at the extremes of life, who cannot access water or have impaired thirst perception, are most prone to this disorder. Thus, infants who lose hypotonic fluids with gastrointestinal ailments and who cannot request water are at risk. Likewise, the elderly with dementia or strokes are in a similar situation, compounded by aging itself being associated with decreased thirst perception. This age group reflects the preponderance of patients admitted with hypernatremia. There is, however, a significant incidence of hospital-acquired hypernatremia caused by unappreciated water losses, osmotic diuresis with hyperalimentation, and the use of loop diuretics. The development of hypernatremia in the hospital is associated with increased mortality and prolonged hospitalization.

KEY POINTS: HYPONATREMIA AND HYPERNATREMIA

1. Abnormalities in serum sodium concentration reflect disturbances in water, not sodium homeostasis. Thus disorders of serum sodium occur with low, normal, or high total body sodium.

2. Although every patient with hypernatremia is hypertonic, not every patient with hyponatremia is hypotonic. Hyponatremia can coexist with normal or even high tonicity as in pseudohyponatremia and translocational hyponatremia.

3. Duration of hyponatremia and the presence of symptoms determine the correction of hyponatremia. In acute symptomatic hyponatremia, increasing serum sodium rapidly with hypertonic saline by 4 to 6 mEq/L may be sufficient to prevent tentorial herniation. In patients with chronic hyponatremia correction limits are 12 mEq/L in 24 hours and 18 mEq/L in 48 hours to decrease the risk for osmotic demyelination. When these are exceeded, serum sodium should be relowered.

4. Hospital-acquired hypernatremia, which is not infrequently hypervolemic, is associated with prolonged hospitalization and increased mortality. This is preventable with attention to water repletion.

22. **What are the symptoms of hypernatremia?**
    The symptoms of hypernatremia are primarily neurologic, resulting in cellular dehydration, which can lead to tears in cerebral vessels. Symptoms include irritability, spasticity, lethargy, and hyper-reflexia. The adaptive response to hypernatremia involves the accumulation of the aforementioned osmolytes, which attenuate brain dehydration and ameliorate symptoms associated with this electrolyte disorder.

23. **How is hypernatremia treated?**
    Hypernatremia, particularly in the elderly and those who acquired it in the hospital, is preventable by proper attention to water repletion. Once established, treatment is based on the etiology of the hypernatremia.

- **Hypovolemic hypernatremia.** Correction of volume deficits takes priority over correction of tonicity in these patients. The restoration of circulatory volume with isotonic saline will restore volume. Thus, in a patient with hypernatremia and hypovolemia, normal saline is the treatment of choice because the sodium is needed to restore extracellular fluid volume. Attention should be given to minimize ongoing loss of hypotonic fluids (either renal or extrarenal) that generated the disorder. Once hemodynamics are stable, attention can be directed to correcting the hypernatremia with hypotonic fluids.
- **Euvolemic hypernatermia.** The treatment of central diabetes insipidus revolves around the replacement of the hormone or drugs that enhance the action of the drug when the disease is partial. The treatment of nephrogenic diabetes insipidus is more challenging (Table 76-2). Gestational diabetes insipidus is treated with DDAVP because this form of the hormone is not cleaved by vasopressinase.
- **Hypervolemic hypernatremia.** These patients represent as much as 30% to 40% of hospital-acquired hypernatremia because they received sodium-containing solutions but an inadequate amount of water to match water losses. This can be reversed by promoting sodium losses with diuretics and repletion with oral or intravenous hypotonic fluids.

24. **How can we estimate water deficits?**
    The amount of water necessary to restore the serum sodium to 140 mEq/L (water deficit) can be calculated with the following equation:

$$\text{Water deficit (L)} = 0.6 \times \text{body weight (kg)} \times \left[1 - \frac{\text{Current plasma sodium}\,(P_{Na})}{140} \right]$$

TABLE 76-2. TREATMENT OF DIABETES INSIPIDUS

	Drug	Dose
Complete central diabetes insipidus	DDAVP	10–20 μg intranasally every 12–24 hours 0.1–0.8 mg orally in divided doses; start with 0.05 mg orally every 12 hours and adjust as needed
Partial central diabetes insipidus	DDAVP	10–20 μg intranasally every 12–24 hours
	Aqueous vasopressin	5–10 U subcutaneously every 4–6 hours
	Chlorpropamide	250–500 mg/day
	Clofibrate	500 mg tid–qid
	Carbamazepine	400–600 mg/day
Nephrogenic diabetes insipidus	Thiazide diuretics	25–50 mg/day
	NSAIDs	Indomethacin 1–2 mg/kg/day
	Amiloride (for lithium-related disease)	5 mg/day
Gestational diabetes insipidus	DDAVP	As above

DDAVP = 1-deamino-8-D-arginine vasopressin, or desmopressin acetate; NSAIDs = nonsteroidal anti-inflammatory drugs.
Modified from Thurman J, Berl T. In Wilcox C (ed.). *Therapy in Nephrology and Hypertension,* 3rd ed. Philadelphia: Saunders, 2008, p. 350.

This formula assumes that 60% of the total body weight is water, a number that should be modified to 50% in women and elderly men. Thus, a 70-kg man who is 60 years old and has a serum sodium of 154 would require 3.5 L of free water:

$$\text{Water deficit} = 0.5 \times 70 \times [1 - 154/140]$$
$$= 35 \times [1 - 1.1]$$
$$= 35 \times -0.1$$
$$= -3.5 \text{ L}$$

This formula is only an estimate, and serum sodium should be monitored frequently. In addition, ongoing water losses also would have to be added to this deficit and repleted.

25. **At what rate should hypernatremia be corrected?**
    It is generally recommended that approximately half of the water losses be corrected in the first 24 hours, but literature supporting such an approach and its safety is lacking. In patients with chronic hypernatremia, a correction of 8 to 10 mmol per 24 hours is probably sufficient. Exceeding this rate could at least theoretically result in the development of cerebral edema. Such a complication, culminating in seizures, coma, and death, has been reported in the pediatric literature but appears to be unusual in older individuals.

BIBLIOGRAPHY

1. Berl T, Parikh C. Disorders of water metabolism. In: Johnson RJ, Feehally J, Floege J (eds.). *Comprehensive Clinical Nephrology*, 4th ed. Philadelphia: Saunders/Elsevier, 2010.
2. Berl T, Schrier RW. Disorders of water homeostasis. In: Schrier RW (ed.). *Renal and Electrolyte Disorders*, 7th ed. Philadelphia: Lippincott Williams & Wilkins, 2010, pp. 1–44.
3. Koenig MA, Bryan M, Lewin JL 3rd, et al. Reversal of transtentorial herniation with hypertonic saline. *Neurology* 2008;70(13):1023–1029.
4. Nguyen MK, Ornekian V, Butch AW, et al. A new method for determining plasma water content: application in pseudohyponatremia. *Am J Physiol Renal Physiol* 2007;292(5):F1652–1656.
5. Waikar SS, Mount DB, Curhan GC. Mortality after hospitalization with mild, moderate, and severe hyponatremia. *Am J Med* 2009;122(9):857–865.

CHAPTER 77

HYPOKALEMIA AND HYPERKALEMIA

Rebecca Moore, MD, and Stuart L. Linas, MD

1. **Describe normal potassium balance.**
   A normal adult has approximately 50 mEq/kg of total body potassium; 98% of that potassium is located in the intracellular space. The body tightly regulates serum potassium concentration at approximately 4 mEq/L. This balance is achieved partially through stool losses (about 5–10 mEq/day) and sweat losses (0–10 mEq/day) but is primarily realized through the kidneys, which appropriately vary potassium secretion based on changes in dietary intake. The average diet contains between 40 and 120 mEq/day of potassium.

2. **Why is potassium balance important?**
   There is a large potassium gradient between the intracellular and extracellular spaces, which is essential for maintaining the cellular membrane resting potential. Regulating this gradient is critical because a difference of as little as 1.5% of intracellular potassium moving into the extracellular space can result in a potentially fatal increase in serum potassium concentration.

3. **What is the primary cellular mechanism that maintains potassium balance?**
   Normal potassium distribution is achieved via the Na-K-ATPase pump located on the cellular membrane. This pump works to keep the intracellular potassium concentration high and the extracellular potassium concentration low. It is regulated by catecholamines, insulin, and the plasma potassium concentration itself.

4. **Why don't serum potassium levels go up when we eat a dietary potassium load (such as a hamburger and soda)?**
   Small increases in serum potassium induce insulin release. Also, when a dietary potassium load is ingested, we also ingest a dietary glucose load, which promotes the release of insulin. Insulin enhances the entry of potassium into skeletal muscle and the liver by increasing the activity of the Na-K-ATPase pump. This results in minimizing the rise in plasma potassium concentration that occurs with the intake of a potassium load.

5. **What factors can cause hypokalemia by shifting potassium into cells?**
   The shift of potassium intracellularly will occur in the following settings: metabolic alkalosis, insulin loading, and beta-2-adrenergic stimulation.

6. **What factors can cause hyperkalemia by shifting potassium out of cells?**
   The shift of potassium extracellularly will occur with acidosis, insulin deficiency, beta-adrenergic blockade, ischemia (or dead cells), exercise, and severe hyperglycemia (and other hyperosmotic states that pull water from cells, thereby increasing cellular potassium, enhancing the gradient to move potassium out of cells, and increasing serum potassium).

7. **What electrocardiogram (ECG) changes occur in patients with hypokalemia?**
   The characteristic changes on ECG seen in hypokalemia include the following: (1) ST segment depression, (2) T-wave flattening, (3) increased U-wave amplitude (waves that occur at the end of the T wave), and (4) ventricular fibrillation.

The progression of ECG changes varies widely from patient to patient so that some patients can present with ventricular fibrillation alone. Thus, continual monitoring of the ECG is required.

8. **What ECG changes occur in patients with hyperkalemia?**
The characteristic ECG changes seen in hyperkalemia progress from peaked T waves initially, followed by lengthening of the PR interval and QRS prolongation, leading to the QRS progressively widening to a "sine wave," which eventually results in cardiac standstill.
As in hypokalemia, the actual potassium concentration associated with the progression of ECG changes varies widely from patient to patient, and continual monitoring of the ECG is essential when managing patients with hyperkalemia.

9. **What are some of the signs and symptoms of hypokalemia?**
In addition to arrhythmias, hypokalemia can induce systemic symptoms. In mild hypokalemia (serum potassium 3.0–3.5 mEq/L), patients are often asymptomatic. As hypokalemia progresses, nonspecific symptoms develop, such as weakness and malaise. When serum potassium drops below 2.0 mEq/L, it can precipitate muscle necrosis and paralysis, causing respiratory failure.

10. **What are some of the signs and symptoms of hyperkalemia?**
Similar to hypokalemia, hyperkalemia can cause systemic symptoms in addition to cardiac arrhythmias. Symptoms usually do not become clinically apparent until serum potassium levels are very high (more than 7.0 mEq/L) and include ascending muscle paralysis progressing to a flaccid paralysis.

11. **What is pseudohyperkalemia and what are some of its causes?**
Pseudohyperkalemia is the elevation of the serum potassium level in the absence of either cell shifts or an increase in total body potassium. It can be present in the setting of thrombocytosis, leukocytosis, and hemolysis. It results from the movement of potassium out of cells during or after the blood sample has been drawn.

12. **How can one determine if an elevated serum potassium is "real"?**
Obtaining a plasma potassium, rather than a serum potassium, will differentiate pseudohyperkalemia from true hyperkalemia.

13. **What factors determine renal potassium excretion?**
Renal potassium excretion is dependent on distal nephron sodium delivery, aldosterone, and urine flow.

14. **How does distal delivery of volume and sodium increase potassium excretion?**
Sodium is reabsorbed in the collecting duct via epithelial sodium channels, which stimulates the basolateral Na-K-ATPase, which in turn facilitates the movement of potassium into the collecting duct (i.e., into the urine) via potassium channels. With poor urine flow or distal sodium delivery, the gradient for potassium to be secreted into the collecting duct is too steep and there is insufficient sodium for uptake by sodium channels.

15. **How does aldosterone effect renal potassium excretion?**
Aldosterone increases renal potassium excretion by acting on principal cells in the collecting duct. Aldosterone stimulates renal uptake of sodium and renal secretion of potassium.

16. **What conditions stimulate release of aldosterone in a normal person?**
Aldosterone is released in response to hypotension and hyperkalemia.

17. **What is the transtubular potassium gradient and how can it be used in the diagnosis of hyperkalemia?**
The transtubular potassium gradient (TTKG) estimates the difference in potassium concentration between the tubular fluid (i.e., urine) at the end of the cortical collecting tubule (CCT) and the plasma. It can be used to estimate the amount of aldosterone activity. In a normal person, the TTKG on a regular diet is 8 or 9, and in the setting of a potassium load, it will rise to higher than 11. In someone with hypoaldosteronism and impaired ability to excrete potassium renally, the TTKG will be low (<7). It can be calculated using this formula:

$$\text{TTKG} = [\text{Urine K} \div (\text{Urine osmolality/Plasma osmolality})] \div \text{Plasma K}$$

18. **How does impaired renal function affect renal potassium excretion?**
The kidney is able secrete potassium normally in patients with impaired renal function until the glomerular filtration rate (GFR) falls to >20% of normal as long as aldosterone secretion and distal sodium delivery are intact.

19. **How do loop or thiazide diuretics cause renal potassium loss?**
Diuretics cause renal potassium loss via several mechanisms, including increased urine flow, increased distal sodium delivery, and aldosterone stimulation from volume depletion.

20. **Which class of diuretics can result in hyperkalemia?**
Sodium channel blockers, such as amiloride and triamterene, can lead to hyperkalemia by blocking sodium reabsorption in the collecting duct, which reduces the electrochemical gradient that favors potassium excretion, thereby inducing hyperkalemia. Aldosterone receptor blockers, such as spironolactone, also can induce hyperkalemia by inhibiting the effect of aldosterone in the collecting duct.

21. **What medications commonly cause hyperkalemia? What is the mechanism?**
See Table 77-1.

22. **Does inhibiting the renin-angiotensin system (RAS) with angiotensin-converting enzyme inhibitors, angiotensin receptor blockers, and aldosterone blockers cause hyperkalemia in patients on dialysis?**
In general, patients with end-stage renal disease (ESRD) receiving dialysis do not have enough renal function to depend on renal potassium excretion to maintain normal serum potassium levels. Rather, they depend on regular dialysis to remove potassium and must watch their dietary intake. Therefore, medications that impair renal potassium excretion do not generally produce hyperkalemia in this population.
However, there appears to be a subset of patients with ESRD who depend heavily on gut elimination of potassium, which may be influenced by RAS inhibition. In these patients, RAS inhibitors may cause hyperkalemia by decreasing fecal potassium excretion.

23. **How should hypokalemia be corrected?**
How one replaces potassium should be based on the severity of hypokalemia, whether the patient is symptomatic, whether normal renal function is present, and whether continued losses are expected. Potassium chloride is generally the preferred compound for repleting potassium (rather than potassium phosphate or potassium citrate) to avoid giving unnecessary phosphate or base to a patient.
If hypokalemia is mild and asymptomatic (>3 mEq/L) and there are no ongoing losses, it is reasonable to use oral replacement with 10 to 20 mEq of potassium chloride two to three times per day and then recheck the potassium level. If the hypokalemia is moderate and asymptomatic (<3.0 mEq/L) and there are no ongoing losses, it is reasonable to give oral potassium chloride 40 to 60 mEq two to three times per day until the potassium is >3.0 mEq/L. If there are ongoing losses present (i.e., diuretics, vomiting, diarrhea), this can be scheduled.

TABLE 77–1. MEDICATIONS THAT CAUSE HYPERKALEMIA	
Medication	Mechanism of Hyperkalemia
Beta blockers	Decrease cellular uptake of potassium
Succinylcholine	Depolarizes cell membranes, making interior charge of cells less negative, reducing the electrical barrier for potassium exit, and allowing leakage of potassium out of cells
Digoxin	Inhibits Na-K-ATPase pump, resulting in impaired cellular uptake of potassium
Spironolactone	Aldosterone antagonist that blunts renal potassium secretion
Amiloride and triamterene	Reduce sodium reabsorption in CCT, which leads to a reduction in the electrical gradient for potassium movement from the intracellular space to the tubular lumen, and decreases the driving force for renal potassium secretion
ACE inhibitors, ARBs, and direct renin inhibitors	Induce a state of hypoaldosteronism
Trimethoprim and pentamidine	Same mechanism as amiloride (competitively inhibit sodium transport channels)
Heparin	Inhibition of adrenal aldosterone production
NSAIDs	Induce a state of relative hyporeninemic hypoaldosteronism; NSAIDs inhibit renal prostaglandin synthesis, which would normally stimulate renal synthesis of renin and the subsequent synthesis of aldosterone

CCT = cortical collecting tubule; ACE = angiotensin-converting enzyme; ARBs = angiotensin receptor blockers; NSAIDs = nonsteroidal anti-inflammatory drugs.

If the patient is symptomatic (or cannot take oral medications) intravenous (IV) potassium chloride should be used for repletion. IV potassium should not be given in a dextrose-containing solution because this will stimulate insulin secretion, driving potassium into cells and potentially worsening the hypokalemia. Additionally, it should not be given at a rate higher than 10 to 20 mEq/hour, and a potassium level should be checked after administration. Many patients will experience peripheral vein irritation with repeated IV potassium repletion and will require placement of a central line.

24. **What is the treatment of choice for life-threatening hyperkalemia?**
Life-threatening hyperkalemia, or hyperkalemia causing ECG changes, requires immediate treatment. Calcium will work within minutes to counteract the cardiac arrhythmias of hyperkalemia; however, it only lasts for minutes, so other, more definitive treatments must be used after this initial life-saving measure. The usual dose is 1000 mg IV of calcium gluconate given over 2 to 3 minutes to a patient receiving constant cardiac monitoring. Alternatively, 500 mg of calcium chloride can be given in the same fashion. The dose of either should be repeated every 5 minutes if there is no change in ECG findings.

KEY POINTS: HYPOKALEMIA AND HYPERKALEMIA

1. In a normal adult, 98% of total body potassium is located in the intracellular space. The body tightly regulates serum (extracellular) potassium concentration at approximately 4 mEq/L.

2. There is a large potassium gradient between the intracellular and extracellular spaces, which is essential for maintaining the cellular membrane resting potential. Regulating this gradient is critical because a small shift of intracellular potassium moving into the extracellular space can result in a potentially fatal increase in serum potassium concentration.

3. Calcium will work within minutes to counteract the cardiac arrhythmias of hyperkalemia; however, it only lasts for minutes, so other, more definitive treatments must be used after this initial life-saving measure.

25. **What other acute treatments can be used for management of severe hyperkalemia?**

    The administration of insulin and glucose will drive potassium into cells without inducing hypoglycemia. The usual dose is 10 mg of regular insulin given with 40 g of glucose given via intravenous bolus. Supplemental glucose should not be given if the patient is already hyperglycemic (glucose >200 mg/dL). Inducing metabolic alkalosis with sodium bicarbonate will also drive potassium intracellularly. This can be accomplished by administering 1 amp of sodium bicarbonate or 45 mEq of sodium bicarbonate. However, the amount of bicarbonate required to induce a metabolic alkalosis varies according to the clinical scenario. Agonizing beta-adrenergic receptors with a beta-2 agonist such as albuterol will also drive potassium intracellularly. The usual dose of albuterol is 10 to 20 mg given via nebulizer over 10 minutes. All of these treatments will move potassium into the intracellular space in approximately 30 to 60 minutes, and the effect will last several hours.

26. **How can one definitively remove potassium from the body?**

    Definitive treatment of hyperkalemia is removing the excess potassium from the body, which can be accomplished by increasing renal excretion of potassium with diuretics, increasing fecal excretion with cation-exchange resins, or mechanically removing it with dialysis.

    The most commonly used cation-exchange resin is sodium polystyrene sulfonate, which is usually orally dosed at 15 to 30 g repeated every 4 to 6 hours for hypokalemic effect. However, when used concomitantly with sorbitol, it has been associated with colonic necrosis, and this combination, which is commercially available, should be avoided.

27. **What are common causes of extrarenal potassium loss?**

    Vomiting and diarrhea are both methods of extrarenal potassium loss and can potentially lead to hypokalemia.

BIBLIOGRAPHY

1. Allon M. Hyperkalemia in end-stage renal disease: Mechanisms and management. *J Am Soc Neph* 1995;6:1134–1142.

2. Allon M, Takeshian A, Shanklin N. Effect of insulin-plus-glucose infusion with or without epinephrine on fasting hyperkalemia. *Kidney Int* 1993;43:212–217.

3. Ethier JH, Kamel KS, Magner PO, et al. The transtubular potassium concentration in patients with hypokalemia and hyperkalemia. *Am J Kidney Dis* 1990;15:309–315.

4. Evans K, Greenberg A. Hyperkalemia: A review. *J Intens Care Med* 2005;20:272–299.

5. Gennari J. Hypokalemia. *New Engl J Med* 1998;330:451–458.

6. Han SW, Won YK, Yi JH, et al. No impact on hyperkalemia with renin-angiotensin system blockades in maintenance haemodialysis patients. *Nephrol Dial Tranplant* 2007;22:1150–1155.

7. Sevastos N, Theossiades G, Archimadritis J. Pseudohyperkalemia in serum: A new insight into an old phenomenon. *Clin Med Res* 2008;6:30–32.

8. Sterns RH, Rojas M, Bernstein P, et al. Ion-exchange resins for the treatment of hyperkalemia: are they safe and effective? *J Am Soc Nephrol* 2010;21(5):733–735.

9. Weiner D, Linas S, Wingo C. Disorders of potassium metabolism. In: Feehally J, Floege J, Johnson RJ (eds.). *Comprehensive Clinical Nephrology*, 3rd ed. Philadelphia: Mosby, 2007, pp. 111-122.

CHAPTER 78

HYPOCALCEMIA AND HYPERCALCEMIA

Stanley Goldfarb, MD, and Lavinia A. Negrea, MD

1. **What are the most common causes of hypocalcemia?**

   Chronic renal failure

   Hypomagnesemia

   Vitamin D deficiency

   Hypoparathyroidism

   Hyperphosphatemia

   Pseudohypoparathyroidism

   Hypoalbuminemia (artifactual)

   Artifactual hypocalcemia (gadolinium interference)

   Drug-induced hypoparathyroidism (cinacalcet)

   Complication of massive transfusion with citrated blood (low ionized calcium)

   Acute severe pancreatitis

2. **What are the clinical manifestations of hypocalcemia?**

   The symptoms of hypocalcemia depend as much on the rate of its occurrence as on the degree of the reduction in plasma calcium. Symptoms include neuromuscular manifestations such as tetany, muscle spasm, cramps, carpopedal spasm, irritability, and seizures. Cardiovascular manifestations include arrhythmias, hypotension, and congestive heart failure.

3. **How does hypoalbuminemia cause hypocalcemia?**

   A reduction in serum albumin will result in a reduction in the total serum calcium, whereas the ionized portion (the physiologically important one) remains normal. A reduction in albumin concentration of 1 g/dL is associated with a fall in total serum calcium concentration of approximately 0.8 mg/dL. It has recently been shown that the measure of serum albumin in patients with advanced renal failure may be unreliable and lead to errors in estimating ionized serum calcium. Therefore, ionized serum calcium should be directly measured if hypocalcemia or hypercalcemia is suspected.

4. **Describe the vitamin D–related causes of hypocalcemia.**

   - Vitamin D deficiency: associated with inadequate exposure to ultraviolet light, poor dietary intake, or malabsorption. Also, vitamin D deficiency may occur in patients with nephrotic syndrome as a result of losses of vitamin D binding protein in the urine.
   - Abnormalities of vitamin D metabolism: either reduced hydroxylation of vitamin D to 25-hydroxyvitamin D in chronic liver diseases or reduced hydroxylation of 25-hydroxyvitamin D to 1,25-dihydroxyvitamin D in renal failure.
   - **Resistance** to the actions of vitamin D: for example, vitamin D–dependent rickets type I (deficiency of renal 1α-hydroxylase) and type II (molecular defects in the vitamin D receptor).
   - **Anticonvulsant use:** associated with decreased levels of 25-hydroxyvitamin D through enhanced hepatic metabolism of 25-hydroxyvitamin D to inactive metabolites.

5. **How does hypomagnesemia cause hypocalcemia?**

   Hypomagnesemia is a common cause of functional hypoparathyroidism, resulting from impaired secretion of parathyroid hormone (PTH) and from resistance to the action of PTH on organs such as bone and kidney.

6. **Explain how hypocalcemia can result from hyperphosphatemia.**

   Hyperphosphatemia can abruptly induce hypocalcemia through an increase in calcium × phosphorus product with subsequent spontaneous precipitation of calcium phosphate salts in soft tissues. This commonly occurs with excessive enteral or parenteral phosphate administration (during treatment of hypophosphatemia) or with massive release of intracellular phosphate in patients with tumor lysis syndrome or acute rhabdomyolysis. It can also occur in advanced kidney disease as hyperphosphatemia develops through defective renal excretion of phosphate.

7. **What factors contribute to hypocalcemia in chronic renal failure?**
The factors responsible for hypocalcemia in chronic renal failure are hyperphosphatemia, decreased levels of 1,25-dihydroxyvitamin D, and skeletal resistance to the calcemic action of PTH. Traditionally, the decreased 1,25-dihydroxyvitamin D levels were attributed to decreased renal mass as kidney disease progressed. Also, the accumulation of the bone derived hormone fibroblast growth factor 23 (FGF-23) in the circulation of patients with advanced kidney disease is also responsible for decreased 1,25-dihydroxyvitamin D levels (FGF-23 reduces the activity of the 1-hydroxylase enzyme in the kidney).

8. **What are some causes of hypoparathyroidism?**
Idiopathic hypoparathyroidism may be a result of absence of the parathyroid glands, branchial dysembryogenesis (DiGeorge syndrome), or a polyglandular autoimmune disorder. Acquired hypoparathyroidism can result from surgery, neck irradiation, or infiltrative disease (hemochromatosis, amyloidosis, thalassemia). The most common cause is hypomagnesemia.

9. **What is pseudohypoparathyroidism?**
In contrast to hypoparathyroidism, in which the synthesis or secretion of PTH is impaired, in pseudohypoparathyroidism, target tissues are unresponsive to the actions of PTH. Chronic hypocalcemia in this disorder leads to hyperplastic parathyroid glands and increased levels of PTH.

10. **Can hypocalcemia be associated with malignant disease?**
Yes. Osteoblastic metastases, most commonly associated with cancer of the prostate or breast, can cause hypocalcemia as a consequence of accelerated bone formation. The osteoblastic lesions are usually evident on plain radiography, and the serum alkaline phosphatase is generally elevated.

11. **What laboratory tests are helpful in the evaluation of hypocalcemia?**
Once true hypocalcemia is confirmed by measuring ionized calcium levels in blood, serum magnesium should be measured to exclude hypomagnesemia. If this is not present, measurement of intact PTH should help differentiate between hypoparathyroidism (low PTH) and conditions associated with elevated PTH levels, such as pseudohypoparathyroidism and vitamin D deficiency. Serum phosphorus is elevated in pseudohypoparathyroidism and decreased in vitamin D deficiency.

12. **What is the treatment for acute symptomatic hypocalcemia?**
Acute symptomatic hypocalcemia requires therapy with intravenous calcium. This can be given as 10–20 mL of calcium gluconate (90 mg of Ca^{++} per 10-mL ampule) infused at no more than 2 mL/min. This should be repeated as needed to keep the patient free of symptoms.

13. **What are the most common causes of hypercalcemia?**
- Hyperparathyroidism
- Malignancy (lung, breast, and stomach cancers and multiple myeloma most common)
- Granulomatous diseases (e.g., sarcoidosis, tuberculosis)
- Thyrotoxicosis
- Immobilization
- Vitamin D intoxication
- Milk-alkali (or calcium alkali) syndrome
- Use of thiazide diuretics in patients with subclinical primary hyperparathyroidism

14. **What are the clinical manifestations of hypercalcemia?**

Common clinical manifestations of hypercalcemia include lethargy, confusion, irritability, stupor, coma, anorexia, nausea, vomiting, constipation, polyuria, and hypertension.

15. **Describe the mechanisms leading to hypercalcemia in primary hyperparathyroidism.**

Primary hyperparathyroidism is the most common cause of hypercalcemia, accounting for more than 50% of all cases. PTH causes hypercalcemia by stimulating osteoclastic bone resorption greater than bone formation and by decreasing renal calcium excretion. PTH also increases 1,25-dihydroxyvitamin D synthesis, which leads to increased calcium absorption from the gut.

16. **What is the association between hypercalcemia and malignancy?**

Malignancy is the second most common cause of hypercalcemia. Humoral hypercalcemia of malignancy refers to hypercalcemia that results from secretion of PTH-related peptide (PTH-rP) by tumors including squamous cell carcinomas of the lung, head, or neck and renal cell carcinoma. PTH-rP mimics the actions of PTH by binding to the same receptor. Other tumors secrete either bone-resorbing cytokines (such as lymphotoxin, interleukin-1, and interleukin-6 in some patients with multiple myeloma) or 1,25-dihydroxyvitamin D (certain lymphomas), with resultant hypercalcemia. In addition to these mechanisms, local osteolytic hypercalcemia is believed to result from resorption by cancer cells, either directly or by secreting osteoclast-activating factors such as prostaglandins.

17. **What are the mechanisms responsible for hypercalcemia in granulomatous disorders?**

Hypercalcemia in sarcoidosis, tuberculosis, and other granulomatous diseases results from increased production of 1,25-hydroxyvitamin D by the macrophage, a prominent constituent of the sarcoid granuloma.

18. **How does thyrotoxicosis lead to hypercalcemia?**

The thyroid hormones thyroxine and tri-iodothyronine stimulate osteoclastic bone resorption.

19. **How does hypercalcemia occur during immobilization?**

Immobilization regularly leads to accelerated bone resorption and hypercalcemia in individuals with high rates of bone turnover (e.g., adolescents on bed rest or patients with Paget's disease). Hypercalcemia is preceded by hypercalciuria, which may lead to renal stones. Hypercalcemia promptly reverses with the resumption of normal weightbearing.

20. **What medications have been associated with hypercalcemia?**

The hypercalcemia of vitamin D intoxication usually develops in vitamin faddists and has gastrointestinal, renal, and skeletal components. Vitamin A intoxication, more commonly seen today with dermatologic or oncologic use of vitamin A analogues, causes hypercalcemia mediated by osteoclast-mediated bone resorption. Excessive oral ingestion of calcium-containing compounds can occasionally result in hypercalcemia. Thiazide diuretics can cause hypercalcemia by increased renal calcium reabsorption, particularly in patients with some underlying defect in calcium metabolism such as excess vitamin D intake or mild primary hyperparathyroidism

21. **What is the milk-alkali syndrome?**

The milk-alkali syndrome consists of hypercalcemia, hyperphosphatemia (although with use of calcium supplements such as calcium carbonate, phosphate binding in the gastrointestinal tract may produce hypophosphatemia), metabolic alkalosis, and renal failure. It was most commonly observed years ago in patients who were treated for peptic ulcer disease with large doses of calcium carbonate antacids and milk. Renal failure was mediated by metastatic calcification of the kidney resulting from excessive calcium and phosphorus absorption. Renal failure accounted for impairment of bicarbonate excretion. Currently it results from the use of calcium supplements in patients seeking to enhance bone formation such as postmenopausal women with osteoporosis.

22. **Which laboratory tests are helpful in the evaluation of hypercalcemia?**
In patients with normal renal function, an elevated serum intact PTH level will diagnose primary hyperparathyroidism in more than 90% of cases. Serum phosphorus is usually decreased in PTH or PTH-rP–mediated hypercalcemias and elevated in 1,25-dihydroxyvitamin D–mediated hypercalcemias. Elevated serum levels of PTH-rP can be helpful in diagnosing hypercalcemia of malignancy. Elevated levels of 1,25-dihydroxyvitamin D are detected in patients with certain lymphomas and granulomatous diseases. Elevated serum levels of 25-hydroxyvitamin D (usually >150 nmol/L) suggest vitamin D intoxication.

KEY POINTS: HYPOCALCEMIA AND HYPERCALCEMIA

1. It has recently been shown that the measure of serum albumin in patients with advanced renal failure may be unreliable and lead to errors in estimating ionized serum calcium. Therefore, ionized serum calcium should be directly measured if hypocalcemia or hypercalcemia is suspected.

2. The modern milk-alkali syndrome results from the use of calcium supplements in patients seeking to enhance bone formation such as postmenopausal women with osteoporosis.

3. The decreased 1,25-dihydroxyvitamin levels in renal failure are a result of the accumulation of fibroblast growth factor 23 in the circulation of patients with advanced kidney disease.

23. **What are the general therapeutic interventions in the management of hypercalcemia?**
In symptomatic patients, general measures that facilitate urinary calcium excretion include administration of intravenous saline, followed by furosemide. The latter is calciuric and helps prevent pulmonary congestion. Patients with impaired renal function who are unable to excrete the sodium load may require hemodialysis against a low calcium bath.

24. **What specific treatment should be used in hypercalcemia associated with granulomatous disease?**
Glucocorticoids are the mainstay of therapy. These agents inhibit the macrophage hydroxylation reaction and prompt a decrease in the circulating levels of 1,25-dihydroxyvitamin D.

25. **What specific treatment should be used in hypercalcemia of malignancy?**
Hypercalcemia of malignancy almost always is associated with increased osteoclastic bone resorption. Osteoclast activity is best inhibited by drugs such as calcitonin (effect often transient) or bisphosphonates (etidronate, pamidronate). Cinacalcet may be used in patients with parathyroid cancer in whom surgical parathyroid resection is not curative.

BIBLIOGRAPHY

1. Cooper MS, Gittoes NJ. Diagnosis and management of hypocalcaemia. *BMJ* 2008;336(7656):1298–1302.

2. Fraser WD. Hyperparathyroidism. *Lancet* 2009;374(9684):145–158.

3. Marx SJ. Hyperparathyroid and hypoparathyroid disorders. *N Engl J Med* 2000;343:1863–1875.

4. Medarov BI. Milk-alkali syndrome. *Mayo Clin Proc* 2009;84(3):261–267.

5. Mundy GR, Edwards JR. PTH-related peptide (PTHrP) in hypercalcemia.*J Am Soc Nephrol* 2008;19(4):672–675.

6. Mundy GR, Reasner CA. Hypercalcemia. In: Jacobson HR, Striker GE, Klahr S (eds.). *The Principles and Practice of Nephrology*, 2nd ed. St. Louis: Mosby, 1995, pp. 977–986.
7. Mundy GR, Reasner CA. Hypocalcemia. In: Jacobson HR, Striker GE, Klahr S (eds.). *The Principles and Practice of Nephrology*, 2nd ed. St. Louis: Mosby, 1995, pp. 971–977.
8. Shane E. Hypercalcemia: Pathogenesis, clinical manifestations, differential diagnosis, and management. In: Favus MJ (ed.). *Primer on the Metabolic Bone Diseases and Disorders of the Mineral Metabolism*, 3rd ed. Philadelphia: Lippincott-Raven, 1996, pp. 177–181.
9. Shane E. Hypocalcemia: Pathogenesis, differential diagnosis, and management. In: Favus MJ (ed.). *Primer on the Metabolic Bone Diseases and Disorders of Mineral Metabolism*, 3rd ed. Philadelphia, Lippincott-Raven, 1996, pp. 217–219.
10. Shoback D. Clinical practice. Hypoparathyroidism. *N Engl J Med* 2008;359(4):391–403.
11. Thomas MK, Demay MB. Vitamin D deficiency and disorders of vitamin D metabolism. *Endocrinol Metab Clin North Am* 2000;29:611–627.
12. Ziegler R. Hypercalcemic crisis. *J Am Soc Nephrol* 2001;12:S3–S9.

DISORDERS OF PHOSPHORUS METABOLISM

Earl H. Rudolph, DO, and Joyce M. Gonin, MD

1. **What is the difference between phosphorus and phosphate, and how are they related?**

   Elemental phosphorus circulates in blood as a constituent of both organic (e.g., phospholipids) and inorganic molecules. Inorganic phosphate refers to ionic species derived either from pyrophosphoric acid (a component of bone) or orthophosphoric acid (H_3PO_4). At a blood pH of 7.4, the molar ratio of $H_2PO_4^-$ to HPO_4^{2-} is 1.4, with an average valence of -1.8. Concentrations of inorganic phosphate are conventionally expressed in terms of elemental phosphorus, where 1 millimole of inorganic phosphate contains 31 mg of elemental phosphorus.

   Phosphate is one of the major constituents of the skeleton, imparting mineral strength to bone. Phosphate also is necessary for most cellular processes. The phosphate bonds of adenosine triphosphate (ATP) store the chemical energy required for virtually all cellular functions. Phosphate also forms the chemical backbone of the nucleic acids DNA and RNA. Phosphate also functions to buffer the pH of bone, blood, and urine.

2. **Describe normal phosphate homeostasis including hormonal influences.**

   Normal adult serum phosphate levels are maintained at ~2.5 to 4.5 mg/dL (~0.80–1.44 mmol/L), although reference values may vary from laboratory to laboratory. The average adult consumes 800 to 1200 mg of phosphate per day, largely in the form of meats and dairy products. Approximately 80% of ingested phosphate is absorbed in the small intestine under the influence of vitamin D, and ~40% is excreted in stool. However, the kidneys are primarily responsible for regulating serum phosphate levels. Normally, 80% to 90% of filtered inorganic phosphate is reabsorbed by the renal proximal tubules. Renal tubular phosphate transport is influenced by several hormones; parathyroid hormone (PTH) and 1,25-dihydroxyvitamin D_3 [1,25-$(OH)_2D_3$] decrease phosphate reabsorption, whereas growth hormone and thyroxine increase phosphate reabsorption. The distribution of phosphate within body compartments also is influenced by acid–base status. For example, respiratory and metabolic alkalosis are accompanied by a decrease in serum phosphate that results from an intracellular shift of phosphate in exchange for organic acids necessary to buffer the alkalosis.

3. **What is the difference between phosphate depletion and hypophosphatemia?**

   Phosphate depletion refers to total body phosphate depletion, whereas hypophosphatemia refers to low serum phosphate levels, which can result from a transcellular shift of phosphate from the extracellular to the intracellular compartment without loss of total body phosphate. Given that multiple factors influence phosphate distribution (e.g., hormones, acid–base status, others), serum phosphate levels, like serum levels of any predominantly intracellular ion, may not necessarily reflect total body stores.

4. **Define hypophosphatemia, and discuss the clinical manifestations and degrees of severity.**

   Hypophosphatemia is defined as a serum phosphate level <2.5 mg/dL (<0.80 mmol/L) and can be further characterized as mild (~2.0–2.5 mg/dL or ~0.64–0.80 mmol/L), moderate

(~1.0–2.0 mg/dL or ~0.32–0.64 mmol/L), or severe (<1.0 mg/dL or <0.32 mmol/L). No specific symptoms suggest hypophosphatemia; rather, symptoms are often nonspecific and depend largely on the cause, duration, and severity. Mild hypophosphatemia is usually asymptomatic regardless of whether it is acute or chronic. Patients may complain of fatigue and weakness; however, whether this is related to the cause or an effect of hypophosphatemia is unclear. Patients with chronic and/or moderate or severe hypophosphatemia are more likely to be symptomatic. Symptoms of severe hypophosphatemia include irritability, confusion, coma, and respiratory difficulty.

5. **What are the causes of hypophosphatemia?**
The main causes of hypophosphatemia are inadequate intake, increased renal excretion, and transcellular shift from the extracellular to the intracellular compartment.

Inadequate phosphate intake alone is an uncommon cause of hypophosphatemia because nearly all foods contain phosphate. However, poor dietary intake can occur with protein-calorie malnutrition and chronic alcoholism. Intestinal malabsorption in the setting of poor dietary intake also can cause hypophosphatemia. Overuse of calcium-, magnesium-, and aluminum-containing antacids also has been reported to cause hypophosphatemia as has overtreatment of hyperphosphatemia with calcium-, sevelamer-, lanthium-, and aluminum-based phosphate binders. Poor dietary intake coupled with an acute increase in phosphate requirement also can cause hypophosphatemia, as occurs in the refeeding syndrome. Although not sufficient to cause hypophosphatemia, vitamin D deficiency can contribute by failing to stimulate intestinal phosphate absorption.

Increased renal phosphate excretion is a common cause of hypophosphatemia. The most common cause of increased renal phosphate excretion is hyperparathyroidism resulting from parathyroid hormone (PTH) inhibition of renal proximal tubule phosphate reabsorption. However, hypophosphatemia is not always present in the setting of hyperparathyroidism and when present is typically mild. Increased renal phosphate excretion also can result from forced saline diuresis, which also inhibits renal proximal tubule phosphate reabsorption and is typically mild. Although not sufficient to cause hypophosphatemia, vitamin D deficiency can contribute by decreasing renal proximal tubule phosphate reabsorption. There are also several genetic and acquired syndromes of phosphate wasting and associated skeletal abnormalities.

Transcellular shift of phosphate from the extracellular to the intracellular compartment alone is an uncommon cause of hypophosphatemia; however, it can exacerbate hypophosphatemia caused by inadequate intake or increased renal excretion. Transcellular shift of phosphate can contribute significantly to hypophosphatemia with refeeding syndrome, hungry bones syndrome, acute respiratory alkalosis, and during treatment of diabetic ketoacidosis.

6. **What is rickets, how can it affect phosphate homeostasis, and what are some of the genetic defects that cause rickets?**
Phosphate wasting can result from genetic or acquired disorders. Many of the genetic disorders of phosphate wasting often manifest in childhood, resulting in bone deformities and short stature (Table 79-1). Rickets is a disease of children and adolescents in which the osteoid of growing bone fails to calcify. The result is a "softening of bones" that may lead to skeletal deformities and fractures. Rickets is among the most common childhood diseases in developing countries as a result of malnutrition during the early stages of childhood. The predominant cause is vitamin D deficiency, but lack of adequate dietary calcium also may lead to rickets. Osteomalacia is the term used to describe a similar condition occurring in adults, also resulting from failure of osteoid to calcify and usually from vitamin D deficiency. Patients with rickets can suffer from skeletal deformities (cranial, spinal, pelvic, and extremity), short stature, bone pain or tenderness, muscle weakness, increased risk of fractures, calcification of tendons, and dental abnormalities. Along with hypocalcemia, hypophosphatemia and phosphaturia are commonly observed, often in conjunction with defects in vitamin D metabolism and sometimes with elevated levels of fibroblast growth factor 23 (FGF-23) and/or PTH. Decreased 1,25-$(OH_2)D_3$ activity and increased PTH activity decrease proximal tubule

TABLE 79-1. GENETIC DISORDERS ASSOCIATED WITH HYPOPHOSPHATEMIA AND CLINICAL RICKETS

Genetic Disorder	Gene Defect and Inheritance	Proposed Mechanism	Clinical Manifestations
X-linked hypophosphatemic rickets	Mutation of *PHEX* gene encoding membrane-bound endopeptidase X-linked dominant	Mutated endopeptidase unable to cleave FGF-23 Elevated FGF-23 decreases sodium-phosphate cotransporter activity	Clinical rickets Hypophosphatemia Inappropriately low 1,25-$(OH_2)D_3$
Autosomal-dominant hypophosphatemic rickets	Mutation of FGF-23 gene Autosomal dominant	Mutated FGF-23 is resistant to degradation by endopeptidase Elevated FGF-23 decreases sodium-phosphate cotransporter activity	Clinical rickets Hypophosphatemia Inappropriately low 1,25-$(OH_2)D_3$
Autosomal-recessive hypophosphatemic rickets	Mutation of *DMP1* gene encoding phospho-protein needed for osteocyte maturation Autosomal recessive	Mutated DMP1 causes elevated FGF-23 levels Elevated FGF-23 decreases sodium-phosphate cotransporter activity	Clinical rickets Hypophosphatemia Inappropriately low 1,25-$(OH_2)D_3$
Hereditary hypophosphatemic rickets with hypercalciuria	Mutation of type 2c sodium-phosphate cotransporter gene Autosomal recessive	Inactivation of type 2c sodium-phosphate cotransporter decreases renal phosphate reabsorption	Clinical rickets Hypophosphatemia Hypercalciuria Elevated 1,25-$(OH_2)D_3$
Vitamin D-resistant rickets type I	Mutation of *CYP27B1* gene encoding renal 1-α-hydroxylase Autosomal recessive	Defect in renal 1-α-hydroxylation of 25-(OH)D Decreased 1,25-$(OH_2)D_3$ activity and increased PTH activity decrease proximal tubule phosphate reabsorption	Clinical rickets Hyperparathyroidism Hypophosphatemia Hypocalcemia Decreased circulating 1,25-$(OH_2)D_3$
Vitamin D-resistant rickets type II	Mutation of the vitamin D receptor gene Autosomal recessive	End-organ resistance to effects of 1,25-$(OH_2)D_3$ Decreased 1,25-$(OH_2)D_3$ activity and increased PTH activity decrease proximal tubule phosphate reabsorption	Clinical rickets, alopecia Hyperparathyroidism Hypophosphatemia Hypocalcemia

1,25-$(OH_2)D_3$ = 1,25-dihydroxyvitamin D_3; 25-(OH)D = 25-hydroxyvitamin D; DMP1 = dentin matrix acidic phosphoprotein 1; FGF-23 = fibroblast growth factor 23.

phosphate reabsorption. Elevated FGF-23 levels are associated with impaired renal phosphate reabsorption resulting from decreased activity of the sodium–phosphate cotransporter.

7. **What is refeeding syndrome?**
Refeeding syndrome is a constellation of metabolic disturbances that can occur as a result of reinstitution of nutrition ("refeeding") in patients who are starved or severely malnourished (e.g., alcoholics, anorexics, bulimics). Typically within 4 days of refeeding, patients can develop fluid and electrolyte disorders, along with neurologic, neuromuscular, cardiac, pulmonary, and hematologic complications. The clinical manifestations can vary widely from confusion to convulsions, coma, and death in severe cases. The syndrome is thought to result largely from a sudden shift from fat to carbohydrate metabolism along with a sudden increase in insulin levels after refeeding, which leads to increased cellular uptake of phosphate and other electrolytes. Intracellular movement of electrolytes, most notably phosphate, occurs along with a decrease in serum potassium, magnesium, glucose, and thiamine. Formation of phosphorylated carbohydrate compounds in the liver and skeletal muscle depletes intracellular ATP and 2,3-diphosphoglycerate (2,3-DPG) in erythrocytes, leading to cellular dysfunction and inadequate delivery of oxygen to the vital organs. Refeeding concurrently increases the basal metabolic rate, which also increases overall oxygen demand, further exacerbating cellular dysfunction. Moreover, increased oxygen demand stimulates the respiratory system, which can make weaning from mechanical ventilation more difficult. Electrolyte and fluid shifts increase cardiac workload and heart rate, which can lead to acute heart failure. Careful electrolyte monitoring and prompt repletion of phosphate, potassium, and magnesium are paramount. Thiamine, vitamin B complex, and multivitamin supplementation also are recommended. Identifying patients at risk and careful renourishment can avoid refeeding syndrome.

8. **How does hypophosphatemia cause rhabdomyolysis?**
Hypophosphatemia can cause rhabdomyolysis as a result of ATP depletion of myocytes and their subsequent inability to maintain cell membrane integrity. Patients in acute alcohol withdrawal are particularly at risk for development of rhabdomyolysis secondary to hypophosphatemia caused by the rapid uptake of phosphate by myocytes. Similarly, rhabdomyolysis also can develop in patients with diabetic ketoacidosis or refeeding syndrome. Once rhabdomyolysis develops, hyperphosphatemia can result from release of a high burden of intracellular phosphate resulting from cell death that is often accompanied by hyperkalemia, hypocalcemia, hyperuricemia, and renal failure.

9. **What is the likely etiology of new-onset hypophosphatemia in the early post-transplant period, and how can calcineurin inhibitors cause hypophosphatemia?**
Hypophosphatemia is a common complication after successful renal transplantation, occurring in up to 80% of patients in the early post-transplant period. Hypophosphatemia that occurs early in the post-transplant period with functional renal allografts is largely a result of increased renal phosphate excretion. Hypophosphatemia in this setting can be multifactorial, including residual secondary hyperparathyroidism, glucocorticoids used in many transplant protocols, and a low vitamin D state. Moreover, persistence of inappropriately high levels of FGF-23, a recently discovered phosphaturic hormone, also may play an important role in post-transplant hypophosphatemia. In some cases, hypophosphatemia may be severe enough to cause profound muscle weakness, including respiratory muscles, which can precipitate respiratory failure or make weaning from mechanical ventilation more difficult. Persistent phosphate depletion also can contribute significantly to post-transplant bone disease. Concurrent changes in serum calcium levels are also common, requiring close monitoring along with phosphate and other electrolytes. Calcineurin inhibitors (e.g., cyclosporine A, tacrolimus, others) also can cause hypophosphatemia by inhibition of the sodium–phosphate cotransporter in the proximal tubule causing phosphaturia and also may inhibit phosphate absorption in the small intestines.

10. **What is the treatment for hypophosphatemia?**
Treat the underlying cause of hypophosphatemia whenever possible. Moreover, anticipating the need for phosphate replacement in patients at risk for hypophosphatemia (e.g., refeeding syndrome-associated hypophosphatemia in patients who are alcoholic, anorexic, bulimic, or otherwise malnourished or starved) is a good approach.

The route of phosphate replacement depends on the severity of hypophosphatemia, functional status of the gastrointestinal tract and the kidneys, and concurrent need for mechanical ventilation. Severe hypophosphatemia can be treated with intravenous replacement therapy (0.08–0.16 mmol/kg) over 2 to 6 hours. Moderate hypophosphatemia can be treated with intravenous replacement therapy (0.08–0.16 mmol/kg) over 2 to 6 hours in patients requiring mechanical ventilation and oral replacement therapy (1000–2000 mg/day) in patients who are not ventilated. Mild hypophosphatemia can be treated with oral replacement therapy (1000 mg/day), whereas very mild hypophosphatemia may be adequately treated with increased dietary phosphate intake alone. Foods high in phosphate include meat, poultry, fish, eggs, dairy products, cereals, beans, and peas.

Approximately 1000 to 2000 mg (32–64 mmol) of phosphate per day for 7 to 14 days is adequate to replenish total body phosphate stores in many cases. Vitamin D replacement also is necessary for patients with deficiency because it enhances intestinal calcium and phosphate absorption; therefore, levels of both should be closely monitored.

Oral phosphate supplements may be adequate for the treatment of many genetic disorders of phosphate wasting, often normalizing serum phosphate levels, and have been reported to decrease bone pain in some cases. Serum phosphate and calcium levels, bone density, and growth should be monitored frequently to ensure adequacy of treatment. Oral phosphate supplements also are useful for the treatment of oncogenic osteomalacia until the tumor can be surgically removed.

11. **What are the side effects and complications of treating hypophosphatemia?**
Oral phosphate supplements are generally well tolerated, except at high doses, which may cause diarrhea. Parenteral phosphate administration is generally reserved for patients who are critically ill, patients with severe hypophosphatemia, or patients with nonfunctional gastrointestinal tracts. Parenteral phosphate administration is more likely to be associated with complications, particularly with too rapid correction or overcorrection, which can cause hypocalcemia, tetany, and hypotension. Other complications include metastatic calcification, hyperkalemia associated with potassium-containing phosphate supplements, hypernatremia associated with sodium-containing phosphate supplements, volume overload, metabolic acidosis, and hyperphosphatemia. To prevent complications, serum phosphate and calcium levels should be monitored frequently to avoid too rapid correction or overcorrection of phosphate and to monitor for hypocalcemia. In general, serum phosphate can be safely corrected by ~1 to 3 mmol/hour.

KEY POINTS: HYPOPHOSPHATEMIA

1. Renal tubular phosphate transport is influenced by several hormones; parathyroid hormone (PTH) and 1,25-dihydroxyvitamin D_3 decrease phosphate reabsorption, whereas growth hormone and thyroxine increase phosphate reabsorption.

2. Hypophosphatemia (<2.5 mg/dL or <0.80 mmol/L) can be caused by inadequate intake, increased renal excretion, and transcellular shift from the extracellular to the intracellular compartment.

3. Treat the underlying cause of hypophosphatemia. The route of phosphate replacement depends on the severity, presence of symptoms, functional status of the gastrointestinal tract, and concurrent need for mechanical ventilation. Vitamin D replacement may be necessary for patients with deficiency.

12. **Define hyperphosphatemia, and discuss the clinical manifestations and degrees of severity.**

Hyperphosphatemia is defined as a serum phosphate >4.5 mg/dL (>1.44 mmol/L) and can be further characterized as mild (~4.5–5.5 mg/dL or ~1.44–1.76 mmol/L), moderate (~5.5–6.5 mg/dL or ~1.76–2.08 mmol/L), or severe (~6.5 mg/dL or ~2.08 mmol/L). The acute clinical manifestations of hyperphosphatemia include hypocalcemia and tetany, which occur most commonly with rapid elevations in serum phosphate levels. Phosphate-induced hypocalcemia is common in both acute and chronic renal failure. Tetany is more likely to develop with acute decreases in ionized calcium levels that sometimes accompany significant changes in serum pH. For example, severe hypocalcemia and tetany have been reported during the early phases of tumor lysis syndrome and rhabdomyolysis. Hyperphosphatemia also causes dysregulation of vitamin D metabolism, PTH activity, and overall calcium homeostasis, causing secondary hyperparathyroidism and renal osteodystrophy. Hyperphosphatemia also can cause soft tissue calcification, which is associated with a high level of mortality.

13. **What are the causes of hyperphosphatemia?**

The main causes of hyperphosphatemia are increased phosphate intake, decreased renal excretion, excess resorption of bone, and transcellular shift or release from the intracellular to the extracellular compartment.

Increased phosphate intake can cause hyperphosphatemia. Administration of intravenous phosphate to treat phosphate depletion, parenteral nutrition, and hypercalcemia can cause hyperphosphatemia. Overuse of oral phosphate supplements and phosphate-containing enemas (e.g., Fleet phospho-soda enemas) also can cause hyperphosphatemia.

Decreased renal phosphate excretion is the most common cause of hyperphosphatemia. The presence of underlying renal insufficiency significantly increases the risk of hyperphosphatemia resulting from decreased phosphate excretion. This can occur in the setting of acute kidney injury, chronic kidney disease, and end-stage renal disease. Defects in renal phosphate excretion in the absence of renal failure can occur in pseudohypoparathyroidism, which is characterized by hyperphosphatemia and hypocalcemia. In pseudohypoparathyroidism, although parathyroid hormone is present, renal proximal tubules are resistant to its actions to decrease phosphate reabsorption, resulting in hyperphosphatemia. Defects in renal phosphate excretion also can occur in tumoral calcinosis, which is characterized by ectopic calcification around large joints as a result of increased renal tubular reabsorption of calcium and phosphate. Hypoparathyroidism and the high levels of growth hormone present in acromegaly also can cause hyperphosphatemia. Bisphosphonates (e.g., alendronate, pamidronate, others) also can cause hyperphosphatemia, possibly by mechanisms that include cellular phosphate redistribution and decreased renal phosphate excretion.

Excess resorption of bone is an under-recognized cause and/or contributor to hyperphosphatemia. Various disorders that stimulate bone resorption have been reported to cause hyperphosphatemia, although the underlying mechanisms are not completely clear.

Transcellular shift or release of phosphate from the intracellular to the extracellular compartment may be caused by conditions associated with increased catabolism or tissue destruction and cell death. Common examples include diabetic ketoacidosis, rhabdomyolysis, tumor lysis syndrome, lactic acidosis associated with systemic infections or tissue hypoxia, fulminant hepatitis, severe hyperthermia, and hematologic malignancies. Rhabdomyolysis may result from either traumatic or nontraumatic myocyte injury resulting in cell death, whereas tumor lysis syndrome results from chemotherapy-induced tumor cell death. Patients with diabetic ketoacidosis often exhibit hyperphosphatemia at presentation despite total body phosphate depletion. Insulin therapy, fluid resuscitation, and treatment of the resultant acidosis can precipitate development of hypophosphatemia, which is actually more reflective of total body phosphate stores. Both conditions can cause release of a high burden of intracellular phosphate and profound increases in serum phosphate that are often accompanied by hyperkalemia, hypocalcemia, hyperuricemia, and renal failure. In lactic acidosis, hyperphosphatemia results from tissue hypoxia and breakdown of ATP to adenosine monophosphate (AMP) with concomitant release of inorganic phosphate. Artifactual hyperphosphatemia also can result from hemolysis during collection or processing of blood samples.

14. **How does phosphate handling change in chronic kidney disease (CKD)?**
Decreased renal excretion of phosphate is the most common cause of hyperphosphatemia. During CKD stages II and III, normophosphatemia is maintained by a progressive reduction in the fraction of filtered phosphate reabsorbed by the tubules and corresponding increase in renal phosphate excretion. However, if the glomerular filtration rate falls below 20 mL/min and dietary intake is sustained, normophosphatemia can no longer be maintained by reduction of tubular reabsorption and hyperphosphatemia develops.

15. **How does hyperphosphatemia affect vitamin D metabolism?**
Hyperphosphatemia inhibits the activity of renal 1α-hydroxylase (also known as 25-(OH) D-1α-hydroxylase), which converts the hepatic prehormone 25-hydroxyvitamin D (also known as calcifediol, calcidiol, 25-hydroxycholecalciferol, or abbreviated 25-(OH)D) to the hormone 1,25-dihydroxyvitamin D_3 (also known as calcitriol, 1,25-dihydroxycholecalciferol, or abbreviated 1,25-$(OH_2)D_3$) in the kidney. The result is decreased serum 1,25-dihydroxyvitamin D_3 levels, which further potentiates hypocalcemia by impairing intestinal calcium absorption and inducing a state of skeletal PTH resistance.

16. **How does hyperphosphatemia cause soft tissue calcification?**
Hyperphosphatemia contributes to an increased calcium–phosphate product (Ca $\times$ P, serum calcium multiplied by serum phosphate), which significantly increases the risk of calcium deposition in soft tissues. Vascular calcification is most often observed in patients with chronic kidney disease, diabetes, and/or severe atherosclerosis and worsens with age. Calcification of the large blood vessels can cause coronary artery disease, peripheral artery disease, hypertension, heart failure, and myocardial infarction. In fact, both vascular calcification and hyperphosphatemia are independent risk factors for cardiovascular disease and mortality. Calcification of smaller peripheral arteries and arterioles can manifest clinically as calciphylaxis (also known as calcific uremic arteriolopathy, abbreviated CUA). Calciphylaxis is a highly morbid syndrome of vascular calcification and skin necrosis resulting from ischemia. This condition most often develops in patients with chronic kidney disease, especially those with end-stage renal disease on dialysis. Prolonged hyperphosphatemia and a calcium–phosphate product (Ca $\times$ P) of >55 mg^2/dL^2 are associated with development of calciphylaxis.

17. **How does hyperphosphatemia cause secondary hyperparathyroidism and renal osteodystrophy (chronic kidney disease-mineral and bone disorder, CKD-MBD)?**
Hyperphosphatemia plays an important role in the development of secondary hyperparathyroidism and renal osteodystrophy by several mechanisms including hyperphosphatemia-induced hypercalcemia, hyperphosphatemia-associated increased expression of transforming growth factor-alpha (TGF-α) and epidermal growth factor receptors (EGF-Rs) in parathyroid chief cells causing hyperplasia, increased PTH secretion, inhibition of vitamin D synthesis, and hyperphosphatemia-induced vascular calcification. In advanced renal failure, PTH-mediated osteolysis may become the predominant factor influencing serum phosphate levels.

18. **What is hypophosphatasia?**
Hypophosphatasia is a rare inherited metabolic bone disorder characterized by bone and teeth demineralization and deficiency of serum and bone alkaline phosphatase activity. Tissue nonspecific alkaline phosphatase (TNSALP) deficiency in osteoblasts and chondrocytes impairs bone mineralization, leading to soft bones manifest as rickets in infants and children or osteomalacia in adults. The TNSALP enzyme normally hydrolyzes several substances, including inorganic pyrophosphate (PPi) and pyridoxal 5'-phosphate (PLP), the principal form of vitamin B_6. When

TNSALP activity is low, inorganic phosphate accumulates and inhibits hydroxyapatite formation (mineralization). PLP (vitamin B_6) must undergo dephosphorylation by the TNSALP enzyme to PL before it can cross the cell membrane. Vitamin B_6 deficiency in the brain can impair neurotransmitter synthesis, which may precipitate seizures. In some cases, deposition of calcium pyrophosphate dehydrate (CPPD) crystals in joints can precipitate pseudogout. The clinical manifestations are highly variable, ranging from a rapidly fatal perinatal variant with severe skeletal hypomineralization and respiratory compromise to a milder progressive osteomalacia that manifests in adults. The diagnosis is based on decreased activity on a serum alkaline phosphatase activity assay (as a result of decreased activity of the TNSALP enzyme) or screening for one of more than 200 known genetic mutations in the *TNSALP* gene. Genetic inheritance is autosomal recessive for the more severe perinatal and infantile forms and either autosomal dominant or recessive in milder forms. The incidence of severe forms is estimated to be 1:100,000. There are currently no approved therapies for hypophosphatasia. Management should focus on palliation of symptoms, maintenance of calcium homeostasis, and orthopedic and dental interventions as appropriate.

19. **What is the treatment for hyperphosphatemia?**
Treat the underlying cause of hyperphosphatemia whenever possible. If it results from increased exogenous phosphate intake, discontinue phosphate replacement or adjust nutrition as necessary and maintain adequate volume status because functional kidneys will readily excrete excess phosphate. If increased serum phosphate is a result of endogenous release, as may occur with tumor lysis syndrome and rhabdomyolysis, again maintain adequate volume status because functional kidneys will readily excrete excess phosphate.

If hyperphosphatemia results from decreased renal phosphate excretion, treatment should include a low-phosphate diet and phosphate binders in an amount necessary to achieve and maintain normophosphatemia. If it results from excess resorption of bone, treat the underlying disease. If it results from a transcellular shift of phosphate from the intracellular to the extracellular compartment, treatment depends on the underlying cause. For example, hyperkalemia associated with diabetic ketoacidosis resolves with insulin, which also stimulates cellular uptake of phosphate.

20. **What are the different types of phosphate binders used in advanced CKD and ESRD and any associated advantages and disadvantages of each?**
Phosphate binders reduce intestinal absorption of phosphate when taken with meals and snacks. Common phosphate binders include calcium, sevelamer, lanthium, and aluminum. Calcium-based phosphate binders (e.g., calcium carbonate, calcium acetate) are effective and inexpensive; however, use may be limited by hypercalcemia. Sevelamer-based phosphate binders are effective but expensive; moreover they are not absorbed and more likely to cause diarrhea. Certain formulations also have been associated with metabolic acidosis (sevelamer hydrochloride), whereas newer formulations reportedly are not (sevelamer carbonate). Sevelamer also has a secondary effect of reducing serum uric acid, which may be beneficial to patients with hyperuricemia, uric acid nephrolithiasis, and gout. Lanthium-based phosphate binders (lanthium carbonate) are useful in patients who cannot tolerate calcium- or sevelamer-based phosphate binders. Notably, lanthium carbonate is among the largest pills manufactured and intended to be chewed, not swallowed whole, but choking has been reported. Aluminum-based phosphate binders (aluminum hydroxide) are highly effective; however, long-term use is associated with aluminum toxicity and deposition in the bones, joints, and brain, which has curtailed their use except for short-term treatment of severe hyperphosphatemia. Although epidemiologic studies failed to establish a link between aluminum exposure and neurologic disorders, concerns that long-term exposure may cause dementia still persist.

Phosphate binders must be ingested with each meal or snack to effectively bind dietary phosphate. Many patients also experience gastrointestinal intolerance (bloating, nausea, vomiting, diarrhea). High dietary phosphate burden also mandates a high pill burden for some phosphate binders. Together, these issues translate into significant patient noncompliance. Route of administration also may become an issue because only certain phosphate binders are available in powder or liquid form. Hyperphosphatemia in patients receiving total parenteral nutrition with concomitant renal failure requires adjustment of the phosphate content of the nutritional formulation.

KEY POINTS: HYPERPHOSPHATEMIA

1. Hyperphosphatemia (>4.5 mg/dL or >1.44 mmol/L) can be caused by increased intake, decreased renal excretion, excess resorption of bone, and transcellular shift or release from the intracellular to the extracellular space.

2. Hyperphosphatemia plays an important role in the development of secondary hyperparathyroidism and renal osteodystrophy and increases the risk of calcium deposition in soft tissues, including large and small blood vessels.

3. Treat the underlying cause of hyperphosphatemia. If hyperphosphatemia is a result of increased exogenous intake, discontinue or decrease intake; if it is a result of increased endogenous release, maintain adequate volume status because functional kidneys will excrete excess phosphate; and if it is a result of decreased renal excretion, treatment should include a low-phosphate diet and phosphate binders if necessary.

BIBLIOGRAPHY

1. Amanzadeh J, Reilly RF Jr. Hypophosphatemia: An evidence-based approach to its clinical consequences and management. *Nat Clin Pract Nephrol* 2006;2:136–148.

2. Bushinsky DA. Disorders of calcium and phosphorus homeostasis. In: Greenberg A, Cheung AK, Coffman TM, et al. (eds.). *Primer on Kidney Diseases*, 5th ed. Philadelphia: Elsevier Saunders, 2009, pp. 120–130.

3. Gaasbeek A, Meinders AE. Hypophosphatemia: An update on its etiology and treatment. *Am J Med* 2005;118:1094–1101.

4. Gattineni J, Baum M. Regulation of phosphate transport by fibroblast growth factor 23 (FGF-23): Implications for disorders of phosphate metabolism. *Pediatr Nephrol* 2010;25:591–601.

5. Hruska KA. Disorders of phosphate balance: Hypophosphatemia hyperphosphatemia. In Lerma EV, Berns JS, Nissenson, AR (eds.). *Current Diagnosis and Treatment: Nephrology & Hypertension*, 1st ed. New York: McGraw-Hill, 2009, pp. 69–78.

6. Levine BS, Kleeman CR, Felsenfeld AJ. The journey from vitamin D-resistant rickets to the regulation of renal phosphate transport. *Clin J Am Soc Nephrol* 2009;4:1866–1877.

7. Liu S, Gupta A, Quarles LD. Emerging role of fibroblast growth factor 23 in a bone-kidney axis regulating systemic phosphate homeostasis and extracellular matrix mineralization. *Curr Opin Nephrol Hypertens* 2007;16:329–335.

8. Malluche HH, Monier-Faugere MC, Herberth J. Bone disease after renal transplantation. *Nat Rev Nephrol* 2010;6:32–40.

9. Mehanna HM, Moledina J, Travis J. Refeeding syndrome: What it is, and how to prevent and treat it. *BMJ* 2008;336:1495–1498.

10. Mornet E. Hypophosphatasia. *Orphanet J Rare Dis* 2007;2:40.

11. Rogers NM, Coates PT. Calcific uraemic arteriolopathy: An update. *Curr Opin Nephrol Hypertens* 2008;17:629–634.

12. Tiosano D, Hochberg Z. Hypophosphatemia: The common denominator of all rickets. *J Bone Miner Metab* 2009;27:392–401.

Acknowledgment

The authors wish to thank Dr. Donald E. Hricik for his contributions to this chapter.

CHAPTER 80

DISORDERS OF MAGNESIUM METABOLISM

Earl H. Rudolph, DO, and Joyce M. Gonin, MD

1. **Describe elemental magnesium and its role in physiologic processes.**
   Magnesium is a predominantly intracellular divalent cation that is the second most abundant intracellular cation (after potassium) and the fourth most common cation in the human body. The molecular weight of magnesium is 24.3 daltons; therefore, 1 mole contains ~24 g of elemental magnesium. Elemental magnesium is conventionally expressed in terms of grams (or milligrams) and serum magnesium is expressed in terms of milligrams per deciliter (where 2.4 mg/dL ≈ 1 mmol/L ≈ 2 mEq/L). The average adult contains ~24 g (≈ 1 mol ≈ 2000 mEq) of magnesium. Approximately 99% of total body magnesium is in the intracellular compartment, and only 1% is in the extracellular compartment. Of intracellular magnesium, ~60% is found in the bone, ~20% in muscle, and ~20% in other soft tissues. Of extracellular magnesium, ~60% to 65% is free, ionized, and biologically active; ~30% is protein bound; and ~5% to 10% is complexed to citrate, phosphate, oxalate, and other anions. The exchange of intracellular and extracellular magnesium occurs at a very slow rate; therefore, acute changes in extracellular magnesium concentrations are not readily compensated. Magnesium is necessary for many cellular processes including enzymatic reactions, regulation of ion channels, and stabilization of membrane structures. Numerous enzymatic reactions require magnesium including those involving adenosine triphosphate (ATP) and energy, nucleic acid, and protein metabolism.

2. **Describe normal magnesium homeostasis including hormonal influences.**
   Normal adult serum magnesium levels are maintained at ~1.7 to 2.3 mg/dL (~0.71–0.96 mmol/L or ~1.4–1.9 mEq/L), although reference values may vary from laboratory to laboratory. The average adult consumes ~300 to 400 mg of magnesium per day, largely in the form of green vegetables, whole grains, meats, and seafood. Some water supplies also can be a significant source of magnesium (i.e., "hard water"). Approximately 30% to 50% of ingested magnesium is absorbed, mostly in the small intestines but some in the colon and rectum. A small amount of magnesium is secreted by the small intestines (~40 mg/day) but is reabsorbed by the colon and rectum (~20 mg/day), resulting in overall net intestinal excretion in stool (~20 mg/day). Transcellular absorption of magnesium in the small intestine is primarily by passive transport, except in the ileum, where absorption is primarily by active transport. Intestinal magnesium absorption does not appear to be significantly influenced by any particular hormone, with the possible exception of vitamin D, which may increase absorption.

   The kidneys are primarily responsible for regulating serum magnesium levels. Normally, ~70% to 80% (~2400 mg) of total serum magnesium if filtered by the kidneys and ~95% to 97% is reabsorbed by the renal tubules, with ~3% to 5% (~120 mg) excreted in urine. When serum magnesium levels are increased, tubular reabsorption can be substantially decreased, such that most of the filtered load is excreted in urine. When serum magnesium levels are decreased, tubular reabsorption can achieve a fractional excretion of magnesium ($FEMg^{2+}$) of <0.5% (~12 mg). Approximately 15% to 25% of magnesium reabsorption occurs in the proximal tubule, ~60% to 70% in the cortical portion of the thick ascending limb of the loop of Henle (TALH), and only ~5% to 10% in the distal convoluted tubule (DCT). There is no magnesium reabsorption in the medullary portion of the TALH.

In the proximal tubule and cortical TALH, magnesium is passively reabsorbed by paracellular transport driven by bulk flow that is dependent on sodium reabsorption. In the cortical TALH, the driving force for magnesium and calcium reabsorption is a positive electrical potential generated in the lumen by sodium and chloride reabsorption via the $Na^+/K^+/2Cl^-$ cotransporter driven by a basolateral membrane Mg^{2+}-dependent Na^+-K^+-ATPase and chloride channel, along with an apical membrane potassium channel. In the cortical TALH, the apical membrane potassium channel and $Na^+/K^+/2Cl^-$ cotransporter can be inhibited by activation of a basolateral membrane Ca^{2+}/Mg^{2+}-sensing receptor (CaSR), which binds both calcium and magnesium. CaSR activation inhibits passive paracellular transport of calcium and magnesium, which are normally reabsorbed at the tight junctions through the same ion channel facilitated by paracellin-1 and claudin-16. In the DCT, magnesium is actively reabsorbed by a transcellular process that is likely mediated by a luminal Mg^{2+}-selective ion channel and a basolateral membrane Na^+/Mg^{2+} exchanger. Although only a small percentage of magnesium is reabsorbed in the DCT, transport is active and therefore an important determinant of final urinary concentration. Activation of the CaSR in the DCT also can decrease calcium and magnesium reabsorption. Unlike other cations (e.g., sodium, potassium, calcium), renal tubular magnesium reabsorption does not appear to be significantly influenced by any particular hormone, although several may exert minor influences.

3. **What is the difference between magnesium depletion and hypomagnesemia?**
Magnesium depletion refers to total body magnesium depletion, whereas hypomagnesemia refers to low serum magnesium levels that can result from a transcellular shift of magnesium from the extracellular to the intracellular compartment, chelation (e.g., by citrate) or saponification (e.g., by triglycerides) of magnesium ions without loss of total body magnesium. Given that multiple factors influence magnesium distribution, serum magnesium levels may not necessarily reflect total body stores, as is the case for any predominantly intracellular ion. Although hypomagnesemia usually indicates total body magnesium depletion, normomagnesemic total body magnesium depletion also can occur and should be considered in patients with unexplained hypokalemia or hypocalcemia, particularly those at risk for hypomagnesemia (e.g., alcoholics, anorexics, patients with diarrhea).

4. **Define hypomagnesemia and discuss the clinical manifestations and degrees of severity.**
Hypomagnesemia is defined as a serum magnesium level <1.7 mg/dL (<0.71 mmol/L or <1.4 mEq/L) and can be further characterized as mild (~1.4–1.7 mg/dL or ~0.58–0.71 mmol/L or ~1.16–1.40 mEq/L), moderate (~1.0–1.4 mg/dL or ~0.41–0.58 mmol/L or ~0.82–1.16 mEq/L) or severe (<1.0 mg/dL or <0.41 mmol/L or <0.82 mEq/L). Mild hypomagnesemia, regardless whether it is acute or chronic, is usually asymptomatic, especially if the onset is insidious. Moderate hypomagnesemia may cause nonspecific symptoms including confusion, depression, and anorexia. Severe hypomagnesemia may cause cardiovascular, neuromuscular, and other electrolyte abnormalities, especially when acute.

Magnesium plays an important role in regulation of cardiac ion channels, including calcium channels and efflux potassium channels. Therefore, when intracellular magnesium concentration is deceased, action potentials may be shortened, which can lead to electrocardiogram changes (e.g., widened QRS complexes, prolonged PR and QT intervals, T-wave abnormalities) and arrhythmias (e.g., torsades de pointes, supraventricular and ventricular arrhythmias) that may be responsive to intravenous magnesium therapy. Hypomagnesemia also can increase the risk of digitalis glycoside toxicity because both magnesium depletion and glycosides can inhibit the Mg^{2+}-dependent Na^+-K^+-ATPase resulting in decreased intracellular potassium. Magnesium also plays an important role in regulation of skeletal muscle contraction and relaxation. Therefore, hypomagnesemia can cause neuromuscular symptoms similar to those caused by hypocalcemia including muscle cramps, weakness, fasciculations, Chvostek's and Trousseau's signs, tetany, and possibly seizures. Hypomagnesemia often coexists with other electrolyte abnormalities, including hypokalemia and hypocalcemia, which may result from the same underlying cause (e.g., diarrhea, diuretics).

5. **What are the causes of hypomagnesemia?**

There are many causes of hypomagnesemia including inadequate intake, increased gastrointestinal loss, increased renal excretion, increased cutaneous loss, transcellular shift from the extracellular to the intracellular compartment, and chelation or saponification of magnesium ions. Complex multifactorial causes of hypomagnesemia also are common in some conditions.

Inadequate magnesium intake alone is an uncommon cause of hypomagnesemia because nearly all foods contain magnesium. However, poor dietary intake can occur with protein-calorie malnutrition and chronic alcoholism. Prolonged administration of low-magnesium or magnesium-free parenteral nutrition or intravenous fluids can cause hypomagnesemia as can an acute increase in magnesium requirement, as occurs in refeeding syndrome.

Increased gastrointestinal loss is a common cause of hypomagnesemia. Although gastrointestinal magnesium loss is negligible under normal circumstances, chronic diarrhea, laxative abuse, fistulas, small bowel resections, and intestinal malabsorption can cause hypomagnesemia. Accordingly, any medication that causes significant diarrhea as a side effect can cause hypomagnesemia. Intestinal malabsorption can be caused by a wide variety of disorders (e.g., inflammatory bowel disease, celiac sprue). Familial hypomagnesemia with secondary hypocalcemia is a rare genetic disorder that causes impaired intestinal absorption and impaired renal reabsorption of magnesium.

Increased renal magnesium excretion is a common cause of hypomagnesemia and can be caused by diuretics, inherited tubular defects, acquired tubular dysfunction, and other electrolyte disorders that cause magnesium wasting. Diuretics are a common cause of increased renal magnesium excretion (see question 8), whereas inherited tubular defects causing hypomagnesemia are rare (see question 11). Acquired tubular dysfunction causing hypomagnesemia is often associated with other medical conditions and accompanied by other electrolyte disorders. Acquired tubular dysfunction is common in polyuric states, with extracellular fluid volume expansion, and as a result of certain medications. Polyuric states, such as with diuretic use, the polyuric phase of acute tubular necrosis, postobstructive diuresis, postrenal transplant, and hyperglycemia from uncontrolled diabetes mellitus (osmotic diuresis) can cause hypomagnesemia. Acquired tubular dysfunction causing hypomagnesemia also can occur with chronic interstitial disease or acute tubular necrosis without polyuria. Extracellular fluid volume expansion resulting from excessive or prolonged normal saline infusion or excessive sodium and water reabsorption, as occurs in primary hyperaldosteronism, can cause hypomagnesemia. Hypercalcemia also can cause hypomagnesemia by a distinct mechanism involving calcium acting through a CaSR in the renal tubules (see question 7). Medications known to cause hypomagnesemia include diuretics (see question 8), aminoglycosides, cisplatin, foscarnet, cyclosporine A, amphotericin B, and pentamidine. Cisplatin-associated hypomagnesemia has been reported in as many as half of patients, is dependent on the cumulative dose, and can persist for months or years after cessation of treatment.

Increased cutaneous magnesium loss also can occur in marathon runners and patients who have had severe burns.

Transcellular shift of magnesium from the extracellular to the intracellular compartment alone is an uncommon cause of hypomagnesemia. However, it can exacerbate hypomagnesemia caused by inadequate intake, increased renal excretion, and increased gastrointestinal loss. Transcellular shift of magnesium also can contribute significantly to hypomagnesemia in patients with hungry bones syndrome, refeeding syndrome, and during treatment of diabetic ketoacidosis (see question 9).

Chelation or saponification of magnesium ions also can cause hypomagnesemia, although total body magnesium does not change. Moreover, the magnesium content of blood may not change as a result of chelation; rather, only the measured fraction of magnesium may change. Hypomagnesemia from chelation by citrate may occur after multiple blood transfusions or when used for anticoagulation, as is sometimes the case with continuous renal replacement therapy (CRRT). Saponification of magnesium ions also can cause hypomagnesemia. For example, in acute pancreatitis fatty acids can absorb magnesium ions in the pancreatic bed.

Complex multifactorial causes of hypomagnesemia are common among patients with chronic alcoholism, uncontrolled diabetes mellitus, starvation or severe malnourishment, or in those who are critically ill.

6. **How can urinary magnesium concentration help differentiate between the causes of hypomagnesemia?**
Once transcellular shift, chelation, and saponification of magnesium ions have been considered, measurement of serum and urinary magnesium concentrations allows for calculation of the fractional excretion of magnesium ($FEMg^{2+}$) to differentiate between renal and extrarenal loss. The $FEMg^{2+} = [UMg^{2+}/(0.7 \times SMg^{2+})]/(UCr/SCr)$, where serum magnesium concentration is multiplied by 0.7 to approximate the ionized portion that is filtered across the glomeruli. $FEMg^{2+} <3\%$ implies renal conservation of magnesium is appropriate in the setting of hypomagnesemia, suggesting an extrarenal cause of hypomagnesemia (e.g., inadequate intake, gastrointestinal loss). In fact, active transport of magnesium in the distal tubules can achieve a $FEMg^{2+} <0.5\%$ to conserve magnesium if necessary. $FEMg^{2+} >3\%$ suggests renal magnesium loss as the cause of hypomagnesemia. Measurement of 24-hour urine magnesium excretion also can be performed, where a 24-hour urine magnesium >1 mmol (>2 mEq or >24.3 mg) suggests total body magnesium depletion.

7. **How can other electrolyte disorders affect magnesium handling by the kidney?**
Serum magnesium concentration is the most important factor influencing renal magnesium reabsorption. Hypomagnesemia increases magnesium reabsorption in the cortical thick ascending limb of the loop of Henle (TALH) and DCT, and hypermagnesemia decreases magnesium reabsorption in these segments. However, other electrolyte disorders also influence magnesium reabsorption.

Hypomagnesemia associated with hypokalemia can be caused by decreased activity of the Mg^{2+}-dependent Na^+-K^+-ATPase in the loop of Henle (and possibly cortical collecting tubules), loop diuretics inhibiting the $Na^+/K^+/2Cl^-$ cotransporter in the loop of Henle, or gastrointestinal loss (e.g., diarrhea), all of which can cause potassium wasting along with further magnesium wasting.

Hypomagnesemia associated with hypocalcemia is likely a result of inhibition of parathyroid hormone (PTH) secretion or skeletal resistance to the effects of PTH, possibly involving inhibition of 1,25-dihydroxyvitamin D_3 (also known as calcitriol, 1,25-dihydroxycholecalciferol, or abbreviated 1,25-(OH_2)D_3) production in the kidney, which further potentiates hypocalcemia by impairing intestinal calcium absorption and contributing to the state of skeletal PTH resistance.

Hypomagnesemia associated with hypercalcemia can result from calcium acting through a basolateral membrane CaSR in the TALH and DCT that can bind both calcium and magnesium, causing decreased reabsorption. CaSR activation inhibits the apical membrane potassium channel and $Na^+/K^+/2Cl^-$ cotransporter, which decreases paracellular transport of calcium and magnesium facilitated by paracellin-1 and claudin-16 at the tight junctions.

Hypomagnesemia associated with hypophosphatemia can be seen in refeeding syndrome in which a constellation of metabolic disturbances can occur as a result of reinstitution of nutrition ("refeeding") in patients who are starved or severely malnourished (e.g., alcoholics, anorexics). The syndrome is thought to result largely from a sudden shift from fat to carbohydrate metabolism along with a sudden increase in insulin levels after refeeding, which leads to increased cellular uptake of magnesium, phosphate, and other electrolytes.

8. **How do diuretics affect magnesium handling by the kidney?**

Diuretics are a common cause of increased renal magnesium wasting. Loop diuretics (e.g., furosemide, torsemide) inhibit the $Na^+/K^+/2Cl^-$ cotransporter in the loop of Henle, which causes loss of the positive electrical potential in the lumen that drives paracellular divalent cation reabsorption, causing both hypomagnesemia and hypocalcemia, with corresponding increases in urinary magnesium and calcium excretion. The mechanism whereby chronic use of thiazide diuretics may cause hypomagnesemia is unclear; however, acute administration of thiazide diuretics may actually increase magnesium reabsorption. Hypomagnesemia caused by loop and thiazide diuretics is often mild because volume contraction increases sodium and water reabsorption in the proximal tubule, which increases magnesium reabsorption in this segment, which tends to attenuate magnesium loss in the cortical thick ascending limb of the loop of Henle (TALH). Moreover, potassium-sparing diuretics (e.g., amiloride) are sometimes used to treat chronic hypomagnesemia refractory to magnesium replacement because they tend to increase magnesium reabsorption in the DCT.

9. **What are the mechanisms that cause transcellular shift of potassium, which can cause or contribute to hypomagnesemia in hungry bones syndrome, in refeeding syndrome, and in patients being treated for diabetic ketoacidosis?**

In all three of these syndromes, transcellular shift of magnesium can cause or contribute to hypomagnesemia. In hungry bones syndrome, some patients with hyperparathyroidism and severe bone disease who undergo parathyroidectomy experience a sudden decrease in PTH that decreases bone reabsorption while allowing a high rate of bone formation to continue. Consequently, these patients also have severe hypocalcemia. In refeeding syndrome, patients who are starved or severely malnourished (e.g., alcoholics, anorexics) develop fluid and electrolyte disorders within days of reinstitution of nutrition, along with neurologic, neuromuscular, cardiac, pulmonary, and hematologic complications thought to result from a sudden increase in insulin levels, which leads to increased cellular uptake of glucose, phosphate, magnesium, and thiamine. Patients being treated for diabetic ketoacidosis with insulin also can have increased cellular uptake of electrolytes, causing hypomagnesemia as described for refeeding syndrome.

10. **Discuss chronic alcoholism, uncontrolled diabetes mellitus, starvation or severe malnourishment, and patients who are critically ill from the perspective of having complex multifactorial causes of hypomagnesemia.**

Hypomagnesemia associated with these conditions has been described as complex multifactorial. Hypomagnesemia associated with chronic alcoholism can be a result of poor dietary intake, increased gastrointestinal loss, increased renal loss, and transcellular shift of magnesium. Increased gastrointestinal loss can occur from vomiting and diarrhea, whereas increased renal loss can be a direct effect of alcohol causing tubular dysfunction, which can persist for weeks after cessation of alcohol use. Chronic alcoholics also are at increased risk of refeeding syndrome as a result of poor nutrition and pancreatitis, both of which can contribute to hypomagnesemia. Increased free fatty acids resulting from pancreatitis can cause saponification of magnesium ions in the pancreatic bed. Hypomagnesemia associated with diabetes mellitus can result from transcellular shift of magnesium in uncontrolled insulin-dependent diabetics with ketoacidosis and/or hyperglycemia-induced osmotic diuresis. Hypomagnesemia in patients who are starved or severely malnourished can result from poor dietary intake and a transcellular shift of magnesium that may occur with refeeding syndrome. Patients who are critically ill can have complex multifactorial hypomagnesemia resulting from any of the aforementioned causes, in addition to diarrhea, diuretics, intravenous fluids, and other medications. Identifying patients at risk for hypomagnesemia from complex multifactorial causes can help avoid complications associated with these conditions. Close monitoring of electrolytes with prompt repletion of magnesium, potassium, and phosphate is paramount. Thiamine, vitamin B complex, multivitamin, and other supplements also may be necessary.

11. **What are some inherited genetic defects in magnesium transport that cause hypomagnesemia?**

Inherited genetic defects in both intestinal and renal magnesium transport can cause hypomagnesemia. Genetic disorders associated with hypomagnesemia are summarized in Table 80-1, including the gene defect, inheritance pattern, proposed mechanism, and some important associated serum and urine electrolyte abnormalities.

12. **What is the treatment for hypomagnesemia?**

Treat the underlying cause of hypomagnesemia whenever possible. Moreover, anticipating the need for magnesium replacement in patients at risk for hypomagnesemia (e.g., patients taking diuretics, refeeding syndrome, treatment of diabetic ketoacidosis) is a good approach. The route of magnesium replacement depends on the severity, presence of symptoms, and functional status of the gastrointestinal tract and kidneys. Severe hypomagnesemia, which may be associated with cardiac, neuromuscular, or other electrolyte abnormalities, can be treated with intravenous replacement therapy (e.g., magnesium sulfate) with an initial bolus of 1 to 2 g (~8–16 mEq) over 15 minutes, followed by continuous infusion of 4 to 6 g (~32–48 mEq) over the next 24 hours, followed by re-evaluation. Moderate hypomagnesemia can be treated by intravenous replacement therapy if symptoms are present or if a parenteral route is otherwise necessary or with oral replacement therapy (e.g., magnesium oxide, magnesium chloride), which is preferred. An initial oral dose of 30 to 60 mEq in three or four divided doses, followed by 0.5 to 1 mEq/kg daily thereafter is reasonable until magnesium is replete. Mild hypomagnesemia can be treated with oral replacement therapy, whereas very mild hypomagnesemia may be adequately treated with increased dietary magnesium intake alone in some cases. Foods high in magnesium include green vegetables, whole grains, meats, and seafood.

Parenteral magnesium administration can result in significant magnesuria because magnesium exchanges very slowly with the intracellular compartment and it can easily overwhelm renal magnesium reabsorption capacity. In fact, as much as 50% of the infused dose may be excreted. For this reason, sustained-release oral replacement is preferred because slow intestinal absorption allows for more sustained serum magnesium levels. Oral replacement should continue for 2 to 3 days after serum magnesium normalizes because of slow intracellular uptake. Some patients require maintenance therapy as a result of chronic losses (e.g., patients receiving diuretic therapy, inherited magnesium wasting disorders). Moreover, patients with chronic potassium wasting on maintenance potassium therapy often require magnesium.

Approximately 0.5 to 1 mEq/kg of magnesium per day for 5 to 7 days is adequate to replenish total body magnesium stores in many cases. Oral magnesium supplements may be adequate for the treatment of the genetic disorders of magnesium wasting, often normalizing serum levels. However, potassium-sparing diuretics (e.g., amiloride) are sometimes used to treat chronic hypomagnesemia refractory to magnesium replacement because they increase magnesium reabsorption in the DCT. Serum potassium, calcium, and phosphate levels also should be monitored during treatment.

13. **What are the side effects and complications of treating hypomagnesemia?**

Oral magnesium supplements are generally well tolerated, except at high doses, which may cause diarrhea. Parenteral magnesium administration is generally reserved for patients who are critically ill, patients with severe hypomagnesemia, or patients with nonfunctional gastrointestinal tracts. Parenteral magnesium is more likely to be associated with complications, particularly with too rapid or overcorrection, which can cause skin flushing, hypocalcemia, loss of deep tendon reflexes, atrioventricular block, and hypotension. To prevent complications, serum magnesium, potassium, calcium, and phosphate levels should be monitored frequently to avoid too rapid correction or overcorrection and to monitor for other electrolyte abnormalities. Magnesium doses may need to be adjusted by 25% to 50% in patients with reduced glomerular filtration rate (GFR).

TABLE 80–1. GENETIC DISORDERS ASSOCIATED WITH HYPOMAGNESEMIA			
Genetic Disorder	Gene Defect/Inheritance	Location/Proposed Mechanism	Other Electrolytes/Urine
Primary intestinal hypomagnesemia	Mutation of TRPM6 Autosomal recessive	Affects the small intestines and DCT Mutated TRPM6 inhibits intestinal absorption and renal reabsorption of Mg^{2+}	Hypocalcemia Normokalemia Hypermagnesuria (or normal)
Isolated dominant hypomagnesemia	Mutation of Na^+-K^+-ATPase Autosomal dominant	Affects the DCT Mutated Na^+-K^+-ATPase inhibits Mg^{2+} reabsorption	Normocalcemia Normokalemia Hypermagnesuria Hypocalciuria
Isolated recessive hypomagnesemia	Mutation unknown Autosomal recessive	Affects the DCT Defect inhibits Mg^{2+} reabsorption	Normocalcemia Normokalemia Hypermagnesuria
Bartter syndrome	Mutation of $Na^+/K^+/2Cl^-$ cotransporter, ROMK1, CLC-Kb, or Barttin Autosomal recessive	Affects the TALH Mutated $Na^+/K^+/2Cl^-$ cotransporter, ROMK1 K^+ channel, or CLC-Kb or Barttin Cl^- channels inhibits Mg^{2+} reabsorption	Hypocalcemia Hypokalemia Hypermagnesuria (or normal) Hypermagnesuria

	Mutation / Inheritance	Mechanism	Findings
Gitelman syndrome	Mutation of NCCT Autosomal recessive	Affects the DCT Mutated NCCT inhibits Mg^{2+} reabsorption	Normocalcemia Hypokalemia Hypermagnesuria Hypocalciuria
Familial hypomagnesemia hypercalciuria	Mutation of paracellin-1 or claudin-16 Autosomal recessive	Affects the TALH Mutated paracellin-1 or claudin-16 inhibits Mg^{2+} reabsorption	Hypocalcemia Hypokalemia (or normal) Hypermagnesuria Hypercalciuria
Autosomal dominant hypoparathyroidism hypocalcemia	Mutation of CaSR Autosomal dominant	Affects the TALH Mutated CaSR is constitutively active inhibiting Ca^{2+} and Mg^{2+} reabsorption	Hypocalcemia Normokalemia Hypermagnesuria Hypermagnesuria

TRPM6 = transient receptor potential ion channel M6; DCT = distal convoluted tubule; ROMK = renal outer medullary potassium channel; CLC-Kb = chloride channel-Kb; TALH = thick ascending limb of the loop of Henle; NCCT = sodium chloride cotransporter; CaSR = Ca^{2+}/Mg^{2+}-sensing receptor.

KEY POINTS: HYPOMAGNESEMIA

1. Approximately 15% to 25% of magnesium reabsorption occurs in the proximal tubule, ~60% to 70% in the thick ascending limb of the loop of Henle, and only ~5% to 10% in the distal convoluted tubule.

2. Hypomagnesemia (<1.7 mg/dL or <0.70 mmol/L or <1.4 mEq/L) can be caused by inadequate intake, increased gastrointestinal loss, increased renal excretion, increased cutaneous loss, transcellular shift from the extracellular to the intracellular compartment, chelation or saponification of magnesium ions, and complex multifactorial causes.

3. Treat the underlying cause of hypomagnesemia. The route of magnesium replacement depends on the severity, presence of symptoms, and functional status of the gastrointestinal tract and kidneys.

14. **Define hypermagnesemia and discuss the clinical manifestations and degrees of severity.**
Hypermagnesemia is defined as a serum magnesium level >2.3 mg/dL (>0.96 mmol/L or >1.9 mEq/L) and can be further characterized as mild (~2.3–4.0 mg/dL or ~0.96–1.64 mmol/L or ~1.9–3.3 mEq/L), moderate (~4.0–7.0 mg/dL or ~1.64–2.88 mmol/L or ~3.3–5.8 mEq/L), or severe (>7.0 mg/dL or >2.88 mmol/L or >5.8 mEq/L). Mild hypermagnesemia is usually asymptomatic regardless of whether it is acute or chronic. Patients with moderate hypomagnesemia may develop skin flushing, nausea, vomiting, mild hyporeflexia, mild hypotension, and electrocardiogram abnormalities. Patients with severe hypermagnesemia may develop loss of deep tendon reflexes, muscle weakness, and severe hypotension. Respiratory failure and cardiac arrest typically do not develop until serum magnesium levels are >10 mg/dL (>4.1 mmol/L or >8.2 mEq/L).

15. **What are the causes of hypermagnesemia?**
The main causes of hypermagnesemia are increased intake, decreased renal excretion, and transcellular shift or release from the intracellular to the extracellular compartment.
Increased magnesium intake can cause hypermagnesemia including overuse of magnesium-containing antacids, laxatives, enemas, and nutritional supplements. Overzealous administration of intravenous magnesium as therapy for hypomagnesemia, severe preeclampsia, or eclampsia and oversupplementation of parenteral nutrition formulations also are common causes. Magnesium should always be used cautiously in patients with impaired renal function.
Decreased renal magnesium excretion is usually necessary for hypermagnesemia to develop because normal kidneys filter ~70% to 80% of total serum magnesium, and when levels are increased, tubular reabsorption can be substantially decreased, such that most of the filtered load is excreted in urine. Hypermagnesemia can develop in patients with acute kidney injury and chronic kidney disease, but typically not until GFR falls below 30 mL/min. Moreover, patients receiving dialysis typically do not develop hypermagnesemia unless they receive a significant magnesium load. Hypermagnesemia can also result from rare inherited tubular defects such as familial hypocalciuric hypercalcemia (see question 16).
Transcellular shift or release of magnesium from the intracellular to the extracellular compartment may be caused by conditions associated with increased tissue destruction and cell death such as rhabdomyolysis or tumor lysis syndrome.

16. **What is familial hypocalciuric hypercalcemia, and how does it cause hypermagnesemia?**
Familial hypocalciuric hypercalcemia (FHH) is characterized by lifelong hypercalcemia with concurrent hypocalciuria; it is also known as familial benign hypercalcemia because it is usually

asymptomatic and does not require treatment. Most cases of FHH are associated with loss-of-function mutations in the CaSR expressed by the parathyroid glands and kidneys. The result is inability of calcium to signal through the CaSR (loss of inhibition) allowing the parathyroid glands to inappropriately produce high levels of PTH in the setting of hypercalcemia. The presence of concurrent hypocalciuria indicates inappropriate retention of calcium by the renal tubules. As a result of mutation of the CaSR, magnesium also may be inappropriately reabsorbed. Routine diagnostic methods do not always allow for clear distinction between FHH and primary hyperparathyroidism, which can be treated with parathyroidectomy, whereas FHH is not; therefore genetic testing may be indicated in some cases.

17. **What is milk-alkali syndrome, and how does it cause hypermagnesemia?**
Milk-alkali syndrome involves the triad of hypercalcemia, metabolic alkalosis, and renal impairment caused by ingestion of excessive amounts of calcium and absorbable alkalizing agent (e.g., sodium bicarbonate, calcium carbonate, magnesium hydroxide). High serum calcium levels and suppression of PTH further increase renal tubule bicarbonate reabsorption. When excessive magnesium-containing antacids are ingested in the setting of renal impairment, hypermagnesemia can develop along with milk-alkali syndrome. It was once somewhat rare, but recent increased use of calcium carbonate for dyspepsia and for calcium supplementation for bone health has caused a resurgence of milk-alkali syndrome, which can be precipitated by ingestion of more than 2 g of calcium per day in some individuals. If untreated, milk-alkali syndrome can lead to metastatic calcification and renal failure.

18. **What is the treatment for hypermagnesemia?**
Treat the underlying cause of hypermagnesemia whenever possible. If it is a result of increased exogenous magnesium intake, discontinue use and/or adjust parenteral nutrition formulation as necessary and maintain adequate volume status because functional kidneys will readily excrete excess magnesium. If increased serum magnesium results from endogenous release, as may occur with tumor lysis syndrome and rhabdomyolysis, again maintain adequate volume status because functional kidneys will readily excrete excess magnesium. If hypermagnesemia results from decreased renal magnesium excretion, treatment should include a low-magnesium diet and/or magnesium supplement dose reduction. If hypermagnesemia is severe or symptomatic, intravenous calcium can transiently antagonize the effects of magnesium. If necessary, dialysis can remove excess magnesium.

KEY POINTS: HYPERMAGNESEMIA

1. Hypermagnesemia (>2.3 mg/dL or >0.95 mmol/L or >1.9 mEq/L) can be caused by increased intake, decreased renal excretion, and transcellular shift or release from the intracellular to the extracellular compartment.

2. Treat the underlying cause of hypermagnesemia. If hypermagnesemia results from increased exogenous intake, discontinue or decrease intake; if it results from increased endogenous release, maintain adequate volume status because functional kidneys will excrete excess magnesium; and if it results from decreased renal excretion, treatment should include a low-magnesium diet and/or magnesium supplement dose reduction.

3. If hypermagnesemia is severe or symptomatic, intravenous calcium can transiently antagonize the effects of magnesium. If necessary, dialysis can remove excess magnesium.

BIBLIOGRAPHY

1. Berns JS. Disorders of magnesium homeostasis. In: Greenberg A, Cheung AK, Coffman TM, et al. (eds.). *Primer on Kidney Diseases*, 5th ed. Philadelphia: Elsevier Saunders, 2009, pp. 131–135.

2. Gunn IR, Gaffney D. Clinical and laboratory features of calcium-sensing receptor disorders: A systematic review. *Ann Clin Biochem* 2004;41:441–458.

3. Knoers NV. Inherited forms of renal hypomagnesemia: an update. *Pediatr Nephrol* 2009;458:679–705.

4. Naderi AS, Reilly RF Jr. Hereditary etiologies of hypomagnesemia. *Nat Clin Pract Nephrol* 2008;4:80–89.

5. Topf JM, Murray PT. Hypomagnesemia and hypermagnesemia. *Rev Endocr Metab Disord* 2003;4:195–206.

6. Waldman M, Kobrin S. Disorders of magnesium balance: Hypomagnesemia & hypermagnesemia. In Lerma EV, Berns JS, Nissenson AR (eds.). *Current Diagnosis and Treatment: Nephrology & Hypertension*, 1st ed. New York: McGraw-Hill, 2009, pp. 79–87.

CHAPTER 81

METABOLIC ACIDOSIS

Kamel S. Kamel, MD, and Mitchell L. Halperin, MD

Because metabolic acidosis is such a large topic, the emphasis will be on "secrets," as is the theme of this book (Table 81-1). This chapter is divided into four sections. We begin with a general introduction, which is followed by a synopsis of major principles of physiology. In the third section, we outline our clinical approach to patients with this heterogeneous group of disorders, which includes the initial steps to recognize and deal with threats to the life of the patient and anticipate and prevent the dangers that may arise during therapy. We conclude in the fourth section with "secrets" related to the specific causes for metabolic acidosis.

GENERAL INTRODUCTION

1. **What is metabolic acidosis?**

   Metabolic acidosis is a process that leads to an increase in the concentration of H^+ and a decrease in the concentration and/or the content of bicarbonate (HCO_3^-) in the extracellular fluid (ECF) compartment. The risks for the patient depend on the underlying disorder responsible for the metabolic acidosis, the ill effects resulting from a high concentration of H^+ (binding of H^+ to intracellular proteins in vital organs [e.g., brain and heart]; see equation 2 in Fig. 81-1), possible dangers associated with the anions that accompany the H^+ load (e.g., chelation of ionized calcium during citric acidosis), and risks from toxins produced in the metabolic process that lead to the production of these acids (e.g., formaldehyde produced during the metabolism of methanol to formic acid or glycoaldehyde produced during metabolism of ethylene glycol to glycolic acid) or as a marker of a serious metabolic threat (e.g., production of pyroglutamic acid because this indicates depletion of the reduced form of glutathione, which compromises the ability to detoxify reactive oxygen species in these patients).

TABLE 81-1. ABBREVIATIONS AND NORMAL VALUES IN PLASMA

pH: 7.40 ± 0.02

[H^+]: 40 ± 2 nmol/L

[HCO_3^-] in plasma (P_{HCO3}): 25 ± 2 mmol/L

Arterial PCO$_2$: 40 ± 2 mm Hg

Brachial venous PCO$_2$: <10 mm Hg higher than the arterial PCO$_2$.

Albumin in plasma ($P_{Albumin}$): 4.0 g/dL or 40 g/L. Accounts for ~16 mEq/L of the anionic charge in plasma.

Anion gap in plasma ($P_{Anion\ gap}$): 12 ± 2 mEq/L (must adjust for the valence from the $P_{Albumin}$)

Henderson equation: $[H^+]$ (nmol/L) $=$ PCO$_2$ (mm Hg) $\times$ (25 or 24)/P_{HCO3}

To make the mathematics easier at the bedside, one can use 25 or 24 as the constant.

---

(1) Acid $\longrightarrow$ $\boxed{H^+}$ + Anion

(2) $\boxed{H^+}$ + Protein$^0 \longrightarrow$ $\boxed{H \cdot Protein^+}$

(3) $\boxed{H^+}$ + $HCO_3^- \longleftrightarrow$ $\boxed{CO_2}$ + H_2O

Figure 81-1. Buffer systems to remove a H$^+$ load. Although equations 2 and 3 describe buffer systems to remove H$^+$ in terms of chemistry of this process, there is a different emphasis in physiologic terms. In this context, flux through equation 2 must be minimized. This occurs if these added H$^+$ are forced to bind to bicarbonate (HCO$_3^-$) by lowering the PCO$_2$ in capillaries of skeletal muscles (equation 3) where this buffer system is most abundant, thereby pulling equation 3 to the right, which lowers the concentration of H$^+$ in plasma and minimizes binding of H$^+$ to intracellular proteins in vital organs (e.g., brain and heart).

There are two other points to emphasize with respect to the concentration of H$^+$ in patients with metabolic acidosis.

- Two major mechanisms can cause a large input of H$^+$, the addition of an acid (see Fig. 81-1, shift in equation 1 from left to right) or the loss of HCO$_3^-$ with sodium (Na$^+$) (NaHCO$_3$) (see Fig. 81-1, shift in equation 3 from right to left).
- To prevent the binding of H$^+$ to proteins in patients with metabolic acidosis, there must be little if any rise in the concentration of H$^+$ in cells (see Fig. 81-1, equation 2). This occurs if these added H$^+$ are forced to bind to HCO$_3^-$ (see Fig. 81-1, equation 3). The mechanism focuses on having a low concentration of carbon dioxide (CO$_2$) in capillaries around skeletal muscle, as shown in the grey shading in Figure 81-1, equation 3.

2. **Must the concentration of HCO$_3^-$ in plasma (P$_{HCO3}$) be low in a patient with metabolic acidosis?**

   It is not a secret that P$_{HCO3}$ may not be low in a patient with metabolic acidosis who has another simultaneous processes that adds HCO$_3^-$ to the ECF compartment (e.g., metabolic alkalosis from the loss of HCl during vomiting, which raises the P$_{HCO3}$). The secret, however, is that there is another mechanism that causes the P$_{HCO3}$ not to be low despite a low content of HCO$_3^-$ in the ECF compartment. In more detail, the P$_{HCO3}$ is the ratio of the *content* of HCO$_3^-$ in the ECF compartment to the ECF volume:

   Concentration of HCO$_3^-$ in the ECF = Content of HCO$_3^-$ in the ECF/ECF volume

   A patient can have metabolic acidosis (i.e., a decreased content of HCO$_3^-$ as a result of the addition of an acid (e.g., in a patient with diabetic ketoacidosis, or DKA) or from a large loss of NaHCO$_3$ (e.g., in a patient with cholera) with a P$_{HCO3}$ that is not appreciably low if the ECF volume is markedly contracted. Hence a patient with a very marked degree of ECF volume contraction can have a P$_{HCO3}$ that is not appreciably low despite the presence of a severe degree of metabolic acidosis (e.g., a patient with diarrhea and a very contracted ECF volume). To detect the presence of metabolic acidosis in a patient with a very low ECF volume, one cannot rely on measurement of the P$_{HCO3}$; rather, a quantitative estimate of the ECF volume is needed, as described later.

   Sample calculation: We use the hematocrit (if the patient does not have preexisting anemia or polycythemia) or the concentration of albumin or total proteins in plasma to obtain a quantitative estimate of the ECF volume and calculate its *content* of HCO$_3^-$. In a normal adult, the usual hematocrit is 0.40; this represents a blood volume of 5 L (2 L of red blood cells [RBC] and 3 L of plasma:

   Hematocrit (0.40) = 2 L RBC/Blood volume (5 L total volume), (2 L RBC + 3 L plasma)

Therefore, when the hematocrit is 0.50, the plasma volume equals the of RBC volume (i.e., 2 L):

Hematocrit (0.50) = (4 L total volume, 2 L RBC L blood volume)

The present blood volume is 4 L and thus the plasma volume is 2 L. Hence the plasma volume is reduced by 1 L from its normal value of 3 L. Ignoring changes in Starling forces for simplicity, the ECF volume likely to be also reduced to approximately two thirds of its normal volume (i.e., reduced by ~33%).

3. **What is the difference between acidemia and acidosis?**
Acidemia simply describes the concentration of H^+ in plasma; thus it includes all conditions where the concentration of H^+ in plasma is higher than the values observed in normal subjects (40 ± 2 nmol/L, or a pH that is less than 7.38). Acidemia has two main causes: a high concentration of H^+ in plasma as a result of a high PCO_2 in arterial blood (called respiratory acidosis) or high concentration of H^+ in plasma from a low P_{HCO3} (called metabolic acidosis). Notwithstanding, acidemia may be absent in some patients who have metabolic acidosis. In more detail, on the one hand, there may be another process than caused the concentration of H^+ in plasma to fall by raising the P_{HCO3} (e.g., the loss of HCl and/or a deficit of NaCl). On the other hand, a lower arterial PCO_2 than expected in response to metabolic acidemia will lower the concentration of H^+ in arterial plasma in a patient with acidosis of metabolic origin (called coexisting respiratory alkalosis).

SYNOPSIS OF THE IMPORTANT PHYSIOLOGY

4. **How is the danger of a high concentration of H^+ minimized in a patient with metabolic acidosis?**
The key issue is that H^+ are "evil" if they bind to intracellular proteins in vital organs (e.g., brain and heart; Fig. 81-2) because this changes their net charge, shape, and possibly their functions (see equation 2 in Fig. 81-1). In this context, proteins are enzymes, transporters, contractile elements, receptors, and structural elements. To minimize binding of H^+ to intracellular proteins and another process that changes this essential function, another process must prevent the concentration of H^+ from rising despite the H^+ load. This function is achieved by buffering the H^+ load by the bicarbonate buffer system because its first step is to have a low PCO_2 in interstitial space and intracellular fluid (ICF) compartment of skeletal muscle (see equation 3 in Fig. 81-1) because this is the organ where the vast majority of the HCO_3^- is present in the body. If the bicarbonate buffer system in skeletal muscle is not removing H^+ in a patient with metabolic acidosis appropriately, acidemia will be more pronounced and more of the H^+ load will be titrated in vital organs (e.g., brain and heart). As shown in equation 3 in Figure 81-1, the bicarbonate buffer system is driven by pull (i.e., by having a lower PCO_2 in the interstitial space and ICF compartment in skeletal muscle).

5. **Which PCO_2 best reflects this "good" buffering of H^+ in skeletal muscle?**
The PCO_2 in capillaries of skeletal muscle reflects the PCO_2 in its cells and interstitial space. Because there is no CO_2 added once blood leaves capillaries and enters veins, the PCO_2 in these capillaries is reflected by the PCO_2 in venous blood draining muscle (e.g., brachial or femoral venous blood) and can be used to provide a measurement of muscle capillary blood PCO_2. Although the *arterial* PCO_2 must be low to have a low PCO_2 in capillaries in skeletal muscle, this alone does not guarantee that this PCO_2 will be low. As detailed later, the PCO_2 in these capillaries is also influenced by the blood flow rate (see Fig. 81-2). The secret here is that if the bicarbonate buffer system (BBS) in skeletal muscle is not effective in a patient with metabolic acidosis, acidemia will be more pronounced and more of the H^+ load will be titrated in vital organs (e.g., brain and heart).

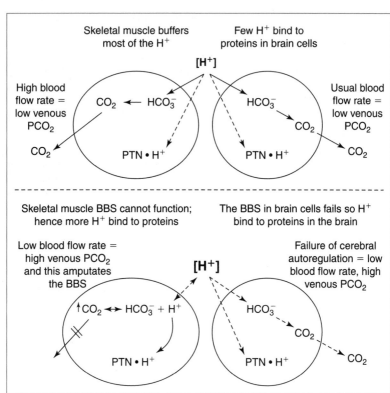

Figure 81-2. Physiology of the bicarbonate buffer system (BBS). Skeletal muscle cells are shown to the left and brain cells to the right; because brain is one twentieth the size of muscle, it has far less intracellular fluid (ICF) and thereby HCO_3^-. When the extracellular fluid (ECF) volume is low, the PCO_2 in the venous blood draining muscle is high. This minimizes the removal buffering of H^+ by the BBS in its ECF and ICF. As a result, the $[H^+]_{plasma}$ rises and more H^+ will be removed in brain cells. As the cerebral blood flow rate is autoregulated, the PCO_2 in the jugular venous blood draining the brain will change minimally and hence the BBS in the brain will still function to titrate the H^+ load. Furthermore, if the degree of ECF volume contraction is severe, cerebral autoregulation fails and the blood flow to the brain falls. Hence, the PCO_2 in brain cells will rise and more H^+ will bind to proteins in brain cells. In contrast, when intravenous saline is administered, blood flow to skeletal muscle rises, its venous PCO_2 should fall, and more H^+ are removed by its BBS. As a result, the $[H^+]_{plasma}$ falls and H^+ will be released from proteins in brain cells.

6. **What are the major reasons for a high capillary PCO_2 during metabolic acidosis?**

   The major clinical settings for failure of the BBS in muscle is/are respiratory suppression, which raises the arterial PCO_2, and thereby the lowest possible value for the capillary PCO_2 and/or a slow blood flow rate to muscle (e.g., from a very contracted effective arterial blood volume). With regard to the latter, at the usual blood flow rate at rest, the brachial venous PCO_2 is 46 mm Hg, whereas the arterial PCO_2 is 40 mm Hg. When the blood flow rate is low and if the same amount of oxygen were to be extracted, more oxygen must be removed from each liter of blood because of the slower blood flow rate. Because ~1 mmol of CO_2 will be formed per mmol of O_2 consumed, there will be little change in the rate of production of CO_2 but much more CO_2 added to each liter of blood flow; thereby there will be a higher PCO_2 in this capillary blood.

7. **What are the benefits and risks to anticipate from an infusion of isotonic saline when there is a high capillary PCO_2 as a result of a slow flow of blood to skeletal muscle?**
Benefits: When enough saline is administered to restore the effective arterial blood volume, this should result in a large fall in PCO_2 in veins draining skeletal muscle. As a result more H^+ will be removed by the BBS in muscle, the concentration of H^+ will fall in plasma, and binding of an appreciable portion of the H^+ load to proteins in vital organs (e.g., brain and heart) will be reversed. Once the blood flow to the brain rises, the PCO_2 in its capillaries will fall and the extra H^+ will no longer be bound to proteins in brain cells. We suggest that enough saline should be given to cause the brachial venous PCO_2 to fall to a value that is less than 10 mm Hg above the arterial PCO_2. This should improve the functions of the vital organs (e.g., the heart and the brain).
Risks to anticipate: These risks may arise in a subset of patients with metabolic acidosis and include a very severe degree of acidemia and the development of pulmonary edema (see the discussion of diarrhea for more discussion of this topic). If these dangers are anticipated, they can be prevented.

CLINICAL ISSUES IN PATIENTS WITH METABOLIC ACIDOSIS

8. **Describe the general approach to metabolic acidosis.**
The diagnostic category of metabolic acidosis is made up of two major subgroups: one where the basis of the disorder is the addition of acids and the other where the basis is a major loss of $NaHCO_3$. The initial steps in our clinical approach to the patient with metabolic acidosis are illustrated in Figure 81-3.
   - *Identify and deal with emergencies.* Although the emergencies may be different within each of the causes for the disorder, we shall deal with threats to life that are specific for each disorder under the heading of "Specific Disorders (page 582)."

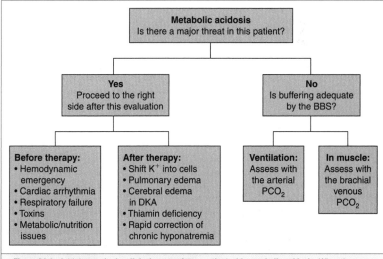

Figure 81-3. Initial steps in the clinical approach to a patient with metabolic acidosis. When the extracellular fluid (ECF) volume is significantly contracted, one must use a definition of metabolic acidosis that is based not only the P_{HCO3}, but also on the content of HCO_3^- in the ECF compartment. Our initial step is to determine threats for the patient that may be present and anticipate those that may develop during therapy *(left side of the flow chart).* The next step is to assess buffering by the bicarbonate buffer system (BBS) in both the ECF and ICF of skeletal muscle by measuring brachial or femoral venous PCO_2.

- *Anticipate and prevent risks that are likely to develop during therapy.* These are summarized in Figure 81-3.
- *Deduce whether there is a risk of excessive binding of H$^+$ to intracellular proteins in vital organs.* If the brachial or femoral venous PCO$_2$ is appreciably higher than 10 mm Hg above arterial PCO$_2$, this indicates that the bicarbonate buffer system in skeletal muscle is not removing the H$^+$ optimally and hence there is a risk of excessive binding of H$^+$ to intracellular proteins in vital organs (e.g., the brain and the heart). Examine the arterial PCO$_2$ and assess the effective arterial blood volume to determine where leverage could be exerted in therapy to lower muscle venous PCO$_2$.

9. **How does one interpret other laboratory studies in the context of metabolic acidosis?**
   A summary of some useful laboratory tests is given in Table 81-2 below.

10. **Is the content of HCO$_3^-$ in ECF compartment low?**
    Calculate the content of HCO$_3^-$ in the ECF compartment (P$_{HCO3}$ × ECF volume) when the ECF volume is appreciably low. The hematocrit or total protein levels in plasma are useful to obtain a quantitative estimate of the ECF volume.

11. **Have new acids accumulated?**
    The presence of new anions in plasma can be detected with the calculation of the P$_{Anion\ gap}$. The baseline value of the P$_{Anion\ gap}$ must be adjusted for the P$_{Albumin}$.

TABLE 81-2. LABORATORY TESTS IN THE DIAGNOSIS OF METABOLIC ACIDOSIS

Question	Parameter Assessed	Tools to Use
Is the content of HCO$_3^-$ low in the ECF?	ECF volume	Hematocrit or total plasma proteins
Have new acids accumulated?	Appearance of new anions in the body or the urine	P$_{anion\ gap}$ Urine anion gap
Are toxic alcohols present?	Detect alcohols as unmeasured osmoles	P$_{Osmolal\ gap}$
Is the renal response to acidemia adequate?	Examine the rate of excretion of NH$_4^+$	Urine osmolal gap
If NH$_4^+$ excretion is high, which anion was excreted?	GI loss of NaHCO$_3$	Urine Cl$^-$ is high
	Acid added, but its new anions are excreted	Urine anion gap
What is the basis for a low rate or excretion of NH$_4^+$?	Low net distal H$^+$ secretion	Urine pH >6.5
	Low NH$_3$ availability	Urine pH ~5.0
	Both defects	Urine pH ~6.0
Where is the defect in H$^+$ secretion?	Distal H$^+$ secretion	PCO$_2$ in alkaline urine
	Proximal H$^+$ secretion	FE$_{HCO3}$, U$_{Citrate}$

ECF = extracellular fluid; GI = gastrointestinal.

New anions in the urine can be detected by calculating the Urine $_{\text{Anion gap}}$ ($U_{Na} + U_K + U_{NH4} - U_{Cl}$); for this calculation, the concentration of NH_4^+ in the urine (U_{NH4}) should be estimated using the urine osmolal gap.

12. **Have toxic alcohols accumulated in the body?**
    Calculate the $P_{\text{Osmolal gap}}$ to reveal whether many new uncharged particles are present in plasma: $P_{\text{Osmolal gap}}$ = measured $P_{osm} - (P_{\text{Glucose}} + P_{\text{Urea}} + 2 P_{Na})$, all in mmol/L units.

13. **In a patient with an increased anion-gap type of metabolic acidosis, what is the cause of overproduction of acids?**
    A list of the causes of metabolic acidosis is provided in Table 81-3. Our clinical approach to the diagnosis of the cause of metabolic acidosis is summarized in Figure 81-4.

TABLE 81-3.   CAUSES OF METABOLIC ACIDOSIS

ACID GAIN

With retention of anions in plasma:

1. L-lactic acidosis

    A. Due predominantly to overproduction of L-lactic acid.

Hypoxic lactic acidosis

Inadequate deliver of O_2 (cardiogenic shock, shunting of blood past organs, e.g., sepsis, or excessive demand for oxygen, e.g., seizures)

Increased production of L-lactic acid in absence of hypoxia

Overproduction of NADH and accumulation of pyruvate in the liver (e.g., metabolism of ethanol plus a deficiency of thiamin)

Decreased pyruvate dehydrogenase activity (e.g., thiamin deficiency, inborn errors of metabolism)

Compromised mitochondrial electron transport system (e.g., cyanide, riboflavin deficiency, inborn errors affecting the electron transport system)

Excessive degree of uncoupling of oxidative phosphorylation (e.g., phenformin)

    B. Due predominantly to reduced removal of L-lactate: liver failure (e.g., severe acute viral hepatitis, shock liver, drugs).

    C. Due to a combination of reduced removal and overproduction of L-lactic acid.

Antiretroviral drugs (inhibition of mitochondrial electron transport plus hepatic steatosis)

Metastatic tumors (especially large tumors with hypoxic areas plus liver involvement)

2. Ketoacidosis (diabetic ketoacidosis, alcoholic ketoacidosis, hypoglycemic ketoacidosis including starvation, ketoacidosis due to a large supply of short-chain fatty acids (i.e., acetic acid from fermentation of poorly absorbed carbohydrate plus inhibition of acetyl-coenzyme A carboxylase)

3. Renal insufficiency (metabolism of dietary sulfur-containing amino acids and decreased renal excretion of NH_4^+)

4. Metabolism of toxic alcohols (e.g., formic acid from metabolism of methanol, glycolic acid, and oxalic acid from metabolism of ethylene glycol)

5. D-lactic acidosis (and other organic acids produced by gastrointestinal bacteria)

6. Pyroglutamic acidosis

Continued

TABLE 81-3. CAUSES OF METABOLIC ACIDOSIS—cont'd

With a high rate of excretion of anions in urine:

1. Glue sniffing (hippuric acid overproduction)
2. Diabetic ketoacidosis with excessive ketonuria

NaHCO₃ LOSS

Direct loss of NaHCO₃:

1. Via the GI tract (e.g., diarrhea, ileus, fistula)
2. Via the urine (proximal renal tubular acidosis or low carbonic anhydrase II or IV activity)

Indirect loss of NaHCO₃ (low urinary NH4⁺ secretion):

1. Low glomerular filtration rate
2. Renal tubular acidosis

   A. Low availability of NH_3 (urine pH ~5) = problem in proximal convoluted tubule (PCT) ammoniagenesis: hyperkalemia, alkaline pH in PCT cells

   B. Defect in net distal H^+ secretion (urine pH often ~7):

H^+ ATPase defect or alkaline α-intercalated cells (a number of autoimmune disorders or disorders with hypergammaglobulinemia, e.g., Sjögren syndrome)

H^+ back-leak (e.g., amphotericin B)

HCO_3 secretion in the collecting ducts (e.g., a molecular defect in the Cl^-/HCO_3^- anion exchanger leading to its mistargeting to the luminal membrane of α-intercalated cells as in some patients with Southeast Asian ovalocytosis)

   C. Problem with both distal H^+ secretion and medullary NH_3 (urine pH ~6): Diseases involving the renal interstitial compartment (e.g., sickle cell disease).

If severe metabolic acidosis with acidemia developed rapidly, suspect that its basis is ingestion of acids, L-lactic acidosis from hypoxia or the ingestion of ethanol in a patient who is thiamin deficient), or explosive diarrhea (e.g., cholera). Metabolic acidosis from overproduction of acids can be detected by finding new anions in the plasma or in the urine (e.g., overproduction of hippuric acid in a patient who sniffs glue with excretion of hippurate anions in the urine). Calculate the plasma osmolal gap to detect the presence of alcohols.

14. **In a patient with hyperchloremic metabolic acidosis (HCMA), is the rate of excretion of NH₄⁺ low enough to be the sole cause of the disorder?**
The expected value for the urinary excretion of NH_4^+ is more than 200 mmol/day in a patient with chronic metabolic acidosis and normal kidney function. The urine osmolal gap ($U_{Osmolal\ gap}$) is the best indirect test to estimate the U_{NH4}, but it is only useful in patients with *chronic* metabolic acidosis. Because NH_4^+ is excreted with an anion, U_{NH4} is half the calculated value of $U_{Osmolal\ gap}$. The $U_{Osmolal\ gap}$ is calculated as shown in the following equations. The concentration of glucose in the urine ($U_{Glucose}$) should be added in patients with hyperglycemia.

$$U_{Osmolal\ gap} = \text{Measured } U_{Osm} - \text{Calculated } U_{Osm}$$

$$\text{Calculated } U_{Osm} = 2\ (U_{Na} + U_K) + U_{Urea} \text{ all in mmol/L}$$

To convert U_{NH4} into an excretion rate, divide it by the concentration of creatinine in the urine ($U_{Creatinine}$). If the ratio of $U_{NH4}/U_{Creatinine}$ is considerably <40 mmol/g creatinine (or <4, in

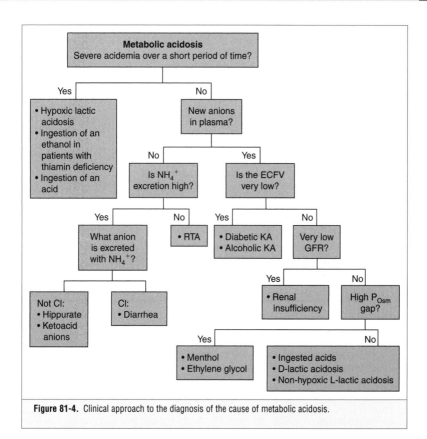

Figure 81-4. Clinical approach to the diagnosis of the cause of metabolic acidosis.

mmol/mmol terms), a low rate of excretion of NH_4^+ is likely to be an important cause of the acidemia. A low rate of excretion of NH_4^+ is the hallmark of a group of diseases called renal tubular acidosis (RTA).

15. **In a patient with HCMA and a high rate of excretion of NH_4^+, what anion accompanied NH_4^+ in the urine?**
In a patient with HCMA and a high rate of excretion of NH_4^+, if the urine anion is Cl^-, the cause of the HCMA is usually loss of $NaHCO_3$ via the GI tract (diarrhoea). In contrast, if the anion is not Cl^-, suspect that the cause of metabolic acidosis is overproduction of an organic acid, the anion of which is excreted in the urine at a very rapid rate (e.g., secreted hippuric acid in the patient with glue sniffing). The presence of a high rate of excretion of organic anions or HCO_3^- (very high urine pH) in the urine can be detected with the calculation of the urine anion gap ($U_{Na} + U_K + U_{NH4} - U_{Cl}$, all in mEq/L terms).

16. **In a patient with HCMA and a low rate of excretion of NH_4^+, what is the basis for a low NH_4^+ excretion rate (Fig. 81-5)?**
The urine pH is most valuable to identify the pathophysiology of the low rate of excretion of NH_4^+. If the urine pH >6.5, the low rate of excretion of NH_4^+ is likely the result of a reduced net rate of distal H^+ secretion. In contrast, if the urine pH ~5, the low rate of excretion of NH_4^+ is usually the result of a disease leading to a diminished production of NH_4^+ in the PCT. However, if urine pH is ~6, there will be a defect that lowers the availability of both H^+ and NH_3 in the lumen of the medullary collecting duct.

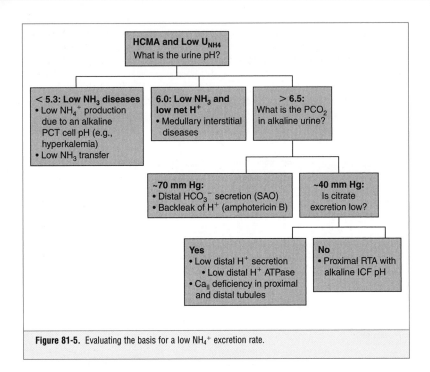

Figure 81-5. Evaluating the basis for a low NH_4^+ excretion rate.

17. **In a patient with HCMA and a low rate of excretion of NH_4^+, is there a defect in H^+ secretion in the proximal tubule?**

A fractional excretion of HCO_3^- that is >15% of it filtered load after giving an $NaHCO_3$ load that increases the P_{HCO3} to ~24 mmol/L indicates a defect in H^+ secretion in the proximal convoluted tubule. This test, however, should not be performed in a patient with hypokalemia until the P_K has been raised to the normal range because of the risk of worsening hypokalemia and inducing a cardiac arrhythmia.

A high rate of excretion of citrate in these patients suggests that there is an alkaline proximal convoluted tubule cell pH as an isolated defect or as a component of a generalized proximal convoluted tubule cell dysfunction (i.e., the Fanconi syndrome).

18. **What is the basis of HCMA in a patient with a low rate of excretion of NH_4^+ and a urine pH >6.5?**

If the urine pH is >6.5, the low rate of excretion of NH_4^+ is a result of a reduced net rate of distal H^+ secretion. To determine the basis of this lesion, measure the PCO_2 in alkaline urine (see Fig. 81-5). Patients with H^+ pump defect (a congenital or an acquired defect resulting from a number of autoimmune or disorders with hypergammaglobulinemia, e.g., Sjögren syndrome) have a PCO_2 in alkaline urine that is close to its value in their arterial blood. In contrast, the PCO_2 in alkaline urine is high in patients with disorders in which HCO_3^- are secreted in the distal nephron (some patients with Southeast Asian ovalocytosis) or if H^+ back-diffuse in the distal nephron (e.g., from drugs such as amphotericin B). A high rate of excretion of citrate in patients with this type of disorder indicates that the underlying lesion also involves the proximal tubule cells (e.g., carbonic anhydrase II deficiency) and/or if acidemia is not present.

19. **How should you correct for the $P_{Anion\ gap}$ for an abnormal $P_{Albumin}$?**

Two pitfalls are related to the $P_{Albumin}$ in the calculation of the $P_{Anion\ gap}$ to detect the addition of new acids by the finding of new anions in plasma. First, in some clinical situations, the $P_{Albumin}$

can be very low (e.g., in patients with cirrhosis of the liver or nephrotic syndrome), whereas in others, the $P_{Albumin}$ can be very high (e.g., a patient with severe diarrhea and a very contracted ECF volume; see the next section of this chapter for more detail). Hence the baseline value for the $P_{Anion\ gap}$ must be adjusted for the $P_{Albumin}$. A rough guide for correcting the baseline value of $P_{Anion\ gap}$ for $P_{Albumin}$ is that at $P_{Albumin}$ of 4.0 g/dL (40 g/L), the $P_{Anion\ gap}$ including the P_K is 16 mEq/L; hence for every 1.0 g/dL (10 g/L) decrease in $P_{Albumin}$, the $P_{Anion\ gap}$ will be lower by ~4 mEq/L. The converse is true for a rise in the $P_{Albumin}$.

20. **Is there a reproducible quantitative relationship between the fall in P_{HCO3} and the rise in the $P_{Anion\ gap}$ in all patients with metabolic acidosis?**

The relationship between the rise in the $P_{Anion\ gap}$ and the fall in the P_{HCO3} is used to detect the presence of coexisting metabolic alkalosis in a patient with metabolic acidosis (i.e., the rise in $P_{Anion\ gap}$ is larger than the fall in P_{HCO3}) and/or the presence of both an acid over-production type and a $NaHCO_3$ loss type of metabolic acidosis (i.e., the rise in $P_{Anion\ gap}$ is smaller than the fall in P_{HCO3}). It must be recognized, however, that this relationship uses *concentration* rather than in *content* terms and therefore will underestimate the magnitude of the HCO_3^- deficit if an appreciable degree of contraction of the ECF volume is present.

For example, a 50-kg patient with diabetic ketoacidosis has a P_{HCO3} of 10 mmol/L and the "expected" 1:1 relationship between the rise in $P_{Anion\ gap}$ and the fall in the P_{HCO3}. Let's assume that this patient had a normal ECF volume of 10 L before DKA developed, but as a result of the glucose-induced osmotic diuresis, his current ECF volume is 8 L. Now, examine Table 81-4, when the fall in the P_{HCO3} and the rise in the concentration of ketoacid anions were equal, to see if indeed the deficit of HCO_3^- is quantitatively equal to the amount of ketoacid anions present in the ECF compartment. In fact, the deficit of HCO_3^- is 170 mmol, but the quantity of new anions in the ECF is only 120 mEq. This discrepancy is only revealed when the contents of HCO_3^- and of the new anions in his ECF volume are calculated. There was another component of the indirect loss of HCO_3^- when ketoacids were added; some of the ketoacid anions were excreted in the urine with Na^+; an indirect form of $NaHCO_3$ loss. This loss of HCO_3^- is not reflected by an increase in $P_{Anion\ gap}$. Hence the rise in $P_{Anion\ gap}$ did not reveal the actual quantity of ketoacids that were added and the fall in P_{HCO3} did not reflect the actual magnitude of the deficit of HCO_3^-. With re-expansion of the ECF volume with the administration of saline, the degree of deficit of HCO_3^- will be become evident because the fall in the $P_{Anion\ gap}$ will not be matched by a rise in the P_{HCO3}. In addition, more ketoacids anions will be lost in urine, as their filtered load is increased with the increase in glomerular filtration rate (GFR) as a result of re-expansion of effective arterial blood volume.

TABLE 81-4. CHANGES IN THE CONTENT OF HCO_3^- AND NEW ANIONS IN THE ECF COMPARTMENT

Condition	ECF Volume	HCO₃⁻ Concentration (mmol/L)	HCO₃⁻ Content (mmol)	KA⁻ Concentration (mmol/L)	KA⁻ Content (mmol)
Normal	10 L	25	250	0	0
DKA	8 L	10	80	15	120
Balance	**−2 L**	—	**170**	—	**−120**

ECF = extracellular fluid; KA⁻, ketoacid anions; DKA = diabetic ketoacidosis.
In these calculations, we ignored changes in the $P_{Albumin}$ for simplicity.

21. **Does the strong ion difference provide an improved way to determine the cause of an acid–base disorder?**

The calculation of the strong ion difference and the $P_{Anion\ gap}$ are used by clinicians to detect the addition of new acids in a patient with metabolic acidosis. Although the strong ion difference is popular with some specialists, the authors do not use it. The advantage of the strong ion difference approach is that its calculation takes into account the net negative charge on $P_{Albumin}$. The calculation of the strong ion difference is complex; this advantage over the calculation of the $P_{Anion\ gap}$ is easily negated if one were to adjust the baseline value of the $P_{Anion\ gap}$ for the $P_{Albumin}$ routinely. Of note, both the strong ion difference and the $P_{Anion\ gap}$ approaches rely on the concentration of HCO_3^- and ignore the content of HCO_3^- in the ECF compartment. Furthermore, as pointed out earlier, an important initial step in the clinical approach in patient with metabolic acidosis is to determine if the BBS in skeletal muscle is functioning effectively to remove the bulk of the added new H^+ and minimize the rise in the concentration of H^+ and thereby the binding of H^+ to intracellular proteins in vital organs such as the brain and the heart; this information can be only obtained by measuring the brachial or the femoral venous PCO_2. This is, however, not part of the usual clinical approach whether clinicians use the strong anion difference or the $P_{Anion\ gap}$, because both approaches rely *solely* on the arterial PCO_2 to assess buffering of H^+ by the bicarbonate buffer system.

SPECIFIC DISORDERS

22. **Discuss diarrhea as a cause of metabolic acidosis.**

Although the case example we use to reveal the "secrets" in the diagnosis and management of patients with this disorder is a patient with cholera, these principles should apply to any other patients with severe diarrhea illness from other causes.

Case: A male, age 25, was healthy prior to developing massive diarrhea 24 hours ago (stool volume was estimated ~5 L) after he drank contaminated water. His blood pressure was 90/60 mm Hg, pulse rate was 110 beats/minutes, and his jugular venous pressure was low. He had no urine output since he arrived in the hospital. Acid–base measurements in arterial blood revealed a pH 7.39, P_{HCO3} 24 mmol/L, and a PCO_2 39 mm Hg; his $P_{Anion\ gap}$ was 24 mEq/L, his hematocrit was 0.60, and his $P_{Albumin}$ was 8.0 g/dL (80 g/L). The concentration of HCO_3^- in diarrhea fluid was 40 mmol/L.

23. **Does this patient have a severe degree of metabolic acidosis?**

There are several ways to decide if metabolic acidosis is present, but not all of them will yield the correct answer for the right reasons.

Laboratory data: If one uses a definition of metabolic acidosis that relies *solely* on concentration terms (pH 7.39, P_{HCO3} 24 mmol/L, and arterial PCO_2 39 mm Hg), the answer would be no. However, because the $P_{Anion\ gap}$ was 24 mEq/L, one might conclude that this patient may have two simultaneous acid–base disorders: metabolic acidosis from added acids and metabolic alkalosis from the very low ECF volume that caused the P_{HCO3} not to fall.

Clinical findings: This patient lost 5 L of diarrhea fluid that each contained 40 mmol of $NaHCO_3$, which means that he lost 200 mmol of HCO_3^- (5 L × 40 mmol/L). Hence he does have a process that led to a serious degree of metabolic acidosis. Moreover, there was no evidence of a gain of HCO_3^- because he did not ingest $NaHCO_3$, there was no history of significant vomiting, and there was no addition of new HCO_3^- by the kidneys because there was little excretion of NH_4^+ (he had little if any urine output). Because the P_{HCO3} reflects the quantity of HCO_3^- in the ECF compartment divided by the ECF volume (see equation in question 2), we need to determine whether there was an *occult* source of HCO_3^- and/or a very large decrease in the ECF volume.

Correlating the clinical and laboratory information: To confirm that there is a deficit of HCO_3^-, its *content* in the ECF compartment must be calculated. The hematocrit of 0.60 provides a quantitative, minimum estimate that his plasma volume was reduced from 3.0 L to ~1.3 L (i.e., >50%). There was probably a greater reduction in his ECF volume (10 L to 4 L) because his $P_{Albumin}$ was 8.0 g/dL (80 g/L and hence there was a greater oncotic pressure to draw interstitial fluid into the intravascular subcompartment of the ECF volume). Therefore it is safe to conclude that he has metabolic acidosis with a large deficit of HCO_3^- in his ECF compartment (24 mmol/L $\times$ 4 L = 96 mmol versus the usual 240 mmol [24 mmol/L $\times$ 10 L]).

24. **What is the basis for the high $P_{Anion\ gap}$?**
One must distinguish between a process leading to a deficit of HCO_3^- (as suggested from history and the measured $NaHCO_3$ loss in diarrhea fluid) and a process that caused the addition of acids (as suggested by the rise in $P_{Anion\ gap}$) because of different implications for therapy. The high $P_{Anion\ gap}$ resulted mainly from a very high $P_{Albumin}$ (because of the profoundly contracted ECF volume) rather than the addition of new acids. This was confirmed because the concentrations of lactate and ketoacid anions in plasma were less than 2 mmol/L.

25. **What dangers should be anticipated when this patient is given a large infusion of isotonic saline?**
   - **A very severe degree of acidemia:** There will be a fall in the P_{HCO3} when a large volume of saline without $NaHCO_3$ is given to a patient who has a very severe degree of ECF volume contraction because this infused solution will lower the P_{HCO3} by dilution. In fact, it is reported that when saline was infused very rapidly, some of these patients with metabolic acidosis owing to $NaHCO_3$ loss from diarrhea and a severe degree of contraction of the effective arterial blood volume developed pulmonary edema before the ECF volume was totally re-expanded. This may be the result of the severe degree of acidemia they developed, which led to the redistribution of blood from the peripheral to the central circulating blood volume. It is important to recognize this complication because pulmonary edema can be prevented and/or treated successfully with an infusion of fluid that contains $NaHCO_3$ (or an anion that can be metabolized quickly to produce HCO_3^-, e.g., citrate or L-lactate). In addition to dilution, two other mechanisms may lead to a more severe degree of acidemia with the infusion of a large amount of saline in these patients.
     - **Loss of more $NaHCO_3$ in diarrhea fluid:** Re-expansion of the "effective" arterial blood volume will increase splanchnic blood flow. This will permit a much larger volume of Na^+ and Cl^- to be secreted in the small intestine. When a large volume of luminal fluid containing Na^+ and Cl^- reaches the colon, more Cl^- will be reabsorbed in exchange for HCO_3^- as compared to the reabsorption of Na^+ in exchange for secreted H^+; hence the loss of $NaHCO_3$ in diarrhea fluid might rise markedly.
     - **Back titration of HCO_3^- by H^+ that were bound to intracellular proteins in muscle:** Because almost the same amount of CO_2 will be produced if the same amount of O_2 is consumed, less CO_2 will be added to each liter of blood. Hence the tissue PCO_2 and the venous PCO_2 will decline. As a result of the decline in PCO_2, the concentration of H^+ in cells will fall, and fewer H^+ will be bound to proteins in cells (see Fig. 81-1, equations 2 and 3). Many of these H^+ that are released will combine with HCO_3^- in the ICF and ECF compartments of muscle and hence the concentration of HCO_3^- in the ECF compartment will decline (see Fig. 82-2).
   - **Hypokalemia:** Despite an important degree of K^+ depletion from loss of K^+ in diarrhea fluid, hypokalemia was not present on admission in this patient presumably because K^+ had shifted out of cells. The mechanism for this K^+ shift was probably a deficiency of insulin, which was the result of inhibition of its release by the α-adrenergic surge in response to the very contracted effective arterial blood (ECF) volume. Hence one should expect a significant drop in the P_K with re-expansion of the ECF volume because this will lead to a fall in circulating α-adrenergic hormone levels and a rise in plasma insulin levels. One should also be aware that the degree of hypokalemia may become more severe with the infusion of $NaHCO_3$, and more aggressive therapy with KCl will likely be needed. If a severe degree of K^+ depletion with hypokalemia develops, bowel motility may diminish to a degree such that intestinal secretions are pooled in the gut and diarrhea is no longer observed.

26. **Does this patient have respiratory acidosis?**

Because the pH and PCO_2 in arterial blood were in the normal range, he does not have a ventilation form of respiratory acidosis. His brachial venous PCO_2, however, was much higher than the usual value of $\sim$6 mm Hg higher than the arterial PCO_2. This is because the blood flow rate to muscle was very low as a result of the significant degree of effective circulating blood volume contraction. Hence more O_2 was extracted from each liter of blood and almost an identical amount of CO_2 was added to capillary blood, raising the muscle venous PCO_2. The higher concentration of CO_2 in interstitial space and in cells of muscles makes the bicarbonate buffer system ineffective in removing the H^+ load (i.e., what we call a tissue form of respiratory acidosis).

27. **Discuss renal tubular acidosis as a cause of metabolic acidosis.**

There are two types of RTA: proximal RTA (type II) and distal RTA (type I). Although both types have a low rate of excretion of NH_4^+, in proximal RTA there is also decreased capacity for the reabsorption of HCO_3^- in the proximal convoluted tubule. The diagnostic category of type III RTA was never clearly defined and did not stand the test of time. Although some authorities use the term type IV RTA to describe the constellation of findings of hyperkalemia and metabolic acidosis resulting from a low rate of excretion of NH_4^+, there are two ways that hyperkalemia and a low rate of excretion of NH_4^+ may coexist. In one, hyperkalemia is responsible for the low rate of excretion of NH_4^+ because hyperkalemia is associated with an alkaline proximal convoluted tubular cell pH, which leads to inhibition of ammoniagenesis. In these patients, if the plasma K^+ is returned to normal, the metabolic acidosis should be corrected. However, in a second subset of patients, hyperkalemia is not the major reason for the low rate of excretion of NH_4^+; rather these patients have medullary interstitial disease causing the low rate of excretion of NH_4^+, which also involves the cortical distal nephron leading to hyperkalemia.

Proximal RTA may present as an isolated defect in reabsorption of HCO_3^- in the proximal convoluted tubule or as a component of a generalized proximal tubule cell dysfunction; Fanconi syndrome, in which in addition to the loss of HCO_3^- in the urine these patients will have glucosuria; aminoaciduria; and increased excretion of urate, phosphate, and citrate. The most common cause of Fanconi syndrome in the pediatric population is cystinosis, whereas common causes in adult population are paraproteinemias and autoimmune disorders. The steps in the clinical approach and differential diagnosis in patients with RTA were outlined in Figure 81-5.

In patients with proximal RTA, treatment with $NaHCO_3$ does not maintain the P_{HCO3} near the normal range because bicarbonaturia ensues as the distal capacity for the reabsorption of HCO_3^- is exceeded. Do not be aggressive with the administration of $NaHCO_3$ because bicarbonaturia may lead to the development of hypokalemia and the alkaline urine pH may increase the risk of formation of calcium phosphate stones. Conversely, $NaHCO_3$ seems to be beneficial in patients with proximal RTA and growth retardation.

In patients with distal RTA from a defect in net distal H^+ secretion, the major threat to the patient on presentation is usually cardiac arrhythmia resulting from hypokalemia. Hypokalemia may also cause respiratory muscle weakness and thus severe acidemia from superimposed respiratory acidosis. $NaHCO_3$ should not be given until enough K^+ is given to raise plasma K^+ to a safe level ($\sim$3 mmol/L). After the P_{HCO3} is corrected, the dose of $NaHCO_3$ needed to maintain P_{HCO3} in the normal range is usually less than 30 to 40 mmol/day (i.e., enough to titrate the acid load produced from the metabolism of sulfur-containing amino acids).

In a subset of patients with hyperkalemia and RTA, correction of hyperkalemia is sufficient to raise the rate of excretion of NH_4^+ and correct the acidosis. In another subset, however, the administration of $NaHCO_3$ as listed previously is needed because hyperkalemia is not the cause of the metabolic acidosis.

28. **Discuss starvation ketoacidosis as a cause of metabolic acidosis.**

The major imperative in this setting is to provide the brain with fuel to oxidize the regeneration of the adenosine triphosphate (ATP) consumed when work is performed in this organ. Its major fuels are glucose in the fed state and ketoacid anions during starvation.

Regulation: When the $P_{Glucose}$ is low, insulin levels in plasma ($P_{Insulin}$) decline because the major stimulus to release insulin from β cells of the pancreas is a high $P_{Glucose}$.

The second major site of regulation is in the liver. When the $P_{Glucose}$ is low, more adrenaline is released, which augments lipolysis in adipose tissue and promotes hepatic ketogenesis by inhibiting acetyl-coenzyme A (CoA) carboxylase, the key enzyme in the conversion of acetyl-CoA to fatty acids. As the concentration of acetyl-CoA rises in hepatocytes, this drives the synthesis of ketoacids.

The degree of acidemia is usually modest (P_{HCO3} ~19 mmol/L with a normal ECF volume so there is a very modest decrease in the content of HCO_3^- in the ECF compartment), although the rate of production of ketoacids may be as high as in a patient with diabetic ketoacidosis. This is because there is a relatively rapid rate of removal of ketoacids in the brain (the $P_{Glucose}$ is low, which permits a higher rate of ketoacid oxidation in the brain) and in the kidneys (GFR is not low so the kidneys will oxidize more fuel [ketoacid anions] to provide the ATP needed to reabsorb the filtered Na^+).

Treatment of starvation ketoacidosis is simply the provision of glucose.

29. **Discuss alcoholic ketoacidosis as a cause of metabolic acidosis.**

The biochemical features of ketoacid formation from ethanol are very similar to those of the physiologic process of ketoacid formation during prolonged fasting; the substrate for acetyl-CoA, however, may be ethanol rather than free fatty acids. As during starvation, for ketoacid production to proceed at a rapid rate, conversion of acetyl-CoA to fatty acids must be inhibited. The adrenergic surge in this setting (perhaps from the acute gastritis and vomiting) leads to inhibition of acetyl-CoA carboxylase, the key enzyme in the conversion of acetyl-CoA to fatty acids.

There is an important difference, however, between ketoacid formation from fatty acids or ethanol as its major substrate. There is a lag period before ketoacids are produced at a rapid rate when long-chain fatty acids are the substrate for ketogenesis but not when ethanol is the substrate; this leads to "rapid ketosis." Another important difference is that the rate of ketoacid removal in brain (sedative effect of alcohol decreases brain oxygen consumption) and the kidneys (low effective arterial blood volume leads to a low GFR and low filtered load of Na^+ and hence less renal work) is diminished in patients with alcoholic ketoacidosis. Nevertheless, the degree of acidemia may not be severe because of the presence of metabolic alkalosis (from vomiting) and/or respiratory alkalosis (hyperventilation from aspiration pneumonia or alcohol withdrawal).

Another aspect of ethanol metabolism in the liver merits emphasis. When ethanol is oxidized in the liver, there is a rise in $NADH:NAD^+$ ratio in hepatocytes. This leads to the conversion of pyruvate to lactate because these two metabolic intermediates can be interconverted by an NAD^+ like dehydrogenase with a very large catalytic capacity. This reduces the rate of formation of glucose from pyruvate and leads to hypoglycemia in the malnourished alcoholic. This high $NADH:NAD^+$ ratio also leads to conversion of acetoacetic acid to β-hydroxybutyric acid, which becomes the major form of ketoacids released from the liver. This leads to less formation of acetone, and hence its odor may not be detected in exhaled air at the bedside. Furthermore, the nitroprusside test, result which is used as a quick assay for ketones, may be falsely negative because it detects acetone and acetoacetate but not β-hydroxybutyrate.

Patients with alcoholic ketoacidosis can be classified into two groups with regard to their clinical presentation. The first group consists of normal subjects who consumed a large amount of ethanol, and the second group consists primarily of chronic alcoholics who had a binge intake of ethanol. The $P_{Glucose}$ on admission may help identify each group because patients in the latter group who are malnourished will usually have hypoglycemia. This point is emphasized because these patients are likely to have other nutritional deficiencies (e.g., thiamine deficiency). It is critical that thiamine (and probably riboflavin) be administered early in therapy in these patients; this will permit aerobic oxidation of glucose in the brain once ketoacids disappear and prevent the development of Wernicke's encephalopathy. These patients are likely also to be K^+ depleted (especially if there is a prolonged history of vomiting) despite normokalemia and perhaps hyperkalemia on presentation because the α-adrenergic surge inhibits the release of insulin and causes K^+ to shift out of cells. Once the effective arterial blood volume is expanded, the α-adrenergic surge disappears, insulin is released, and K^+ move back into cells. Do not wait for hypokalemia to develop before administering KCl.

No specific therapy is needed for ketoacidosis because excessive production of ketoacids ceases once the alcohol disappears. Furthermore, utilization of ketoacids by the brain (as ethanol level falls) and the kidney (as GFR improves) increases. Therapy with $NaHCO_3$ is not needed in most cases (and may be dangerous if the patient is K^+ depleted).

30. **Discuss diabetic ketoacidosis as a cause of metabolic acidosis.**
    Although there are many aspects in diagnosis and management of patients with DKA that are worthy of discussion, the secret to emphasize is how to minimize the risk of development of cerebral edema (CE). CE occurs in very young patients and is responsible for mortality or significant morbidity in ~1 of 150 children treated for DKA even in the best pediatric medical centers. CE occurs more commonly during the first episode of DKA, which is often more severe, possibly because of the long delay in making the diagnosis. CE usually becomes evident, with little warning, 5 to 15 hours after therapy is instituted.

    This is a clinical diagnosis—it should be suspected if a headache or vomiting develops, if there is unexpected deterioration in neurologic status, or if there is an unexpected rise in blood pressure and a fall in heart rate. Therefore these patients should be admitted to a unit where they can be observed closely because therapy must be instituted without delay to minimize the risk of permanent brain damage.

    Because a gain of water in the skull leads to a rise in intracranial pressure, and because the intracellular volume is the largest intracranial compartment, measures must be taken to prevent cell swelling. Said another way, one must prevent a fall in the effective osmolality in plasma ($P_{Effective\ osm}$). Because the most common cause for a large fall in the $P_{Effective\ osm}$ is the large decrease in the $P_{Glucose}$ early during therapy, the P_{Na} must rise by one half of the fall in the $P_{Glucose}$ to prevent a fall in the $P_{Effective\ osm}$) (Fig. 81-6).

    Our secret is with concern to an "occult" factor that may contribute to the development of this complication. Although stomach emptying is usually slow in the patient with a high $P_{Glucose}$, it is a source of an infusion of water with or without glucose but with few electrolytes. Although this is more likely to occur once the $P_{Glucose}$ has decreased, it may also occur at other times.

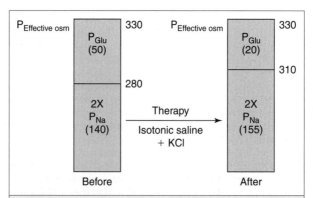

Figure 81-6. Defense of the effective osmolality of plasma. A rise in the P_{Na} is needed to prevent a fall in the $P_{Effective\ Osm}$ when there is a fall in the $P_{Glucose}$. If the P_{Na} on admission is close to 140 mmol/L, the P_{Na} should rise to 155 mmol/L when the $P_{Glucose}$ falls from 50 mmol/L (900 mg/dL) to 20 mmol/L (360 mg/dL) to maintain a constant $P_{Effective\ Osm}$.

31. **What are the clues to suggest that there was an occult stomach emptying?**
     When subjects drink a beverage that contains sugar to quench their thirst, some of this glucose (and water) will remain in the stomach because hyperglycemia slows stomach emptying. This will represent a gain of water after this fluid is absorbed and its glucose is removed by metabolic means. The following observations, however, are clues that stomach emptying and absorption of a sugar-containing solution occurred in a patient with hyperglycemia. However, a fall in $P_{Effective\ osm}$ may suggest that stomach emptying and absorption of water has occurred.
     - A rise in $P_{Glucose}$ in the absence of an infusion of solutions containing glucose or a precursor of glucose, such as L-lactate
     - A sudden large rise in the urine output as a result of a glucose-induced osmotic diuresis
     - Absence of a sufficient fall in $P_{Glucose}$ despite the excretion of glucose in the urine

32. **What therapy should be given if cerebral edema is suspected?**
     Because there is such a high mortality and morbidity rate once CE develops as a result of brain herniation, one must draw water out of the skull. This means that the patient must be given a rapid intravenous infusion of hypertonic saline, using the clinical response as the guide to further therapy. Do not send the patient for imaging studies because the cerebral edema can worsen very quickly. Be aware because the stomach may contain fluid that will become hypotonic after it is absorbed and the glucose is removed by metabolic means.

33. **Discuss toxin-induced metabolic acidosis.**
     Ingestion of methanol propanediol or ethylene glycol should be suspected in a patient with metabolic acidosis, an elevated $P_{Anion\ gap}$, and no obvious cause for these findings, especially if the ECF volume is not significantly contracted. Failure to make this diagnosis can be devastating. If ingestion of these alcohols is suspected, one must calculate the $P_{Osmolal\ gap}$. If this value is considerably greater than 20 mOsm/kg H_2O, and because it is the products of the metabolism of these toxic alcohols that create the danger rather than the parent compounds, administer ethanol to prevent their metabolism until the facts become clear by direct measurements of the level of these alcohols in plasma.

     Fomepizole, an inhibitor of alcohol dehydrogenase, has been used in treatment of patients with methanol or ethylene glycol poisoning instead of the administration of ethanol. Although fomepizole is easy to dose and administer and side effects are rare, its main disadvantage is its high cost.

     The principal use of isopropanol is as a topical antiseptic; it is the major constituent of rubbing alcohol. This 3-carbon alcohol is with the $\beta-OH$ group on the middle carbon. When oxidized by hepatic NAD^+-linked alcohol dehydrogenase, the alcohol group is converted to a keto group forming acetone:

     $$Isopropyl\ alcohol + NAD^+ \rightarrow Acetone + NADH + H^+$$

     Thus there is no accumulation of H^+ in this metabolic process. The acetone is volatile and has a characteristic fruity odor; it reacts with the Ketostix reagent yielding a positive test for ketones, which in the absence of metabolic acidosis, a high value for the plasma osmolal gap should lead the clinicians to the correct diagnosis.

     No toxic effects can be attributed to acetone. Patients should be managed in a similar fashion to patients with ethanol overdose. Endotracheal intubation should be considered to avoid aspiration pneumonia if there is concern about the patient's ability to protect the airway. Hemodialysis is rarely indicated except in patients with massive ingestion who are hemodynamically unstable despite aggressive supportive measures.

     Propane 1,2-diol (propylene glycol) is commonly used as a diluent for many intravenous drug preparations (e.g., lorazepam, which may be used in large doses as a sedative in the Intensive Care Unit and to treat delirium tremens). It is also used as solvents for other drugs like cough medicine and at times without proper labeling. When given in large quantities, this alcohol can be detected by finding a large $P_{Osmolal\ gap}$. The danger associated with its use is that one of its metabolites is an aldehyde, which is in general very toxic.

34. **What type of metabolic acidosis develops in patients who receive propane 1,2-diol?**
Propane 1,2-diol is a 50:50 mixture of D and L isoforms. Approximately 40% of the administered dose is excreted unchanged in the urine, whereas 60% is metabolized in the liver by alcohol dehydrogenase to lactaldehyde. L-lactaldehyde is then metabolized by aldehyde dehydrogenase to L-lactic acid (Fig. 81-7). D-lactaldehyde, however, is not a good substrate for aldehyde dehydrogenase. Therefore, it accumulates and leads to many of the toxic effects observed in this setting. D-lactaldehyde can be metabolized in the liver via an alternate pathway that uses reduced glutathione (GSH) as a cofactor to D-lactic acid. Because D-lactic acid is metabolized much slower than L-lactic acid, the acid that accumulates is principally D-lactic acid. The most important step in therapy is to stop the formation of D-lactaldehyde by giving ethanol or fomepizole. This must be followed up by removal of propane 1,2-diol by hemodialysis.

35. **A large muscular man with a long history of alcohol abuse was perfectly well until he drank a solution containing an unknown substance ~6 hours ago. In the past hour, he began to feel very unwell. He denied blood loss, excessive sweating, vomiting, or appreciable diarrhea. His clinical condition deteriorated very quickly. On admission to hospital, his blood pressure was 80/50 mm Hg, pulse rate was 150 beats/minute, jugular venous pressure was very low, and respirations were rapid and deep. His electrocardiogram revealed changes resulting from hyperkalemia. Laboratory data are provided in Table 81-5. Shortly after he was given intravenous calcium gluconate for the emergency**

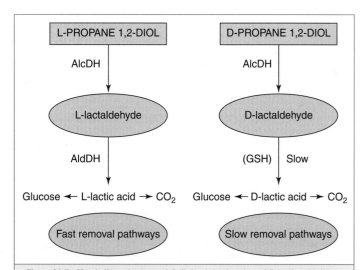

Figure 81-7. Metabolism of propane 1,2-diol to L-lactic acid and D-lactic acid. When a large quantity of propane 1,2-diol is ingested, the body is presented with a racemic mixture. Both the L-form *(shown to the left of the vertical dashed line)* and the D-form *(shown to the right of the vertical dashed line)* are substrates for alcohol dehydrogenase (AlcDH); hence their metabolism occurs in the liver. The products are L-lactaldehyde and D-lactaldehyde, which are substrates for aldehyde dehydrogenase (AldDH), but the D-form is a much poorer substrate and the D-lactaldehyde accumulates and is responsible for most of the toxicity. The cofactors, NAD^+ and NADH, are not shown for simplicity.

TABLE 81–5. LABORATORY DATA

pH = 7.20 (64 [H^+] nmol/L)	**Na^+** = 143 mmol/L
PCO_2 (arterial) = 25 mm Hg	**K^+** = 6.3 mmol/L
HCO_3^- = 11 mmol/L	**Cl^-** = 99 mmol/L
Glucose = 180 mg/dL (10 mmol/L)	**Albumin** = 4.5 g/dL (45 g/L)
Creatinine = 1.8 mg/dL (160 μmol/L)	**Blood urea nitrogen (urea)** = 8.4 mg/dL
Calcium (total) = 10 mg/dL (2.5 mmol/L)	(3.0 mmol/L)
	L-lactate = 2.0 mmol/L

treatment of hyperkalemia, his blood pressure rose and he felt much better. Judging from the time frame, which acid accumulated?

In this type of metabolic acidosis the conjugate base of the acid is a greater threat to survival than the newly added H^+. The "secret" in this context is that the anion or conjugate base of the acid may have important properties that dominate the clinical picture. The only acid that is made endogenously at a very rapid rate is L-lactic acid during hypoxia. The $P_{L\text{-lactate}}$ was not elevated in blood by a sufficient degree (only 2 mmol/L) for this diagnosis, so this is not the correct final diagnosis. Therefore the most likely etiology is that he ingested an acid. Now let us see if we can deduce which acid was ingested from the properties of its anion.

36. **Why did his blood pressure fall so precipitously?**
Blood pressure is a direct function of cardiac output and peripheral vascular resistance. Cardiac output is directly related to the heart rate and stroke volume. Because his heart rate was rapid, one should look for a process that could compromise his stroke volume and/or possibly lower his peripheral resistance. Because he did not have evidence of blood loss, sepsis, or a disorder that can cause salt deficiency (e.g., a history of vomiting, diarrhea), suspect that there is a problem with contractility of his heart and/or the vasoconstrictor tone of his blood vessels. One factor that is essential for contractility is ionized calcium. Therefore it is possible that the new anion might have removed ionized calcium. Because citrate chelates ionized calcium (e.g., this is why citrate is used to prevent coagulation of the blood), this patient may have ingested citric acid. As part of the emergency treatment of hyperkalemia, he was given a bolus of a calcium salt. This corrected the low concentration of ionized calcium in plasma, and hence his myocardial contractility increased, as did his peripheral vascular resistance. This was another piece of the puzzle that alerted his physicians to the possibility that this patient may have ingested citric acid. This was confirmed later when the composition of the ingested solution became known.

37. **Why did he have an elevated P_K?**
A less negative intracellular voltage will cause K^+ to shift out of cells (Fig. 81-8). One possible mechanism for this to occur in this patient who ingested citric acid is if the Cl^-/HCO_3^- anion exchanger in cell membrane of skeletal muscle was activated (probably by a fall in the concentration of HCO_3^- in the ECF compartment). Although this is an electroneutral pathway, it will result in a higher concentration of intracellular Cl^-; this and the negative voltage inside the cell will force Cl^- to exit cells through open Cl^- channels in cell membrane down their electrochemical gradient. This exit of Cl^- should diminish the degree of negative intracellular voltage so K^+ can exit from cells if K^+ channels are open.

38. **Under what circumstances will the ingestion of ethanol cause a serious degree of L-lactic acidosis?**
Fast production of L-lactic acid occurs when there is an inadequate delivery of oxygen to tissues to meet their demands for ATP regeneration. This usually occurs during vigorous muscle work (e.g., a sprint or a grand mal seizure) or when systemic hemodynamics is severely

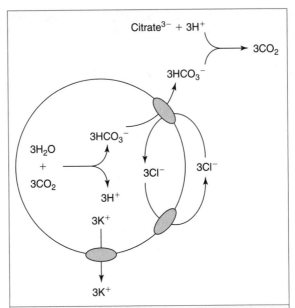

Figure 81-8. Shift of K^+ out of cells in patients with metabolic acidosis as a result of citric acid accumulation. The circle depicts the cell membrane. When there is a H^+ load with anions that cannot enter cells readily (e.g., citric acid), the fall in the P_{HCO3} leads to more flux through the HCO_3^-/Cl^- anion exchanger, which accelerates the electroneutral exit of HCO_3^- from, along with the entry of Cl^- into cells. The subsequent exit of Cl^- via Cl^- ion channels decreases the net negative intracellular voltage, leading to the exit of K^+ and HCO_3^- from cells, the former via K^+ ion channels.

compromised. Slower forms of L-lactic acidosis occur when the usual rate of L-lactic acid removal is diminished. A steady-state L-lactic acidosis will develop but requires that there is a high concentration of L-lactate in plasma ($P_{L-lactate}$). The major reason for this pathophysiology is a marked decrease in liver mass or a compromised metabolism of pyruvate resulting from lower activities of the major enzymes that catalyze pyruvate metabolism: pyruvate dehydrogenase (PDH) or pyruvate carboxylase. A diminished activity of PDH may be result from less amount of the enzyme, the absence of one of its essential cofactors (e.g., vitamin B_1 or thiamin), or the presence of inhibitors of PDH activity such as the products of oxidation of fat-derived fuels (e.g., high ATP or low ADP [adenosine diphosphate], high acetyl-CoA or low CoASH, or high NADH or low NAD^+). Similarly, low activity of pyruvate carboxylase or the availability of its cofactor, biotin, can lead to the need for higher levels of pyruvate (and hence L-lactate) in liver cells to permit the conversion of pyruvate to glucose or glycogen.

39. **What is the biomedical basis for very rapid rates of production of L-lactic acid?**
The secret to understand this pathophysiology is that there are two substrates for glycolysis (glucose and ADP). In addition, the availability of ADP controls the rate of conversion of glucose to pyruvate/L-lactate:

$$Work + ATP \rightarrow ADP + H^+$$

$$Glucose + ADP + NAD^+ \rightarrow Pyruvate + ATP + NADH$$

Hence fast L-lactic acid production depends on having high levels of ADP. This in turn is a result of performing more biological work or in settings where oxidative phosphorylation in mitochondria is compromised by low delivery of oxygen, by defects in the TCA (tricarboxylic acid, or citrate) cycle or the electron transport system, or by uncoupling of oxidative phosphorylation such that fuel and oxygen consumption are in fact increased but *less* ADP is converted to ATP during mitochondrial metabolism.

40. **What factor other than the concentration of pyruvate will increase the production of L-lactic acid?**
As shown in this equation, NADH is the other substrate for L-lactate dehydrogenase:

$$\text{Ethanol} + \text{NAD}^+ \rightarrow \text{Acetate} + \text{NADH}$$

Hence the combination of a high concentration of pyruvate and a high concentration of NADH will result in a very large accumulation of L-lactic acid:

$$\text{Pyruvate} + \text{NADH} \rightarrow \text{L-Lactate} + \text{NAD}^+$$

Therefore, when the only lesion is thiamin deficiency, this will only cause a small elevation in the $P_{L\text{-lactate}}$. Similarly, high rates of oxidation ethanol will result in a high concentration of NADH but only a modest rise in the rate of L-lactic acid production and $P_{L\text{-lactate}}$ of ~4 to 5 mmol/L. Notwithstanding, when a patient who is thiamin deficient consumes a large amount of ethanol, a very severe degree of L-lactic acidosis may develop.

Treatment with thiamin or a blocker of alcohol dehydrogenase (e.g., fomepizole) alone may not have a dramatic effect to ameliorate the severity of the L-lactic acidosis. In contrast, using both therapeutic options could result in the desired rapid correction of this acid–base disorder.

41. **What is the basis of chronic L-lactic acidosis in patients who are malnourished?**
   - **Thiamin deficiency:** Thiamin (vitamin B_1) deficiency is not uncommon in chronic alcoholics. Lack of this cofactor compromises the metabolic removal of pyruvate because it is a component of the active form of PDH. In this setting there is an accumulation of L-lactic acid. Of greater importance, because the oxidation of glucose via PDH must occur in the brain, these patients need therapy with thiamin at the outset to prevent the development of Wernicke-Korsakoff encephalopathy.
   - **Riboflavin deficiency:** Other patients may develop lactic acidosis if they are deficient in riboflavin (vitamin B_2), a necessary cofactor for the conversion of ADP to ATP in mitochondria. This is more likely if the patient is taking a tricyclic antidepressant drug, because this class of drugs prevents the formation of the active form of riboflavin. Large doses of riboflavin should be administered to have adequate levels of ATP in cells.

42. **Discuss metformin-induced L-lactic acidosis.**
Metformin is used in many patients with type 2 diabetes mellitus for glycemic control. Its major mode of action is to uncouple oxidative phosphorylation (it carries H^+ across the inner mitochondrial membrane, which decreases the rate of regeneration of ATP by mitochondria). Nevertheless, because it is not very soluble in lipids, it is a weak uncoupler and hence rarely (in the absence of an acute overdose) is the sole cause of lactic acidosis. However, its "grandfather" phenformin is a much stronger uncoupler because it is much more soluble in the lipid in the inner membranes of hepatic mitochondria and, as such it prevented the conversion of ADP + Pi to ATP when oxygen was consumed. Because ADP + Pi are the other substrates for glycolysis, there is much more L-lactic acid formed than can be removed by metabolic means:

$$\text{Work} + \text{ATP}^{4-} \rightarrow \text{ADP}^{3-} + \text{Pi}^{2-} + \text{H}^+$$

$$\text{Glucose} + \text{ADP}^{3-} + \text{Pi}^{2-} + \text{H}^+ \rightarrow 2\ \text{L-lactate}$$

$$\text{L-lactate} + \text{O}_2 + \text{NADH} \rightarrow \text{NAD}^+$$

The current recommendation is not to use metformin in patients with renal insufficiency with a serum creatinine of 1.4 mg/dL (124 umol/L) in women or 1.5 mg dL (132 umol/L) in men. Data suggest that this recommendation is widely disregarded by physicians. The fact that the incidence of lactic acidosis remains extremely low calls for re-evaluation of these recommendations.

43. **Discuss D-lactic acidosis.**

Bacteria are normally segregated from dietary sugar by GI "geography"; they are primarily in the colon and glucose is absorbed in the jejunum. Disruption of this geographic separation of bacteria and glucose is the major factor in the development of D-lactic acidosis. Altered bacterial flora (e.g., from antibiotic therapy) may migrate up to and proliferate in the small intestine. Certain sugars (e.g., fructose) that are poorly absorbed in the small intestine may be delivered to the colon when their intake is high. Decreased bowel motility (e.g., blind loops, drugs) increases the contact time for bacteria and sugar and, as a result, more organic acids may be produced. In addition, antacids or drugs that inhibit gastric H^+ secretion may lead to a higher pH that is more favorable for bacterial growth and metabolism.

Organic acids, noxious alcohols, aldehydes, amines, and mercaptans produced during fermentation may lead to many of the central nervous system symptoms that are observed in this disorder.

Humans metabolize D-lactate more slowly than L-lactate. D-lactate may also be excreted in the urine, and hence the rise in the $P_{Anion\ gap}$ may be lower than expected as judged from the fall in P_{HCO3}.

The usual laboratory test for "lactate" detects L-lactate but not D-lactate. Hence a specific assay for D-lactate must be performed to confirm the diagnosis.

Treatment should be directed at the gastrointestinal (GI) problem. The oral intake of fructose and complex carbohydrates should be decreased. Antacids should be avoided and drugs that diminish GI motility should be stopped. Poorly absorbed antibiotics (e.g., vancomycin) could be used to change the bacterial flora. Insulin may be helpful by lowering the rate of oxidation of fatty acids and hence permitting a higher rate of oxidation of organic acids.

44. **What is the danger in patients who have high levels of pyroglutamic acid?**

This is an example of a metabolic threat in patients with metabolic acidosis, where the latter is simply a marker of a more serious underlying disorder. In this condition, the threat to life results from depletion of glutathione and hence compromised ability to detoxify reactive oxygen species. Metabolic acidosis is a "red flag" that warns the physician about this pathophysiology. Repletion of glutathione by administering N-acetyl cysteine may be an option for therapy in these patients. In theory, one might also wish to administer riboflavin because flavin nucleotides are cofactors for glutathione reductase.

45. **Can you summarize the approach to metabolic acidosis?**
   - Initial steps in the diagnostic approach in a patient with metabolic acidosis include the following:
     1. Identify and deal with emergencies; at times one may need to know the etiology to institute this therapy.
     2. Anticipate and prevent risks that are likely to develop during therapy (see Table 81-2).
     3. Deduce whether there is a risk of excessive binding of H^+ to intracellular proteins in vital organs (the brain and the heart).
   - Two major amendments are needed to the traditional approach to the patient with metabolic acidosis:
     1. **One should not rely solely on concentration terms to determine if metabolic acidosis is present when the ECF volume is contracted.** Rather, a quantitative estimate of the ECF volume is needed to calculate its *content* of HCO_3^- in this setting. Use the hematocrit to calculate the plasma volume and thereby to calculate the content of HCO_3^- in the ECF compartment, especially if this latter volume may be contracted.

2. **One must assess the effectiveness of the bicarbonate buffer system.** When the bicarbonate buffer system is compromised in skeletal muscle, more H^+ will bind to proteins in cells of vital organs (e.g., brain, heart) and this may compromise their essential functions. One should not rely solely on the arterial PCO_2 for this assessment. Rather, the brachial or femoral venous PCO_2 reflects the capillary PCO_2 in that drainage bed, and this is required to evaluate the effectiveness of the vast bulk of this buffer system to remove added H^+.

- **Determine whether the basis of the metabolic acidosis is a result of added acids and/or a deficit of $NaHCO_3$:** Look for new anions in plasma (high $P_{Anion\ gap}$ adjusted for the $P_{Albumin}$) and urine (high urine anion gap) and assess the rate of excretion of NH_4^+. At times the new anions may cause serious other problems (e.g., chelation of ionized calcium by citrate anions).

- **Assess the rate of excretion of NH_4^+:** The major renal response in chronic metabolic acidosis is a high rate of excretion of NH_4^+. The urine osmolal gap provides the best indirect test to detect very high urinary NH_4^+ concentration.

KEY POINTS: METABOLIC ACIDOSIS

1. The diagnostic category of metabolic acidosis is made up of two major subgroups: one where the basis of the disorder is the addition of acids, and the other where the basis is a major loss of $NaHCO_3$.

2. When the extracellular fluid (ECF) volume is significantly contracted, one must use a definition of metabolic acidosis that is based not only the $PHCO_3$, but also on the content of HCO_3^- in the ECF compartment.

3. In patients with proximal renal tubular acidosis (RTA), one should not be too aggressive with the administration of $NaHCO_3$ because bicarbonaturia may lead to the development of hypokalemia and the alkaline urine pH may increase the risk of formation of calcium phosphate stones. In patients with distal RTA from a defect in net distal H^+ secretion, the major threat to the patient on presentation is usually cardiac arrhythmia from hypokalemia.

4. The current recommendation not to use metformin in patients with renal insufficiency with a serum creatinine of 1.4 mg/dL (124 umol/L) in women or 1.5 mg dL (132 umol/L) in men is widely disregarded by most physicians because the incidence of lactic acidosis remains extremely low; because it is not very soluble in lipids, it is a weak uncoupler of oxidative phosphorylation and hence rarely (in the absence of an acute overdose) is the sole cause of lactic acidosis.

BIBLIOGRAPHY

1. Carlisle EJF, Donnelly S, Vasuvattakul S, et al. Glue sniffing and distal renal tubular acidosis: Sticking to the facts. *JASN* 1991;1:1019-1027.

2. Davids MR, Edoute Y, Jungas RL, Cheema-Dhadli S, Halperin ML. Facilitating an understanding of integrative physiology: Emphasis on the composition of body fluid compartments. *Can J Physiol Pharmacol* 2002;80:835–850.

3. Dyck RF, Asthana S, Kalra J, West ML Massey, L. A modification of the urine osmolal gap: an improved method for estimating urine ammonium. *Amer J Nephrol* 1990;10:359–362.

4. Fenves AZ, Kirkpatrick HM, Patel VV, Sweetman L, Emmett M. Increased anion gap metabolic acidosis as a result of 5-oxyproline (pyroglutamic acid): a role for acetaminophen. *Clin JASN* 2006;1:441–447.

5. Gowrishankar M, Kamel KS, Halperin ML. Buffering of a H^1 load; A 'brain-protein-centered' view. *J Amer Soc Nephrol* 2007;18:2278–2280.

6. Halperin ML, Kamel KS. Some observations on the clinical approach to patients with metabolic acidosis. *J Am Soc Nephrol* 2010;21:894–897.

7. Halperin ML, Kamel KS, Goldstein MB. *Fluid, Electrolyte and Acid-Base Physiology: A Problem-Based Approach*. Philadelphia: Elsevier, 2010.

8. Halperin ML, Kamel, KS, Maccari, C, et al. Strategies to reduce the danger of cerebral edema in a pediatric patient with diabetic ketoacidosis. *Pediatric Diabetes* 2006;7:191–195.

9. Halperin ML, Margolis BL, Robinson LA, H et al. The urine osmolal gap: a clue to estimate urine ammonium in 'hybrid' types of metabolic acidosis. *Clin Invest Med* 1988;11:198–202.

10. Kamel KS, Briceno LF, Santos MI, et al. A new classification for renal defects in net acid excretion. *Am J Kidney Dis* 1997;29:126–136.

11. Kamel KS, Halperin ML. An improved approach to the patient with metabolic acidosis: A need for four amendments. *Clin Nephrology* 2006;65:S76–S85.

12. Kamel KS, Halperin F, Cheema-Dhadli S, Halperin ML. Anion gap: Do the anions restricted to the intravascular space have modifications in their valence? *Nephron* 1996;73:382–389.

13. Kamel KS, Lin S-H, Cheema-Dhadli S, Marliss EB, Halperin ML. Prolonged total fasting: a feast for the integrative physiologist. *Kidney Int* 1998;53:531–539.

14. Kraut J, Madias N. Serum anion gap: its uses and limitations in clinical medicine. *Clin J Am Soc Nephrol* 2007;2:162–174.

15. Oh MS, ML Halperin ML. Toxin-induced metabolic acidosis. In *Acid-Base Disorders and their Treatment*. Eds: Genari FJ, Adrogue HJ, Galla JH, Madias NE. 2004, Marcel Decker Inc Publisher, Boston MA, USA, pp. 377–409.

16. Rastegar A. Clinical utility of Stewart's method in diagnosis and management of acid-base disorders. *Clin JASN* 2009;4:1267–1274.

17. Shull PD, Rapoport J. Life-threatening metabolic acidosis caused by alcohol abuse. *Nature Reviews Nephrology* 2010;6:555–558.

METABOLIC ALKALOSIS

Mitchell L. Halperin, MD, and Kamel S. Kamel, MD

CHAPTER 82

DIAGNOSIS

1. **What are the hallmarks for the diagnosis of metabolic alkalosis?**
    The diagnostic criteria for this condition are a high concentration of bicarbonate (HCO_3^-) in plasma (P_{HCO3}) and a low concentration of H^+ (or high pH) in plasma. Although one might suspect that a large input of $NaHCO_3$ could lead to a high P_{HCO3}, this will not cause metabolic alkalosis because the kidneys will excrete sodium (Na^+) and HCO_3^- or potential HCO_3^- very quickly with the exception of conditions such as renal insufficiency.

2. **Is there a tubular maximum for the renal reabsorption of filtered HCO_3^-?**
    Under normal conditions, the kidneys reabsorb >90% of filtered HCO_3^- in the proximal convoluted tubule. The stimuli for this process are the ambient level of angiotensin II and the usual pH in cells of the proximal convoluted tubule. Hence, to inhibit this reabsorption of HCO_3^-, the effective arterial blood volume must be expanded (e.g., create a positive balance for Na^+) to diminish the release of angiotensin II and/or the pH in the cells of the proximal convoluted tubule must rise. Bearing this in mind, we shall examine the conditions that were present in the experimental studies that were interpreted to indicate that there is a renal threshold for the reabsorption of HCO_3^- by the kidneys.

    - **Data to suggest that there is a renal threshold for the reabsorption of HCO_3^- by the kidneys:** In the seminal experiments, the infusion of $NaHCO_3$ was large enough to expand the extracellular fluid (ECF) volume sufficiently to diminish circulating levels of angiotensin II and to raise the pH in cells of the proximal convoluted tubule. Hence the two physiologic stimuli for the proximal reabsorption of HCO_3^- were removed. Rather than relate these findings to the physiology, the conclusion was that there is a tubular maximum for the renal reabsorption of HCO_3^-.

    - **Data to suggest that there is not a renal threshold for the reabsorption of HCO_3^-:** The design of these experiments was to avoid a large expansion of the ECF volume while creating a positive balance of $NaHCO_3$. Even though the P_{HCO3} rose, there was little bicarbonaturia and hence a tubular maximum for the renal reabsorption of $NaHCO_3$ was not observed. In support of this view, the range for the P_{HCO3} is from 22 to 31 mmol/L in normal subjects consuming a typical Western diet, and there is no appreciable bicarbonaturia at the upper range values for the P_{HCO3}, despite much higher filtered loads for HCO_3^-, because the glomerular filtration rate (GFR) is relatively constant throughout the day.

    In summary, the enthusiasm for a T_m for HCO_3^- reabsorption in the proximal convoluted tubule is based on data from experimental conditions, which amputated the usual stimuli for the reabsorption of filtered HCO_3^-. In addition, an infusion of $NaHCO_3$ does not represent an important physiologic setting. Based on the above interpretation of the physiology, there need not be a special message delivered to the kidneys to provide a stimulus to increase the reabsorption of filtered HCO_3^- in patients with chronic metabolic alkalosis.

    Two other points merit emphasis. First, a steady state with metabolic alkalosis can be achieved when the blood pH rises sufficiently to overcome the stimulatory actions of angiotensin

II of the reabsorption of HCO_3^- in cells of the proximal convoluted tubule. Second, the excretion of potential HCO_3^- in the form of organic anions such as citrate is augmented by a high pH in cells of the proximal convoluted tubule.

3. **How does hypokalemia affect the excretion of HCO_3^-?**
Because this electrolyte disorder is accompanied by lower pH in cells of the proximal convoluted tubule, there is activation of the Na^+/H^+ exchanger in the luminal membrane of this nephron segment (NHE3) and thereby there is augmented secretion of H^+ in this nephron segment. As a result, more $NaHCO_3$ is reabsorbed in the proximal convoluted tubule during hypokalemia.

4. **What mechanisms may lead to a rise in the P_{HCO3}?**
Because concentrations have numerators and denominators, the P_{HCO3} will rise when there is a net addition of HCO_3^- to the ECF compartment and/or when the volume of the ECF compartment declines (Fig. 82-1):

$$P_{HCO3} = \text{Content of } HCO_3^-/\text{ECF volume}$$

5. **How is HCO_3^- added to the body?**
Three processes add new HCO_3^- to the body
   1. **Generation of HCO_3^- via loss of HCl.** This occurs most commonly when the HCl that is secreted in the stomach is lost via vomiting or nasogastric suction (Fig. 82-2). Hence these conditions represent one of the most common clinical causes of metabolic alkalosis.
   2. **Generation of new HCO_3^- via loss of NH_4Cl.** A second cause of a high P_{HCO3} is the generation of new HCO_3^- by the kidneys, which occurs when ammonium ion (NH_4^+) production and excretion is stimulated:

$$\text{Glutamine}^0 \rightarrow 2\ NH_4^+ + 2\ HCO_3^-$$

In a patient with metabolic alkalosis, the stimulus is the presence of a low pH in cells of the proximal tubule (e.g., during hypokalemia). The latter is commonly due a result of the use or abuse of diuretics. In this setting, reabsorption of HCO_3^- in the proximal convoluted tubule is stimulated. In addition, angiotensin II levels may be elevated because of a decrease in the effective arterial blood volume.

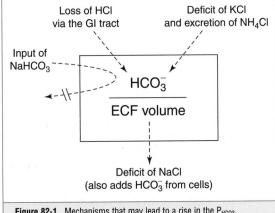

Figure 82-1. Mechanisms that may lead to a rise in the P_{HCO3}.

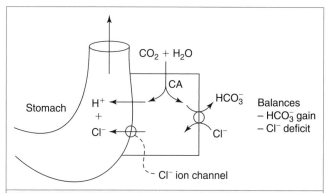

Figure 82-2. Electroneutrality during the deficit of HCl. The stylized structure is the stomach with a parietal cell on its right-hand border. In this cell, $CO_2 + H_2O$ are converted to H^+ and HCO_3^- by a reaction catalyzed by carbonic anhydrase (CA). H^+ are secreted into the lumen of the stomach by the H^+/K^+-ATPase, whereas K^+ recycle back into the parietal cell (not shown for simplicity). Cl^- from the extracellular fluid compartment enter parietal cells on the basolateral Cl^-/HCO_3^- anion exchanger; Cl^- enter the lumen of the stomach via Cl^- ion channels. Overall, there is a loss of Cl^- and a gain of HCO_3^- in the body. Thus there is also electroneutrality in all compartments.

3. **Generation of new HCO_3^- by skeletal muscle cells.** In states with a low effective arterial blood volume and a slow blood flow to muscles, there is a higher PCO_2 in capillary blood. Because CO_2 must diffuse from cells to capillaries, this means that the PCO_2 in cells must also be high in this setting. As shown in Figure 82-3, this high PCO_2 will drive its conversion to H^+ and HCO_3^- in skeletal muscle cells. The H^+ bind to proteins in cells while the HCO_3^- exit on the Cl^-/HCO_3^- anion exchanger, which raises the P_{HCO3}. This condition will persist as long as the blood flow rate to muscles remains low.

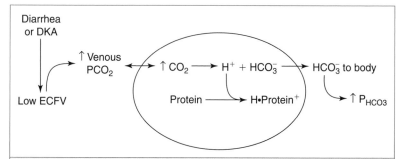

Figure 82-3. Generation of new HCO_3^- in skeletal muscle when there is a deficit of NaCl. The oval represents a cell membrane containing HCO_3^- and protein buffer systems. When the effective arterial blood volume is contracted, the rate of blood flow is reduced. The subsequent extraction of most of the O_2 from each liter of blood flowing through the capillaries raises both the capillary and the intracellular fluid PCO_2 (*left portion of the figure*). The higher PCO_2 in the interstitial fluid and in these cells drives the synthesis of H^+ and HCO_3^-; the H^+ bind to intracellular proteins while the HCO_3^- is exported to the ECF (*right portion of the figure*). The net result is a rise in the P_{HCO3}. After the infusion of enough saline, there is a decline in capillary and, thereby, the PCO_2 in cells. When these events are reversed, there will be a fall in the P_{HCO3}.

6. **What causes the contraction of the ECF volume?**
When there is a *deficit of NaCl* without a simultaneous loss of $NaHCO_3$, the content of HCO_3^- in the ECF compartment does not change, but the P_{HCO3} rises because the denominator of the content of HCO_3^-/ECF volume (see equation in question 4) is diminished. This contraction type of metabolic alkalosis is particularly important when there is a large decrease in the ECF volume (e.g., in patients with massive diarrhea or when diuretics are given to patients with congestive heart failure).

PATHOPHYSIOLOGY

7. **Are the abnormalities in metabolic alkalosis restricted to the ECF compartment?**
No. There are abnormalities in both the ECF and ICF compartments in patients with metabolic alkalosis. The primary stimulus for these changes largely arises secondary to deficits of compounds that contain Cl^-. In a small number of patients, there will be a positive balance for $NaHCO_3$, but in these patients, hypokalemia plays a central role. To understand the pathophysiology, one must examine how electroneutrality and balance were achieved in the ECF and intracellular fluid (ICF) compartments and in the urine.

8. **What is the impact of a deficit of H^+ and Cl^- (i.e., HCl)?**
The only example with sufficient data to understand the impact of this deficit is the selective removal of H^+ and Cl^- from the stomach in seminal experiments performed by Schwartz and Kassirer. The design had unique elements in that the subjects consumed little if any compounds containing Cl^-. We shall describe the events while the deficit develops and later when a new steady state developed (Table 82-1).
   Events while the deficit of HCl develops (called the drainage period):
   - **Process:** As shown in line 1 in Table 82-1, there is a deficit of 200 mmol of Cl^- without a deficit of Na^+ or K^+. Based on electroneutrality, this likely represents a deficit of 200 mmol of H^+. Hence there is a net gain of 200 mmol of HCO_3^- in the body, alkalemia, and a higher P_{HCO3}.
   - **Balances:** There were no important changes in Na^+ or in K^+ balance. Hence there were no important changes in the ICF compartment, merely a loss of Cl^- and an equivalent gain of HCO_3^- in the ECF compartment.
   - **Electroneutrality:** When HCl is lost, there is electroneutrality in the lumen of the stomach (equivalent to a loss of H^+ and Cl^-), in cells of the stomach (net loss of CO_2), and in the ECF compartment (loss of 1 Cl^- per gain of 1 HCO_3^-, see Fig. 82-2).
   - **Therapy:** When the deficit is HCl, one could in theory give HCl to the patient. Alternatively, one could give NaCl because the expanded ECF volume will result in the excretion of the administered Na^+ with the extra HCO_3^- that was present in the ECF compartment. The administered Cl^- will be retained. Thus therapy executed an exchange of HCO_3^- (loss) for Cl (gain) in a 1:1 stoichiometry, and this should correct the disorder.

TABLE 82-1. BALANCE DATA IN THE SELECTIVE DEPLETION OF HCL MODEL OF METABOLIC ALKALOSIS					
	BALANCE DATA			**BLOOD**	
Setting	Na^+ (mmol)	K^+ (mmol)	Cl^- (mmol)	pH	P_{HCO3}
Normal	0	0	0	7.40	25
Drainage	0	0	−200	7.47	37
Post-drainage period	0	−200	0	7.46	37
Therapy with NaCl	+800	0	+800	7.40	25

Events in the steady state following a deficit of HCl (post-drainage period):

Process: There is a net loss of 200 mmol of K^+ without Cl^- or HCO_3^- (the urine did not contain HCO_3^- because its pH was close to 6.0). The K^+ loss from the ICF compartment was likely accompanied by a gain of H^+. The source of these H^+ was from H_2SO_4 formed when dietary sulphur-containing amino acids were oxidized (Fig. 82-4):

$$\text{Sulfur-containing amino acids}^0 \rightarrow \text{Urea} + CO_2 + 2\,H^+ + SO_4^{2-}$$

The sulphate anions (SO_4^{2-}) were excreted in the urine with K^+ rather than NH_4^+ because of alkalemia. This excretion of K^+ will decline when hypokalemia develops and it augments the excretion of NH_4^+. Because there were no obvious changes in the ECF volume and the Na-K-ATPase of cells in the body will excrete Na^+ when its concentration rises in their ICF, we suspect that these cells gain predominantly H^+ rather than Na^+ when K^+ was lost.

Balance: The overall balance has changed from a deficit of HCl to one of KCl over a matter of days with no change in the plasma pH and P_{HCO3}. If the ICF rather than the ECF were sampled, the disorder would be called K^+ deficiency and metabolic acidosis owing to the gain of H^+. This is strikingly different from the name of the disorder defined from sampling the ECF compartment where the acid–base term is metabolic alkalosis.

Electroneutrality: As shown in Figure 82-4, there is electroneutrality in the ECF compartment, the ICF compartment, and the urine.

Therapy: Once the deficit becomes KCl, one should give enough KCl to replace this deficit. Giving NaCl does not correct the deficit of KCl acutely. Nevertheless, if there was K^+ in the diet, ultimately this K^+ would be retained and the extra Na^+ in the body would be excreted, because the expanded ECF volume will augment the excretion of the retained Na^+ once the deficit of K^+ is restored.

9. **In total body terms, is there a positive balance of HCO_3^- in the selective loss of HCl model of metabolic alkalosis?"**

Before answering this question, one must appreciate that the major fate of added HCO_3^- is to react with H^+, forming CO_2, which is exhaled via the lungs:

$$HCO_3^- + H^+ \leftrightarrow H_2CO_3 \leftrightarrow CO_2 + H_2O$$

Because the deficits of Cl^- and K^+ were equal, the gain of HCO_3^- in the ECF compartment was equal to the gain of H^+ in the ICF compartment. Accordingly, there is no overall change in balance of HCO_3^-, but there are opposing acid–base abnormalities in the ECF and ICF compartments.

10. **What are the diagnostic hallmarks of metabolic alkalosis resulting from depletion of HCl?**

Because of the deficit of Cl^-, the urine should be virtually free of Cl^-. Despite a contracted ECF volume, Na^+ may be excreted if the urine contains anions other than Cl^-. In this latter setting, the urine may contain K^+ even though the patient has chronic hypokalemia. If there

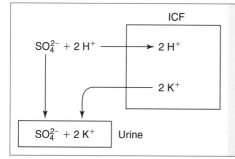

Figure 82-4. Balance of cations in the intracellular fluid (ICF) compartment during the deficit of KCl. The large square represents the ICF compartment, which contains the vast bulk of body K^+. When the deficit of KCl develops, K^+ are excreted in the urine with an anion other than Cl^- *(represented by the rectangle in the lower left portion of the diagram)*. This anion is SO_4^{2-}, which was produced with H^+ during the oxidation of sulfur-containing amino acids to yield H_2SO_4. For electroneutrality in the ICF compartment, the shift of K^+ out of cells was accompanied by a shift of H^+ in cells.

has been a very recent bout of vomiting, the urine may contain HCO_3^- and have a pH that is distinctly greater than 6.0. Hence these additional findings to the low urine Cl^--concentration provide a bigger picture of the pathophysiology in a patient who has a deficit of HCl.

11. **What is the appropriate renal response to a deficit of KCl?**
Ideally, the kidney should limit further losses of K^+ and Cl^-. The ideal response would be to retain the extra HCO_3^- in the ECF compartment because if HCO_3^- were excreted, metabolic acidosis would develop once the ECF volume is re-expanded and H^+ shift out of cells (i.e., a total body deficit of HCO_3^- would be present). Moreover, a cation would also be excreted. If this cation were K^+, a more severe degree of K^+ deficiency and hypokalemia would develop, and this could provoke a cardiac arrhythmia. The ECF volume would be contracted if Na^+ were excreted with the HCO_3^-, phosphate excretion, a fall in citrate excretion owing to a high concentration of H^+ in cells of the proximal convoluted tubule, and thereby an increased risk of forming $CaHPO_4$ kidney stones.

12. **What is the pathophysiology of metabolic alkalosis in patients with primary high mineralocorticoid activity?**
In this setting, there is an initial positive balance of NaCl as a result of actions of mineralocorticoids. The next step is the excretion of K^+ along with some of the Cl^- that was retained. The resulting deficit of K^+ acidifies proximal convoluted tubular cells and thereby results in the retention of some of the dietary alkali (i.e., lower excretion of citrate) and in an increased rate of excretion NH_4^+, and both lead to the development of a higher P_{HCO3}. In total body terms, there is a net gain of $NaHCO_3$. Although balance data are not available in these patients, it is likely that the loss of K^+ from ICF was accompanied by a gain of some Na^+ in ICF compartment. Once the P_{HCO3} rises sufficiently to return the ICF pH toward its normal value, these patients can achieve acid–base balance by excreting the appropriate amounts of NH_4^+ and organic anions in the urine, as dictated by their dietary intake but at a higher P_{HCO3}. A list of specific disorders is provided in Table 82-2.

13. **What is the result of a deficit of NaCl?**
The deficit of Na^+ and Cl^- can lead to a higher P_{HCO3} for two reasons. The first reason is a fall in the denominator of the ratio of HCO_3^- to ECF volume (see equation in question 4). The reason for this fall is that the major function of Na^+ is to retain water in the ECF compartment. The second reason for a higher P_{HCO3} is the generation of new HCO_3^- in skeletal muscle because the blood flow declines appreciably to this organ for hemodynamic reasons, although there is no increase in the extraction of oxygen, more oxygen will be extracted per liter of blood flow. This oxygen is converted to CO_2, which leads to a high capillary PCO_2 and thereby a higher intracellular PCO_2 (see Fig. 82-3).

CLINICAL APPROACH

14. **Is metabolic alkalosis a specific acid–base diagnosis?**
The simple answer is no. Metabolic alkalosis represents a heterogeneous group of disorders that have in common a high P_{HCO3} and a low concentration of H^+ (or high pH) in plasma. This constellation of findings can be seen in a number of different pathophysiologic entities (see Table 82-2). Hence metabolic alkalosis is not a final diagnosis.
There is also no one-size-fits-all strategy for therapy of patients with this group of disorders. Nevertheless, certain questions can be answered to help with the decisions with respect to therapy.

15. **What is the most reliable way to perform a quantitative analysis of the ECF volume in patients with metabolic alkalosis?**
Because accurate quantitative data about the ECF volume cannot be obtained by the physical examination, the hematocrit or total protein level in plasma can be used to obtain this information.

TABLE 82-2.   CAUSES OF METABOLIC ALKALOSIS

Causes usually associated with a contracted effective arterial blood volume:
- Low U_{Cl} (unless a diuretic is acting)
  - Loss of gastric secretions (e.g., vomiting, nasogastric suction)
  - Remote use of diuretics
  - Delivery of Na^+ to CCD with non-reabsorbed anions plus a reason for avid Na^+ reabsorption
  - Post-hypercapnic states
  - Loss of H^+ and Cl^- via lower gastrointestinal tract (e.g., congenital disorder with Cl^- loss in diarrhea, acquired forms of DRA)
- Persistent high U_{Cl}
  - Current diuretic use
  - Endogenous diuretics (occupancy of the CaSR in the thick ascending limb of the loop of Henle, inborn errors affecting transporters of Na^+ and/or Cl^- in the nephron, e.g., Bartter's syndrome or Gitelman's syndrome)

Causes associated with an expanded extracellular fluid volume and possibly hypertension:
- Disorders with primary enhanced mineralocorticoid activity causing hypokalemia
  - Primary aldosteronism
  - Secondary hyperaldosteronism (e.g., renal artery stenosis, malignant hypertension, renin-producing tumor)
  - Disorders with cortisol acting as a mineralocorticoid (e.g., apparent mineralocorticoid excess syndrome, licorice ingestion, adrenocorticotropic hormone produced by a tumor)
  - Disorders with constitutively active ENaC in the CCD (e.g., Liddle's syndrome)
  - Large reduction in glomerular filtration rate plus a source of $NaHCO_3$

U_{Cl} = concentration of Cl^- in the urine; CCD = cortical collecting duct; DRA = down-regulated in adenoma/adenocarcinoma; CaSR = calcium-sensing receptor.

The hematocrit or the concentration of hemoglobin in blood will rise when there are more red blood cells and/or fewer liters of plasma. If one ignores the Starling forces across capillaries, the changes in the plasma volume will reflect alterations in the ECF volume. The hematocrit on admission provides helpful information to guide initial decisions about intravenous fluid therapy and to decide when to slow down this infusion rate.

For example, assume that the hematocrit is 0.40 and the blood volume is 5 L. Therefore the plasma volume will be 3 L and volume of red blood cells (RBC) is 2 L:

Hematocrit (0.4) = RBC volume (2 L)/plasma volume (3 L) + RBC volume (2 L)

If the hematocrit on admission is 0.60 in a patient who does not have polycythemia, the new plasma volume can be calculated as follows:

Hematocrit of 0.6 = RBC volume (2 L)/Blood volume (X L)

On rearranging this equation, 0.6 X = 2.0 L and X is 3.3 L. Because 2 of these liters are red blood cells, the remaining volume is the plasma volume (3.3 L − 2.0 L = 1.33 L). Thus the plasma volume has fallen from 3 L to 1.33 L and, by inference, the ECF volume is reduced to 44% of its normal volume (i.e., 100 × 1.33 L/3.0 L = 44%). Because hematocrit values of 0.6 can be seen in patients with diabetic ketoacidosis or in states with severe diarrhea (e.g., cholera), the measured P_{HCO3} will be more than two-fold higher than in a similar patient who did not have such a contracted ECF volume.

16. **What is the optimal clinical approach to the patient with metabolic alkalosis?**
    Our approach to the patient with metabolic alkalosis is provided in Figure 82-5. The first step is to rule out the common causes of metabolic alkalosis: vomiting and use of diuretics. Although this may be evident from the clinical history, some patients may deny the intake of diuretics or previous vomiting. Examining the urine electrolytes is particularly helpful to suspect this diagnosis. We begin with the concentration of Cl^- in the urine (U_{Cl})—a very low U_{Cl} is expected when there is a deficit of HCl and/or NaCl, but the recent intake of diuretics will cause the excretion of Na^+ and Cl^-. The U_{Na} may be high if there is a recent episode of vomiting. If the U_{Cl} is not low, assessment of effective arterial blood volume and blood pressure help separate patients with disorders of high primary mineralocorticoid activity (effective arterial blood volume is not low, presence of hypertension) from those with Bartter's-like syndromes (effective arterial blood volume is low, absence of hypertension). Serial measurements of U_{Cl} in spot urine samples are helpful to separate patients with Bartter's or Gitelman's syndromes (persistently high U_{Cl}) from those with diuretic abuse (intermittently high U_{Cl}).

17. **What is the major differential diagnosis in a patient who has metabolic alkalosis, a urine Cl^- concentration that is not low, and a contracted ECF volume?**
    In this setting, one must look for the basis for a deficit of HCl, KCl, and/or NaCl. In addition, there will be a renal problem in the conservation of Cl^- (see Table 82-2). The most common cause is the chronic use of diuretics. In this setting, some urine samples but not others may

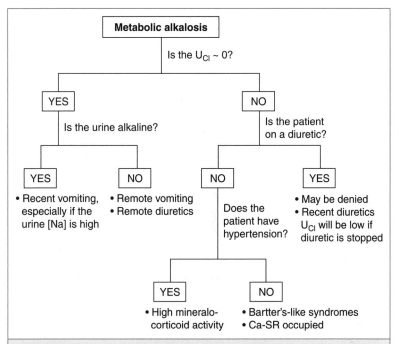

Figure 82-5. Clinical approach to the patient with metabolic alkalosis. The U_{Cl} should be close to nil if the cause of metabolic alkalosis is vomiting or the remote use of diuretics. If the U_{Cl} is not low, an assessment of "effective" arterial blood volume and blood pressure helps separate patients with disorders of high primary mineralocorticoid activity from those with Bartter's-like syndromes. CaSR = calcium sensing receptor in thick ascending limb of the loop of Henle.

have high Cl^- concentration. However, if the urine always has a high Cl^- concentration, look for chronic rise of diuretics or an inborn error that causes a reduced reabsorption of Na^+ and Cl^- such as Bartter's syndrome or Gitelman's syndrome. There is also one other group of causes to exclude—the presence of a drug, cation, or cationic protein that binds to the calcium sensing receptor (Ca-SR) in the basolateral membrane of the thick ascending limb of the loop of Henle. The major ligands for the Ca-SR are a high concentration of ionized calcium in plasma, cationic antibiotics such as gentamicin, and circulating cationic proteins as seen in immunologic disorders or with disorders such as multiple myeloma. A clue for the latter condition is a lower than expected value for the anion gap in plasma adjusted for the concentration of albumin in plasma (i.e., -3 to -4 mEq/L per reduction of 1 g of albumin/dL or per 10 g of albumin/L).

18. **What is the major differential diagnosis in a patient who has metabolic alkalosis, a urine Cl^- concentration that is not low, and an ECF volume that is not contracted?**
    The usual causes are patients with conditions accompanied by high mineralocorticoid activity (see Table 82-2). Clues to suspect these disorders include the causes of the metabolic alkalosis, hypokalemia, and hypertension. The associated hypokalemia is important in the pathophysiology in these patients. Because of the high mineralocorticoid activity or a constitutively active ENaC, principal cells of the cortical distal nephron are poised to reabsorb Na^+. Initially Na^+ and Cl^- are retained, and hence the ECF volume will be expanded. Subsequently, K^+ will be lost in the urine with Cl^- if these cells have open K^+ channel in their luminal membrane and if Na^+ is reabsorbed faster than Cl^-. The net effect is that hypokalemia will lead to an acidified proximal tubule cell, which results in the excretion of more NH_4^+ with Cl^- and the retention of dietary alkali (low excretion of potential HCO_3^-, i.e., organic anions). Overall, the body continues to have a surplus of Na^+, but some of the retained Cl^- are excreted in the urine (with NH_4^+) and therefore are replaced with HCO_3^-. The ICF compartment has a deficit of K^+. Although balance data are not usually available, the cation that is retained in the ICF is likely to be Na^+ and possibly some H^+.

KEY POINTS: METABOLIC ALKALOSIS

1. Concentrations have numerators and denominators. Thus the $PHCO_3$ will rise when the content of HCO_3^- increases and/or when the volume of the extracellular fluid (ECF) compartment declines. Hence metabolic alkalosis represents a heterogeneous group of disorders.

2. Support for a T_m for HCO_3^- reabsorption in the proximal convoluted tubule is derived from data from the infusion of $Na^+ + HCO_3^-$, but this is not an important physiologic setting.

3. Classification of the common forms of metabolic alkalosis should be based on deficits of HCl, KCl, and/or NaCl (i.e., do not focus only on Cl^- deficiency because this is a partial description of the pathophysiology).

4. Hypokalemia plays a central role in the pathophysiology of metabolic alkalosis as a result of high mineralocorticoid actions.

5. Measuring the concentration of Cl^- in the urine is an excellent first step in the clinical approach to patients with metabolic acidosis.

6. A quantitative estimate of the degree of contraction of the ECF volume is helpful because it will indicate the magnitude of the deficit or surplus of HCO_3^- in the ECF compartment.

7. There is no one-size-fits-all strategy for therapy of patients with this heterogeneous group of disorders.

BIBLIOGRAPHY

1. Cheema-Dhadli S, Lin S-H, Halperin ML. Mechanisms used to dispose of a progressively increasing alkali load in the rat. *Am J Physiol* 2002;282:F1049–F1055.

2. Cogan MG. Angiotensin II: A powerful controller of sodium transport in the early proximal tubule. *Hypertension* 1990;15:451–458.

3. Gowrishankar M, Kamel KS, Halperin ML. Buffering of a H^+ load; A "brain-protein-centered" view. *J Am Soc Nephrol* 2007;18:2278–2280.

4. Hebert SC. Extracellular calcium-sensing receptor: Implications for calcium and magnesium handling in the kidney. *Kidney Int* 1996;50:2129–2139.

5. Kassirer JP, Schwartz WB. The response of normal man to selective depletion of hydrochloric acid. *Am J Med* 1996;40:10–18.

6. Purkerson ML, Lubowitz H, White RW, et al. On the influence of extracellular fluid volume expansion on bicarbonate reabsorption in the rat. *J Clin Invest* 1969;48:1754–1760.

7. Scheich A, Donnelly S, Cheema-Dhadli S, et al. Does saline 'correct' the abnormal mass balance in metabolic alkalosis associated with chloride-depletion in the rat. *Clin Invest Med* 1994;17:448–460.

8. Simpson D. Citrate excretion: A window on renal metabolism. *Am J Physiol* 1983;244:F223–F234.

9. Zalunardo N, Lemaire M, Davids MR, et al. Acidosis in a patient with cholera: A need to redefine concepts. *QJM* 2004;97:681–696.

CHAPTER 83

RESPIRATORY ACID–BASE DISORDERS

Biff F. Palmer, MD

1. **What is the role of the respiratory system in acid–base balance?**
   The lungs serve to defend pH by altering alveolar ventilation, which controls the pCO_2 of body fluids. An increase in nonvolatile acid production lowers blood pH and HCO_3 concentration (metabolic acidosis). The lungs respond to this fall in pH by lowering the pCO_2 (compensatory respiratory alkalosis). As a result, the fall in blood pH will be less than would have occurred in the absence of respiratory compensation. The opposite happens with metabolic alkalosis. If the fractional change in CO_2 tension were similar to that in HCO_3 concentration, blood pH would not change. However, respiratory compensations generally do not return blood pH to normal; thus the fractional change in CO_2 tension will be less than that in HCO_3 concentration.

   The contribution of the respiratory tract in maintaining acid–base homeostasis becomes obvious in view of the large amount of daily cellular CO_2 production. Each day approximately 15,000 mmol of CO_2 are produced by cellular metabolism. Under physiologic conditions CO_2 produced during cellular metabolism matches CO_2 excretion by the lungs and arterial CO_2 tension ($PaCO_2$) is maintained relatively constant between 35 and 45 mm Hg. Even during exercise, when the amount of CO_2 production increases many fold per unit of time, the respiratory system is able to maintain acid–base balance by increasing minute ventilation.

2. **What are the primary physiologic stimuli that regulate respiration?**
   Arterial hypoxemia and hypercapnia have been recognized as the main physiologic stimuli to respiration. Changes in $PaCO_2$ are sensed as cerebral interstitial pH changes in the chemosensitive areas of the medulla. Changes in arterial oxygen tension are sensed by chemoreceptors in the carotid bodies, which are located close to the carotid artery bifurcation. Among these two, the medullary chemoreceptors are more sensitive and respond to subtle CO_2 tension changes as low as 1 mm Hg with stimulation of the respiratory drive. Because of the sensitive regulatory mechanism of medullary chemoreceptors, hypercapnia is almost always a result of ineffective alveolar ventilation and not a result of increased metabolic $PaCO_2$ production.

3. **What are the causes of respiratory acidosis?**
   The development of respiratory acidosis is usually multifactorial. Major causes of CO_2 retention include diseases or malfunction within any element of the respiratory system, including the central and peripheral nervous systems, the respiratory muscles, the thoracic cage, the pleural space, the airways, and the lung parenchyma. The following six factors should be considered in the differential diagnosis of acute and chronic respiratory acidosis:
   - **Increased CO_2 production:** Increased levels of CO_2 can be found in physiologic and pathophysiologic settings. Physical activity, shivering, fever, hyperthyroidism, and prolonged seizure activity can lead to increased CO_2 production. Yet increased metabolic CO_2 production alone rarely leads to hypercapnia. Chemosensitive areas of the medulla respond to elevated CO_2 levels, which are sensed as interstitial pH changes, by increasing the respiratory drive. The large ventilatory reserve of most patients allows alveolar ventilation to increase in proportion to the amount of additional CO_2 produced. Increased production can only play a role in the pathophysiology of respiratory acidosis when alveolar ventilation is fixed as in a patient receiving controlled mechanical ventilation.

- The administration of large amounts of carbohydrates to a patient who is mechanically ventilated can lead to increased CO_2 production, particularly when glycogen stores are replete. In this setting pyruvate generated from the metabolism of glucose coupled with acetylcoenzyme A leads to increased lipogenesis. The shunting of these metabolites toward fatty acid synthesis increases the activity of the tricarboxylic acid cycle with resultant increased generation of CO_2.
- **Inhibition of the medullary respiratory center:** Anesthetics, sedatives, and opiates cause hypercapnia by decreasing the respiratory drive. Patients with chronic hypercapnia may develop worsening hypercapnia and respiratory failure if they use high flow rates of supplemental oxygen because hypoxemia serves as an important stimulus for respiratory drive in these patients.
- **Disorders of the respiratory muscles and chest wall:** Electrolyte disturbances such as severe hypokalemia or hypophosphatemia may lead to hypercapnia secondary to muscle weakness. Neurologic diseases like spinal cord injury, myasthenia gravis, Guillain-Barré syndrome, poliomyelitis, amyotrophic lateral sclerosis, and multiple sclerosis are other causes that may lead to hypercapnia as a result of respiratory muscle weakness.
- **Airway obstruction:** Hypercapnia can result in the setting of acute upper airway obstruction with foreign bodies, as frequently observed in the pediatric age range or with vomitus in patients who cannot control their airways because of altered mental status, unconsciousness, or neurologic diseases.
- **Disorders affecting gas exchange across the pulmonary capillary:** Any clinical disorder that impairs gas exchange in the alveoli can lead to hypoxemia and hypercapnia. Exacerbation of underlying lung disease, acute pulmonary edema, pneumonia, and adult respiratory distress syndrome are the most common causes.
- **Mechanical ventilation:** In the intensive care setting patients who are mechanically ventilated can develop primary respiratory acidosis if the ventilator settings do not allow proper exhalation of CO_2. Increasing the respiratory rate or the tidal volume both increases alveolar ventilation and corrects primary hypercapnia.

4. **What are the clinical manifestations of respiratory acidosis?**
   Acute respiratory acidosis manifests with a variety of neurologic symptoms. The severity of symptoms depends on the magnitude of hypercapnia and hypoxemia and the rapidity with which the respiratory acidosis develops. All patients with hypercapnia will also be hypoxemic when breathing room air as a result of decreased oxygen uptake. In disease states hypoxemia often occurs earlier and is more prominent than hypercapnia because CO_2 diffuses much more rapidly across the alveolar capillaries than does oxygen. In the setting of parenchymal disease of the lung, there is also preferential ventilation of less involved areas allowing for more CO_2 excretion. Additional oxygen cannot be taken up because hemoglobin is nearly saturated in these areas.

   Hypercapnic encephalopathy is a clinical syndrome that usually starts with irritability, headache, mental cloudiness, apathy, confusion, anxiety, and restlessness and can progress to asterixis, transient psychosis, delirium, somnolence, and coma. Papilledema and other manifestations of increased intracranial pressure that are collectively named pseudotumor cerebri are occasionally observed in patients with either acute or chronic hypercapnia. The increase in intracranial pressure is in part a result of cerebral vasodilation resulting from acidemia. Acute respiratory acidosis is typically much more symptomatic than is acute metabolic acidosis because CO_2 diffuses and equilibrates across the blood–brain barrier much more rapidly than does HCO_3 resulting in a more rapid fall in cerebral spinal fluid and cerebral interstitial pH.

   Severe respiratory acidosis may have life-threatening effects on the cardiovascular system. Severe hypercapnia can lead to decreased myocardial contractility, arrhythmias, and peripheral vasodilatation, particularly when the blood pH falls to <7.1.

5. **What compensatory mechanisms take place in acute respiratory acidosis?**
   Acute hypercapnia is associated with several effects that lead to an immediate small rise in the serum HCO_3 concentration. First, the decrease in pH that accompanies acute respiratory acidosis

increases H^+ binding to albumin. This effect will cause a fall in the anion gap and a slight rise in the serum HCO_3 concentration. Second, a small amount of H^+ enters parenchymal cells in exchange for Na^+ and K^+, also contributing to a small increase in extracellular HCO_3 concentration. Third, the high CO_2 tension is immediately transmitted into red blood cells, where in the presence of carbonic anhydrase, H_2CO_3 is generated. This acid disassociates and the H^+ binds to hemoglobin, leaving HCO_3 in the cytoplasm of the red cell. Hemoglobin can bind a considerable amount of H^+ as a result of the rich histidine content of the molecule. As the HCO_3 concentration rises, it exits from the cell in exchange for plasma Cl^-, a process termed the red cell HCO_3-Cl^- shift. The net effect of these changes is that in acute respiratory acidosis the plasma HCO_3 concentration increases by 1 mmol/l for each 10 mm Hg elevation in $PaCO_2$.

6. **What compensatory mechanisms take place in chronic respiratory acidosis?**
    In chronic respiratory acidosis the increase in plasma HCO_3 concentration is higher as a result of compensatory renal mechanisms. The chronic elevation in CO_2 leads to intracellular acidosis in proximal tubular cells, increasing H^+ secretion and resulting in accelerated HCO_3 reabsorption. The retention of $NaHCO_3$ leads to slight expansion of the extracellular fluid compartment and causes increased renal excretion of NaCl so as to return volume back to normal. The net effect is an increase in serum HCO_3 and decreased Cl^- concentration. In chronic respiratory acidosis there is a 3.5 mEq/L increase in HCO_3 for each 10 mm Hg elevation in $PaCO_2$. Higher or lower plasma HCO_3 concentrations suggest the presence of mixed respiratory and metabolic acid–base disorders.

7. **What is the treatment for acute respiratory acidosis?**
    The mainstay of treatment in acute respiratory acidosis is to recognize and treat the underlying cause whenever possible. Patients with acute respiratory acidosis are primarily at risk of hypoxemia rather than hypercapnia or acidemia. Thus, immediate therapeutic efforts should focus on establishing and securing a patent airway to provide adequate oxygenation. If the patient is in a coma, severely obtunded, extremely hypercapnic ($PaCO_2$ >80 mm Hg), or severely acidemic (blood pH <7.10), assisted ventilation should be initiated promptly. In emergency situations the clinician should provide a high inspired oxygen tension to all patients with acute respiratory acidosis; concerns that this measure will further depress ventilation are unfounded. Indeed, maximal PaO_2 levels must be assured for those found apneic, in cardiac arrest, or unconscious from carbon monoxide poisoning.

8. **Is there a role for $NaHCO_3$ in the treatment of respiratory acidosis?**
    Although the primary aim of therapy is to restore ventilation in acute respiratory acidosis, the administration of $NaHCO_3$ may allow the pH to be partially corrected in settings where the pCO_2 cannot be rapidly corrected. In patients with status asthmaticus, a lower ventilatory rate and peak inspiratory pressure may be required to minimize barotrauma to the lung but at the expense of a persistently higher pCO_2. Small amounts of $NaHCO_3$ can help prevent excessive falls in blood pH in this setting. The downside of such therapy is infusion of $NaHCO_3$ can result in increased CO_2 production, causing a further increase in pCO_2 when ventilation cannot be increased.

9. **What are the treatment considerations in patients with chronic respiratory acidosis?**
    Patients with chronic respiratory acidosis suffer from hypoxemia in addition to hypercapnia. The primary therapeutic goal in these patients is to ensure adequate oxygenation. Unfortunately, in most cases the underlying disease cannot be removed. The appropriate treatment of chronic respiratory acidosis depends on the underlying disease. Clinicians should be careful in prescribing drugs, which might suppress the central ventilatory drive.
        Excessive oxygen should be avoided because it might lead to worsening hypoventilation. Chronic respiratory acidosis is accompanied by a progressive insensitivity to the stimulatory effect of CO_2 and hypoxemia becomes an increasingly important factor in driving ventilation. In general, the hypoxic drive to ventilation remains adequate as long as the PaO_2 does not exceed 60 mm Hg. Oxygen flow rates of 2 L/min by nasal canula deliver an inspired oxygen

concentration of 23% to 28% and improve PaO_2 values to levels of 50 to 60 mm Hg in many patients with chronic respiratory failure. Use of continuous low-flow oxygen therapy is indicated in patients with severe hypoxemia (PaO_2 less than 55 mm Hg) because it has been shown to diminish the severity of cor pulmonale and improve the quality of life.

10. **What is posthypercapnic metabolic alkalosis?**
Many patients with chronic respiratory acidosis have an underlying lung disease and are at risk of developing worsening hypercapnia and hypoxia during episodes of acute worsening of pulmonary functions as with the development of pneumonia. In case mechanical ventilation is required to ensure adequate ventilation, care should be taken to lower the $PaCO_2$ carefully and slowly because there is the risk of overshooting alkalemia because of the presence of a high HCO_3. The kidneys must excrete the HCO_3 to normalize the acid–base status. This excretion will not occur when effective arterial blood volume is reduced either because of salt depletion owing to restricted intake or diuretic therapy or a salt-retentive state such as heart failure and cirrhosis. Under such circumstances increased proximal reabsorption of HCO_3 prevents renal HCO_3 clearance despite the fall in pCO_2. Chronic respiratory acidosis is converted to metabolic alkalosis in a process called posthypercapnic metabolic alkalosis. A high pH in the central nervous system can lead to severe neurologic abnormalities such as seizure and coma.

11. **What is the role of acetazolamide in patients with chronic respiratory acidosis?**
Correction of the superimposed metabolic alkalosis can usually be achieved with saline and discontinuation of loop diuretics if they are being utilized. In patients with edema with heart failure this is not possible and acetazolamide may have to be used to correct the alkalosis.
Acetazolamide inhibits HCO_3 reabsorption because of its ability to inhibit luminal carbonic anhydrase. This enzyme normally catalyzes the dehydration of carbonic acid (produced when filtered bicarbonate reacts with secreted H^+) to water and CO_2, thereby maintaining a favorable concentration gradient for further H^+ secretion. The uncatalyzed dehydration of carbonic acid occurs very slowly. By inhibiting the activity of this enzyme, acetazolamide allows for the concentration of luminal carbonic acid to increase. The resultant increase in H^+ concentration creates an unfavorable concentration gradient for further H^+ secretion. Because of the lipid solubility of acetazolamide, inhibition of intracellular carbonic anhydrase may also contribute to the impairment in proximal HCO_3 reabsorption. Inhibition of the intracellular enzyme will decrease the supply of H^+ available for the secretory process. In either case, decreased secretion of H^+ will inhibit reabsorption of filtered HCO_3 and thus cause the kidney to at least partially correct the metabolic alkalosis. The magnitude of the bicarbonaturia is directly related to the serum HCO_3 concentration. As the HCO_3 concentration falls, the clinical effectiveness of the drug declines in a parallel fashion. As a result, only rarely does the plasma HCO_3 concentration return to normal.
A potential problem associated with use of carbonic anhydrase inhibitors in patients with lung disease is a worsening of hypercapnia. Carbonic anhydrase is normally present within red blood cells and is involved in CO_2 movement into red cells in peripheral tissues and movement from red cells into the alveoli in the lungs. Thus carbonic anhydrase inhibition can prevent red cell uptake of pCO_2 in peripheral tissues and can prevent pCO_2 release in the lung. The latter can lead to an increase in pCO_2 of the arterial blood, whereas the former leads to an even further increase in pCO_2 in peripheral tissues. Generally, patients with normal lungs can respond to this by increasing respiration and preventing the increase in the pCO_2 of the arterial blood. However, patients with lung disease cannot respond adequately, and further increases in arterial pCO_2 and even larger increases in tissue pCO_2 may be dangerous to the patient.

12. **What is respiratory alkalosis?**
Primary respiratory alkalosis results from hypocapnia and is defined by a $PaCO_2$ of >35 mm Hg in the setting of alkalemia. Primary respiratory alkalosis needs to be differentiated from secondary hypocapnia, which is a compensatory mechanism in the setting of primary metabolic acidosis. An increase in alveolar ventilation relative to CO_2 production gives rise to respiratory alkalosis.

Because changes in CO_2 production are negligible, almost all cases of hypocapnia result from increased CO_2 elimination, which is the equivalent of increased alveolar hyperventilation.

13. **What is the etiology of respiratory alkalosis?**

In the large majority of cases, primary hypocapnia reflects pulmonary hyperventilation as a result of increased ventilatory drive. The latter might result from signals arising from the lung, the peripheral chemoreceptors (carotid and aortic), the brain-stem chemoreceptors, or influences originating in other centers of the brain. The response to CO_2 of the brain-stem chemoreceptors can be augmented by systemic diseases (e.g., sepsis, liver disease), pharmacologic agents, anxiety, volition, and other influences. Hypoxemia is a major stimulus to pulmonary ventilation, but PaO_2 values less than 60 mm Hg are required to elicit this effect consistently.

Primary hypocapnia is probably the most frequent acid–base disturbance encountered. In patients who are critically ill, its presence might be a grave prognostic sign, especially if pCO_2 levels are below 20 and 25 mm Hg. Furthermore, respiratory alkalosis is the most common acid–base abnormality in patients hospitalized in intensive care units, occurring either as the simple disorder or as a component of mixed disturbances.

Hepatic failure is a common and important cause of primary hypocapnia. The severity of hypocapnia correlates with the level of blood ammonia and has prognostic significance. Systemic infections arising from gram-positive and gram-negative bacteria are also a major cause of respiratory alkalosis. Direct stimulation of central chemoreceptors by bacterial toxins from gram-negative organisms accounts, at least in part, for the hyperventilation observed in some patients with sepsis. Thus, unexplained respiratory alkalosis in a hospitalized patient calls for evaluation for the presence of gram-negative sepsis. The presence of respiratory alkalosis can be an important clue to the presence of salicylate intoxication. High progesterone levels (pregnancy) can also cause respiratory alkalosis.

14. **What are the clinical manifestations of respiratory alkalosis?**

Mild respiratory alkalosis causes lightheadedness, palpitations, and paresthesias of the extremities and the circumoral area. Acute hypocapnia decreases cerebral blood flow and produces decreased acidity in all body fluids and hypocalcemia, hypokalemia, and a pH-induced shift of oxyhemoglobin dissociation curve; all these alterations have been implicated as determinants of the clinical manifestations of this acid–base disorder. The acute hypocapnia-induced reduction in cerebral blood flow might reach values lower than 50% of normal, resulting in an increased lactate output by the brain from cerebral hypoxia. A reduction in intracranial pressure, which is generally not harmful, and electroencephalographic changes consisting of generalized slowing and high-voltage waves are also present in acute respiratory alkalosis. The effects of acute hypocapnia on the cerebral circulation have been used in the treatment of brain edema resulting from neurosurgical procedures, head trauma, meningitis, and encephalitis. Unfortunately, the hypocapnia-induced reduction in intracranial pressure is short-lasting, and blood flow returns to normal in sustained hypocapnia.

Hypocapnia leads to alkalemia, which causes binding of free calcium to albumin in the blood. Thus, patients with acute respiratory alkalosis might present clinically in a similar way to patients with hypocalcemia. Chvostek's and Trousseau's sign are well-known clinical tests that can be occasionally elicited in patients with acute respiratory alkalosis.

The cardiovascular manifestations of respiratory alkalosis might be also prominent. A major reduction in cardiac output accompanied by arteriolar vasoconstriction, tissue hypoperfusion, and a large increment in plasma lactate frequently is attributed to severe acute hypocapnia. This syndrome is typically observed in surgical patients under general anesthesia or those having depression of the central nervous system and receiving mechanical respiratory assistance; in all likelihood, it reflects the effects of passive hyperventilation. Normal volunteers with active hyperventilation do not develop clinical manifestations of coronary insufficiency or cardiac arrhythmias. Patients with ischemic heart disease might occasionally develop cardiac arrhythmias, ischemic electrocardiographic changes, and even angina pectoris during acute hypocapnia.

None of the previously described hemodynamic effects seem to be present in uncomplicated chronic hypocapnia.

15. **How does one make the diagnosis of respiratory alkalosis?**
The diagnosis of respiratory alkalosis is made by evaluating the patient's history, performing a physical examination, and obtaining laboratory data including a blood gas analysis. Tachypnea or Kussmaul breathing can be detected on physical examination and can be the first clue to the presence of a primary respiratory alkalosis or a compensatory respiratory mechanism in the setting of a primary metabolic acidosis. To assess if a respiratory alkalosis is adequately compensated, a detailed history needs to be obtained.

Changes in serum electrolytes can aid in the diagnosis of respiratory alkalosis. An acute fall in pCO_2 causes plasma and red blood cell CO_2 tensions to fall. In response, albumin and other non-HCO_3 buffers release H^+ to decrease the plasma HCO_3 concentration. Within red cells the fall in pCO_2 causes hemoglobin to release H^+ and red blood cell HCO_3 concentration also falls. Plasma HCO_3 will enter the red cell in exchange for Cl^-. This HCO_3-Cl^- shift accounts for the small initial compensatory response in acute respiratory alkalosis in which the HCO_3 concentration falls by 2 mEq/L for every 10 mm Hg decrease in pCO_2.

In chronic respiratory alkalosis the renal HCO_3 reabsorptive capacity decreases and there is a transient HCO_3 diuresis. This process takes 2 to 3 days to become fully manifest. Once a new steady state is achieved, the HCO_3 concentration will have decreased by 5 mEq/L for each 10 mm Hg fall in pCO_2. A higher or lower value for the plasma HCO_3 concentration suggests the presence of an additional metabolic disorder.

To defend extracellular fluid volume in the setting of increased urinary loss of $NaHCO_3$, the kidney retains NaCl. These changes are reflected in the serum electrolytes of patients with chronic respiratory alkalosis in which the Cl^- is typically increased with respect to the serum Na^+ concentration. Another characteristic finding is an increase of 3 to 5 mEq/L in the serum anion gap. The increased gap is a result of the greater fixed-negative charge on serum albumin and an increase in serum lactate concentration. Lactate production is increased because of a stimulatory effect of high pH on phosphofructokinase, the rate-limiting step in the glycolytic pathway.

KEY POINTS: RESPIRATORY ACID-BASE DISORDERS

1. Major causes of CO_2 retention include diseases or malfunction within any element of the respiratory system, including the central and peripheral nervous systems, the respiratory muscles, the thoracic cage, the pleural space, the airways, and the lung parenchyma.

2. Chronic respiratory acidosis is accompanied by a progressive insensitivity to the stimulatory effect of CO_2 and hypoxemia becomes an increasingly important factor in driving ventilation. Excessive oxygen should be avoided because it might lead to worsening hypoventilation.

3. A potential problem that is associated with use of carbonic anhydrase inhibitors in patients with lung disease is a worsening of hypercapnia.

4. Respiratory alkalosis is the most common acid–base abnormality in patients hospitalized in intensive care units, occurring either as the simple disorder or as a component of mixed disturbances.

5. Acute hypocapnia decreases cerebral blood flow and produces decreased acidity in all body fluids and hypocalcemia, hypokalemia, and a pH-induced shift of oxyhemoglobin dissociation curve; all these alterations have been implicated as determinants of the clinical manifestations of this acid–base disorder.

6. Once a new steady state is achieved the HCO_3 concentration will have decreased by 5 mEq/L for each 10 mm Hg fall in pCO_2. A higher or lower value for the plasma HCO_3 concentration suggests the presence of an additional metabolic disorder.

16. **What is the treatment of respiratory alkalosis?**
Primary respiratory alkalosis is treated by correcting the underlying cause. A patient with anxiety–hyperventilation syndrome should be treated by providing reassurance. Rebreathing into a paper bag or any other closed system will cause the pCO_2 to increase with each breath taken and lead to a partial correction of hypocapnia and improvement of symptoms. In the rare case where there is no response to conservative management, sedatives can be used.

BIBLIOGRAPHY

1. Laffey J, Kavanagh B. Hypocapnia. *N Engl J Med* 2002;4;347:43–53.
2. Morris C, Low J. Metabolic acidosis in the critically ill: Part 1. Classification and pathophysiology. *Anesthesia* 2008;63:294–301.
3. Morris C, Low J. Metabolic acidosis in the critically ill: Part 2. Causes and treatment. *Anesthesia* 2008;63:396–411.
4. Palmer BF. Approach to fluid and electrolyte disorders and acid-base problems. *Prim Care Clin Office Pract* 2008;35:195–213.
5. Palmer BF, Alpern RJ. Metabolic alkalosis. *J Am Soc Nephrol* 1997;8:1462–1469.
6. Palmer BF, Sterns R. Fluid, electrolyte and acid-base disturbances. *NephSAP* 2009;8:70–165.

CHAPTER 84

NEPHROLOGY BEGINNINGS

Garabed Eknoyan, MD

1. **Why does the history of nephrology matter?**

   "To understand a science it is necessary to know its history," said August Comte (1798–1857), founder of modern sociology. With its roots in sociology, this saying evolved into what is now known as the theory of path dependence, which explains how the set of decisions one faces for any given new circumstance is determined and limited by the decisions one has made in the past, even though past circumstances may no longer be directly relevant to present ones. This almost intuitively self-evident truth of social behavior applies to the science of decision-making in general and has led to three Nobel Prizes, the last of which was awarded in 2008 to Paul Krugman (born 1953), professor of Economics at Princeton University and an op-ed columnist for the *New York Times.*

   An oft-quoted and good illustration of path dependence is afforded by QWERTY, or the sequence in which the first six letters appear on the keyboard of every computer. The sequencing of the QWERTY letters was necessary for the mechanical operation of the original typewriters with hand-driven keypads but is obsolete for use in current computer technology. Another example of path dependence from our own discipline is the continued use of pH, based on a negative logarithmic unit, in acid–base measurements, where it would be so much simpler to express them in hydrogen ion concentration in nanomoles, a unit that was still not defined at the time pH was introduced in 1917.

   To sum it up with a relevant quote from a contemporary of Auguste Comte, John Quincy Adams (1767–1848): "We have come to understand that we are who we are is also who we were." In essence, history matters because it has an enduring influence, and knowledge of the history of ideas is important if we want to know how or why we make our daily decisions in what has become the discipline of nephrology.

   Magnusson L, Ottosson J (eds.). *The Evolution of Path Dependence.* Northampton: Edward Elgar Publishing, 2009.

   Peacock M. Path dependence in the production of scientific knowledge. *Social Epistemol* 2009;23:105–124

2. **When did nephrology emerge as a medical specialty?**

   Words involving the Greek root *nephros* for the kidney have been used for centuries. The word "nephrology" as a discipline for the study of the kidney in health and disease came into use in the opening decades of the 19th century but did not actually enter the parlance of medicine until the middle of the 20th century, at which time several events contributed to the emergence of nephrology as a medical specialty. First was the continued and increasing number of published articles on kidney function that had been prompted by the World War II medical effort to study shock, climatic adaptation, renal clearance of drugs, and hemodynamics. Second was technological advances that were of direct clinical relevance to kidney disease, specifically dialysis, renal transplantation, and kidney biopsy.

   The first physician to call himself a "nephrologist," as one who specializes in diseases of the kidney, was Arthur Arnold Osman (1893–1972) in 1945, who went on to help found the U.K. Renal Association in 1950 and served as its first president for the next 6 years. The Italian *Società Italiana di Nefrologia* was founded thereafter in 1957, and the French *Société de Nephrologie* was founded in 1959. The first medical publication devoted to the discipline, *Minerva Nefrologica,* appeared in Italy in 1957. As the number of physiologists, pathologists, and clinicians interested in the kidney increased, the membership of these societies increased and new national organizations were established. In 1960 the first international meeting of nephrologists was held in Evian, leading to the establishment of the International Society of Nephrology in 1961 and the launching of its first official journal, *Nephron,* in 1964. The American Society of Nephrology was founded in 1966, and its official journal, the *Journal of the American Society of Nephrology,* was published in 1990. The rest is history.

Eknoyan G. Kidney disease: Wherefore, whence, and whereto? *Kidney Int* 2007;71:473–475.

Robinson RR, Richet G. The International Society of Nephrology: A forty year history. *Kidney Int (Suppl)* 2001;19:S1–S100.

Schreiner G. Evolution of nephrology. The caldron of its organizations. *Am J Nephrol* 1999;19:295–303.

3. **When was the first artificial kidney used in humans?**
   Thomas Graham (1805–1869), a physical chemist whose seminal work on osmotic forces of fluids paved the way to hemodialysis, has been dubbed the father of modern dialysis. His studies on the behavior of biological fluids across a semipermeable membrane presaged the development of an artificial kidney and formulated the scientific basis of clinical dialysis: specifically that blood from a patient flowing in a semipermeable membrane that is in contact with an electrolyte solution (dialysate) allowed for the diffusion of small molecules from blood into the dialysate. The first use of dialysis in vivo, so called vividiffusion, was in rabbits and dogs by John Jacob Abel (1857–1928) and his associates at Johns Hopkins in 1912 and 1913. Tentative attempts at dialysis of humans were undertaken by Georg Haas (1886–1971) in Giessen in the 1920s, using collodion membranes and hirudin as anticoagulant that had been used by Abel. Collodion and hirudin had to be prepared fresh, were not standardized, were difficult to sterilize, and quickly led to the abandonment of clinical dialysis. Practical dialysis became possible in the early 1940s as a result of two new substances: cellulose acetate (cellophane) and the anticoagulant heparin. Three early pioneers to use the new membrane and anticoagulant in dialysis were Gordon Murray (1884–1972), Niels Alwall (1906–1986), and Willem Kolff (1911–2009), but it was Kolff working in Kampen under the tensions and difficult conditions of war-torn Holland who achieved the first clinically successful hemodialysis in humans. Kolff's so called "rotating drum hemodialyzer" was a wooden, pumpless drum, wrapped 30 times with 130 feet of cellophane tubing (connected to the circulation) immersed in a ceramic bathtub containing a saline solution. Beginning in 1942, Kolff experimented with his artificial kidney. His first 16 patients never recovered and went on to succumb in kidney failure. Only 2.5 years later did his first patient, Sofia Schafstadt, survive. Ironically, she had been a Nazi collaborator who was actually imprisoned. She had cholecystitis, developed septicemia, and was treated with one of the recently available sulfonamides. Her acute renal failure was a result of sulfonamide crystal precipitation in the tubules, a common side effect of these early wonder antibacterial drugs then in use.

Cameron JS. *History of Treatment of Renal Failure by Dialysis.* Oxford: Oxford University Press, 2002, pp. 74–94.

Eknoyan G. The wonderful apparatus of John Jacob Abel called the "artificial kidney." *Semin Dial* 2009;22:287–296.

Gottschalk CW, Fellner SK. History of the science of dialysis. *Am J Nephrol* 1997;17:289–298.

4. **Who was the first patient to benefit from chronic maintenance hemodialysis?**
   The artificial kidney introduced after World War II remained experimental and was used mainly in exploratory attempts to sustain the lives of selected patients with acute renal failure through the 1950s. The need for repeated access to the circulation limited the use of hemodialysis to the short term only in patients with acute renal failure. Even in patients with acute renal failure with delayed recovery, prolonged dialysis presented insurmountable problems that led to its abandonment before kidney function had recovered. The breakthrough came in March 1960, when Belding Scribner (1921–2003), a nephrologist, and Wayne Quinton (1929–), an engineer, working in Seattle developed the so-called Quinton-Scribner shunt using Teflon, which had

become available recently and was being used to coat implantable cardiac pacemakers. Shortly thereafter, the shunt was modified to be made from more flexible silicone tubing with Teflon tips inserted into the radial vasculature. The first patient to benefit from this new device was Clyde Shields (1921–1971), a 39-year-old Boeing machinist. In April 1960 Scribner took Clyde to the annual meeting of the American Society for Artificial Internal Organs (ASAIO) in Atlantic City, New Jersey for a private showing of the shunt. The news traveled with lightening speed and suddenly, long-term hemodialysis became possible. For the first time in medicine, technology and creativity allowed the replacement of the functions of a vital body organ. Literally overnight, repeated hemodialysis allowed survival from the otherwise-fatal disease described by Richard Bright (1789–1858) some 150 years earlier. Clyde Shields survived 11 years on dialysis, succumbing to a myocardial infarction in 1971.

Blagg CR. The early history of dialysis for chronic renal failure in the United States. A view from Seattle. *Am J Kidney Dis* 2007;49:482–496.

Cameron JS. *History of Treatment of Renal Failure by Dialysis.* Oxford: Oxford University Press, 2002, pp. 187–199.

Peitzman SJ. Nephrology in the United States from Osler to the artificial kidney. *Ann Intern Med* 1986;105:937–946.

5. When were the first kidney biopsies performed?

Biopsies of the kidney on the operating table were performed by surgeons through the first decades of the 20th century for various reasons. They were first systematically studied in subjects undergoing dorsolumbar sympathectomy for hypertension. Percutaneous needle biopsy of the kidney was introduced after the successful use of cutting needles in liver biopsy. Nils Alwall (1904–1986) of Lund performed the first systematic needle kidney biopsies in 1944. An early death of a patient after biopsy led him to abandon the technique. He did not publish his results until 1952. In the meantime, Poul Iversen (1889–1966) and Claus Brun (1914–) of Copenhagen began using the technique in 1949. The initial needles, known as Vim-Silverman needles, were a modification of the liver biopsy cutting-edge needles. Apart from the skill needed in handling these needles, positioning of the kidney presented a major challenge in those early days. Improved imaging and renal ultrasound together with new disposable needles and then biopsy gun needles have changed that. The first international meeting on kidney biopsies was held in 1961, and organizations to discuss renal pathology were precursors of the Renal Pathology societies that emerged thereafter.

Cameron JS, Hicks J. The introduction of renal biopsy into nephrology from 1901–1961: A paradigm of the forming of nephrology by technology. *Am J Nephrol* 1999;17:347–358.

Kark RM. The development of percutaneous renal biopsy in man. *Am J Kidney Dis* 1990;16:585–589.

6. Why the complexity of acid–base balance?

Variable notions of acid and alkali have been part of medicine since antiquity. The concept of acidity and alkalinity were well known from their sensory perception, either gustatory from their taste or visual from the color changes they produced in certain dyes. Their taste is what provided their nomenclature. Acids tasted sour, hence the origin of the term "acid" from the Latin *acere* (sour), and its prototype the taste of acetic acid in vinegar, still known in Italian as *aceto*. Alkali, referring to that of the ash of charred wood or plants, whose principal constituent is potassium carbonate, is derived from the Arabic, *al-qali*.

Early chemical studies in the 17th century by Johann Glauber (1607–1673) working in Amsterdam identified salts that resulted from the union of various acids and bases and ascribed disease to disturbances in their balance in the body. With methodologic advances in chemical measurement, it was then recognized that blood is alkaline and the urine is acid. One of the earliest studies on urinary acid and base constituents was published in 1812 by John Jacob Brezilius (1770–1843), considered one of the founding fathers of chemistry. Interest in acid–base balance grew thereafter but remained descriptive in the main. The theory of electrolyte dissociation in aqueous solutions and the presence of hydrogen ions in acids and hydroxyl ions in bases proposed by Svante Arrhenius (1885–1927) in 1887 were instrumental in the subsequent development of concepts of acid–base solutions and buffers. For his contributions Arrhenius was awarded the 1903 Nobel Prize in Chemistry. Refinements in the instrumentation to measure the concentration of hydrogen and hydroxyl ions provided much of the advances in acid–base balance that followed. Research was stimulated by epidemics of cholera and subsequently diabetic ketoacidosis by such pioneers in renal physiology as Bernhard Naunyn (1839–1925), Lawrence Henderson (1878–1942), and Donald Van Slyke (1883–1971).

In 1911 Henderson introduced an equation for evaluating the buffering properties of weak acids and bases from their dissociation constant. The logarithmic transformation of Henderson's equation by Karl Hasselbach (1874–1962) in 1917 yielded what is known now as the Henderson-Hasselbach equation. The fundamental importance of this mathematic equation in the subsequent elucidation of acid–base disorders notwithstanding, its complexity remains the principal cause of the difficulty encountered by most in understanding acid–base disorders. As mentioned in the introductory question of this section on path dependence, the use of hydrogen ion concentration expressed in nanomoles would resolve much of the difficulty associated with the continued, but unnecessary, use of the negative logarithmic expression of pH.

Structured studies in acid–base homeostasis and the role of the kidney in maintaining acid–base balance were undertaken during the period between the two World Wars. The role of the kidney in the process was elucidated in the 1940s to a great extent by the studies of Robert F. Pitts (1908–1977) and his associates at Cornell University.

Astrup P, Severinghaus W. *The History of Blood Gases, Acids, and Bases.* Copenhagen: Munksgaard, 1986.

Rector FC. Acidification of urine. In: Gottschalk CW, Berliner RW, Giebisch GH (eds.). *Renal Physiology: People and Ideas.* Bethesda, MD: American Physiological Society, 1987, pp. 353–374.

Smogorzewski MJ. Historical perspectives on the role of the kidney in acid-base regulation. *J Nephrol* 2009;22(Suppl 14):S108–S114.

7. **When was the first successful kidney transplant performed?**
Experimental allotransplants and xenotransplants of the kidney in animals were begun in the latter half of the 19th century. By the opening decades of the 20th century, unsuccessful attempts at xenotransplantation in humans were undertaken in Vienna by Emerich Ullman (1861–1937), who transplanted a pig kidney in the elbow of a young woman with uremia, and in Lyon by Mathieu Jaboulay (1860–1913), who transplanted a sheep kidney in one patient and a pig kidney in another. The first cadaveric kidney transplant was performed on April 3, 1933 in Kiev by Yuri Voronoy (1895–1961), who transplanted the kidney from a 60-year-old woman who had died from head injury to a 26-year-old woman with acute renal failure from mercury poisoning, a common cause of kidney injury at the time. The patient died 48 hours later.

Technical difficulties and the lack of an understanding of the immunologic basis of organ rejection hampered these early efforts at organ transplantation. Their respective study and partial resolution resulted in two Nobel Awards in Physiology and Medicine: the first in 1912 to Alexis Carrel (1873–1944) and the second in 1960 to Peter Medawar (1915–1987). The first documented kidney transplant in the United States was performed on June 17, 1950 on a 44-year-old woman with polycystic kidney disease in Evergreen Park, Illinois. The kidney was rejected. The first successful kidney transplant was performed in Boston by a team led by John P. Merrill (1917–1984) and Joseph Murray (b. 1919), who on December 23, 1954 transplanted a kidney from one identical twin, Ronald Herrick, to his brother, Richard. This was before chronic maintenance hemodialysis became feasible and generated considerable interest and excitement for the future treatment of kidney failure.

Richard Herrick recovered kidney function, married the recovery room nurse who had cared for him after the transplant, had two children, and enjoyed good health until his death in March 1963. In 1990 Joseph Murray received the Nobel Prize in Physiology and Medicine, the third to be granted for work on transplantation.

Carrel A. Transplantation in mass of the kidneys. *J Exp Med* 1908;10:98–141.

Merrill JP, Murray JE, Harrison JH, Guild WR. Successful homotransplantations of the human kidney between identical twins. *JAMA* 1956;160:277–282.

Morris PJ. Transplantation—A medical miracle of the 20th century. *New Engl J Med* 2004;351:2678–2680.

Nagy J. A note on the early history of renal transplantation: Enrich (Imre) Ullmann. *Am J Nephrol* 1999;19:346–349.

8. **What is the origin of the term "uremia"?**

   Much of our understanding of the pathophysiology of diseases comes from the analysis of body fluids that were being introduced into medicine in the 19th century. These early biochemical studies were instrumental in shaping much of the subsequent nomenclature and progress in the study of diseases in general and that of the end-stage kidney disease described by Richard Bright (1789–1858) at about that time, in particular.

   Large volumes were necessary for the rather crude analytic methods available then, and it was generally easier to use the readily accessible and substantial quantities of urine rather than blood. Of the various chemical substances that were identified in the urine, it was probably that of urea that contributed most to what followed. In 1799 François Fourcroy (1755–1809) and Nicolas Vaquelin (1763–1829) already had isolated pure urea salts. By 1817 the properties, appearance, and chemical reactions of urea were described by William Prout (1785–1850), who alluded to its presence in the blood. Shortly thereafter, in 1828 Friederich Wöhler (1800–1882) synthesized urea from two inorganic molecules, ammonia and cyanic acid, which prompted him to write triumphantly: "I can make urea without the use of kidney, either man or dog." This was a major breakthrough and turning point in the history of science that placed the notion of vitalism, which had dominated medical theory theretofore, to rest and validated the chemical approach to biology that was to launch the new basic sciences of organic chemistry and biochemistry. Wöhler's discovery literally coincided with the description of Bright's disease. Within a year, Robert Christison (1797–1882) reported increased urea levels in the serum of patients with Bright's disease, which by 1847 led to the introduction by Pierre Piorry (1794–1879) of the term *urémie* (uremia), literally urine in the blood, to describe patients with high blood urea levels.

   Over the years, uremia has come to encompass all the clinical manifestations of the failing kidneys. The sole role of urea to account for the symptom complex of patients with advanced kidney disease was questioned from the outset. George Johnson (1818–1896), a contemporary of Richard Bright and a prominent authority on kidney disease who described the microscopic changes of Bright's disease, wrote in 1852, "It is in the highest degree probable that urea is a poisonous agent, but we have no proof that it is more so than other urinary constituents which must be retained or accumulated in the blood, when the kidneys are so much disorganized as they are often found to be." Nevertheless, the uremia of Piorry remains in use to this day as a rather vague and catch-all medical term used to refer to abnormalities of kidney failure that remain unexplained and presumed to result from some as-yet-elusive chemical product that should have been excreted by the kidneys.

   Of note, it was the continued studies of urea that were to provide much of the experimental and theoretic concepts that led to the discovery of the artificial kidney. Indeed, it was studies on the diffusion and osmotic properties of urea by Thomas Graham (1805–1869) that laid the very conceptual foundations of hemodialysis, and it is the proportional clearance of urea from the body by dialysis (urea reduction ratio, URR) that now provides a measure of the adequacy of artificial kidneys in treating patients with kidney failure.

Kinne-Safran E, Kinne RKH. Vitalism and synthesis of urea: From Friedrich Wöhler to Hans A. Krebs. *Am J Nephrol* 1999;19:290–294.

Peitzman SJ. Dropsy, dialysis, transplant. A short history of failing kidneys. Baltimore: Johns Hopkins University Press, 2007.

Richet G. Early history of uremia. *Kidney Int* 1988;33:1013–1015.

9. **What is the origin of the term "nephrotic syndrome"?**

   "Nephrotic syndrome" as a diagnostic term came into use in the 1920s to describe the triad of heavy proteinuria, hypoalbuminemia, and edema, usually with associated dyslipidemia and lipiduria. The common presenting symptom of edema, once called dropsy, has an ancient history. Actually, it was the association of dropsy with proteinuria that established the link of edema with kidney disease and launched the discipline that was to become nephrology. Dropsy, or the accumulation of fluid, was regarded as a separate disease until the end of the 18th century. Its association with cirrhosis of the liver was well known in antiquity, and its association with kidney disease was also described, particularly in patients with oliguria, but its association with diseases of the heart was indirect and generally ascribed to the broader concept of diseases of the chest, when fluid was detected in the lungs or pleural space of some patients with dropsy. Two landmark publications laid the foundations that were to clarify the role of the kidneys and the heart in dropsy, their inter-relationships in health and disease, and ultimately the identification of edema as a symptom of underlying diseases rather than a disease itself.

First was the publication in 1785 of *An Account of the Foxglove and Some of its Medical Uses* by William Withering (1741–1799), who showed that the administration of an infusion of the leaves of foxglove (*digitalis purpurea*) produced a diuresis and an amelioration of dropsical symptoms. It was obvious from the outset, including a third of the cases reported by Withering, however, that not all patients with dropsy responded to the infusion and that some of the nonresponders who died while taking the infusion were suffering from cirrhosis of the liver with ascites. No comment was made of the kidney of some of these nonresponders. The determination of the other principal cause of dropsy (kidney) had to await a second landmark publication in 1827 of the *Reports of Medical Cases* by Richard Bright (1789–1858), which contained his description of end-stage kidneys and led to the distinction of dropsy as a result of kidney disease by the presence of heat-coagulable albuminous material in the urine. The link of dropsy with hypoalbuminemia was suspected shortly thereafter from the low specific gravity of the serum of patients with Bright's disease who had the heaviest albuminuria reported by Robert Christison (1799–1882) of Edinburgh in 1829 but had to await improved chemical methods to define it as hypoalbuminemia.

Even though it was clear from the outset that kidney disease is not always associated with dropsy or albuminuria, Bright's disease soon came to be accepted as a diagnostic term for albuminuric kidney disease. It was studies to differentiate the various renal lesions of Bright's disease and the quantification of their associated proteinuria that determined the course of subsequent events in the emergence of nephrology. Richard Bright had described three principal types of the gross appearance of the kidneys he reported: (1) a hard, small (one half normal size) kidney with cysts; (2) a soft, mottled, yellowish-grey kidney of normal size; and (3) a swollen large (twice normal size) soft pale kidney. It was the latter, which was associated with anasarca and heavier proteinuria, that ultimately came to be associated with nephrotic syndrome. The descriptive morphologic term "nephrosis," probably derived from the German *nephrotische,* was introduced in 1905 by Friedrich von Müller (1858–1941), a pathologist working in Munich, to differentiate the microscopic lesions of these large kidneys from those of the inflammatory lesions of "nephritis." The subsequent grouping of the common clinical manifestations of the various renal lesions of nephrosis under the term "syndrome of nephrosis," "nephrosis syndrome," and "nephrotic syndrome" were introduced between 1924 and 1929 in the writings of Henry A. Christian (1876–1951) of Boston. Of those, nephrotic syndrome received the better acceptance and entered medical parlance thereafter.

Cameron JS. The nephrotic syndrome: A historical review. In: Cameron JS, Glassock, RJ (eds.). *The Nephrotic Syndrome.* New York: Marcel Dekker, Inc., 1988, pp. 3–56.

Cameron JS, Hicks J. The origin and development of the concept of a "nephrotic syndrome." *Am J Nephrol* 2002;22:240–247.

Christian HA. What is nephrosis? *New Engl J Med* 1933;208:129–131.

Peitzman SJ. *Dropsy, Dialysis, Transplant. A Short History of Failing Kidneys.* Baltimore: Johns Hopkins University Press, 2007.

10. **Name an early and eminent pioneer nephrologist and his famous patient.**
Thomas Addis (1881–1949), a pioneer in nephrology, was one of the first clinicians to systematize the study of kidney disease, quantify the cellular (especially red blood cells) constituents of the urine sediment, use the recently developed clearance technique to

determine kidney function, and introduce dietary treatment for those with kidney failure. His book, titled *Glomerular Nephritis: Diagnosis and Treatment*, published in 1948, remains a reference worth perusal by anyone seriously interested in the beginnings of clinical nephrology. His most famous patient was the double Nobel laureate for Chemistry and Peace, Linus Pauling (1901–1994), who Addis treated with a protein-restricted diet. Shortly before his death, Addis resigned from the American Medical Association because he refused to contribute to its campaign against President Truman's national plan for health insurance.

The heritage of Addis is best summed in one of his sayings, "When the patient dies the kidneys go to the pathologist, but when he lives the urine is ours. It can provide us day by day, month by month, and year by year, with a serial story of the major events going on within the kidney." This is a statement that deserves to be remembered and propagated daily by every nephrologist.

Blagg CR. Thomas Addis, 1881–1949, clinical scientist, hematologist, and pioneering nephrologist. A brief biography. *J Nephrol* 2009;22:S115–S119.

Lemley KV, Pauling L. Thomas Addis: July 27, 1881–June 4, 1949. *Biogr Mem Natl Acad Sci* 1994;63:3–46.

Peitzman SJ. Thomas Addis (1881–1949): Mixing patients, rats, and politics. *Kidney Int* 1990;37:831–840.

INDEX